SJ ALLE·ZEIT·WACH 1842

"More may be done towards the preservation of the health and lives of seamen than is commonly imagined; and it is a matter not only of humanity and duty, but of interest and policy."*

Sir Gilbert Blane

* Observations on the Diseases of Seamen, 1789

Handbook of Nautical Medicine

Edited by:
W. H. G. Goethe · E. N. Watson · D. T. Jones

With 38 Figures and 12 Tables

Springer-Verlag
Berlin Heidelberg New York Tokyo 1984

Professor Dr. W. Hartmut G. Goethe
Scientific Director

Bernhard-Nocht-Institut für Schiffs- und
Tropenkrankheiten, Abt. für Schiffahrtsmedizin,
Bernhard-Nocht-Straße 74, 2000 Hamburg 4/FRG

Dr. E. Norton Watson

formerly Chief Medical Officer
General Council of British Shipping,
London/UK

The Late Dr. Dilwyn T. Jones
formerly Medical Officer Health
Port and City of London/UK

ISBN-13:978-3-642-69417-2 e-ISBN-13:978-3-642-69415-8
DOI: 10.1007/978-3-642-69415-8

Library of Congress Cataloging in Publication Data. Main entry under title:
Handbook of nautical medicine.
Bibliography: p. Includes index.
1. Medicine, Naval-Handbooks, manuals, etc. I. Goethe, W. H. G. (W. Hartmut G.), 1923 - II. Watson, E. N. (E. Norton), 1921 - III. Jones, D. T. (Dilwyn T.), 1927–1982 [DNLM: 1. Naval medicine-Handbooks. VG 460 H236]
RC986.H29 1984 616.9'8024 84-1211

Softcover reprint of the hardcover 1st edition 1984

2119/3020-543210

Contributors

Anderson, W. R., MD,
Anderson Medical Group, Inc., San Pedro, California 90731, USA

Backhaus, A., Dr. med., OMD,
Port and Airport Health Authorities, Hamburg, FRG

Bäter, H., Dr. med. dent.,
Lauenburg/Elbe, FRG

Ball, Th.,
Bernhard-Nocht-Institute for Nautical and Tropical Diseases,
Department of Nautical Medicine, Hamburg, FRG

El Batawi, M. A., Prof. Dr. med.,
Chief Medical Officer, Office of Occupational Medicine, WHO, Geneva, Switzerland

Boehm, H., Professor, Dr. rer. nat., Dipl.-Psych.,
Nautical School, Bremen, FRG

Cox, R. A. F., MA, MB, BChir, MFOM,
Medical Director, Phillips Petroleum Company Europe-Africa, London, UK

Dolmierski, R., Professor, Dr. med.,
Director Institute of Maritime and Tropical Medicine, Gdynia, Poland

Duffy, J. C., Professor Dr.,
Assistant Surgeon General, Office of the Surgeon General U. S. Public Health Service, Rockville, Md, USA

Ebert, H., OMR Doz. Dr. sc. med.,
Medical Service of the Transport System of the GDR, Rostock, GDR

Gardner, A. Ward, MD, FRCPI, FFOM (Ireland), FFOM (London), DIH,
Esso Medical Centre, Fawley, Southampton, UK

Goethe, W. H. G., Professor Dr. med.,
Scientific Director
Bernhard-Nocht-Institute for Nautical and Tropical Diseases,
Department of Nautical Medicine, Hamburg, FRG

Harrington, J. M., Professor, MSc, MD, FRCP, FFOM,
The University of Birmingham, Institute of Occupational Health, Birmingham, UK

Herrmann, R., Dipl.-Ing.,
Bernhard-Nocht-Institute for Nautical and Tropical Diseases,
Department of Nautical Medicine, Hamburg, FRG

Huisman, J., Professor Dr. med.,
Chief Department for Communicable Diseases and Hygiene, Municipal Public Health Service, Rotterdam, Netherlands

Ivergård, T., PhD, ScD,
Scandinavian Airlines System (SAS), Stockholm, Sweden

Jamall, O. A., FRCS (Edin.)
Consultant Orthopaedic Surgeon, Dreadnought Seamen's Hospital, Greenwich, London, UK

The Late D. T. Jones, BSc, MB, BCh, MFCM, DCH Eng, DPH,
formerly Medical Officer of Health, Port and City of London, UK

Low, A., Dr. med.
Bernhard-Nocht-Institute for Nautical and Tropical Diseases,
Department of Nautical Medicine, Hamburg, FRG

Milton-Thompson, G. J., Surgeon Commodore, QHP, FRCP,
Deputy Medical Director General (Naval), Ministry of Defence, London, UK

Naeve, W., Professor, Dr. med.,
Forensic Medical Service, Hamburg, FRG

Ohashi, N., Senior Research Fellow,
Maritime Labour Research Institute, Tokyo, Japan

Oliver, P. O., RD, MD, FFOM RCP, DPH, DIH,
Group Medical Director, Cunard Steam-Ship Company, Southampton, UK

Pettersen, J. W. E., B. Sc. (Eng.)
Principal Research Engineer, Det Norske Veritas, Høvik, Oslo, Norway

Renfrew, R. R., MB, ChB, MFOM,
Medical Officer, Fish Docks Medical Services, Grimsby, UK

Shafran, L., MD, Dr. med. sc.
Branch of the Institute of Watertransport Hygiene, Toxicological Laboratory, Odessa, USSR

Sobol, Z., Dr. Ing.,
Institute of Maritime and Tropical Medicine, Head of Department of Transport Hygiene and Environment Protection, Gdynia, Poland

Schadewaldt, H., Professor Dr. med.,
Director of the Institute for History of Medicine of the University of Düsseldorf, FRG

Stenko, J. M., Professor Dr. med.,
Director Scientific Research Institute of Water Transportation and Hygiene, Moscow, USSR

Tenfjord, O. W., MD, DPH,
The Medical Office for Seamen, Oslo, Norway

Tortori-Donati, B., Professor Dr.,
Finmare, Medical Department, Genova, Italy

Vollum, D., FRCP, DCH,
Consultant Dermatologist, Lewisham Hospital, London, UK

Vuksanović, P., Dr. med. Dr. sc.,
Head of Public Health Service, Medical Center “Blažo Orlandić”, Bar, Yugoslavia

Watson, E. N., MRCS Eng, LRCP (Lond), MFOM RCP,
formerly Chief Medical Officer General Council of British Shipping, London, UK

Williams, J. G., Surgeon Commander, MSc, MRCP,
Professor of Naval Medicine, Royal Naval Hospital, Haslar, Gosport, UK

Zorn, E., Priv. Doz. Dr. med. Dr. sc.,
formerly Senior Scientist
Bernhard-Nocht-Institute for Nautical and Tropical Diseases,
Department of Nautical Medicine, Hamburg, FRG

Foreword

International cooperation on the health of seafarers began many years ago. As early as 1921, an international convention regarding this matter was presented to governments of maritime countries for ratification. The First World Health Assembly, in 1948, recommended that WHO should establish, with the International Labour Office, a Joint Committee on the hygiene of seafarers. The first session of this Committee, held in 1949, defined the problems affecting the health of seamen and made a number of recommendations.

In the opinion of this Joint Committee, the health of seamen called for international attention for a number of reasons. By the nature of his work, the seafarer is obliged to travel from country to country and is exposed to great variations of climate and also to any disease that may be prevalent in the port of call. He may therefore become a carrier of disease, so that the protection of his health is of importance not only to himself and the other members of the crew but also to the populations of other countries he visits. Yet, on account of the nature of his employment, it is difficult to provide the seafarer with the same standard of health care that is generally available to other sections of the population.

At the time of the opening session of the Joint Committee, the following factors were of most importance to the seafarer's health: medical examinations, medicine chests on board, accomodation and food supplies on board, hospital treatment, rehabilitation and social welfare. The Committee made recommendations aimed at finding solutions to problems in these areas. Also, proposals were made regarding the control of tuberculosis and venereal diseases among seamen.

In 1954, the Joint ILO/WHO Committee met for the second time and suggested the minimal list of medicaments which should be contained in a ship's medicine chest. It also discussed the model scheme of diagnosis, treatment and other control procedures in venereal infections, reviewed the diagnostic and therapeutic measures for these infections in a number of large ports throughout the world and discussed the medical examinations of seamen to detect tuberculosis.

During the third meeting of the Committee, in 1961, it was realized that it had been difficult to present a definite picture of seafarers' health problems as very little accurate or reliable data had been available. Not all countries were able to give precise employment statistics regarding seafarers. Even fewer countries were able to provide an age group structure of their merchant navy personnel. Without such information, no morbidity study was possible. Also, there was considerable variation in the problems encountered between various countries owing to different geographical and social conditions.

A further step in expanding the international cooperation on the health of seafarers was the *WHO International Medical Guide for Ships,* published in 1967.

Following the resolution of the World Health Assembly, WHO Pilot Health Centres for Seafarers were designated in Gdynia, Poland and Auckland, New Zealand in order to collect international data on morbidity and accidents among seafarers, to conduct research related to their health, to provide medical and dental services for seamen and fishermen and to conduct postgraduate training in maritime medicine. In 1975, the Department of Nautical Medicine, Hamburg, was also designated by WHO.

The fifth (1973) and sixth (1981) sessions of the Joint Committee in Geneva dealt with medical and first-aid training for ship personnel, preventive care of teeth and mouth and emergency dental facilities for seamen in ports, medical examination of crew members of tankers carrying bulk chemicals, existing medical centres for seamen, immersion hypothermia, recording of medical examinations and treatment of seafarers and the updating of the *International Medical Guide for Ships*. In 1982, in collaboration with the Centre in Gdynia, this Guide was updated and the new edition will be published by WHO in 1984.

With developments in the world shipping industry during recent years – the introduction of new types of ships and new technologies – the pattern of the health problems of seafarers has changed. Infectious diseases have become less important (in fact, smallpox was completely eradicated from the world in 1976). One of the new problems has been their exposure to the dangers connected with carrying chemical cargoes in bulk. This new challenge has been met by experts and by international organizations. In 1973, the *Medical First Aid Guide for Use in Accidents Involving Dangerous Goods* was published by IMCO. Other problems include the effect of environmental stress on the seafarer's health the psychosocial aspects of work on-board ship, the need always to maintain high standards of health on modern, highly automated ships, on which the number of crew has decreased compared with standards existing in the 1960s and 1970s, and also the need to introduce the telemetric system of exchanging health information from ship to shore-based hospitals.

All these and many other problems still need to be studied and answers found through the combined efforts of shipowners, seafarers, scientists and experts in maritime medicine.

For all of them, the *Handbook of Nautical Medicine* will be an excellent source of up-to-date information on all relevant subjects. It will also provide a source of inspiration for further research and efforts to improve the environmental conditions on board ships which influence the health of seamen and to improve the health services provided for them, both at sea and on shore.

The Handbook is an important contribution to international cooperation on the health of seamen. Experts, invited by the editors and representing a number of well-known research centres on maritime medicine from eleven countries, have presented here a wide range of subjects clearly and concisely, indicating appropriate directions for further research.

Dr. M. A. El Batawi
Chief Medical Officer
Office of Occupational Health
WHO, Geneva

Preface

Over recent decades the shape of the shipping industry has changed considerably in response to the pressures exerted by changing international patterns of trade together with the swings of fortune in national economies. Many of the traditional maritime countries have suffered a decline in their fleets while over the same period there has been a corresponding increment in those of emerging countries. The competition for available cargoes in depressed world markets has been intense. However, the international trade in exports from and imports to countries throughout the world is still largely dependent upon transport by sea. This has been responsible for the continued growth of the shipping industry as a whole, despite the loss of passengers to air and land travel, which has resulted in the severe decline in the number of passenger liners. Indeed, it is estimated that there is a total world strength in excess of 70000 ships registered within the fleets of over 70 maritime countries.

A direct consequence of heightened competition in international sea trade has been the impetus given to continuing advances in ship design, technology and cargo handling. This has led to the development of larger, faster ships manned by fewer crew and spending much less time in port. In many countries the average cargo ship carries only 20 crew members and this complement has been reduced still further by some shipping companies. The advent of container ships and other highly specialised types, such as carriers of bulk chemicals, liquified gas, oil and ore, has brought additional attendant problems for both seafarers and the occupational doctors concerned with health and welfare.

The unfortunate impact of these commercial changes has been that nowadays, with the exception of certain eastern European countries, few doctors are carried by merchant ships and, regrettably, just as few are employed in full-time practice in maritime organisations and shipping company offices ashore. This is a matter for continuing concern because, although living standards on ships have improved, it has yet to be shown that these have produced a commensurate improvement in the health of crew members. It is quite possible to argue that the reduction of hard physical work in conjunction with plentiful rich food and cheap tobacco and alcohol has had a deleterious effect. Furthermore, the almost universal trend towards single cabins for all crew members is not always psychologically beneficial.

It is true that a carefully selected smaller crew should result in a higher average standard of health on board irrespective of a possible healthier environment. The drawback is unfortunately that given a smaller crew, there is less reserve to cushion the effect of interim illness among crew members. Therefore, the pre-employment medical examination should be made even more stringent to exclude anyone who has a condition, or pre-condition, which might develop into unfitness for work at any time in the future. It is almost universally agreed that medical examinations of such crucial importance are best carried out by doctors who have long personal experience in the industry.

When to all this is added the increase in the number and complexity of dangerous cargoes, it is seen that the burden of clinical and preventive medicine which falls upon the shoulders of the smaller number of nautical medicine specialists is very great and will remain so in the foreseeable future. Despite all the changes, the seafarer is still one of the most medically deprived of workers. Although working in an industry which is becoming more and more technologically and commercially advanced, he is still almost totally divorced from any form of fully qualified medical care during his time at sea, and when he comes ashore he may find it very difficult to locate a doctor in hospital or general practice who has any knowledge or experience of nautical medicine.

It is apparent that there is a field of fascinating work for young doctors who would like to combine medical practice with an opportunity to see more of ships and the sea but, in view of the smaller number of doctors already in the field, where can these young doctors, and the doctors ashore who see a seafarer only occasionally, look for information and opinion based upon experience?

We see that as one of the functions of this book. Each of the authors is an expert in his own field, with long experience of the care of seafarers, and we should like to express to each of them our grateful thanks for the time they have given from their already over-busy lives. As appropriate to an industry which enjoys so much international co-operation in its practices and procedures, the authors have been chosen to give as much varied national participation as possible. However, it should be accepted that the individual contributions reflect not only personal concepts of nautical medicine but also the prevailing practices in the countries of origin. The chapters must be seen as such, with the understanding that both therapy and practice vary from country to country. In this respect the editors decided to include at the end of each chapter a comprehensive list of references greater than usual. It is our sincere wish that this Handbook will represent not only an up-to-date account of nautical medicine but also a useful guide to the future reading from international sources, which is necessary if progress is to be maintained in the development of this often neglected speciality.

The editing of a book compiled from the work of authors from so many countries presents inevitable difficulties but none greater that the task of reconciling the differing versions of the English language which make up the international lingua franca of today. In this we wish to express our profound gratitude to the copy-editing staff of the publishers who have assisted us and also to the authors, who have accepted with goodwill the changes to their original texts.

W. H. G. Goethe · E. N. Watson · D. T. Jones

Table of Contents

2 The Seafarer's Environment

5 Special Fields in Nautical Medicine

1 Introduction to Nautical Medicine

1.1 The History of Nautical Medicine

H. Schadewaldt and W. H. G. Goethe

1.1.1 A Medical View of the Development of Shipbuilding and Navigation

From early times, doctors have had to deal with the special problems associated with seafaring, as in the past, much more so than today, sailors were exposed on their often months-long voyages to dangers which hardly existed in the same form on land. For this reason, promoted by a relatively small number of ship's surgeons from the most diverse countries and backgrounds, a specific area developed within medicine some time before there was any talk of specialization. A wide range of valuable treatises from the sixteenth century onwards stemmed from "medicina nautica".

In the history of seafaring, as in the development of nautical medicine, three periods can be distinguished: a) the age of manpower (oars), b) the use of the wind (sail), and c) the employment of engines (steam, oil, and now nuclear power).

The first period extended from the dawn of humanity to approximately the middle of the fifteenth century. In general, no one strayed far from the coast, and only a few seafarers, such as the Phoenicians, with their knowledge of the stars, and the daring Vikings had the confidence to venture onto the open seas.

A direct crossing of the Mediterranean was therefore the exception; the preference was for "hopping" from island to island. Unbroken voyages were limited to 8–10 days; even the sometimes sizeable seagoing vessels could carry provisions for only 1 or 2 weeks. The southern climate made no great demands regarding the standard of quarters for the crews, most of whom were slaves to whose well-being hardly any attention was paid. Open ships of up to 50–200 t (tons) were the rule, although the Greeks, Phoenicians and Romans also had covered ships of up to 2000 t in their war fleets to accommodate large boarding parties. Without exception, ships were built of wood. Sails were used mostly on merchant ships.

The Phoenicians long had a monopoly of sea trade, which led them as early as 850 B.C. to Spain and Britain, but the Greeks were the experts in naval warfare. This is indicated by the fact that even later in the Roman navy, large galleys with three and four banks of oars were called triremes and tetraremes, and most of the crew members as well as many captains and ship's surgeons were Greeks.

Around 1480 Martin Behaim (1459–1507) began trying to adapt astrolabes to navigation, and in 1492 he completed his first globe, now at the German National Museum in Nuremberg. In the same year came Columbus' discovery of America, which ushered in the second period of navigation.

From then on, everything depended on building seaworthy deep sea vessels capable of crossing the ocean. Crews had to be enlarged because the greater size of the sails and rigging necessitated more hands. Besides the gun-crew needed to man the cannon (often 40–60), boarding parties were taken who could also be used on land in the New World. On top of this, illnesses and accidents among the crew during the monthslong, unbroken voyage had to be allowed for. When one considers that, on technical grounds, the size of the ships was usually limited to 300–500 tons, and that sufficient water and provisions for the lengthy crossings had to be carried, one can imagine how excessively cramped it was on board. These conditions were for the most part to blame for making this period of seafaring history the most tragic chapter in nautical medicine.

This era's voyages of exploration, e.g. the discovery of the sea route to India by Vasco da Gama (1469–1529) in 1498 and the first circumnavigation of the globe under the command of Fernão de Magalhães (c. 1480–1521) in the years 1519–1522, claimed many lives.

In the course of the long voyages – the journey to America by sail could last anything from 23 days to 23 weeks – the planking became porous, especially as the feverish shipbuilding activity after the discovery of the New World led to the frequent use of green, badly seasoned wood. In addition, the wood was attacked by the notorious shipworm, teredo navalis, which belongs to the family Teredinidae. The result was that below the waterline it was continually damp. In the bilge, the lowest part of the ship, water always gathered and mixed with the ballast sand to form a sludge. At that time there were still absolutely no sanitary facilities; in bad weather, leftovers, urine and excrement were tossed into the bilge, where rats and other vermin prospered. An infernal stench resulted, and this putrefying muck was often the source of devastating epidemics. All possible processes were used to prevent ships from leaking – charring the outer surface of the hull, treating it with ferrous sulphate, tarring (still practised today), lining the inner surface of the hull with a second layer of wood, pumping out the bilge – but all had their disadvantages. Only copper-sheathing, introduced in 1758, brought an improvement.

For a long time it was the French and Italian custom to keep the bodies of those who had died on board in the bilge for later burial on land. The now usual burial at sea was first introduced on English ships and may be principally traced back to considerations of hygiene. It was only when it became normal to use blocks of iron instead of sand for ballast, to wash the bilge out regularly with seawater, and to provide toilets and ventilation facilities on board that this source of many serious diseases was eliminated.

For the reasons mentioned above, the numerical size of crews was very large in comparison with that of modern ship, e.g. the East India Company's ship "Dragon" of 600 t had 300 people on board. The sleeping accommodation was usually particularly bad. Until the year 1772, when the famous world voyager Captain James Cook (1728–1779) introduced the three-watch system, there were only two watches. Only enough sleeping space was provided for the men not on duty, in the form of plank beds that were intended for four men, but often had to do for six. On slave and convict ships conditions were even more catastrophic. The door was open for the spread of venereal and other infections and for homosexual excesses.

The hammock, today a symbol of life at sea, was a Caribbean gift to the seaman, brought back to Europe by Columbus' crew from the West Indies, where the natives wove *hamacas* (hence the English name) which could be hung one over the other and did not let the occupant fall out even with the motion at sea – an ideal form of bed in view of the great shortage of space. This practical innovation was introduced into the Royal Navy by Queen Elizabeth in 1597 and adopted on the warships and merchant vessels of all other nations soon thereafter. There was still only one hammock for every two men. Anyone who wanted one for himself had to get it, and as usual, at the evening "Pfeifen und Lunten aus" (lights out), the seaman's signal to go to bed, it was the strongest who could get the best spot by a hatch or a ventilator; there are said to have been pitched brawls.

The third period of seafaring history shows friendlier aspects. In 1777 James Watt (1736–1819) built the first usable steam engine, and 11 years later Patrick Miller (1731–1819) and William Symington (1763–1831) constructed the first small steamboats, long before Robert Fulton's (1765–1815) steamship made her maiden voyage on the Hudson. Of course, shipbuilders and -owners had no great trust in the newfangled engine, and for security retained all the sails and rigging. For this reason, the early steamships had even bigger crews. A new category of seaman came into existence: the stoker.

The decisive advantages of mechanization were the shortening of time at sea and the relative independence from wind and weather. Questions of water and provisions no longer took first place, and a replacement crew was no longer necessary, particularly as medical examination of all new recruits had in the meantime been introduced in all the navies of the world. New engineering and sanitary problems arose, however; space had to be made for the engine and the paddle wheels – the propeller was not generally introduced until 1847 – and coal and water for the engine had to be carried. On top of that there was the overwhelming heat in the engine room to combat, which was the cause of many heatstrokes and was particularly unpleasant in the tropics. The stokers' washing facilities had to be improved, and special attention had to be paid to the ventilation systems.

With the introduction of iron ships, from about 1840, some problems were solved at a stroke, but others were intensified. While it had previously been impossible on technical grounds to build ships with a displacement of more than 3 000 tons, size was now no longer limited; this relieved the acute shortage of space, especially on merchantmen. It became unnecessary to carry ballast, the ships were more manoeuvrable, and finally, leaky wooden hulls, with all their attendant evils, became a thing of the past.

However, it soon became unpleasantly obvious that iron was a good conductor of heat. In summer the new ships were unbearably hot, particularly in the engine room – temperatures of up to 75 °C were measured on French ships – and in winter or in the north terribly cold, the steam heating introduced first on German ships proving insufficient. The result was a conspicuous increase in colds and chills, to which the condensation gathering on the cold iron must have contributed. This problem was tackled with cork or wood panelling and absorbent paint. Nowadays the air-conditioning units on merchant vessels and warships do not allow such variations in temperature. The original engines were not insulated and caused considerable vibration, thereby greatly increasing the incidence of seasickness.

With the introduction of armour-plated ships (e.g. the Gloire, 1859), the pattern of injuries in sea battles changed. Whereas sabre slashes, bullet wounds and wood-splinter injuries had previously been in the forefront, now burns and inhalation of poisonous fumes became common, in the battle of Skagerrak accounting for as many as 25% of all injuries. The installation of bulkheads to make the armoured ships not so easily sinkable forced changes in the methods of ventilation and in the accomodation of the wounded.

The sick bay – commonly called the "cockpit" in the British navy – was formerly accommodated above the waterline in the bow, often separated only by a sailcloth curtain from the crew quarters, and was naturally very vulnerable in battle. For example, in the Russo-Japanese war, a direct hit on a Japanese ship during the battle of Tschuschima (1905) destroyed the only dressing station and killed both doctors and all the stretcher bearers. Therefore, later ships were equipped with two or more sick bays under the armoured deck, as far amidships as possible, in order to prevent a complete loss of medical facilities.

The great shortening in the duration of voyages after the opening of the Suez and Panama canals (1869 and 1914), as well as international disease control measures, made a decisive contribution to the reduction of morbidity and mortality at sea to today's levels, not significantly higher than on land. The effect of the introduction of steamships can be illustrated by the following example: In a 12000-strong French expeditionary force to China in 1859, mortality was only half as high among those accommodated on 13 steamships as in those on six sailing ships.

In earlier centuries crews were a mixture of all possible positive and negative elements. Next to adventurers and runaway adolescents could be found sensitive natures attracted to the seafaring experience. Emigrants and naturalists, ex-army officers and revolutionaries filled the ranks of officers and crew. In England, for example, convicts were pressed into service, preferring to go to sea rather than spend their lives at forced labour in a quarry. If there was a shortage of seamen, the Royal Navy in particular did not shy away from a sort of slaving expedition, the press-gang rounding up the drinkers from the nearest quayside inns and dragging them on board to serve the king. It is no wonder, then, that iron discipline was needed to keep this motley crowd in check. The infamous cat-o'-nine-tails, consisting of nine finger-thick knotted thongs or ropes, was no invention of any writer of sea adventures, but was for centuries a harsh reality. The French navy was the first to abolish corporal punishment in 1848, followed in 1850 by Sardinia and, although not until 1866, by Britain. The ship's doctor had an important role to play in this punishment; indeed, he often had to carry out the whipping himself, since he could best judge what was reasonable in each individual case. From 1830 onwards the captain could pass such sentences only with the consent of the ship's doctor, whose position had by then improved to the extent that he no longer had to perform the degrading duty himself. Midshipmen were also subject to such punishment, the only difference being that they were beaten with a rope, in which a red cloth was weaved. Also barbaric was the punishment of nailing cut-throats to the mainmast by their hands. However, the worst which could happen to a sailor was the infamous keelhauling, which some poor souls did not survive. The offender was tied to a rope, thrown from the mast, and dragged under the keel to the other side of the ship. This inhuman punishment was abolished as a result of the influence of the French Revolution and the repeated intervention of many ship's doctors.

1.1.2 Hygiene

1.1.2.1 Diet

The Barcelona Ordinance (1258) laid down a victualling scale containing salt, meat, bread, vegetables, oil, wine and water. It is therefore reasonable to say that a mediaeval seaman in the Mediterranean at that time was probably better fed and quartered than his 18th Century counterpart.

How important a complete, well-balanced diet was for health at sea is shown by the prevalence of scurvy although other avitaminoses were also common. During the Russo-Japanese war, 31% of the Japanese sailors suffered from beri-beri. The cases of hemeralopia which occurred on British ships in 1768 were mostly healed by the addition of mashed carrot to the diet.

There were three main reasons for the unsatisfactory nature of the supplies taken on board in earlier times: the inadequate knowledge of nutritional physiology, the lack of sufficient means of preservation, and the uncertain duration of the voyage, often with no chance of replenishing the provisions en route.

At sea as on land, the greatest worth was attached to bread and meat. As only salted meat and fish could be taken on longer voyages, they made up the main part of the daily ration. When captains or unscrupulous shipping agents wanted to spend as little as possible, they bought half-rotten or otherwise spoiled meat, the taste being disguised by heavy salting. The bread was no better. Fresh bread was first baked on board ship around 1880; before then the men had to be content with the so-called ship's biscuit, which incidentally was already known to the ancient Romans, who called it "panis nauticus". On lengthier voyages the constant wet conditions reduced it to crumbs, on which the assorted vermin on board – worms, cockroaches, mice, rats – did very well, not without leaving their filth behind. Half-starved sailors must have forced down some revolting meals on long journeys. Besides bread and meat, other provisions carried were oil, butter, cheese and pulses. The French and the Spaniards took onions and garlic, to which is attributed the fact that they had a lower rate of scurvy than English seamen. The Dutch, for their part, placed great value on sauerkraut, which later, on Captain Cook's advice, was adopted by the British as an anti-scurvy measure.

Alcohol played a very important part in life at sea, and when one considers the seaman's daily ration, in the form of beer, brandy, rum or wine, one must conclude that many were drunk every day. This high consumption is understandable in view of the continually cold and wet conditions, and the alcohol was also sometimes intended as a safe substitute for contaminated water.

The constant drinking on board often led to disputes and violence, the most inveterate ruffians eventually being put in irons and making the acquaintance of the cat-o'-nine-tails. For this reason, in 1740 the British admiral Edward Vernon (1684–1757) ordered the official rum ration, the "king's allowance" or "necessity", to be mixed with three parts of water and have sugar added. The admiral, little liked for this order, always wore a jacket made of the coarse material grogram, and hence acquired the nickname "Old Grog", from which the name of the drink came. His creation has since attained greater popularity. A second modern drink with a naval origin, although the ingredients differ, is the "flip", a mixture of rum and small beer. The name stems from the joke that after drinking several glasses one could fly over the mainmast.

On English and German ships beer, which was reputed to have antiscorbutic properties, was preferred. In the main, however, it was small beer, which was consumed on board ship at the rate of 4–5 l per crew member per day; French seamen preferred to drink between 0.5 and 1 l of wine a day. In all navies a substantial quantity of brandy, rum or arrack, varying from 0.25 to 0.5 l was consumed daily. There was often a greater supply of alcohol than of drinking water. The Spanish Armada, for example, carried 57000 l of water, but 82000 l of wine. It was not until 1823 that alcohol at breakfast was replaced by tea or cocoa in the British navy, and by coffee in the French, although there had been the alternative of oat or barley gruel if anyone wanted to forgo his morning beer or wine. The results of this alcohol abuse were inevitable; whereas among land forces delirium tremens accounted for 2.8‰ of all sickness, in the British navy, even after 1830, the figure was 18.1‰.

In the eighteenth century the weekly food ration for a sailor in the Royal Navy, to give one example, consisted of 2 kg of beef, 1 kg of pork, 1.5 kg of peas, 1.5 kg of oatmeal, 180 g of butter, 360 g of cheese, condiments and possibly fish, with 0.5 kg of ship's biscuit each day. This made up about 3700 calories a day, enough for a man doing heavy manual work, but lacking in vegetables. Beginning in 1757, adopting James Lind's suggestions, the meat ration was cut, and cabbage, cucumber, and occasionally fruit and vinegar were added to the diet. In very rough weather cooking was sometimes impossible, so the crew had to eat their rations raw and cold. From these times comes the well-known sailor's meal Labskaus (the name stems from Norwegian), in which for simplicity the meat, fish, peas, carrots, cucumbers and condiments were cooked together in one pot, originally with flour, later with potatoes. Even with the ship pitching and rolling, the ship's cook could still just manage.

The food available became more varied thanks to the preserving methods invented by the Swiss-French cook Nicolas Appert (c. 1750–1841) in 1806. They were tested by the French navy in the same year, and from 1830 onwards the use of preserved foodstuffs was widespread at sea. Dried carrots, dried potatoes, and vegetable meal were first used in 1850, Liebig's meat extract in 1865, and in 1866 condensed milk was introduced for infants on passenger ships. "Portable soups", blocks of compressed soup ingredients and flour, had been known as early as 1757 and were taken by Captain Cook on his voyages. From 1853 onwards there were "cereal stones" with beer wort, from which a tasty beer substitute could be made.

The development of refrigeration units ended centuries of problems for captain, ship's doctor and cook. Any kind of food could now be taken to any part of the world, and the reduction in time needed for any given voyage has also helped to ensure that in modern times food on board ship hardly ever runs short. What in earlier times was at best possible only for monarchs and the nobility, namely to have fresh fish or poultry available at sea, is today taken for granted by every passenger on a liner.

1.1.2.2 Water Supply

The supply of drinking water without doubt posed a greater problem than the transport of food. The Greeks and Romans carried their modest stock of water in goatskins or leather bags. Later, larger wooden barrels came into use, but again and again it was found that the water went bad, became cloudy, tasted revolting, and caused many infections. Strangely, this disgusting liquid often cleared and tasted relatively good after about 3 weeks at sea. Now we know that the acid sulphur salts in the water were reduced by organic compounds in the wood to hydrogen sulphide, which, along with the putrefactive bacteria, was then used by the flourishing algae which gathered at the bottom of the barrel, with the result that the water became clear again. For many years there was truth in the old sailor's rule that water must be allowed to go bad three times before it could be drunk with impunity. The countermeasures recommended were sulphurization of the barrels and charring and painting of the inside surface. Beginning in 1800, deodorizing with charcoal and powdered lime and filtration assumed prominence. In 1815 iron water tanks were introduced, eliminating many problems.

The water ration was very low, only 0.25–0.5 litre per day, and had to do for washing (including clothing) as well as drinking. Even in the tropics it was raised to only a litre or so. According to modern calculations one should allow at least 5–6 litres.

Naturally, the attempts to gain drinking water during the voyage began very early. The most primitive method was the collection of rainwater in large sails, an inadequate process in areas of low rainfall. The disgusting taste was improved by the immersion in the water of glowing-hot iron rods.

Another method, appropriate for arctic and antarctic regions, was the melting of ice, first reported in 1671. Captain Cook supplied a great proportion of his water needs in this way. Icebergs were preferred as the source. Cook observed the very frequent occurrence of sore throat after consumption of such water, and from a modern viewpoint these may have been the first epidemics of Pfeiffer's glandular fever described at sea.

The greatest significance was attached to

attempts to obtain fresh water from seawater. The first attempted distillation is attributed in legend to Saint Basil (born c. 330), who was cast away on an island after a shipwreck. He is said to have boiled seawater and caught the steam in sponges, thereby saving himself from death by thirst.

The world has Andres a Laguna (1499–1560), personal physician to Emperor Charles V (1519–1566), to thank for the rediscovery of this process. Other experimenters attempted distillation with the addition of chemicals, Sir Richard Hawkins, for one, in 1588, with lunar caustic, lime and boneblack, and Hauton in 1670 with alkalis. In 1717 Hubert Gautier (1660–1737) constructed a distillation apparatus, but it was unusable in heavy seas because the newly won fresh water then got mixed with the remaining seawater again. Many others occupied themselves with this problem until around 1770, when both Lind and Pierre Poissonnier (1720–1798) constructed workable devices and the dispute over who had been first attracted public interest. Although Lind was the first who strove to manage without the addition of chemicals, Poissonnier's apparatus was undoubtedly more practical. Quite wrongly, the ship's doctor George James Irvine (1722–1798) was credited with invention of the seawater distillation process, and in 1772 he received a prize which had been put up by the British Parliament.

In 1817, Balthasar Sage (1740–1824) claimed that distilled water was harmful, but the untenability of this theory was proved by an experiment in which 60 slaves were put on a small island without natural water and given only distilled water to drink. Sage was not altogether wrong, however, in that on French ships the distilled water flowed through lead pipes, often leading to lead colic, the so-called coliques sèches des pays chauds. The cause was first recognized in 1837 by Alexandre Ségond (1799–1841). The problem did not arise on English ships, as the receptacles and pipes contained hardly any lead.

One further point worth mentioning is that seawater was long held to be unsuitable for putting out fires; the urine of the crew was therefore collected in large casks for this purpose.

1.1.2.3 Ventilation

On Greek and Roman, and later on Venetian and Genoese, galleys ventilation was no problem. The vessels were mostly open or had a 'tween deck which let in sufficient air. It was first around 1500, with the construction of more decks, the larger crews, and the building in of gun ports, that artificial ventilation of the lower decks became necessary. Around the middle of the nineteenth century the arrangement of bulkheads on armour-plated ships placed further demands on the ventilation system. In World War I it was shown how crucial this problem was for the crew members in the armoured turrets, many of whom died not after a direct hit, but as a result of inhaling poisonous fumes. The lower parts of the ship, especially the bilge, were very unhealthy. The English surgeon Tobias Smollett (1721–1771) describes the conditions as they then were:

> We descended by divers ladders to a space as dark as a dungeon, which I understood was immersed several feet under water, being immediately above the hold: I had no sooner approached this dismal gulph, than my nose was saluted with an intolerable stench of putrified cheese, and rancid butter, that issued from an apartment at the foot of the ladder, resembling a chandler's shop, ...

Around the same time, in 1748, carpenters working on bilge pumps are known to have asphyxiated, and they were certainly not the only victims.

The oldest kind of ventilator was the wind sail. An improvement on this was the wind tube, through which the air could travel to the lower decks. Such systems were of course useless when there was no wind. The first attempts at artificial ventilation go back to the first half of the eighteenth century. In 1734, Jean Théophile Desaguliers built a machine that worked on the principle of the fan. The man who operated the machine became known as the ventilator, a name later transferred to the machine itself. In 1741, Stephen Hales (1677–1761) suggested a system based on the principle of the bellows, the bad air being pumped out of the room through one tube, fresh air in through another. A small respirator, two "ass's ears" which the seaman working in the bilge could put on, was made on the same principle, but had hardly any practical significance. Around 1745, Samuel Sutton constructed a ventilation system of tubes connected to the fireplace in the ship's galley. The hot air was supposed to draw off the unhealthy vapours, but the system could not be used in heavy seas, when all doors, companionways and portholes were closed and the fire had to be put out. Finally, no further attempts were made, not least out of fear of the scorbutic sea air, until the coming of steam power enabled the technical solution of the problem (which will not be discussed here).

1.1.2.4 Cleanliness, Heating and Lighting

In contrast to modern warships or merchant vessels, which the visitor always finds spick-and-span, the cleanliness on earlier ships left a lot to be desired. To blame were the crowded conditions on board and the scarcity of fresh water. Until the Age of Enlightenment the captain and officers did not bother themselves with these problems; they hardly took the trouble to go from their cabins on the upper deck to the crew's dark, cramped, stifling quarters. Soap was unknown on board ship until 1787, when Sir Gilbert Blane (1749–1834) introduced it into the British navy, each man getting half a pound of soft soap a week. The fresh water was still reserved for drinking, and as before, the crew's ragged clothes were changed only when they were nearly falling off. The upper deck was washed regularly with salt water; the lower decks, which dried badly, hardly ever. At most, juniper or pine branches were burnt in the bilge.

Things were just as bad with the heating. On wooden ships there was always the danger of fire, one of the reasons why chewing tobacco so quickly gained popularity among sailors. Even on whaling ships the men tried to warm themselves only in a makeshift way, using red-hot cannonballs. The first iron stoves were used on Captain Cook's expeditions, but served mainly to dry out the eternally wet bilge. It is no wonder that "heating from inside" with strong alcoholic drinks was so popular. Often the flint and tinder or the pinewood kindling needed for starting the fires were soaked through, and the cook anxiously watched over the only fire on board. The honour of having introduced steam heating – an obvious development on steam-powered ships – belongs to the navy of the North German Confederation. The first trials began in 1856, and the method was later adopted by all navies.

Lighting was for long a problem as well. The crew tried in a rough and ready way to light the nearly always dark living quarters with wretched little oil lamps, but these naturally went out in heavy seas. Their place was later taken by stearin candles. It was a great step forward when in 1822, on the French ship of the line "Jean Bart", portholes were first added to the gun ports, which were closed in bad weather. This meant that some light entered the lower decks the whole day long, regardless of the weather. The introduction of electric lighting solved all the problems at a stroke.

1.1.2.5 Clothing

Whereas land troops started wearing uniforms in the time of Gustavus II Adolph of Sweden (1594–1632), this was not normal among navies until much later. Everyone knew all the others on board, and direct contact with the enemy through boarding became ever rarer. The crew wore what they liked or what they had. Often enough they were quite inadequately equipped, or had squandered their hiring-on fee in taverns ashore and couldn't afford a change of clothes. Occasionally a captain would demand that his crew should have some kind of uniform, but more than likely this was to avoid having unsuitably dressed men begging for warmer clothes on the high seas and for preventing desertion.

The first uniform regulation for officers, however, came from King James I (1566–1625) in 1603, and with time this became the rule. The traditional blue of navies throughout the world is supposed to trace its origin to the Duke of Bedford, who at the British court in 1746 wore a blue jacket which pleased the king so much that he determined to introduce it for his valued naval officers. Blue had already been made the colour for medical officers, at least on land, under the prince elector Georg Wilhelm of Brandenburg (1595–1640) in 1631. In 1748 blue uniforms were officially prescribed for officers in the British navy, but the ship's doctors continued to wear civilian clothes. It was in the French navy in 1767 that the doctors first got colourful uniforms; the blue first appeared in 1798, during the French Revolution. In the meantime, in 1776, the American navy had introduced uniforms for its ship's doctors, although this measure seems not to have been popular, as a special decree made failure to wear the uniform punishable by dismissal. The German navy furnished its doctors with uniforms on the English pattern in 1849, 1 year after it was founded. Nevertheless, even the doctors with officer's rank were differentiated from other porte-épée officers, the absence of the sword-knot being a clear indication of their lower position. Among the crew it had become an established nautical custom to wear a wide collar, still today called the sailor's collar, to protect their oiled pigtails. Almost all navies adopted the collar as it was in the British navy at the time of the Napoleonic Wars, the black or deep-blue ground representing the death of Nelson and the three white stripes standing for his three naval victories at St. Vincent, Aboukir and Trafalgar.

In many navies the staff of Aesculapius has become the specific emblem of the ship's doctor. The practical-minded Americans replaced the staff (which in Prussia was conferred on naval doctors in 1868) with the letters MD (medicinae doctor) and later with an oak leaf. Peru (and the American army) chose the staff of Hermes (the so-called caduceus, or kerykeion), mistaking its significance. The Brazilian navy uses the stethoscope as emblem for its doctors. Many countries, Great Britain and France among them, now prefer to use a particular colour, especially green or crimson, as a background for the insignia of rank.

1.1.3 Quarantine

The history of quarantine begins in the fourteenth century in Venice. As early as 1348 there were "health inspectors", whose duty it was to visit suspected ships and enforce any disinfection measures that were necessary, and then in 1374 the harbour was closed to ships from plague areas. The period of quarantine was at first only 10 days, but was soon increased to 30, as in Ragusa in 1377, and then to 40 (hence the name), as in Marseille in 1383. The term of 40 days "quaranta dies" was not chosen arbitrarily, but represented the long-established boundary between acute and chronic illnesses. Since the infectious diseases were all considered acute, 40 days would always suffice.

The first isolation ward, enabling better supervision, was built on an island off Venice in 1403, followed in 1450 by similar institutions in Zara and Ragusa. The second significant Mediterranean sea power, Genoa, followed suit in 1467. From 1665 onwards, ships' "health certificates" served to alleviate the problems incurred by the growth in sea traffic; the penalty for falsification was death. Contaminated ships had to be either completely fumigated or simply burnt.

Various international conferences, the first in 1838 and one of the last in 1920, have laid down details of length and type of quarantine. Nowadays, radio communication enables rapid clearance on board by virtue of its rapid transmission of comprehensive information on epidemics all over the world, but passengers and crew on a ship flying the yellow flag still may go ashore only when cleared by the port medical officer.

1.1.4 Diseases at Sea

An example of an early provision made for sick seafarers is contained in the Judgments of Oléron (c. 1194) upon which code northern European maritime law was founded. The Judgments stipulated that if a sick sailor had to be put ashore the Master must provide lodgings, light, rations and either engage a nurse or put a ship's servant ashore to attend him.

During the long voyages by sail in the fifteenth to nineteenth centuries, diseases often occurred at sea which were only seldom observed in the ship's country of origin, such as scurvy or the various tropical diseases, and obviously seasickness was seen only on board ship. Other typical conditions included the occupational diseases contracted while the seamen worked in the rigging, or later in the engine-room, and all sorts of injuries and burns from engagements with the enemy. Without doubt, tuberculosis, various skin conditions and venereal infections also played a special role, although they could not be said to be typical seamen's diseases.

The surviving statistics on morbidity and mortality on board ship are shocking, showing that contemporary voyagers' reports were not exaggerated and that up to the nineteenth century more seamen died as a result of illness than from wounds received in hostilities. Vasco da Gama's crew was not the only one to suffer catastrophic losses. For example, in 1506 a Spanish vessel lost 123 of its approximately 360 men within 2 months, mostly to malaria. Sir Francis Drake (c. 1540–1596) lost almost 600 of the 2300 men under his command in 1585, and a few years later, in 1589, the story was repeated, probably as a result of scurvy; this time half of the 1200 men died and hardly a quarter were fit for duty. Of the 680 men under Sir James Lancaster (died 1618) on his voyage to the East Indies in 1600, 180 were dead before the beginning of the return trip and half did not see England again. Particularly tragic was the fate of the English ship "Gloucester", which in 1617 lost 626 of its 961 men! Especially high losses were suffered aboard vessels in the yellow fever areas of West Africa and Central America, sometimes the entire crew, including the doctor, dying and having to be replaced. Sometimes the insidious disease would first manifest itself at sea, leading in southern waters and in the cramped conditions on board the wooden ships – ideal breeding conditions for Stegomyia – to devastating epidemics. No wonder serious researchers assume that sailing vessels whose crews were dead could have been the model for the legend of the Flying Dutchman.

However, two examples can be brought to show that even in those times, suitable means were sometimes used to combat this extremely high mortality. In 1759, Admiral Edward Hawke (1705–1787) of England led a fleet of 14000 men so successfully that only 20 men had to be disembarked, although some of the ships had crews 700 or 800 strong. His squadron was always followed by a tender carrying fresh provisions, and on the one occasion when bad weather prevented the tender from sailing the number of cases of illness rose sharply.

Even more impressive are the figures from Captain Cook's round-the-world expeditions. He personally took charge of the medical care, rations, and general hygiene on the ships in his command. On his first voyage to the Pacific (1768) 23 of the 85 crew members on the flagship died, but on the second (1772–1775) it was only four of 81 men during a journey of 6000 nautical miles. Three perished in accidents, leaving only one single victim of illness.

The British navy was very early in keeping precise records of deaths, from which we learn that in the years 1780–1783, during the sea fighting in the West Indies, 1148 of the 21608 men were lost in engagements with the enemy, but 3200 – well over twice as many – as a result of illness. Thanks to the endeavours of Lind, Blane and Trotter, the three most important British ship's doctors, mortality had decreased markedly by the turn of the century. In 1760 the rate was still as high as 125‰, but by 1810 it had sunk to 50‰–40‰, and by 1878 to 6.7‰. However, this was still higher than the remarkably low German rate of 3‰, which did not go up even in World War II, when the figure was only 2.55‰, compared with the 2.38‰ who died through enemy action. The relationship had therefore undergone a fundamental change, particularly impressive evidence of the work of ship's doctors. Losses in the merchant marine at this time were still at the much higher level of 10‰. Notifications of illness and sickbay admissions also decreased. In 1779, 24266 of the 70000 members of the Royal Navy, i.e. one in three, were sent to the sick bay, but in 1810 it was only 9965 of 145000, a ratio of 1:14.

The statistics that Lind gave in 1760 for the British naval hospital Haslar, where he was in charge, may also be interesting. Over a 2-year period, the 5743 patients admitted included those with the following diagnoses:

Fever	2174
Scurvy	1146
Consumption	360
Rheumatism	350
Dysentery and other fluxes	245
Complaints of old injuries	80
Cutaneous diseases	73
Ague or intermittent fever (malaria?)	67

No other condition formed a significant proportion of the total.

The improvement in medical care also affected the treatment of injuries sustained in battle, but the new, long-range, large-calibre guns caused much greater devastation than the old direct rain of cannonballs. Shrapnel wounds from explosive shells increased dramatically, and burns and smoke inhalation were common. Some British statistics also speak eloquently here (see Table 1).

1.1.4.1 Scurvy

In ancient times scurvy was hardly known; for example, Homer's Odyssey, the greatest sea epic in the history of literature, contains no mention of it. The first reports come from the distant north in the tenth century. Indeed, the name itself (old German Scharbock, Latin scorbutus) is said by some to come from the old Norse skyrbjur (skyr = sour milk, bjur = oedema), though according to others it can be traced back to the Slavonic scorb (disease). In any case, the long-used specialist term "morbus saxonicus" indicates a northern origin. The disease was certainly known to the Norsemen who around the year 1000 crossed to Greenland and Iceland. There are reports of high-ranking people, e.g. a bishop, who to everybody's astonishment lost their teeth early in life. The oft-mentioned swelling of the legs raises the possibility of the concurrent appearance of beri-beri, and purpura was frequently described. On the crusade led by Louis IX of France (1226–1270) in the year 1250, scurvy appeared in the south.

The disease first became of crucial importance at sea after the discovery of America. True, it had affected the crew of the Venetian merchant Pedro Quirino when their galleon was stranded in the waters between Norway and Iceland, but it was the account of Vasco da Gama's 1497–1498 voyage to the East Indies by the Portuguese poet Luis Vaz de Camões (1524–1580), the epic poem entitled "Os Lusiadas", describing the explorer's experiences, which presented the horrors of this new disease to a

Table 1. Casualties in four great sea battles

Year	Battle	Men	Casualties		
			Injuries	Deaths	%
1797	Camperdown	8221	622	203	10.03
1798	Nile	7985	678	218	11.22
1805	Trafalgar	17772	1242	449	9.51
1916	Skagerrak	60000	674	6014	11.14

wider public. Before then the only people on land acquainted with scurvy were the inhabitants of besieged cities.

A second catastrophe of similar proportions was described by Jacques Cartier (1491–1557), who on the way to Newfoundland had to spend the winter 1535–1536 on his ship in the St. Lawrence River. Only three of the 110 members of his crew remained healthy, and 25 died. Most of those on board, probably misled by the ecchymoses, were convinced that the disease was a kind of plague. After unsuccessfully trying every possible remedy, they followed the advice of the local Indians and ate the tips of the needles of the thuja tree, with the result that many recovered. The tree became known as the arbor vitae, and the needle tips of pine trees formed a part of the treatment of scurvy for centuries thereafter.

In 1541, Johannes Echt (born before 1515) gave what is said to be the first scientific description of scurvy in his book "De scorbuto vel scorbutica passione Epitome". He considered the malady to be infectious and based on tainted blood, in his time a natural conclusion.

In 1564 followed the Dutch doctor Boudewjn Ronsse's (1525–1597) volume "De magnis Hippocratis lienibus Pliniique stomacace ac sceletyrbe, seu vulgo dicto scorbuto libellus", regarded for many years as the standard work. Ronsse traced the illness back to the turbulent, cold sea air, and was repeatedly cited by serious doctors when they wanted to prove the damaging potential of artificial ventilation.

Over the years, the most varied theories were proposed to explain the origin of this disease, which appeared infectious but could be quickly and certainly cured when the patient was back on land. Without doubt, scurvy was often mistaken for the lues, rheumatism or gout, or, under the name of "purpura nautica", confused with infectious exanthemas. Felix Platter (1536–1614) was convinced in 1608 that scurvy had been brought back from America along with the lues. Around 1650, the doctor Abraham Leonard Vrolingh regarded it as a "disease of decay" and prescribed preparations against mould. Steven Blankaart (1650–1704) set against this theory the hypothesis of the thickening of the blood through acids, sugar and cold, and discarded lemon juice in favour of alkali, coffee and tea. In 1675 Verbrugge believed that the purpura could be relieved by the sinking of the thick humours of the blood and prescribed fresh vegetables. Cornelis Bontekoe (1640–1685) attributed a great range of diseases to scurvy, including cancer. Many authors suspected a dyscrasia of the humours (to take one example from as late as 1789 William Cullen (1710–1790) assumed a dissolution of the humours), and climatic influences, the cold wet conditions on board and the unseasoned wood from which the ships were constructed were all blamed. Due attention was first paid to nutrition in the nineteenth century, and even then the treatments proposed were as numerous as the theories mentioned above. Salt and salt meat were given preference, but other suggestions included alkalis or acids, particularly dilute phosphoric acid, and electuaries and distillations of the most varied materials – Bontekoe, for instance, created an "elixier antiscorbuticum" out of cinnamon, cloves, orange peel and oil of vitriol.

The beneficial effect of fresh vegetables was recognized at an early stage through practical experience. Around 1560, the doctor Franz Joël I (1508–1579), from Greifswald, learned from sailors that watercress (Nasturtium officinale) was an antiscorbutic. In northern regions a big role was played by the spoonwort (Cochlearia), also referred to as scurvy grass, which may have saved the lives of some very ill people. Horseradish and mustard grass were widely used, and later Pierre Seignette (1660–1719) discovered the antiscorbutic property of mustard during a siege. Pine beer, prepared from needles and cones, was very popular for this kind of illness. The advice to bury scurvy sufferers up to the neck in the ground for one day after coming ashore is an interesting curiosity. More sensible was the 1844 recommendation for the patients to eat potatoes. Sauerkraut and cider, pomegranate and chicken broth were all prescribed. The evidence of the antiscorbutic effect of a seawater cure must have led Czar Peter the Great (1672–1725) to recommend that his seamen's children should regularly drink salt water.

A strange but successful treatment was that used by travellers to Greenland who were trapped in the ice by the Arctic winter; they drank the fresh blood of whales and seals. This idea was taken up in the scientific literature in 1683, C. Dellon (1649–1709) recommending guinea pig blood as an antiscorbutic. In 1696, Archibald Pittcairne (1652–1713) advised against the then usual blood-letting, suggesting in contrast transfusions of animal blood.

The causal therapy, intake of fresh orange or lemon juice, may have been known very early. At any rate, it was described around 1450 in "Tractatus de limonibus", a translation by Andrea Alpago of the work of Ibn-al-Baitār (1197–1248). Oranges and lemons were known in northern Europe from 1290 onwards, but the knowledge of their antiscorbutic properties must have been lost. In 1564, the same year in which Ronsse's work appeared, this knowledge was accidentally rediscovered by shipwrecked Dutch sailors. They drifted on the ocean, scurvy began to spread; the provisions were exhausted, and in desperation they ate the oranges which had been taken on board only as delicacies. To everyone's great surprise, the scurvy sufferers recovered. Ronsse made incidental mention of the favourable effect of oranges, and one may assume that, directly or indirectly, he had come to know of this involuntary experiment. This knowledge was never completely lost, but not even the recommendations of such learned men as Felix Platter (1536–1614), John Woodall (1556–1643) and Thomas Sydenham (1624–1689) led to the stocking of this simple remedy on board all ships. Thousands upon thousands of seamen died wretchedly of scurvy over the next 200 years before this policy was generally adopted.

A few progressive ship's captains used this knowledge; for instance, we learn that on the flagship of Admiral Sir James Lancaster's expedition in 1601 three teaspoons of lemon juice formed part of the daily ration. The result was that hardly anyone contracted scurvy, whereas the crews of the other ships in the fleet suffered terribly.

It was James Lind's brilliant experiments on board the "Salisbury" in the year 1747 which ushered in the new era of the battle against scurvy. Probably for the first time in medical history he used a control group, in that he gave his preparation (already established as effective) to one part of the crew but not to the other members living under the same conditions. In a preliminary experiment he tested all possible antiscorbutics recommended in his day on groups of two; only lemon juice and, to a minor degree, cider were found effective. In the main experiment the treated crew members remained scurvy free; the untreated were affected and could quickly be cured with small amounts of lemon juice. Lind summarized his experience in "A Treatise of the Scurvy" (1753).

At that time lemons were naturally very expensive, and on long voyages with large crews sufficient stocks took up a lot of space. Attempts were therefore made to replace lemon juice with the cheaper but equally effective lime juice. Only after a long time, however, was it recognized that lime juice, in contrast to lemon juice, loses its antiscorbutic properties very quickly in storage. Efforts were then made to prepare the lemon juice on land by adding sugar and boiling it down. Although Jacob Zahalon (1630–1693) had already established in 1683 that boiling decreased the antiscorbutic properties of fresh juices and vegetables, it was not until 1785 that Blane won recognition for this fact. Under his influence, the use of lemon juice and the carrying of fresh fruit was obligatory in the navy from 1795 onwards. Unfortunately it did not become compulsary in the merchant marine until 1865. Captain Cook had not believed in the effect of lemon juice because he had boiled it. In the French navy the giving out of lemon juice was first officially introduced in 1856, and in the German navy the first regulations on the subject date from 1855, although the food on German warships was previously very varied and scurvy was rare. Unfortunately it was believed, under the influence of Trotter, that lemon juice could be replaced by citric acid, an error that was only cleared up in 1928 with the discovery of vitamin C.

The introduction of lemon juice as a remedy, and a little later as a prophylactic, had undreamed-of results. Whereas scurvy had previously crippled whole fleets – for example the Spanish Armada in 1588 – it was now hardly significant. According to Admiral Sir Richard Hawkins (1562–1622), at least 10000 men died of scurvy in his 10 years of office, and even in the year 1780, 1457 scurvy sufferers lay in the British naval hospital Haslar. However, after the introduction of lemon juice as a prophylactic, only two cases were recorded during the entire period from 1806 to 1810. Blane could rightly say to the Admiralty: "Fifty oranges or limes mean one sailor more".

One more example of the paramount importance of lemon juice in the prevention of scurvy is provided by the Arctic expedition of 1850–1853. When after 2 years the lemon juice ran out, more than 80% of the crew got scurvy. The ship's surgeon, Alexander Armstrong (1818–1899), carried out what was probably the very first autopsy ever on board ship, on the body of one of the victims, without contributing much to the clarification of the pathology of the disease.

1.1.4.2 Tropical Diseases

Seafarers were the first to come into contact with the tropical diseases of the New World, so it is not surprising that ship's doctors wrote most of the early books on the subject. One can say without exaggeration that tropical medicine originated in nautical medicine. Until well into the nineteenth century, most colonial doctors were from the navy.

Yellow Fever

One of the unwelcome gifts from the newly discovered continents was yellow fever, which had travelled from West Africa and the Congo, particularly to the West Indies, where it spread widely and for centuries infected whole fleets. By the middle of the nineteenth century there were over 150 different names for the disease. Whether the well-known term "ship's typhus" meant typhoid or yellow fever cannot now be determined with any certainty. What is beyond doubt is that many varied diseases were confused with yellow fever, e.g. malignant malaria, blackwater fever and hepatic amoebiasis. In 1847, an official edict laid down for the British navy the choice between only three terms instead of this great variety: febris intermittens (malaria), febris remittens (malaria or typhus, phlebotomus fever, etc.) and febris maligna (yellow fever). For more than a century yellow fever was held not to be infectious, because there was no further spread when the ships returned to northern waters. It could not be known that the disease-carrying gnats needed a certain ambient temperature to be able to develop. As late as 1829, two British ship's doctors thought they had proved that yellow fever was non-infectious by means of an heroic experiment on themselves; they drank the vomited bile of a patient and scratched it into their skin, without becoming ill. A similar experiment had been carried out by several French ship's doctors some years previously.

The statistics spoke clearly against this view. In 1585, Drake lost 750 of his 2300 men to yellow fever alone, and his own death (1596) was a result of the disease. In Santo Domingo, 208 of 300 doctors died in 1802, and the mortality of the ship's doctors in these waters stood at over 60%. Crews frequently had to be completely replaced within 3 months. On the west coast of Africa, where the slave trade flourished, an average of a third of the white crew members fell victim to yellow fever. As late as 1845 the ship "Eclair" lost 74 of 120 men within a short time in this area.

The English marine doctor James L. Donnet (1817–1905) differentiated yellow fever clearly from malaria, but it was not until 1881–1901 that Carlos Finlay (1833–1915) and Walter Reed (1851–1902) clarified the transmission by Stegomyia calopus. Only then was it possible to build the Panama Canal (1910–1914), as the region was plague ridden with yellow fever.

There was no effective therapy for yellow fever. From time to time it was assumed that the harmful matter must come from the bilges, so these were fumigated and disinfected as well as possible. Some believed in the prophylactic effect of blood-letting, which the ship's doctor had to carry out when the equator was crossed. Otherwise the only help was flight back to northern latitudes, where every epidemic vanished instantly.

With the advent of iron ships the gnats were largely robbed of their breeding ground, and today the use of preventive vaccination means that the disease presents no great problems at sea.

Malaria

The English naval doctors Lind and Blane recognized that malaria rarely occurred at more than a certain distance from land, and suggested that ships in hazardous regions should not berth in harbour, but should lay anchor in the roads before sunset. On the same grounds it was recommended not to set up hospitals on land in the tropics, but to accommodate the sick on hospital ships. These suggestions were still followed by the Allies in 1943 during the building of bases in the Pacific; every evening the construction workers were shipped a few miles out to sea. Hardly anyone fell victim to malaria.

Cinchona bark was not to be found in most ships' medicine chests for many years after it was known on land. It was first around 1780 that it was administered in wine. In 1803, Lord Nelson (1758–1805) ordered all ships in his Mediterranean fleet to carry cinchona bark.

1.1.4.3 Other Diseases

Among other infectious diseases, plague played an important role in earlier centuries and, as mentioned above, was the main reason for one of the most significant hygiene measures, quarantine. Probably less well-known is the fact that Indian coal-trimmers very seldom contracted plague, because they rubbed their bodies with oil to protect themselves from the heat and sun, a practice which largely kept the rat fleas away.

It was similar with another well-known seamen's disease, typhus, the significance of which was for centuries disguised by the losses from scurvy, yellow fever and malaria. It was plain to be seen that the slaves shipped from Africa to America were much less vulnerable. Today we know that this can be traced back to their scanty clothing, which offered the transmitting lice much less shelter. The typhus lice were often carried onto ships in their home ports, especially in the ragged clothing of those forced on board to serve in the crew. Here, too, it was Lind who, in exemplary fashion, saw to it that freshly enlisted sailors were first taken onto a quarantine ship, bathed, and given new clothing. In this way a continual source of infection was sealed off.

1.1.4.4 Seasickness

The earliest treatment for seasickness is to be found in the "Lilium medicinae", written in 1303 by Bernhard von Gordon (died c. 1318). He recommended fresh air and the sniffing of toasted, vinegar-soaked bread, advised against eating vegetables, and gave the difficult-to-follow suggestion of holding the head high and moving it with the rolling of the ship. The first descriptions of this disorder, which may affect anyone on board, come from the time of the Crusades. People of rank carried special containers around with them into which to vomit; the remaining voyagers had to empty their stomachs overboard, or in heavy seas into buckets, barrels or the bilge.

In the poem "The Pilgrim's Sea Voyage", which appeared during the reign of Henry VI of England (1422–1471), the main symptoms were accurately portrayed: nausea, vomiting, debility, and heart and stomach complaints. François Rabelais (1494–1553) may have known the illness at first hand, but in any case, he gave a graphic description in his picaresque novel "Gargantua and Pantagruel". Meister Johann Dietz (1665–1738), the German-Dutch surgeon, reported his own experience:

"There was misery and anxiety. There was not one, even 30 years at sea, who was not deathly seasick. I no longer knew who and where I was, quite foolish, with constant vomiting and incontinence, salvo honore".

Heinrich Heine (1797–1856) wrote a poem entitled "Seasickness". Leo Slezak (1873–1946) and the writer Jerome K. Jerome (1858–1927) also reported their own dismal experiences.

Remedies were advanced by the thousands, and more than one charlatan filled his pockets. Sniffing at pomegranates or quinces; consumption of rose syrup, hyssop and raw opium; henbane, nutmeg blossoms and boiled lentils; all kinds of confections and elixirs, some for external use: all were recommended. The strangest pieces of advice were given, such as the setting of cupping-glasses over the stomach area, or boating before a sea voyage for general acclimatization to the movements of a ship.

Even though the nausea was not dangerous and claimed no lives, the numerous remedies show what great importance was attached, also in earlier times, to this most typical of nautical ailments.

1.1.4.5 Venereal Diseases

Sexual infections were always rife on board ship, largely as a result of the weeks alone and the free-and-easy conditions in port. The course of the diseases, however, varied not in the least from that on land. Worthy of note, though, is the infection of whole islands and regions, mostly by seamen. Captain Cook also set an example in this respect, strictly forbidding sexually infected crew members to go ashore.

A great step forward, in 1891, was the introduction by the German naval doctor Walther Uthemann (1863–1944) of obligatory prophylactic treatment, later adopted by all the navies of the civilized world.

It can be mentioned briefly that the English ship's doctor Trotter viewed gonorrhoea and syphilis as different diseases before their definitive separation by Philippe Ricord (1800–1889). Trotter wrote in 1797: "The lues, I think, never produces gonorrhoea".

References

Blane, G.: Observations on the diseases incident to seamen. London: J. Cooper 1785.

Cockburn, W.: An account of the nature, causes, symptoms and cure of distempers that are incident in seafaring people. London: Newman 1696.

Fonssagrives, J.-B.: Traité d'hygiène navale. Paris: Baillière 1877.

Forget, C.: Médecine navale, ou nouveaux éléments d'hygiène, de pathologie et de thérapeutique médico-chirurgicales, a l'usage des officiers de santé de la marine d'état et du commerce. Vols. 1 and 2. Paris: Baillière 1832.

Friedel, C.: Die Krankheiten in der Marine. Geographisch und statistisch nach den Reports on the Health of the Royal Navy. Berlin: Enslin 1866.

Keevil, J. J., C. Lloyd and J. L. S. Coulter: Medicine and navy 1200–1900. Vols. 1–4. Edinburgh: Livingstone 1957–1963.

Keraudren, P.-F.: Mémoire sur les causes des maladies des marins et sur les soins à prendre pour conserver leur santé dans les ports et à la mer. Paris 1817.

Larsen, O.: Schiff und Seuche 1795–1799. Ein medizinischer Beitrag zur historischen Kenntnis der Gesundheitsverhältnisse an Bord dänisch-norwegischer Kriegsschiffe auf den Fahrten nach Dänisch-Westindien. Oslo: Universitetsforlaget 1968.

Le Roy de Méricourt, A.: Die Fortschritte der Schiffshygiene. Transl. by H. Krumpholz Pola 1876.

Lind, J.: An essay on the most effectual means of preserving the health of seamen, in the Royal Navy. Containing directions proper for all those who undertake long voyages at sea, or reside in unhealthy situations. With cautions necessary for the preservation of such persons as attend the sick in fevers. 2nd edn. London: Millar 1762.

Lind, J.: A treatise of the scurvey. Edinburgh: Murray and Cochran 1753.

Mirra, G.: Medicina navale. Padova: Piccin Editore 1961.

Nocht, B.: Vorlesungen für Schiffsärzte der Handelsmarine über Schiffshygiene, Schiffs- und Tropenkrankheiten. Leipzig: Thieme 1906.

Ramazzini, B.: De nautarum et remigum morbis. In: B. Ramazzini: De morbis artificum diatriba cum supplemento. [1713]. Reprint: Rome 1953.

Roddis, L. H.: A short history of nautical medicine. Ann. med. Hist. *3*, 3, 203–247; *3*, 4, 326–352; *3*, 5, 418–447 (1941).

Rouppe, L.: De morbis navigantium, liber unus. [Leiden]: Theodorus Haak 1764.

Ruge, R.: Geschichte der Schiffshygiene. In: Handbuch der Gesundheitspflege an Bord von Kriegsschiffen. Vol. 1: Allgemeine Gesundheitspflege. Eds.: M. zur Verth, E. Bentmann, E. Dirksen et al. Jena: Fischer 1914. pp. 3–68.

Ruge, R.: Schiffsärztliches aus dem 17. und 18. Jahrhundert. Marine-Rundschau *10*, 1011–1041, 1232–1248, 1376–1411 (1900).

Schadewaldt, H.: Zur Geschichte der Verkehrsmedizin unter besonderer Berücksichtigung der Schiffahrtsmedizin. In: Handbuch der Verkehrsmedizin. Eds.: K. and H. J. Wagner. Berlin, Heidelberg, New York: Springer 1968. pp. 1–34.

Schadewaldt, H.: Der Schiffsarzt. Ciba-Z. *7*, 76, 2502–2536 (1955).

Smollet, T.: The adventures of Roderick Random. Oxford: Oxford University Press 1979.

Trotter, Th.: Medicina nautica: an essay on the diseases of seamen. London: Cadell u. Davies 1797–1803.

Turnbull, W.: The naval surgeon. London: R. Philipps 1806.

Woodall, J.: The surgions mate, or a treatise discovering faithfully and plainely the due contents of the surgions chest, the uses of the instruments, the vertues and operations of the medicines, the cures of the most frequent diseases at sea. London: Griffin 1617.

1.2 The Ship's Doctor Yesterday and Today

H. Schadewaldt, W. H. G. Goethe

1.2.1 Greek and Roman Age

In view of the great importance that navigation had for the peoples of the Mediterranean, it is not surprising that ship's doctors are mentioned in various literary sources of the ancient world. The earliest reference is found in a document falsely attributed to Hippocrates: The council of the Athenian fleet deliberated about whether to send a naval doctor on an expedition led by Alcibiades (ca. 450–404 B.C.).

On a marble slab dating from the first century B.C. and found near Constantinople, the crew members of a trireme are recorded in Greek. Listed among the ship's staff, along with captain, navigator and others, is an "iatrós". A tomb in the area of Naples is dedicated to a Roman, M. Satrius Longinus, who was a ship's doctor on board the "Cupido" during the reign of the emperor Hadrian (117–138 A.D.). To date, some more tomb inscriptions of ship's doctors in the service of Rome are known; several of them were Roman and three were Greek. What is unusual is that they were always referred to as "medici duplicarii", which can only mean that they received double pay. Never was a doctor in the army so designated. It is also striking that all of them entered the navy when they were very young, at 20 or 21 years, and that even then there must have been specialists on board, for Galen (129–199 A.D.) expressly mentions an eye doctor, Axios, who served with the Roman fleet in Britain and who compounded a salve from cinnabar which was universally valued in his day. A precursor to the naval medical officer corps of today can be seen in the groups and guilds into which ship's doctors were organized – perhaps to perform religious ceremonies. Even the "naval staff doctor, retired" existed then, for one inscription refers to a "quondam medicus duplicarius".

It can be assumed that for every trireme with a crew of 200 in the mighty Roman fleet – during the reign of Septimus Severus (193–211) it numbered 30000 men – there was a ship's surgeon. His position, however, was quite low. As a "miles" he was at the level of the enlisted men, or of the non-commissioned officers, at best. The better pay is explained today as having been an inducement to join the navy. Naval doctors enjoyed certain privileges as well. Like members of the present-day Red Cross they were "immunes", that is, free from military duties, and if they had given up a private practice they had the "ius restitutionis", the right to compensation.

In Byzantine times as well, there must have been ship's doctors, as Paul of Aegina (seventh century A.D.) proposes that doctors at sea be given written instructions to take along.

1.2.2 The Middle Age and Venice

Until the thirteenth century nothing more is mentioned about ship's doctors. It is quite clear from an order issued by Eleanor of Aquitaine (ca. 1122–1204), wife of Louis VII of France and later of Henry II of England, who had experienced first-hand the suffering of the sick on board during one of the Crusades, that there was no medical care on the ships. She obliged all captains under her authority to have all wounded or sick persons taken ashore and cared for there.

Later on, in an exceptional case, a captain was instructed by his superiors to take a doctor on board: around 1300 a certain "Master Gualtieri" is mentioned as surgeon of the Venetian galleys. He must have been either highly esteemed or quite poor, as he was issued an entire year's salary in advance. Among the files of the Venetian archives there are a number of documents which point to the existence of doctors on board ships.

The first of these decrees is a decision by the High Council of Venice, dated 3 July 1322, to the effect that "unus medicus phisicus mittatur cum istis galeis pro servitio mercatorem et hominum galearum". In 1369 doctors were mentioned among the staff members, and later appeared directly after the commander on the list of personnel on board. In a resolution of 14 February 1411 two ship's doctors were deemed necessary by the Venetian senate: "Teneantur habere ... ad expensas galearum et duos medicos, unum phisicum et unum ciru- siem ...". Up to this time, naval physicians were highly respected; the surgeon was also regarded as "medicus", and so-called barbierotti worked only as assistants, under the direction of university-trained surgeons who had been examined by experienced city and port physicians before embarkation. There was apparently no lack of surgeons who wanted to go to sea; indeed, there were provisos limiting the filling of vacancies on board, due to the huge demand.

In later years the standard and reputation of ship's doctors declined considerably. Up to the seventeenth century fully educated physicians were the exception. Their position was filled by ship's surgeons, some of whom were industrious, studious and talented "Masters". Others, however, were flawed characters, indolent scholars, "barbers" who had broken the law, quacks of all types and men of a decidedly adventurous nature. As every last hand was needed on a sailing ship, it often happened that, instead of an experienced doctor with a good reputation, a less-educated man was signed on, who could also be used in an emergency to hoist the sails or in expeditions on land. The surgeon was often hired with the express instruction to shave crew members once a week, the captain, however, daily. He had to serve as veterinary surgeon as well. Many a commander preferred to practise quackery himself, rather than spend the money for a ship's doctor: As late as 1798 an English captain expelled from his ship a surgeon who had been engaged by the state, believing that he, himself, knew all that was necessary. Some years earlier, an English admiral had refused to stop his ship in heavy seas to rescue a surgeon who had fallen overboard, because he "was useless on board anyway".

1.2.3 The Age of the Explorers

On his voyage around the Cape of Good Hope, Vasco da Gama hadn't a single person on board with medical training; of the 150 men on his flagship, 55 died. Magellan embarked with five ships and a 265-man crew, taking along a surgeon and three barbers. Only his flagship, the "Victoria", reached home in 1522, with a skeleton crew of 18 men. Magellan and his ship's doctor died en route, as well as two of the barbers; the third barber had the good fortune to see his homeland again, and wrote a shocking report of this first voyage around the world. In 1574 there were one barber and one assistant on board a 100-ton corvette; in 1637 as many as six surgeons were available for the 666-man crew of the "Couronne". There were also six surgeons captured along with the 646 men of a privateer in 1657. Even in those days the surgeons appear to have received better treatment; in any case, the chronicler stresses the fact that they were accommodated in a separate cabin. The first evidence of military rank for ship's doctors in the English navy appears in 1512, during the reign of Henry VIII (1509–1547), when the terms "surgeon" and "surgeon's mate" were introduced. The rank of "surgeon"exists even today in the British and American navies; the "surgeon's mate" became an "assistant surgeon" in 1828, a complete university education having been made a requirement for this position in the British navy as early as 1809.

It was up to the captain to decide who was employed as ship's doctor; it was also the captain who paid his salary, usually calculated as head-money per crew member. There were often bonuses in addition: a premium for each crew member who returned healthy. It wasn't until the seventeenth century that government boards took over the payment of doctors' fees. A year's pay for a doctor in England at the time of James I (1566–1625) amounted to £ 200; surgeons received only half of this sum. Until the nineteenth century sailors had to cover the costs of treatment for venereal diseases themselves; presumably, this was a source of not inconsiderable income for poorly paid ship's doctors. The fact that, for this reason, many sailors might not place themselves under medical treatment until it was too late was not appreciated until the Age of Enlightenment. Toward the end of the eighteenth century free treatment was offered for these diseases, too.

Experienced and well-educated surgeons went to sea on Dutch ships even before the Dutch East India Company was founded. From 1610 on, ship's doctors were required to pass an examination given in Middelburg by two sworn town physicians and two town surgeons before they could be engaged. There was a rigorous governmental inspection of the instrumentarium and the medicine bag, both of which the candidate had to provide; ship's doctors who did not conscientiously fulfil their duties were occasionally dismissed without notice. From 1600 to 1625, 114 surgeons and three physicians were hired for the Company. An academy for the further education of ship's doctors was founded in Batavia (now Djakarta) in 1685, so that surgeons on ships lying in port could make use of their time to add to their medical knowledge. Quite early, ship's doctors were ranked equally with officers, and, if they were university trained, they had the right to be addressed as "Sinjeur"; if they were surgeons they received the title "Meester".

Barbers, who usually had a very low level of education, nevertheless occupied a special position on the whaling ships in the seventeenth century. As did their counterparts in ancient Rome, they received double pay if, in addition to performing their surgical duties, they kept the log books and lists, supervised the issuing of rations, and in particular saw to it that the services of worship, celebrated by the captain, were regularly attended.

1.2.4 French Naval Medicine

The view gradually gained acceptance in all countries that – particularly on long voyages – medical care should not be left up to the captain or the shipowner, but rather that laws were necessary to guarantee adequate medical treatment for crew and passengers. On this point, France was ahead of all other seafaring nations. As early as 1628, an article was adopted into the statutes of the surgeons' guild of Marseille requiring an examination before the *chirurgiens jurés* prior to embarkation. A royal decree of 1655 forbade the employment of medically trained persons who had not been examined. In 1681 appeared the famous *„Grande Ordonnance de la Marine"* by the French minister of the navy Jean-Baptiste Colbert (1619–1683), which also dealt with problems of health on shipboard. From 1668 on, the examination for ship's surgeons was held centrally by the *"premier chirurgien du Roi"* or his representative, and no longer by the local guild of barber-surgeons. All the same, there were sundry abuses under Louis XIV (1643–1715): many a certificate was obtained with a bribe. Beginning in 1673, an oath had to be sworn that the surgeon in question would not leave his ship before the end of the voyage, and that he would take no sick sailors on board. In the first 8 years following the promulgation of these regulations 41 diplomas were issued. In contrast, from 1684 to 1692 117 examinations were held; these must have been quite easy, as there is no known case of a candidate who failed. In 1717, as a result of the growing corruption, a new naval decree was made under Louis XV (1715–1774), whereby the examiners were to be appointed in future by the "Admiral de France", a nonmedical authority. In 1746 the "École maritime de chirurgie, d'anatomie et de médecine pratique" was founded in Marseille; it was closed after a short time, opened again in 1777, then closed permanently at the time of the revolution. The school admitted 14-year-old boys who could read, write and – shave. The sons of ship's surgeons had preference. In striking contrast to the efforts that were made to produce well-trained ship's doctors is the fact that in the period up to the revolution the name is known of only one naval physician in France with a doctorate.

1.2.5 British Naval Medicine

In England Henry VIII had established a "Navy Board" which had only an advisory function. In 1588 this authority entrusted four physicians with the supervision of the fleet. Outstanding among them was William Gilbert (1540–1603), who later became personal physician to Queen Elizabeth and president of the Royal College of Physicians. He won great honour for his treatment of the diseases that broke out on board ship.

Medical care in the navy improved considerably after this period. By 1805 only fully qualified physicians were accepted for service with the Royal Navy. In the merchant marine, on the other hand, medical services were often performed by questionable characters. This was particularly true on the numerous convict ships sailing between England and Australia, and on the emigrant ships sailing to America. For example, there were "ship's doctors" who were penalized for selling the rations designated for the sick and letting the prisoners starve, to the extent that they didn't report the death of fellow-prisoners to whom they were chained, in order to have the benefit of their scanty rations. Other "doctors" acted as pimps on ships carrying female prisoners, in this way – and in macabre contrast to their professional duty – promoting generalized venereal infection on board. For this reason special laws for emigrant ships were issued around 1830, and the "Passengers Act" followed in 1849, containing precise figures on the proportion of doctors to passengers on board and regulations covering the medicines to be taken along. There was to be one doctor for every 50 passengers on long voyages, and the power to decide whether a sailor was fit for duty was transferred to the ship's doctor. He was also entrusted with certain public health duties especially in foreign ports, and medical reports were required from him at specified intervals. In the navy daily sick bulletins were introduced, with detailed descriptions of the cases treated. A number of such reports are still available in various English archives; they are no different in structure from our present-day case histories. As of 1838 the younger naval physicians were still not admitted to the officers' mess, but in 1859 the British navy followed the French example: in France as early as 1793 all physicians were given equal rank with officers, and even the youngest surgeons occupied the rank of a junior physician (an aspirant). The American navy, founded in 1775, raised its ship's doctors to the rank of officer in 1828; until then they had been equal to the lower commissioned deck officers. A young navy, the

German Federal, founded in 1848, did require of its candidates a licence to practise and a doctoral degree, but only the Imperial German navy founded in 1871 had its own naval medical officer corps in 1896, and only after the First World War did naval doctors receive rank equal on all points to that of the other naval officers. In the Austro-Hungarian Empire the separation from the army medical officer corps was made in 1855, and even Italy, in 1861, was far ahead of Germany in this respect.

It is remarkable that with the establishment of the North American navy in 1775 four ship's doctors were employed, who, however, held no service rank. Military ranks were first introduced in 1871, and it was still later that the rank of the naval doctor was adjusted to correlate with that of the other officers.

1.2.6 The Ship's Doctor, the Pharmacist and the Medicine Chest

Pharmacists were an exception on board up until the French Revolution, although in ancient times they belonged to the navy. Under the Romans surgeons held the same rank as the highest non-commissioned officers. They were often recruited from among former Greek and Arab slaves, and received Roman citizenship after serving for a specified amount of time. In all probability, however, they prepared the medicaments for the ships on land, and did not go to sea themselves.

Later on, people made do with medicine chests which were carried on long sailing voyages. Two such chests are preserved at the Wellcome Historical Medical Museum in London; they held instruments and numerous medications compounded from more or less beneficial ingredients. Among other medications there were purgatives and emetics, theriaca and substances made with terra sigillata, the tusks of elephants or the horn of the legendary unicorn, bezoar and viper oil.

In France these medicine chests were inspected by the most senior surgeons and pharmacists of the port before the ships set out, but never by the same pharmacist who had delivered the supplies. The inspection was set for the third to last day before embarkation to avoid any kinds of irregularities.

Dieppe was one of the places where a medicine-chest industry sprang up in the seventeenth century, producing standardized chests in various sizes. It did good business, for Colbert's naval legislation of 1668 stipulated that every ship that put to sea for an extended period had to take along a medicine chest.

By 1778 the contents of such chests had become modernized. A British ship's doctor, for example, suggested the following medicaments: cinchona, cascarilla, ipecac, tartar emetic, white antimony glance, opium, laudanum, magnesium sulfuricum, potassium bitartrate, mercurial ointment, calomel, ammonium carbonate, spirit of vitriol, gum arabic and various vesicating plasters. A comprehensive description of ship's apothecary chests during the era of sailing ships can be found in Müller [11].

A great many ship's doctors performed services that went far beyond the medical care on board. Only a few of the doctors are mentioned here, who – ahead of their time – made decisive contributions, not only in their special fields, but also in other disciplines of the natural sciences.

1.2.7 Medical Guides and Famous Ship's Doctors

Many a doctor who went to sea tried, by means of treatises and monographs, to pass on the knowledge gained during long, eventful voyages, or to make new findings generally available to other colleagues. The oldest surviving accounts of this type are probably the health regimens drawn up for high-ranking gentlemen by their personal physicians. Just such a manual is preserved in the state library in Kassel, along with the travel diary of the landgrave Wilhelm I the elder of Hesse (1466–1515), who sailed to Palestine in 1491–1492. In it, wearing scarlet robes was recommended to ward off dysentery; the gentlemen were supposed to take live animals in cages on board, as experience had shown that the nutrition was inadequate and the provisions often spoiled; finally, they were advised to take wrapped urinals and spittoons with lids as it is well known that there were still no toilets at that time.

The "Raiß Büchlin", or *Reise Büchlein* (travel diary) by Georg Pictorius (ca. 1500–1569), which appeared in Straßburg in 1557, can be regarded as the first manual of nautical medicine. It was primarily instructions for captains and navigators, but it included an appendix with the heading "wie sich auff dem Möre oder andern Wasser zu schicken" (i. e. "how to adapt to the sea or other waters").

A second, similar treatise was written not by a physician, but by an English poet and courtier, George Whetstone (1544–1587); his work on nautical medicine and the tropical diseases then known was published posthumously in 1598. Incidentally, Whetstone's strikingly prescient advice for dysentery, which was suffered frequently on board ships, was first to administer a purgative, then to give red wine and rice water, and to apply a mustard plaster to the body. The first work on tropical medicine in general, and on medicinal herbs of India in particular, stems from a Portuguese ship's doctor, Garcia del Huerto (ab Orta) (1490–1570), who lived for a long time in Goa, and is regarded as the first to have described the Rauwolfia serpentina, whose root plays such a large role in the treasury of modern medicines. His „Coloquios dos simples e drogas há causas medicinais da India“ appeared in Goa in 1563.

John Woodall (1556–1643) was also an author with previous medical training; he was a ship's doctor with the Dutch East India Company and published his "Surgeon's Mate" in London in 1617. He was one of the first to recommend lemon juice for scurvy. "An Account of the Nature, Causes, Symptoms and Cure of the Distempers that are incident to Seafaring People", by William Cockburn (1669–1739) appeared in London in 1696. In "The Navy-Surgeon", published in London in 1734 by John Atkins (1685–1757), the African sleeping sickness is described for the first time in English; this was much earlier than the description by Thomas Masterman Winterbottom (1765/66–1859), whose report from Sierra Leone in 1830 was long regarded as the first.

The eighteenth century was the age of the "classics of nautical medicine": In 1753 James Lind (1716–1794) published "A Treatise of the Scurvy"; in 1757, the basic work on ship's hygiene, "An Essay on the Most Effectual Means of Preserving the Health of Seamen in the Royal Navy"; and in 1768, a paper on tropical medicine entitled "An Essay on Diseases Incidental in Europeans in Hot Climates". In 1785 followed the "Observations on the Diseases incident to Seamen" by Sir Gilbert Blane (1749–1834), who had great success in getting Lind's demands with regard to hygiene carried out in the Royal Navy. In 1797 came "Medicina nautica" by Thomas Trotter (1761–1832), who was at that time a doctor with the British fleet. The first American work on nautical medicine was written in 1808 by Edward Cutbush (1772–1843).

The name of one ship's doctor is probably universally known, that of Thomas Dover (1662–1742), who became famous during his lifetime through a series of adventures. In 1732 he published the still authoritative work "Pulvis Ipecacuanhae opiatus", and he owed the establishment of his eminent London practice to his successful privateering expeditions in southern waters. He was the owner of two ships; today he would be called a pirate. In 1709, on a three-year sea voyage, he rescued the shipwrecked sailor Alexander Selkirk (1676–1721) from the lonely Juan Fernandez Island. Selkirk's story was the inspiration for the 1719 novel "Robinson Crusoe" by Daniel Defoe (1660–1731).

A number of places on the map are named in honour of the ship's doctors who discovered them: the Bass Strait is named after George Bass (1771–later than 1802), who proved that Tasmania was not part of the mainland; Elliot's Cove, after the surgeon's mate who was shipwrecked during a voyage of exploration in 1740 and died after long privation; and Capes Richardson and Armstrong, after two respected English naval physicians.

The Edinburgh clinician William Cullen (1712–1790); the biologist Thomas Huxley (1825–1895), founder of neuropathology; Charles Darwin (1809–1882), who went to sea as a medical student – he never took a medical examination; the nautical and tropical physician Bernhard Nocht (1857–1945), after whom the Institute for Nautical and Tropical Diseases in Hamburg was named in 1942; the naval medical corps captain Eduard Hoffmann (born 1837), one of the reorganizers of the medical-surgical academy in Tokyo; his colleague Führmann, who as early as 1872 detected malaria plasmodia in blood, but misinterpreted them; the bacteriologists Albert Calmette (1863–1933), Georg Gaffky (1850–1918) and August Gärtner (1848–1934): all are well-known medical men who spent decisive periods of their lives as ship's doctors. And even the celebrated Rudolf Virchow (1821–1902) was of the opinion that

> for a young man who, along with amassing a rich store of empirical knowledge, has also trained in the practise of autopsy and of epicritic examination, a long sea voyage ... [is] an invaluable opportunity to do his own work and to reflect more deeply.

The final important phase in the work of ship's doctors covers over 100 years, from the mid-nineteenth century to the mid-twentieth. During this period the ever-larger, fast passenger and emigrant ships plied the oceans. The most renowned stretches were Europe–North America, Europe–South America, Europe–East Asia and Europe–Southeast Asia. From the middle of the nineteenth century onward, almost all of the important shipping countries had regulations covering the carriage of ship's doctors. In the absence of regulations, the competition between the large shipping companies forced them to keep relatively good medical facilities on board and to carry ship's doctors. On the great passenger ships of the European and North American shipping lines there were excellently equipped ship's hospitals, operating and consulting rooms, and – quite early on – X-ray equipment. Crew members were cared for by one to five ship's doctors and by male and female nurses. Even though there were no longer academies for ship's doctors, as during the seventeenth and eighteenth centuries in France, the occupation of ship's doctor was recognized and was often pursued as a field of specialization for many years. The Institute for Nautical and Tropical Diseases founded in Hamburg in 1900 held its own courses for ship's doctors. Its director Nocht published his own textbook, "Vorlesungen für Schiffsärzte" (Lectures for Ship's Doctors) [13]; he wrote in the foreword:

> A modern passenger ship is a very complex organism. For the young ship's doctor everywhere it is exceptionally difficult to make quick and correct judgements about hygienic conditions on board and the peculiar characteristics of the crew and passengers, and to get a clear idea at the outset of his own position, the range of his duties, and the resources available to him for fulfilling them.

The book clearly illustrates the problems of that time; infectious diseases, particularly the diseases subject to quarantine such as plague, yellow fever, smallpox and cholera, as well as typhus, amoebic dysentery, malaria, filariasis and trypanosomiasis are the centre of discussion. Among the deficiency diseases beriberi is dealt with in detail, although scurvy is no longer important. A substantial chapter is devoted to ship's hygiene, with special regard to water supply and disinfection.

Another book widely read by ship's doctors was "The Ship Surgeon's Handbook", by Vavasour Elder [19]. It contains classic descriptions of the problems faced by ship's doctors, some of which are still valid for today, even if the current ailments of passengers and crew members may have changed.

> No thought is ever given by the travelling public to his responsibilities, medical and moral, in dealing with an epidemic disease which may, perhaps, attack the whole ship; his anxiety in case of enteric fever or pneumonia, where careful nursing, almost the whole essence of treatment, is practically unobtainable unless a trained nurse happens to be among the passengers, and volunteers her services; his doubts in case of probable malingering, knowing full well that if he makes a mistake in either direction his reputation among the crew is gone; the decision as to the exact point at which a slightly sick man must be laid off duty – all these are unknown and unseen, consequently unappreciated... He is in a position of spendid isolation, having no one on board in sympathy with his work. In fact, the very exercise of his duty at times antagonizes all other departments in so far as their own work is concerned. Moreover, none of these will share any blame attaching to the results of his attempts to satisfy everybody ... A ship-surgeon lives on possibilities. The whole gamut of medicine, surgery and midwifery lies within his sphere, and may arise at any moment calling for prompt measures. The following record of a day's work while taking 1,600 emigrants to Australia may be of interest. It included one normal labour, a compound fracture of tibia and a dislocation of shoulder (the weather was bad at the time), three dental extractions, four abscesses incised, in addition to routine surgery hours, and with diphtheria and scarlet fever both prevalent in epidemic form. This is not quoted as being typical of an ordinary day's work at sea, but more as illustrating the various possibilities at any given moment...

In 1937, in one of the last books to appear along these lines, the editor Kortenhaus collected all the regulations that were relevant to the ship's doctor and the port doctor of his day [14].

Each of the major passenger shipping lines had its own instructions and rules for the ship's doctors and other medical personnel it employed. Even the few shipping companies of today that still operate passenger liners have similar regulations. From them can be gained an impression of the extremely broad area of operations, usually described in plain, dry language. For instance, the booklet *Duties and Responsibilities of Ship's Surgeon, Nurses, and Hospital Attendant,* published in 1969 by the Moore-McCormack Line for the medical personnel on its passenger ships, contains, among others, the following instructions:

> The ship's surgeon as a staff officer is in charge of the medical department of the vessel. He is responsible for the physical welfare of the crew and passengers and is in direct charge of the treatment and care of all sick and injured persons on board ... The ship's surgeon should at all times remember that he is a physician and that his actions may easily be the subject of discussion by passengers ... The surgeon shall consider himself on duty at all times and shall not leave the ship at any foreign port without notifying the master ... [Sherlock 15].

1.2.8 The Ship's Doctor in Recent Decades and Nowadays

The large passenger liners experienced an upswing once again at the end of the 1940s and in the 1950s, following the Second World War. However, they disappeared from the oceans rather quickly at the beginning of the 1960s. As had already happened in the 1920s and 1930s, various large shipping companies switched increasingly to the running of freighters and passenger ships as so-called combination ships. According to their size, these ships had crews numbering between 50 and 80 men and women and carried up to 100 passengers. The occupation of ship's doctor also experienced an upswing once more with this change, although rarely any longer as a long-term commitment; it was much more usual for a doctor to make only a few trips, or even just one. Medically relevant descriptions of the occupation of ship's doctor are becoming increasingly rare. On the other hand, various publications by ship's doctors have achieved belletristic quality (Xadow [20]).

In the late 1960s and the 1970s the great passenger liners vanished altogether from the seas; passenger transport is now handled by the airlines. One form of passenger shipping has survived – however, with considerably smaller ships: the cruise. It has become a speciality. Whereas passengers used the huge liners, and to some extent the combination ships, only as a means of transportation, to get from one part of the world to the other – particularly at the time of mass emigration – the cruise passenger travels purely for enjoyment, or luxury. The make-up of the passengers has changed accordingly. Almost all cruise lines have abolished passenger classes; the only differences now are among cabin prices, but all passengers have the same recreation area on board and receive the same menu. The average age of the cruise passenger has risen quite considerably. On many trips, 90% of the passengers are over 60 years old.

The peculiar characteristics of the travellers are so distinctive that the term "cruise medicine" has already found its way into the literature of nautical medicine (Jäger [7, 8]). Carter [2] goes into the matter of "shipboard medicine on package cruises" in detail. He writes:

> Cheap package cruises have become very popular in Great Britain, but the ships used for these cruises are often not suitable for elderly, handicapped, and mentally unfit people. The cruises run to very tight schedules with many strenuous shore excursions, and do not necessarily constitute restful holidays at sea. Many passengers who embark on these cruises are suffering from pre-existing diseases, which may become exacerbated during the voyage ...

Taking the entire world into consideration, only a few ships today sail with a ship's doctor. There are no longer any fully trained doctors on the freighters of the western industrialized countries, or on those of the developing countries. On these ships, health care is provided by the ship's officers, or, in the case of a few shipping companies, by medical assistants (male or female nurses, enfermeros, paramedics). Since, with only a few exceptions, the combination ships have practically disappeared, ship's doctors can be found only on the passenger-cruise ships or on a few special ships. Ships of the Eastern-Bloc countries, especially of the Soviet Union, Poland and the German Democratic Republic, still carry doctors on freighters with large crews. However, as the average crew size has dropped sharply even in these countries, it can be anticipated that on these ships as well the health of the crew will soon be looked after only by ship's officers or paramedical personnel.

Ship's doctors are still to be found, however, on some special ships, particularly fishery protection vessels, fishing factory and processing boats, research ships and cable laying ships. These vessels carry doctors because of their large crews or their scope of duties. The fishery protection vessels resemble small, specially equipped hospital ships, with the best facilities for operative and conservative treatment on board (Goethe [3]; Kaerger [9]; Naumann [12]).

"In the eyes of the public, the life of a ship-surgeon is commonly invested with glamourous and pleasurable surroundings and circumstances of all sorts" (Meighan [10]). This is an unfortunate, but widespread, error. Even if the doctor on a passenger ship has to play, more or less voluntarily, a certain social role, on neither passenger ships nor fishery protection or research vessels does he have an easy, comfortable life. A ship's doctor who takes his job seriously is required to have a good knowledge of general medicine, as well as experience with minor and intermediate surgery and radiography. Some knowledge of dentistry is also necessary; at the very least, a ship's doctor is expected to be able to extract teeth. He must be capable of treating fractures or injuries, of performing appendectomies, and possibly even of treating a perforated or bleeding stomach ulcer on his own – all this without the facilities of a large hospital, and often with inadequate assistance, or none at all. Nevertheless, an experienced ship's doctor avoids operations as far as possible. The fact that the ship's doctor is left entirely to his own resources in diagnosis and treatment constitutes an essential reality. A doctor from a developed country is not used to such circumstances. The junior doctor at a hospital has many colleagues, the department head, and the director; moreover, there is a great variety of special wards. In private practice there are specialists in every field, and hospitals to which a doctor can refer cases which he cannot handle himself. None of these are available at sea. Every ship's doctor is his or her own assistant, department head and director. There are no specialists whom one can consult. Even if one decides to ask the ship's management to put in at the next port, one must care for the patient oneself until that port is reached – and this can often take many days. Moreover, the captain will be most unwilling to put in at a port not on the planned route, as this could entail heavy financial losses. The ship's doctor is expected to be able to handle all illnesses or accidents on board. A country doctor, or one in a less developed country, is used to working completely on his own, and would be able to cope more easily with such demands. Beyond the purely medical sphere, a ship's doctor must be a person with a large amount of self-confidence, diplomatic talent in his dealing with the idiosyncrasies of the sailors, passengers and the authorities, and last but not least, must have a good knowledge of languages (Goethe [4]). An essential feature of the ship's doctor's job is independent, responsible decision-making (Unger and Ebert [18]).

The ship's doctor plays a major role on board in lowering morbidity among seamen. Slutzker and Balakirev [16] especially point out the possibilities of improving the health of the crew through therapeutic and preventive measures, as well as through sanitation.

The ship's doctor must always make do with the medicaments, instruments and equipment at hand. Things that are lacking must often be improvised; this is an art that every successful ship's doctor must acquire quickly (Heits and Fischer [6]).

The equipment that a ship's doctor finds on board corresponds to the regulations either of the country whose flag his ship flies or of his shipping company. Many countries with a shipping industry have stipulations regarding medications, medical equipment and instruments, as well as the rooms required, for ships which, according to their regulations, must have a doctor. Some shipping countries, however, have no regulations governing the equipment of ship's hospitals and operating and consulting rooms. In these countries it is left to the shipping companies to provide the ship's doctor with an adequate supply of instruments and other necessary equipment. As experiences in international shipping show, this problem is not always perfectly solved, although good shipping companies endeavour – if only because of competition – to have a competent ship's doctor on board and to provide the proper equipment.

In general, the ship's doctor can expect to find a consulting room and a separate operating room. These rooms should be equipped with the necessary apparatus for diagnosis, sterilization and operative treatment, including dental care. A good ship's pharmacy, sufficiently provided with modern medicaments, is especially important. A lack of instruments and apparatus can be compensated for by experience and improvisation; a lack of medication, and particularly of bandaging material, cannot. Equipment today should include an efficient X-ray unit for pictures of bones, an ECG machine, and a small laboratory. In addition, one or several – according to the number of passengers and crew on board – sick-rooms are necessary in the immediate vicinity of the consulting and operating rooms.

In a review of the accomplishments of radiography in the fishing fleet and the merchant marine of the German Democratic Republic, Grimmer and Arlt [5] provide evidence for the fact that shipboard X-ray apparatus is not useless equipment, but rather an indispensable diagnostic aid.

In their discussion of the medical equipment on Italian passenger ships, Tortori-Donati and Giannico [17] point out that passenger ships should also have a morgue, or at least refrigeration rooms, for preserving the bodies of people who die on board.

Faced with the wishes of many handicapped cruise passengers, some shipping lines already provide wheel chairs suitable for use on shipboard. Of late, even dialysis machines can be found on some cruise ships; Behrmann [1] reports on very successful experiences with a special cruise for dialysis patients.

The future development of the occupation of ship's doctor is still uncertain. Presumably, the size of crews on freighters will be further reduced in the next few years – in spite of high unemployment rates on land and the population growth in the developing countries, whose unemployed are searching for work. Even the increasing number of doctors in the developed industrial countries will not bring ship's doctors back on board, because crews have become too small. Only special ships – such as fish-processing vessels, fishing fleets and research ships – will still be provided with medical care by a ship's doctor. In the face of worldwide air traffic and its efficiency, the passenger ship as a means of transportation will probably not make a comeback. What will remain, and possibly gain increasing importance, is the cruise, even as a mass phenomenon. Here the ship's doctor will have a place, even in the future.

References[1]

1. Bermann, G.: Medizinische Erfahrungen während einer Kreuzfahrt mit Dialysepatienten. Dtsch. Ärztebl. *78,* 4, 132 (1981).
2. Carter, J.W.: Shipboard medicine on package cruises. Brit. med. J. 1, 553–556 (1972).
3. Goethe, H.: Wesen und Aufgabe des ärztlichen Dienstes im deutschen Fischereischutz. Zbl. Verkehrsmed. *1,* 3, 189–194 (1955).
4. Goethe, H.: Der Schiffsarzt. Hippokrates *34, 8,* 321–328 (1963).
5. Grimmer, G. and H.C. Arlt: Röntgendiagnostik auf Schiffen aus der Sicht des Schiffsarztes. Verk.-Med. *26,* 5, 193–195 (1979).
6. Heits, E. and M. Fischer: Einführung in die schiffsärztliche Tätigkeit. Chemische Fabrik G. Robisch (ed) München: Hearl [1960].
7. Jäger, H.: Kreuzfahrtmedizin. Bordärztliche Erfahrungen auf modernen Passagierschiffen. Ther. d. Gegenw. *118,* 4, 616–631 (1979).
8. Jäger, H.: Kreuzfahrtmedizin. Ärztliche Betreuung von Besatzung und Passagieren auf See. Z. Allg. Med. 56, 942–948 (1980).
9. Kaerger, E.: Die medizinische Betreuung der deutschen Hochseefischerei. In: Fischereischutzboote und Fischereiforschungsschiffe der Bundesrepublik Deutschland – Aufgaben und Tätigkeiten von 1948 bis 1981, Ed. Bundesministerium für Ernährung, Landwirtschaft und Forsten. Bonn, Hamburg 1982. pp. 57–75.
10. Meighan, J.S.: The ship-surgeon's life. Practitioner 170, 506–511 (1953).
11. Müller, I.: Untersuchungen zur Arzneimittelversorgung an Bord vom Beginn der Entdekkungsreisen bis zur Einführung der Dampfschiffahrt. Dissertation, University of Düsseldorf, 1969.
12. Naumann, P.: Die ärztliche Betreuung der Deutschen Hochseefischereiflotte auf See. Z. ärztl. Fortbild. *51,* 23, 1049–1059 (1957).
13. Nocht, B.: Vorlesungen für Schiffsärzte der Handelsmarine über Schiffshygiene, Schiffs- und Tropenkrankheiten. Leipzig: Thieme 1906.
14. Der Schiffs- und Hafenarzt. Ein Leitfaden für Ärzte und Seeleute. Ed. F. Kortenhaus. Jena: Fischer 1937.
15. Sherlock, P.: Duties and responsibilities of ship's surgeon, nurses and hospital attendant. Moore-McCormack Lines, Inc., Medical Department Manual 1969.
16. Slutzker, D.S. and E.M. Balakirev: The role of a ship's doctor in lowering morbidity among seamen. In: III International Symposiom on Ma-

1 For further references regarding the historical aspect, see the references to Chapt. 1.1.

rine Medicine, Leningrad, 1968. Eds. E. P. Sergeev at al. Moscow 1969. pp. 164–166.
17. Tortori-Donati, B. and L. Giannico: Practice of medical profession on board passenger ships, remarks on equipment and activity of the medical department of the liners and on morbidity on board. In: III International Symposium on Marine Medicine, Leningrad, 1968. Eds. E. P. Sergeev et al. Moscow 1969. pp 189–196.
18. Unger, J. E. and H. Ebert: Schiffsarzt heute. Verk.-Med. *29*, 3, 115–119 (1982).
19. Vavasour Elder, A.: The ship surgeon's handbook. London: Baillière, Tindall & Cox 1926.
20. Xadow, Ch.: Whisky, Haut & Serum. ... Aus dem Tagebuch eines Schiffsarztes. Herford: Koehlers 1974.

1.3 The Ship's Medical Centre and Medicine Chest

A. Backhaus

Since men first travelled long distances on land and sea they have found it necessary to carry medical equipment (Ewald [18]; Goethe [27]; Larsen [54, 55]; Schadewaldt [82, 83, 85]; Volbehr [104, 105]). The aforementioned papers document the ingenuity applied at various times in history in deciding the type of equipment according to prevailing medical knowledge and theories. Few countries then enforced strict regulations for their ships. Nowadays however, most countries have recommendations and regulations governing the medical equipment on their ships. These requirements change to take account of developments in medical science. Consequently, fundamental questions as well as aspects of medical assistance on board will be discussed below (Fischer [19, 20]; Halm [32]; [76]; Ram [79]; White [107]).

1.3.1 Shipbuilding

The design of small ships with a small crew makes no provision for a special room or place for medical care. A necessary factor to be taken into account for larger ships is how far a ship will usually be from shore, i.e. from medical assistance in a port. An additional factor is the use for which the ship has been built. This parameter is of prime importance in shipbuilding when medical provisions have to be considered (Angelov et al. [1]; Koch [48]; Milcheva et al. [69]; [74]; [81]; Schmidt and Kludas [87]; Sobol and Krynicki [94]; Staton [97]; Vinkovetski and Krivenda [103]). All ships carrying dangerous cargo, especially tankers and chemical tankers, should have a sick-bay and a sufficiently large room for medical examination and treatment. This room should contain a bath and a shower, the facilities to perform infusions, suitable equipment for cleaning and rinsing the eyes and good means of temperature regulation for severely burnt patients. There must be provision for administering oxygen. The supervision of the patient is vital, and an emergency bell that could be used by a semiconscious person should be considered.

Other high-risk vessels and structures are dredgers, excavators, cranes, drilling platforms and drilling platform supply boats. These must have a treatment room; since they are not far from shore or from helicopter landing places, there is no need for a sick-bay. Today, most ships of this type have a treatment room, but this room should be large and should have an examination couch that has access from all sides, a chair for the treatment of eye, ear and mouth, facilities for carrying out infusions, a telephone link with the shore, an emergency alarm, a sufficient water supply, a bath and a shower. The minimum size should be 20 m^2, including the bath and shower.

Statutory safety regulations demand less of the fishing fleet than of the merchant fleet (Krynicki [52]; Sobol and Żurawiecki [93]). Small fishing boats usually put to sea in the evening and returned in the morning. This type of fishing has ended in the industrial countries but is still to be found in other parts of the world. Nowadays, there are different methods of fishing, for example, large factory ships that process the

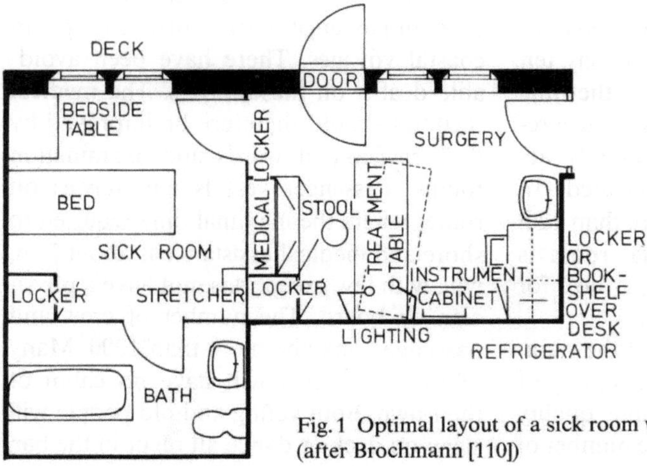

Fig. 1 Optimal layout of a sick room with treatment room. (after Brochmann [110])

catch brought to them by a fleet of smaller fishing boats. The accident risk, especially in side and stern trawlers but even in fish processing on board a ship, is high. The statistics and reports indicate just how dangerous the work is.

Many small fishing boats have only three to five crew members; often there is no covered accommodation for a stretcher case and the casualty is kept in the open on deck. If the ship is big enough, there should be accommodation for treating an injured person and a ward sufficiently equipped for a minimum of two people. If a fishing boat has to leave the fishing grounds to land an injured person at the nearest port, the diversion is more expensive than the best medical equipment. Several countries provide fishing protection vessels with good medical facilities and even a ship's doctor. Cargo ships not carrying dangerous cargo and engaged solely in coastal trade need only a place to carry out first aid – a separate room is preferable. The location of the nearest port with medical assistance should be taken into account, for there are regions in the world where there are ports without medical facilities.

Fig. 1 shows an optimal layout of sick room (ship's hospital) and a room for diagnosis and treatment (surgery) for all types of ships.

1.3.2 Number of Crew

The number of the crew is generally taken into consideration when deciding the extent of medical provisions [2]. According to German regulations there must be a doctor if there are more than 75 people on board. For ships without a doctor the ship's medicine chest (*International Medical Guide for Ships*, [35]) is based on one of two scales: (a) for up to 40 people and (b) for more than 40 people.

There are numerous different national regulations with very diverse parameters concerning the number of the crew. How significant is this "number of crew" parameter? In a crew of 20 one seafarer with heart failure or a fracture of the spine needs the same assistance as one person among 2000 crew members and passengers on a cruise liner. However, the probability of such a case may correspond statistically to the number of people on board. This is true, for example, for heart failure and cancer of the lung. But is it realistic for accidents? A small ship under pressure to earn money may well be a place where accidents occur in spite of a small number of crew. Of course, a small ship transporting cargo could not be constructed to have a medical centre of 40 m^2, which would be used infrequently.

The economic point of view may be an essential one, but if the statistical probability of accidents and diseases among, say, ten crew members is considered and the time to the next port with medical assistance regarded, the following internationally acknowledged fact can be appreciated: In voyages near the coast, not more than 12 h from a port of call, no special room is needed for medical treatment; a box for medical equipment is sufficient.

The essential parameter is not the number of crew members but the possibility of medical assistance of reasonable quality from shore. Today we expect the number of crew to be as small as possible. Ships near a coast with ports providing good medical assistance are sufficiently equipped if they have a place for first-aid treatment and a box or a small cupboard for the medical equipment.

1.3.3 Vessels Engaged in Deep Sea Voyages

If a ship is more than 24 h from medical assistance, be this at sea or in regions with no hospitals or emergency stations ashore, it should have a room for examination and treatment (Krynicki [52]). There should be an examination bed to which there is clear access from all sides, and a locker to store the necessary medicines. There should be a sick-bay for two people with an emergency bell and/or telephone, WC, bathroom and natural light.

1.3.3.1 Passenger Vessels

Passenger ships, even if small, have many more people on board than cargo ships. Most crew members on a cargo ship are under 40 years of age, in contrast to the passengers on a liner, which may include babies and elderly people. The crew of a cargo ship will be checked regarding their fitness for duty at sea. There are virtually no regulations to prevent a sick person boarding a passenger vessel. The regulations have generally neglected these facts even for passenger ferries solely engaged in coastal voyages. There have been avoidable deaths on these ferries. The medical facilities should therefore be improved by the provision of wards and examination rooms. Passenger vessels and ferries on routes where the maximal time required to shore and medical assistance is about 24 h, will, with few exceptions, not have a physician on board. The number of crew and passengers may be more than 1000. Many of the passengers will have no cabin of their own. Both young and old people will sleep on deck or dance all night in the bar. There may be many children, even babies, on board. On a luxury ship every passenger will have his own cabin and is likely to stay there if he falls ill. On the ferries in coastal waters, there must be sufficient room for sick or injured persons, including drunken or mentally disturbed passengers.

Until now, national and international regulations have not considered this point. Luxury vessels have generally more rooms and wards for patients than necessary, but ferries and similar ships often do not have even an emergency room for first aid. On these ships there should be:

1. A room for first aid, large enough to have an examination bed with access from all sides, washing facilities and adequate lighting and a locker for medicine, bandages etc.; the door way should be large enough for a patient on a stretcher to be brought into and out of the room.
2. Two rooms for patients (female or male) with sanitary facilities, emergency bell and natural light. One room should be equipped for a mentally disturbed or drunken person. The room should be lockable from the outside and there should be an observation window to permit supervision from outside whenever the patient is not accompanied by an attendant. The content of the room should be such that nothing can be used by the patient to injure himself.

Passenger vessels engaged in deep sea voyages of more than 24 hours duration – including pilgrim ships of Asiatic and Arabian countries and coastal ships undertaking very long voyages – should have very good medical facilities. General regulations provide a basic outfit, but the company must consider the necessity of special medical provisions for passengers suffering from a known condition, e.g. persons requiring treatment after heart failure, diabetics and even very occasionally patients requiring dialysis of the kidney; it is also necessary to take into account a prevalence of persons over the age of 60 years, special dangers involved in excursions and tropical diseases. A great deal of space is needed to provide for medical care [33]:

1. Accommodation of the staff: As the patient must be attended day and night, the number of staff has to be considered; the minimum is one doctor and two female and one male nurse.
2. Large waiting room; for national, religious and social reasons two rooms would be preferable.
3. Room for a receptionist/secretary, for appointments, for case histories, bills etc.
4. Laboratory with the means of developing X-rays.
5. Doctor's examination room.
6. First-aid room and treatment room.
7. Room for operations (Chapman [12]; Ulrich [101]; Volkov [106]).
8. Facilities for X-ray and electrocardiogram (ECG) examinations.
9. Wards: one for females and one for males (with two beds each); one for emergency cases (with monitor ECG, oxygen); one spare room with four beds; one room for medicine, bandages etc.; one room for dentistry; one room for the mentally ill and/or drunk; room/facilities for sewage, garbage and infected material; direct telephone link with radio room; sufficient space and access for transportation of a patient from deck and cabin to helicopter landing place.

1.3.4 Doctor on Board

Nowadays, ships rarely carry a doctor. One or two decades ago, there were a lot of 'combined' ships, with both passengers and cargo, with a doctor on board. Cruising passenger ships have a doctor, as may cargo ships of a few countries following the example of the Soviet Union, if there is a large crew on board. The following is the experience of the Port Health Authority, Hamburg, during the past 10 years.

1.3.4.1 Cruise Ships

The number of crew and passengers is usually more than 1000. The doctor has 10–50 patients a day. They have 0–4 serious cases in 4 weeks and one fatal case in 3 months. The doctor and nurses are necessary.

1.3.4.2 Cargo Ships

Normally, the doctor has reported that there has been no dangerous disease on board; the captain thinks that the doctor has a good and quiet life on board. But this is not always the case. There may be several cases of accidents with severe bleeding, malaria or meningitis. In some cases the doctor has had to give medical advice and assistance to other ships.

The overall situation of the ship has to be considered. If it is going to be far from shore for a long time or if there are special risks involved, a doctor should be available.

1.3.5 The Ship's Medicine Chest

Every ship, even small ships and those covering short distances, should have a minimum supply. But what is the necessary minimum? ([2]; [7]; Brenning [9]; [10]; [11]; [13]; [17]; [23]; Goede-Oudegeest [26]; [34]; [35]; [42]; [43]; [51]; [60]; [61]; [62]; [64]; [65]; [67]; [68]; Milcheva et al. [69]; Nocht [71]; [73]; Onnen [75]; [76]; [80]; [81]; Serdarević et al. [88]; Sherlock [89]; [90]; [91]; [92]; Sobol and Krynicki [94]; [95]; [96]; Staton

[97]; Stjepanović [98]; Urner and Staton [102]). This question is linked with another: Should a ship be supplied with effective medicines normally used by a doctor, considering that there will be no person on board who has any medical training (or at best somebody with only a minimum of training)? But if the medical chest contains only less effective medicines, what should be done on board in case of emergency? This problem is complicated by the very different rules, regulations and laws in different countries, concerning the administration of medicine. However, a shipowner or a master must be aware of his national regulations (Ebert [16]; Grewe [28]; Klepatski [47]). A list of suitable medicines is recommended in the *International Medical Guide for Ships* [35] and in the IMO's *Medical First Aid Guide for use in Accidents Involving Dangerous Goods* [66]. Many seafaring countries have issued medical scales for their own ships. These may differ considerably in the number and kind of medicines and other supplies.

1.3.5.1 Ships Carrying Dangerous Cargo

Irrespective of the size of a ship or the number of crew members, medicine must be available for immediate treatment and in sufficient quantity for the first hours. Experience proves that many types of dangerous cargo may be carried in a particular ship. So the medical outfit should be standardised and include all known antidotes and medicine for basic treatment of poisoning. There are international schedules of the IMO which should be observed [66]: Included are: atropine injection, polyethylene glycol (*minimum* 2000 ml), amyl nitrite for inhalation, a strong sedative such as diazepam for injection, oxygen equipment, strong analeptics for injection, analgesic eyedrops, sufficient water supply, means of eyewashing, radio and knowledge of sources of specific information. In addition to these contents, methyl prednisolone aerosol for inhalation and methyl prednisolone for injection should be carried. The author is of the opinion that infusion equipment is necessary as well.

1.3.5.2 High-Risk Vessels

There are special problems involved in diving owing to the work being carried out under high pressure, but the medical supplies should be the same as in ships on long voyages. Technical assistance, good connection by telephone and radio with the shore, optimal stretcher equipment, helicopter landing places and other technical facilities are more essential than medicines. Severe burning of large areas of the skin may occur. This means more than usual quantities of: dressings for burns, special preparations for applying to the skin, large aluminium-backed dressings, infusions in large quantities (not less than 10000 ml) antibiotic ointments and analgesics for long-term treatment. For all high-risk vessels the medical outfit must be at least of the standard of that in cargo vessels engaged in foreign-going voyages.

1.3.5.3 Fishing Vessels

The crew of fishing boats are, as previously pointed out, particularly exposed to a high risk of accidental injury. They should be well equipped [72]. On fishing boats which spend months far from land and still farther from a hospital, at sea in bad weather and with the crew carrying out hard work, the equipment should be the same as on cargo vessels engaged in deep sea voyages (see below). However, even this equipment is a minimum. If the fishing vessel is a fish factory ship, it should carry a doctor and be equipped to a medical scale similar to that of a passenger ship. Some adjustment to the scale would be important because the crew of a fish factory ship are more exposed to accidents and infections. Correspondingly, it is unnecessary to carry medicines for geriatric treatment.

The fish factory ships work in conjunction with a fleet of small fishing boats. The central medical equipment should be on the former. Thus, the equipment for the fishing boats may be restricted to first-aid kits, i.e. the same as the equipment for cargo vessels solely engaged in coastal trade. If a fishing vessel carries out both the fishing and the processing and has no doctor on board, it should be equipped according to the medical scale of ships engaged in deep sea voyages, but must have in addition the equipment appropriate for high-risk ships. The probability of many minor accidents will be high. The supply should be: elastic bandages; increased supply of splints for finger, arm and leg; special splints that can be applied with little knowledge of first-aid, e.g. inflatable splints; special adhesive plaster for large areas of the body; and stretchers, floatable and capable of being picked up by helicopter. The transportation of a patient in a rough sea to another ship or helicopter is not difficult, but is dangerous.

1.3.5.4 Vessels Solely Engaged in Coastal Regions

On board ships that work close to the shore, accidents and illnesses may happen but accidents are the main risk. The medical supply should include: bandages, elastic bandages, adhesive plaster of two sizes, dressings for burns, splints, ointment for burns, antibiotic ointment and tight bandages for stopping haemorrhages if surgical assistance is not available. There may be cases of headache, stomach trouble, seasickness and sunburn; the simplest equipment here will suffice. The supply should comprise, for example, ten tablets analgesic and ten tablets sedative. Whether medicine should be provided for serious conditions such as cardiovascular trouble and heart failure is doubtful and depends on the medical training of the officer.

1.3.5.5 Vessels on Deep Sea Voyages

The distribution of diseases on board ships ([3]; Borchgrevink et al. [8]; [21]; [22]; [23]; [24]; [25]; [36]; [37]; [38]; [40]; [45]; Larsen [55, 57]; Nocht [71]; [77]; [78]) and the reports of ships' medical officers (Gruhnwald [29]; Klepatski [47]; Leach [58]; Low [63]; Schaefer [86]; Tortori-Donati [100]) may be used as a basis in compiling a list of medical scales. According to international statistics (see Chap. 3.1), experience in the Port Health Authority, Hamburg, and discussions with many medical specialists, the sequence and frequency seem to be similar. The sequence in general is as follows:

1. Injury;
2. Diseases of the digestive system;
3. Diseases of the respiratory system;
4. Diseases of the musculoskeletal system and connective tissue;
5. Diseases of the nervous system and sense organs;
6. Diseases of the skin and subcutaneous tissue;
7. Symptoms, signs and ill-defined conditions;
8. Diseases of the circulatory system;
9. Diseases of the genito-urinary system;
10. Infections and parasitic diseases;
11. Mental disorders;
12. Endocrine, nutritional and immunity disorders;
13. Neoplasms;
14. Diseases of blood and blood-forming organs;

Disease ranked 1 to 4 amount to 70% of all diagnoses (according to ICD = International Classification of Diseases).

The ships' officers in charge of the medical duties on board who were questioned by the port medical officers said experience on board shows that there are three groups of medicine that ought to be better supplied:

1. Medicines for common colds;
2. Medicines for contusions, sprains etc.;
3. Medicines for so-called rheumatic complaints, e.g. lumbago and myalgia;

These comments correspond closely with the sequence of diseases. Regarding the compilation of relevant medical scales for these ships, another consideration may be useful, i.e. which medicines and other supplies are necessary for:

(a) Accidents;
(b) Diseases which occur frequently;
(c) Diseases which occur seldom but may endanger the life of the patient if not treated.

All deep sea cargo vessels may sometimes carry dangerous goods as additional cargo. In that case they must be equipped according to the recommendations in 1.3.5.1.

Medical scales are discussed below with reference to the above list (a)–(c) concerning the frequencies of accidents and disorders.

1.3.5.6 Accidents (see also Chap. 3.2)

Stretcher

The stretcher must be able to be carried from the deck or place of accommodation to the treatment room and ward and back to the deck, must be able to fit into the narrow spaces of the engine room and the staircases, must be transportable into the cargo holds, must be capable of being picked up by helicopter or crane, should keep the patient comfortable and protect him from injury and ideally should be floatable. The stretcher should cover the body from head to foot and provide protection for the whole length of the body, that is a minimum length of 200 cm. The shoulder and pelvis must be covered, i. e. a minimum width of 80 cm. A wider stretcher would be better, but ship's doorways and staircases are a restricting factor. The stretcher must prevent movement of broken bones, including the spine, i. e. it must be well stabilised and adaptable to the form of the human body. It should be possible to secure violent alcohol-intoxicated persons to the stretcher safely and in such a way that they cannot move. There is always a compromise between desirability and practicality, but the more one is aware of the different uses of a stretcher, the better may be its performance in practice.

Splints

Industry manufactures an enormous assortment of splints, specialised for every purpose. On ships, there should be as few types as possible. The ability to use splints is more essential than having specialised types available. There should be one small size, which can be adapted for different uses on arms and hands, and a special splint for fingers is useful. There should be a larger size splint for legs, which may also be used for phlebitis. For suspected fracture of the spine, the stretcher may be used as the splint. The material of the splint should not be affected by moisture or extreme temperatures. Some synthetic materials are damaged by very high as well as by very low temperatures. *Minimum:* two sizes, 3 of each.

Bandages

There should be sufficient bandages of different sizes including triangular bandages. As the crew do not undergo long training in first aid, the roller bandages should be elastic or semi-elastic. Special bandages for fingers and for the head have been found to be useful. Sizes of the bandages should be:

1. Normal and semi-elastic: 2, 6 and 10 cm × 5 m (*minimum* number: ten normal and ten semi-elastic)
2. Elastic: 6 and 10 cm × 8 m (*minimum* number: ten)

Adhesive Plaster/Bandages

Adhesive plaster should be as bland and as little irritating to the skin as possible (Zorn [108]; *minimum:* two sizes 2.5 cm × 5 m and 5 cm × 5 m (ten of each). Elastic adhesive bandages are necessary, especially for sprains and fractured ribs; two sizes: 6 cm × 8 m and 12 cm × 8 m, *minimum* five of each. A large quantity of adhesive plaster with dressings for wounds is required in *at least* two sizes: 2.5 cm × 5 m and 5.0 cm × 5 m (*minimum* five of each). Special adhesive strips to cover small bleeding wounds will be necessary. All these adhesive plasters must be packed for use in the tropics.

Dressings for burns

The equipment for treating burns should keep pace with the latest methods of treatment: the therapy has changed and is still changing. There should be special dressings for burns in small and very large sizes as well as dressings backed by aluminium or a similar material to cover the whole body or to be laid as a sheet under the patient. The *minimum* should be 25 dressings covering an area of 10 × 10 cm and 5 dressings covering an area of 50 × 50 cm.

Sterile cotton wool is frequently used and five to ten packages of about 100 g should be on hand.

The list below points out only some articles that should be considered in the light of medical experience on ships.

Disinfectant Lotion

This will be used widely. It should be non-irritating and available in several small containers, not in one large one. It must be able to withstand a long storage time and conditions in the tropics. Some disinfectant lotions may colour the skin so that the application can be controlled. *Minimum* 5 × 100 ml.

Ointments

1. Various types with pH 5	*minimum* 5 × 20 g
2. For contusions and sprains	*minimum* 5 × 20 g
3. For haematomas	*minimum* 2 × 20 g
4. Antibiotic	*minimum* 2 × 20 g
5. Activating regeneration	*minimum* 1 × 20 g
6. For burns	*minimum* 5 × 20 g
7. With camomile or azulene	*minimum* 5 × 20 g

Powder

1. Non-reactive type with, for example, camomile or azulene	*minimum* 2 × 50 g
2. Antibiotic	*minimum* 2 × 50 g

Local Anaesthetic Injection

Local anaesthetic should have an effect within a short time and give rise to as little allergic reaction as possible; *minimum* 50 ml.

Instruments

1. Forceps, plain, dressing	*minimum* two
2. Forceps, toothed, dissecting	*minimum* one
3. Forceps, splinter	*minimum* one
4. Scissors, small	*minimum* one
5. Scissors, large	*minimum* one
6. Michel clips and applicator	*minimum* one
7. Holder for needle	*minimum* one
8. Atraumatic needle with catgut or silk	*minimum* two sizes, ten of each

Some countries require that the first-aid equipment on ships includes plaster of Paris bandages. It seems that these plaster bandages are never used. They may be of use if there is someone on board who has had special training in how to apply them, but in general they cannot be reommended. If not used for a long time, they will lose their self-hardening quality.

1.3.5.7 Common Cold

There are many different forms of general cold which will rarely need to be exactly diagnosed by the ship's medical officer. The treatment is usually immediate and mainly symptomatic.

1. Decongestant drops for the nose	*minimum* 2 × 10 ml
2. Tablets, anaesthetic and disinfectant for the throat	*minimum* 50 tablets

3. Ointment for the chest with aromatic ingredients such as eucalyptus	*minimum* 2×20 g
4. Cough medicine (liquid or tablets)	*minimum* 500 ml or 50 tablets
5. Common cold remedies in large quantities	

Liquid medicine or tablets for spastic bronchitis and tablets to diminish the swelling of mucous membranes, especially in the sinuses and nose, might also be useful. In the case of shivering and high temperature, antibiotics should be used and the possibility of malaria considered. Seamen are generally fond of camomile for washing the mouth and throat and for inhalation. *Minimum:* lotio camomile in concentrated form 100 ml.

1.3.5.8 Gonorrhoea and Other Venereal Diseases

Modern therapy is by antibiotics, but the question of a specific antibiotic for gonorrhoea remains. Spectinomycin should be on board as it has a quick and specific effect and allergic reaction to it is rarely seen; *minimum* 10×2 g. Trichomoniasis will very seldom be suspected if there are no women on board. As the therapy is not urgent, no medicine is recommended. See also sections on antibiotics and penicillin.

Syphilis should not be treated on board without the advice of a doctor.

1.3.5.9 Skin Diseases

A hydrous wool fat ointment of pH 5, *minimum* 5×20 g, and a talc dusting powder, *minimum* 5×50 g, should be used first and must be on board in sufficient quantity. Also recommended are: antipruritic ointment without cortisone, *minimum* 2×20 g, ointment for furunculosis and abscesses, e.g. with ichthyol or salicyl, *minimum* 2×20 g, and an ointment containing antibiotic and cortisone in low strength, *minimum* 5×20 g. Skin diseases occur frequently, and the quantity of medicine must be in accordance with the number of crew members and should be sufficient for long-term treatment. Three times the minimum quantity is recommended.

1.3.5.10 Dental Complaints

Material to refill cavities, *minimum* 2×2 g, and an antiseptic lotion to be administered on cotton wool to a tooth cavity, *minimum* 10 ml, are required. Paradentosis is still frequent, chiefly on fishing vessels, and could be treated by tablets or lotions for sore throat.

Some dental instruments should be available:

For cleaning cavities	*minimum* one
For filling cavities	*minimum* one
Dental mirror	*minimum* one
Dental forceps	*minimum* one pair

No untrained person should extract a tooth that is not affected by paradentosis, but if the tooth is nearly falling out through paradentosis or suppuration, dental forceps can be used to extract it. Odontotomy of a tooth with abscess would be of much help, but it cannot be done by a person without experience on a moving ship. Dental drills are not recommended.

1.3.5.11 Stomach and Intestinal Complaints

A suitable range of medicine should be carried to deal with disorders ranging from a mild stomach upset to a serious abdominal condition. The following medicines are recommended: tea of camomile or azulene, *minimum* 100 ml in concentrated form; tablets for heartburn or hyperacidity of the stomach, *minimum* 50 tablets; tablets against gastritis or suspected ulcer, with antispasmodic effect, *minimum* 50 tablets.

In some countries tablets containing enzymes are included in the ship's medicine chest. It seems they are taken very seldom and only by persons who have had them prescribed by their doctor at home. They are therefore unnecessary on board.

Charcoal for diarrhoea is widely used and should be on board as tablets or in granulate form, *minimum* 100 tablets. There should, however, be medicine available in case of painful diarrhoea that cannot be stopped by charcoal. In ships of many nations, opium or morphine in liquid form is used for this purpose. It does not seem to be necessary, but many doctors and ship's officers request this kind of medicine. There have been no reported cases of addiction in consequence of this usage, but there are other sufficiently effective drugs. Every year, new antidiarrhetic drugs are being developed; nevertheless opium and morphine are still in use and still to be found in some ships' medical chests. The conclusion must be that there should be some form of effective antidiarrhetic medicine on board, but it is open to discussion as to whether this should be opium or its derivatives; *minimum* 20 tablets.

Cases of salmonella and amoebiasis may occur. Diarrhoea with blood in the excrement must be treated on shore by a specialist. Amoebiasis must not be treated on the basis of suspicion only but must be investigated on shore.

1.3.5.12 Diseases of Muscles and Joints

This includes different forms of illness such as rheumatism, myalgia, arthritis and ischialgia. On board there should be: analgesic and counter-irritant ointment, *minimum* 2 × 20 g; acetylsalicylic acid, codeine, paracetamol phenylbutazone or similar tablets, *minimum* 20 tablets; counter-irritant plaster, *minimum* five. These will be used frequently.

1.3.5.13 Eye Trouble

On board there should be: Undine for eyewashing, *minimum* one; analgesic eye drops without cocaine, *minimum* one bottle; antibiotic eyedrops, *minimum* one bottle; antibiotic and analgesic ointment for the eyes, *minimum* one bottle. Neither drops nor ointment with cortisone, nor eyeshields, are recommended. For contamination by certain chemicals, polyethylene glycol 400 may be used for eyewashing, *minimum* 500 ml.

1.3.5.14 Kidney and Bladder Complaints

If antibiotics are contra-indicated, an antiseptic and analgesic infusion of certain herbs e.g. fol. uvaeursi may be sufficient. It could be prepared from a concentrate, *minimum* 100 ml.

For urinary and gall-bladder stones, see "Analgesics", and for infections with an increase in temperature, see "Antibiotics".

1.3.5.15 Mycosis

Mycosis is more frequent than statistics indicate. The number of infections by fungi is still increasing. Different strains of fungus give rise to disease, so there should be two or three different fungicides. Fungicides should be in liquid, ointment and powder form, *minimum* five bottles each. The quantity should be in accordance with the number of crew members and the need for long-term treatment.

1.3.5.16 Ear Trouble

There should be on board analgesic and anti-inflammatory eardrops, *minimum* one bottle, and antibiotic eardrops, *minimum* one bottle.

It has proved very useful to have an otoscope on board and the person in charge to be trained to use it. The diagnosis of cerumen, inflammation and abscesses can be made by a layman if he has received instruction in this field. If an ear syringe is on board, it should be of small size or made of rubber to prevent damage when washing out the auditory canal.

1.3.5.17 Burns

In addition to what is listed under "Accidents" and "Skin Diseases", paraffin gauze dressing is necessary, *minimum* 10 cm × 10 cm, five each, as well as paraffin gauze backed by metallic foil in large size, *minimum* 10 cm × 10 cm, ten each. (see also 1.3.6.3 and 1.3.6.5).

1.3.5.18 Lice, Pediculosis

Liquid, spray and powder forms have all proved effective. The liquid form of the current most effective insecticide may be the best. It should not be administered to the eye or to an open wound or sore; *minimum* 250 ml.

1.3.5.19 Constipation

The use of castor oil is old fashioned, though it is still found on many ships. The demand for and the use of laxatives differ from country to country. Laxative might be necessary to treat poisoning. A liquid paraffin emulsion may be used as a laxative and in many cases of poisoning; *minimum* 200 ml.

1.3.5.20 Haemorrhoids

Generally, the patient has brought a supply of the remedy on board when he is suffering from haemorrhoids. The incidence of 0.9% refers only to those persons who were symptom-free until coming on board or who forgot to bring their medicine. On board there should be an ointment with applicator for haemorrhoids, *minimum* 20 g, and suppositories for haemorrhoids with haemostyptic ingredients, *minimum* ten.

1.3.5.21 Nervous Complaints

Different nations have a wide variety of sedatives. It is best to limit those carried aboard ship to several effective varieties. Diazepam is the usual choice. Tablets of 2 or 5 mg and ampoules of 10 mg are necessary; *minimum* 20 × 2 g tablets, 20 × 5 g tablets, 10 × 10 g ampoules.

The anticonvulsant effect is important in cases of poisoning and epilepsy. The use of hypnotics on board is debatable. The unusual periods of work and rest, the change of time and climate and the motion of the ship are all factors that disturb sleep. However, at any time a situation of extreme danger may arise, and the use of long-acting barbiturates causing drowsiness may therefore be hazardous. If a crew member has difficulty in falling asleep, a sedative will be sufficient in most cases. If a hypnotic is added to the ship's medicine chest, it should be effective and have a short-term activity. Barbiturates with short-term activities may be appropriate if not taken with alcohol; *minimum* ten tablets. The possibility of suicide must be considered. The number of tablets available should not be sufficient to cause death if taken all together.

1.3.5.22 Scabies

An antiscabietic ointment should be on board ship; *minimum* 500 ml. The instructions for use should be clear and sufficient.

1.3.5.23 Kinetosis

Seasickness pills and suppositories are in every ships' medical equipment. They are generally given to passengers or novice seamen. A crew member who suffers from kinetosis usually has his own medicine, which he believes to be effective. A really effective medicine against seasickness causes drowsiness and cannot be recommended if the seafarer has to work. A sedative is sufficient to bring about sleep. The rolling of the ship may cause fatigue and drowsiness without the typical symptoms of seasickness, nausea and vomiting. The kinetotic effect may impair alertness and activity (Kohfahl [49, 50]). Even for psychological reasons, there should be tablets and suppositories against kinetosis, but the quantity may be small; *minimum* 20 tablets, ten suppositories.

1.3.5.24 Psychosis/Alcoholism (see also 1.3.5.21)

A suitable sedative should be given as first treatment. However, one effective drug for cases of alcoholic and psychotic hallucination and for aggressive persons that can be administered even when the subjects are in a state of extreme excitement will also be needed. Diazepam or a similar drug could be injected. At the moment, the only alternative is haloperidol, which is tasteless and odourless and can be given as liquid in most beverages. It will rarely be used but must be on board in sufficient quantity; *minimum* 20 ml haloperidol solution 2 mg in 1 ml.

1.3.5.25 Abscesses

See "Skin Diseases".

1.3.5.26 Hepatitis

Every medicine chest has vitamin tablets; the centuries of avitaminosis, especially on seagoing ships, have passed. Today avitaminosis caused by lack of fresh food is a rarity; rather it is caused by alcoholism. Vitamins are the only medicine to be given for hepatitis. If, in an emergency case of acute hepatic failure, cortisone has to be given under radio advice, the cortisone in the basic medical equipment will be sufficient. For hepatitis, alcoholism and colds, multivitamin tablets may be added to the equipment. There has been no evidence of excessive use of these vitamins on board; *minimum* 50 multivitamin tablets.

1.3.5.27 Diabetes

Specific therapy, e.g. insulin, should only be given by a doctor. But for the diagnosis, the medicine chest should contain diagnostic strips for detecting glucose in the urine. To our knowledge, every year there has been one case of diabetes in which the patient was less than 30 years old and ignorant of his condition. It should be routine practice on board ship to use the strips for diagnosis. It would be an advantage to use combination strips for glucose, albumin, blood (erythrocytes), urobilin and pH.

1.3.5.28 Miscarriage

For bleeding in miscarriage, an ergot derivative in ampoules should be included in the medicine chest, *minimum* ten ampoules.

1.3.5.29 Epilepsy

In general it will not be necessary to carry anti-epileptic medicines on board because most countries will not allow epileptics to be employed at sea. If a seafarer should suffer a first fit while at sea, preventive therapy could be achieved with one of the sedatives (see nervous complaints).

1.3.5.30 Asthma

Asthma is a rarity, but it does occur. In all investigated cases, the patients had had previous attacks. However, considering the toxic effect of, for example, dangerous goods, toxic spastic bronchitis and oedema of the lungs could occur. Aerosols with adrenaline or adrenaline compounds and cortisone or cortisone compounds should be added to the medical equipment; *minimum* one aerosol.

In the remainder of this chapter, consideration is given to important groups of medicines and indications, and to various other diverse factors.

1.3.6 Other Medical Supplies

1.3.6.1 Medicines for Diseases of the Heart and Cardiovascular System

Regular medical examinations in most countries perhaps diminish the incidence of cardiovascular diseases on board. Nevertheless, cases of angina pectoris, coronary thrombosis and heart failure do occur. Suitable medicines for these conditions should be carried, but digitalis or antihypertensive drugs should not be included. However, a sphygmomanometer will provide useful information that may be transmitted to a doctor on shore giving radiomedical advice. According to our experience the sphygmomanometers were very successfully used on board and radiomedical advice was easier for the doctor.

The fundamental point here is: everything should be done to improve the diagnosis of cardiovascular conditions on board ship as far as modern technical instruments allow. The same applies to the prophylaxis, e.g. by regular medical examination. Medicine in liquid form and ampoules for the treatment of fainting and low blood pressure, e.g. noradrenaline, should be available; *minimum* 20 ml liquid, ten ampoules. A drug for angina pectoris symptoms (e.g. glyceryl trinitrate) is necessary; *minimum* 20 tablets.

1.3.6.2 Analgesics

Here there are three indications and one question.

1. Analgesic tablets are needed for the group of "normal" pains, e.g. headache; *minimum* 50 tablets.
2. Analgesics with a spasmolytic effect are required. Colic pain is sometimes connected with vomiting, so suppositories must be available in addition to tablets; *minimum* 20 tablets, ten suppositories.
3. Injections for severe pain should be available, *minimum* five ampoules.

Are morphine or morphine derivatives necessary? There are analgesics with effects comparable to morphine, e.g. pentazocine, but they are pharmacologically similar to morphine. There has been no reported abuse of morphine or morphine compounds on board ships and a ship on a long voyage should be equipped with a very potent analgesic. The local regulations concerning opiates must be taken into consideration, but if possible, the medical equipment should include a potent morphine derivative. Severe accidents, urinary and gall-bladder calculi are indications for effective analgesia, not only because of the pain but also to prevent shock. We should select those derivatives that have the least effect on blood pressure and respiration.

Should there be a medicine for migraine? Some schedules have special medicines for hemicrania. According to the reports from ship's officers, they have not been used. Those suffering from migraine usually have their own medicine. It may be that a first attack of migraine is suffered on board but it would rarely be diagnosed. There is no need for medicine against migraine to be on board.

1.3.6.3 Antibiotics

Whoever has followed the development and discussion of antibiotics in the last 30 years will hesitate to give advice on their use in ships. There is both the effect and the side-effect to be considered. The side-effect, the allergic reaction, could be more dangerous and difficult to deal with on board than on shore. So far there is no evidence of a dangerous allergic reaction having occurred on board ship but this does not imply that the use of antibiotics on ship will always be without danger. The increasing total number of allergic and anaphylactic reactions to penicillin indicates that we ought to discontinue using it at sea, but considering the beneficial effects and the number of cases treated without side-effects, we are reluctant to do so.

From general experience on the administration of antibiotics the following is often recommended: injection for gonorrhoea, e.g. spectinomycin, *minimum* ten ampoules; sulphonamides for inflammation of throat and lungs, *minimum* 50 tablets; and wide-spectrum antibiotics, e.g. tetracycline, for those cases not responding to penicillin or spectinomycin, *minimum* 20 tablets/1 g. Based on this experience, we would propose the following: Spectinomycin is the most specific remedy for gonorrhoea, practically no resistance or allergic reactions having been reported to date. Both may develop in time. Penicillin is effective and specific not only to gonorrhoea; it gives rise to more resistance and more allergic side-effects. In most countries it is cheaper than spectinomycin. On board there should be: spectinomycin, *minimum* ten ampoules; penicillin, *minimum* 4,000,000 I.U., ten ampoules.

There are other available antibiotics, e.g. cephalosporin, but these should not be used without specific indications. Sulphonamides for treating a wide range of conditions should be in the medical chest in tablet form, *minimum* 40 tablets. Antibiotics such as tablets or capsules of the wide-spectrum type may be of use in special situations, e.g. prophylactically after severe burning or poisoning, for infections resistant to injection of penicillin or sulphonamides, for diarrhoea thought to be caused by salmonella or cholera, for chancroid and for lymphogranuloma.

1.3.6.4 Cortisone

Research in the medical use of cortisone is developing every day. One cortisone derivative should be available for injection. For cases of allergic reaction, insect, fish or snake bites, poisoning, acute hepatitis etc., an effective cortisone derivative in ampoules must be on board; *minimum* five ampoules/1000 mg. Tablets of cortisone derivative are rarely used. There may be indications, e.g. cases of poisoning and asthmatic allergic reaction, for a prolonged treatment by tablets of cortisone derivatives. These tablets complete the equipment, but they are not absolutely necessary (20 tablets are recommended).

1.3.6.5 Infusions

It is obvious that in some cases an infusion saves a life (Ivanov [44]). However, very many infusions given in hospital, in an ambulance or in a helicopter do no harm but are not really life saving.

There may be cases of severe burning, extreme bleeding, poisoning etc. on board in which only an intravenous infusion might be life saving. However, even a doctor sometimes has difficulties in giving an intravenous infusion in an emergency; the problems facing a lay person in charge of medical care are thus far greater. There are infusions that can be administered subcutaneously, but they are less effective. The question is whether there should be infusions for intravenous use only, which in an emergency may well be useless (*minimum* 5×500 ml), infusions for subcutaneous application, the effectiveness of which is very uncertain, or both infusions. In the latter case, will the person in charge, in the confusion of the emergency, choose the right one? The conclusion is inevitable: The infusion which can save lives in a few cases is only possible if the training of the person responsible for medical care is sufficiently high. The first priority is training, the second is equipment.

1.3.6.6 Disinfectant

There may be incidents of infected potable water. There are different means, such as Cl^-, Ag^-, O_3 and ultraviolet rays, of killing bacteria in water supplies. From experience, Cl^-, administered as a chemical powder, is the best one. It is obtainable in every port as a powder or hypochlorite solution. It can be detected by smell. If too much is added to the water, the taste will be bad, but it can do no physical harm. To add Ag^- would also be effective, but it is not possible to determine whether too much has been added; Ag^-, even in high concentrations, is tasteless and odourless. *Minimum:* The ship should be equipped with a Cl^- donator sufficient for about 15 tons of potable water. There may be infected rooms and sanitary installations. A disinfectant for walls, furniture and sanitary installations should be available. Different products such as formaldehyde or quaternary ammonium salt (QAC) could be employed for this purpose. If they are administered in the right way, i.e. correct concentration at the right time, they will be effective. However, the training in disinfection is more important then the type of disinfectant.

Research has proved bacterial contamination to be present in many pantries, kitchens and provision stores. Regular disinfection once a week or twice a month would prevent infections and diarrhoea. In kitchens, provision stores and pantries, however, the disinfectant used should not have a bad odour or taste. Quaternary ammonium salt seems to be suitable for this purpose.

Conclusion: Recommended are (a) a disinfectant for potable water, *minimum* Cl^- for 15 tons; (b) a disinfectant for rooms, kitchen and sanitary installations, *minimum* 1 000 ml in concentrate.

1.3.6.7 Injection Syringes and Needles

Injection syringes and needles should be used once only (Zorn [108]). If a ship is equipped with syringes that have glass bodies and metal plungers, there must be facilities for sterilising this equipment; however, bearing the dangers of hepatitis and haemorrhagic fever in mind, it is doubtful whether sterilisation can be completely guaranteed. Disposable instruments, primarily injection needles and syringes, should be preferred. Though expensive, they will be cheaper than a sterilisation system. The *minimum* is: injection syringe, disposable 20 × 2 ml, 20 × 5 ml and 10 × 10 ml; injection needles, disposable small size and large size (50 of each).

1.3.7 Control of Medical Chest

The best medical equipment is ineffective if it is not controlled with regard to quantity and quality. As long ago as 1790 the USA copied a regulation of Great Britain, that every ship should be provided with a chest of medicines, "put up by some apothecary of known reputation, and accompanied by directions for administering the same; and the said medicines shall be examined by the same or other apothecary, at least once every year, and supplied with fresh medicines to replace those that have been used up or spoiled" (Urner and Staton [102]).

These principles have stood the test of time and are valid for the future. The medicines should be supplied by a pharmacy of good reputation with experience of the problems on board a ship. The medicine chest should be inspected by a company doctor, a port health medical officer or an other specialist regularly, or at least once a year. The expiry date should be marked distinctly on the medicine containers.

1.3.8 Definition of Medicaments

The definition of the medicaments to be used should take into consideration two difficulties: a) if the definition is too vague, it is possible that simply the cheapest and least effective medicament may be taken on board; b) if the definition is too strict, including the chemical formula, it may become obsolete within a short time. The best solution seems to be to provide a general definition of every feature related to the purpose of the medicine, the method of administration and the quantity to be administered. It would be desirable for there to be a specified list that could be changed, i.e. brought up to date, by a small group of specialists without much bureaucratic difficulty, e.g. every 5 years. However, the ways in which laws or regulations are promulgated in some countries do not permit this system. In this case, a definition of the use of the medicament including all details must be given.

In some countries, the pharmacist cannot supply a ship with medicine without a prescription from a doctor. The law, promulgated by the government, stipulating that certain medicines be in the medical chest can replace the prescription of a doctor. This means that the list of the legal regulations must have the same accuracy and detail as the prescription of the physician. There is no general answer to the problem of equipping a ship with medical provisions. But if the shipowner or captain is aware of these difficulties regarding the legal rules and regulations, an acceptable answer may be found.

1.3.9 Training

1.3.9.1 Doctor on Board (see also Chap. 1.2)

There is no problem with regard to training if a doctor is on board. Having a doctor on board was the rule in former times (Nocht [71]) and is still the practice of some countries, which follow the practice of the So-

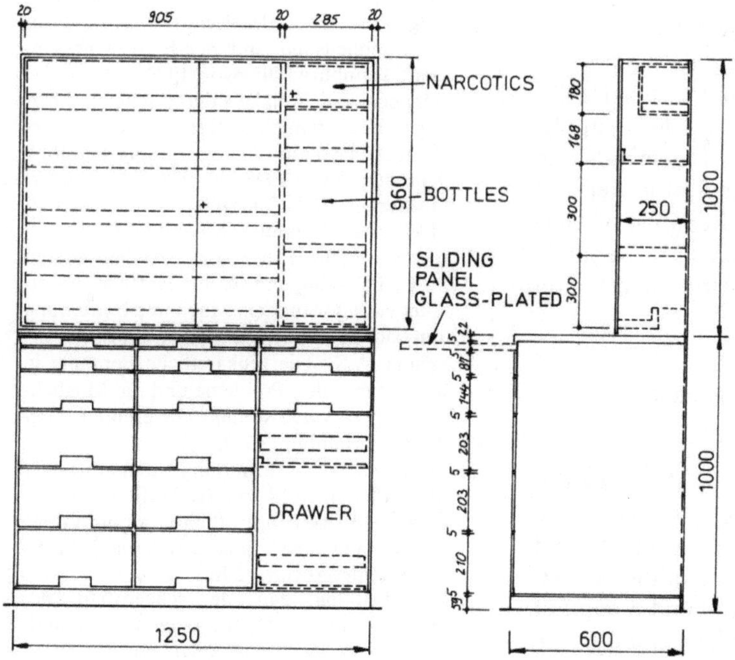

Fig. 2 Medical Locker [2]

viet Union, where for long voyages a doctor is obligatory. Special training for the doctor is very rarely given. This special training is becoming more and more necessary nowadays. We have many specialised physicians who are trained in hospitals with modern and ultramodern equipment from X-ray facilities to well-equipped laboratories. They are not, however, trained to do their job in the environment of a ship almost without technical assistance. Nevertheless, even if a ship is equipped with X-ray facilities, electrocardiograph and laboratory, this equipment will rarely need to be used. The ship cannot be equipped therefore with the modern diagnostic instruments for economic as well as for practical reasons. The doctor must be trained to carry out his diagnosis and therapy without the help of these facilities. Soon it may become difficult to find a medical teacher to train him. This is and will remain a very important question.

1.3.9.2 No Doctor on Board (see also Chap. 1.4)

If the medical chest is to be used as effectively as possible, the person who will use it must be correspondingly highly trained. This training should enable the person in charge to make a correct diagnosis, to give treatment as advised in the medical guide on board ship and to make the necessary observations which will assist a radiomedical adviser ashore. An important aspect of the training will be competence in first aid and emergency treatment. There may be little opportunity for practical experience and it is essential that refresher courses be arranged at regular intervals (Backhaus [6]; Ebert et al. [15]; [24]; [25]; [30]; Hager [31]; [35]; [36]; [37]; [38]; [39]; [40]; [41]; [46]; [53]; [59]; [70]; Staton [97]).

1.3.10 Medical Locker

It will be helpful for the personnel in charge and it will save a great deal of money if there is a standardised medical locker on board (Fig. 2). Every medicament and every piece of equipment will have its place such that it can be checked by the personnel in charge and the pharmacist or Health Authority responsible for medical supply. The rotation of personnel demands the standardisation of the medical locker and equipment [e.g. Federal Republic of Germany [2]; German Democratic Republic (Ebert et al. [15]); USA (Urner and Staton [102])].

1.3.11 Radio Advice (see also Chap. 1.4)

The doctor responsible for providing radio advice to ships should be informed of the standard of the equipment available and the state of medical training of the personnel. He must also have at hand a copy of the relevant National Medical Guide or the International Medical Guide for Ships if he is dealing with a foreign ship.

1.3.12 Conclusion

Medical equipment has improved the medical assistance possible on board ship. This equipment could become more effective if the distribution of diseases occurring at sea and the experience of medical care on ships, which is increasing every year, are taken into account. The possibilities of diagnosis by modern techniques must be considered, but medical assistance has to be given by personnel trained with regard to the necessities and possibilities on board and this fact will always impose limitations.

References

1. Angelov, B., K. Kiryakov and P. Polonov: Equipment of medicine cabinets on ships. In: III. International Symposium on Marine Medicine, Leningrad, 1968. Moscow 1969, pp. 166–168.
2. Anleitung zur Gesundheitspflege. 1. Verordnung über die Krankenfürsorge auf Kauffahrteischiffen. 2. Anleitung zur Gesundheitspflege auf Kauffahrteischiffen. Ed.: Bundesgesundheitsamt and See-Berufsgenossenschaft. Hamburg: Dingwort 1972.
3. Aufgaben und Tätigkeit der Fischereischutzboote (Fischereihilfsschiffe) und der Fischereiforschungsschiffe der Bundesrepublik Deutschland von 1948 bis 1968. Ed.: Bundesministerium für Ernährung, Landwirtschaft und Forsten. Hamburg: Moehlke 1969.
4. Ausrüstung für Fähre von 1000 Passagieren bei Berücksichtigung akuter Notfälle, Fahrtdauer etwa 36 Stunden. Maximale Entfernung vom nächsten Hafen 6 Stunden. 1969.
5. Azzuqa, A. S.: Die funkärztliche Beratung in der Seefahrt, ihre Probleme und die Möglichkeiten ihrer Verbesserung. Dissertation, University of Hamburg 1979.
6. Backhaus, A.: Erprobung diagnostischer Hilfsmittel an Bord von Seeschiffen. Lecture. Meeting "L'assistenza sanitaria a bordo delle navi senza medico". Societá Italiana di Medicina Sociale. Ancona, 2 July 1977.
7. Bekendmaking aan de scheepvaart no. 168/1981 (Lijst van genees- en verbandmiddelen en verplegingsartikelen en aanwijzing van de handleiding voor het gebruik van die middelen). Ed.: Scheepvaartinspectie, Rijswijk, 28 Oct. 1981. Nederlandse Staatscourant No. 218, 12 Nov. 1981.
8. Borchgrevink, Chr. F., E. Dahl, J. Klafstad et al.: Sykdomsbildet hos sjöfolk – helsetjenesten til sjös. Ed.: Institutt for almenmedisin. Oslo: Norges Teknisk-naturvitenskapelige Forskningsraad 1980. (System for Sikkert Skip. Report 80/1)
9. Brenning, M.: Ueber sanitäre Missstände auf Schiffen der deutschen Handelsmarine. Medicinische Woche *18*, 278, 137–141 (1905).
10. Brodske ljekarne. Tablica broj 3. [Ship's medicine chests]. Ed.: Ministarstvo pomorstva FNRJ. No. 2189. Split 5 March 1952
11. Contents of medicine chests on board ship and medical advice by radio to ships at sea. Preparatory Technical Maritime Conference. London, 1956. Geneva: ILO 1956.
12. Chapman, C.: A useful instrument table when operating at sea and for small operating theatres ashore. J. roy. nav. med. Serv. *64*, 1, 20–21 (1978).
13. Medicinali, oggetti di medicatura e utensili di cui debbono essere provviste le navi mercantili senza medico di bordo. Ministerial decree, 21 May 1976. Gazzetta Ufficiale della Repubblica Italiana 182, 5431–5447 (1976).
14. Dotação de medicamentos para um periodo de 90 dias. Medical equipment-list for Brazilian ships.
15. Ebert, H., J. Warncke, K.-D. Fischer et al.: Gesundheitsschutz an Bord. Leitfaden für Ka-

pitäne und Schiffsoffiziere. Berlin: VEB Verlag Volk und Gesundheit 1980.

16. Ebert, H.: Die Gewährleistung des Gesundheitsschutzes auf Seeschiffen ohne Arzt, unter den Bedingungen und den sich abzeichnenden Entwicklungstendenzen im Zusammenhang mit dem wissenschaftlich-technischen Fortschritt in der Schiffahrt der DDR. Dissertation, University of Rostock 1979.
17. Einführung der Vorschrift über Mitnahme von Medikamenten und med. Ausrüstung in Frankreich, Dänemark und England. StAH: Medizinalkollegium, II, F2 Vol. I, p. 38.
18. Ewald, M.: Ausrüstung von Seeschiffen mit Arzneimitteln in der Zeit zwischen dem 16. und Anfang des 19. Jahrhunderts. Personal Communication 1971.
19. Fischer, K.-D.: Hafen-Apotheke und medizinische Schiffsversorgung. In: Medizinische Betreuung an Land und auf See. Ed.: Medizinischer Dienst des Verkehrswesens der DDR, Direktion Rostock. Rostock 1969, pp. 21–22.
20. Fischer, K.-D.: Die medizinische Schiffsausrüstung in Praxis und Lehre. In: V. Internationales Symposium über Schiffahrtsmedizin, Rostock, 29–31 Oct. 1972. Ed.: Medizinischer Dienst des Verkehrswesens der DDR. Rostock 1973, pp. 93–101
21. Fischereischutzboote und Fischereiforschungsschiffe der Bundesrepublik Deutschland - Aufgaben und Tätigkeiten von 1948 bis 1975. Ed.: Bundesministerium für Ernährung, Landwirtschaft und Forsten. Hamburg: Moehlke 1975.
22. Fischereischutzboote und Fischereiforschungsschiffe der Bundesrepublik Deutschland - Aufgaben und Tätigkeiten von 1948 bis 1981. Ed.: Bundesministerium für Ernährung, Landwirtschaft und Forsten. Hamburg: Moehlke 1982.
23. Fortegnelser over skibsmedicinkisters indhold (jfr. handelsministeriets bekendtgørelse, 31 July 1974, om skibes forsyning med laegemidler m. v.). Appendix to: Laegebog for söfarende. 2nd ed. Viborg: Nörhaven Bogtrykkeri 1976.
24. Fourth International Symposium on Marine Medicine, Varna, 15–17 Oct. 1970
25. Fragen der Schiffahrtsmedizin. Vorträge aus dem Internationalen Symposion, Heiligendamm, 28–31 March 1963. Ed.: E. Kersten. Sonderheft des Medizinischen Dienstes des Verkehrswesens II.
26. Goede-Oudegeest, W. J.: Farmacie aan boord. Omnia Praescribendi Gratia *34*, 27–31 (1968).
27. Goethe, H.: Schiffahrtsmedizin und Tropenhygiene. In: Taschenbuch der praktischen Medizin. Ed.: G. Schettler. Stuttgart: Thieme 1980. pp. 1184–1205.
28. Grewe, H.-E.: Apothekenausrüstung in der Seeschiffahrt. Lecture. 7. Sitzung d. gemeinsamen Beirats f. Verkehrsmedizin. 24 March 1971.
29. Gruhnwald, R.: Die medizinische Versorgung an Bord aus der Sicht des Schiffsoffiziers, unter besonderer Berücksichtigung der Ausbildung in der Gesundheitspflege. Hamburg, Fachhochschule Hamburg, Department of Navigation 1980.
30. Guia sanitaria a bordo. Madrid: Instituto Social de la Marina 1976.
31. Hager, G.: Die Grundausbildung von Schiffsoffizieren zu Behandlung von Augenerkrankungen und die dazu notwendige Standardausrüstung auf Seeschiffen. In: Fragen der Schiffahrtsmedizin. Vorträge aus dem Internationalen Symposion, Heiligendamm, 28–31 March 1963. Ed.: E. Kersten. Sonderheft des Medizinischen Dienstes des Verkehrswesens II. pp. 159–164.
32. Halm, W.: Schiffsapotheke, Medikamente und Medikamentenverluste an Bord. In: Fortbildungslehrgang über Fragen der Verkehrsmedizin und Verkehrspsychologie, 10–15 Feb. 1964. Sonderheft des Medizinischen Dienstes des Verkehrswesens der DDR III. pp. 379–392.
33. Hospital auf A-Deck (Deck 4). In: Kreuzfahrtschiff "Europa". Erbaut von der Bremer Vulkan AG Schiffbau und Maschinenfabrik, Bremen-Vegesack. Hansa *118* [Sonderausgabe MS "Europa"], 37 (1981).
34. Inhalt der Schiffsapotheken und funkärztliche Beratung der Schiffe auf See. Internationale Arbeitskonferenz, 41st Meeting 1958. Genf: ILO 1957.
35. International medical guide for ships. Eds.: ILO, IMCO, WHO. Geneva: WHO 1967.
36. II International Symposium of Maritime Medicine. Gdańsk-Gdynia, 16–19 Sept. 1965. Lectures and Reports. Bull. Inst. mar. Med. Gdansk *17*, 3 (1966).
37. III International Symposium on Marine Medicine. Leningrad 1968. Eds.: E. P. Sergeev et al. Moscow 1969.
38. V Internationales Symposium über Schiffahrtsmedizin, Rostock 19–21 Oct. 1972. Rostock: Medizinischer Dienst des Verkehrswesens der DDR 1973.
39. VI International Symposium on Maritime Medicine Gdańsk, 17–19 Oct. 1974. Reports. Bull. Inst. mar. trop. Med. Gdynia *25*, *2/3/4* (1974).
40. VII International Symposium on Marine Medicine 23–30 Sept. 1976, Odessa. Ed.: U. M. Stenko. Moscow 1976.
41. VIII International Symposium on Marine Medicine - Abstracts, Varna, 24–28 Oct. 1978.
42. Inventario del materiale sanitario. Ed.: Italia di Navigazione. Genoa 1976.
43. Inventory and requisition for medical sup-

plies. (U.S.-Medical equipment list). Revised Sept. 1956.

44. Ivanov, V. N.: Izgotovlenie sterilnykh rastvorov v apteke gospitalya flota. [Preparation of sterile solvents in ship hospitals' pharmacies]. Voen.-med. Zh. *8*, 86 (1969).
45. Jahresberichte des hafen- und flughafenärztlichen Dienstes. Hamburg 1973/74, 1975, 1976/77, 1978/79.
46. Joint ILO/WHO committee on the health of seafarers. Sixth report. Geneva: ILO/WHO 1981.
47. Klepatski, O. A.: O nekotorykh pokazatelyakh raboty sudovykh ambulatori vo vremya plavaniya. [Some notes on the use of ship's medicine chests during sea voyages]. Zdravookhr. Ross. Fed. *15*, 29–33 (1971).
48. Koch, W.: Konstruktive Vorschläge zur Einrichtung und Ausrüstung des Hospitaltraktes auf Schiffen. Lecture. Meeting Verband deutscher Schiffswerften (Architekten), 29 Jan. 1970.
49. Kohfahl, M.: Sind Sie wirklich nie seekrank? Boote *10*, 35–36 (1981).
50. Kohfahl, M.: Seekrankheit. Lecture. Seminar "Sicherheit auf See". Landesseglerverband Bremen 17–18 Nov. 1979
51. Kontrollbok för svenskt skeppsapotek. Sjöbo: Nordvall 1966.
52. Krynicki, A.: Analysis of the utilization of hospital beds of merchant and fishing vessels. Bull. Inst. mar. Med. Gdańsk *23*, 3/4, 131–137 (1972).
53. Laegebog for søfarende. Eds.: C.J. Møllenbach and A. Mahneke. Viborg: Nørhaven Bogtrykkeri 1976.
54. Larsen, Ø.: Medisinsk journalmateriale fra 1700-tallet som utgangspunkt for historiske undersökelser. Sydsvenska Medicinhistoriska Sällskapets Årsskrift 1968.
55. Larsen, Ø.: Med sjøfolks helse som siktepunkt. Det sjøfartsmedisinske institutt i Hamburg. Liv. og helse *38*, 174–177 (1971).
56. Larsen, Ø.: Schiff und Seuche 1795–1799. Ein medizinischer Beitrag zur historischen Kenntnis der Gesundheitsverhältnisse an Bord dänisch-norwegischer Kriegsschiffe auf den Fahrten nach Dänisch-Westindien. Oslo: Universitetsforlaget 1968.
57. Larsen, Ø.: Schiffsarztjournale dänisch-norwegischer Kriegsschiffe aus der Zeit vor 1814, die im Reichsarchiv von Kopenhagen aufbewahrt werden. Eine Quellenübersicht. Oslo: Universitetsforlagets Trykningssentral 1967.
58. Leach, R. D.: The medicine of ocean yacht racing. Brit. med. J. *2*, 6154, 1771–1773 (1978).
59. Leach, H.: The ship captain's medical guide. London: Simpkin, Marshall 1879.
60. Legislação de interesse para a marinha mercante. Junta Nacional da Marinha Mercante, Lisbon 1964.
61. List of medical products suggested by C.I.R.M. Vessels lacking medical facilities. Boll. ann. C.I.R.M., pp. 11–12 (1975).
62. Liste der medizinischen Schiffsausrüstungen für Seeschiffe der Deutschen Demokratischen Republik (gemäß § 3 der Anordnung über den Gesundheitsschutz an Bord von Seeschiffen, 23 Jan. 1963. GBl. II. p. 64. Medizinischer Dienst des Verkehrswesens Direktion Schifffahrt, Rostock. Rostock 1964.
63. Low, A.: Bericht über die schiffahrtsmedizinischen Untersuchungen an Bord des Segelschiffes "Amphitrite" (Clipper Verein e. V.) im Verlauf der 70. Reise vom 2. bis zum 15. Juli 1977 in der Ostsee. Hamburg 1977.
64. Medical allowance list – CG 344. Part 2. Vessels class 2 A, 2 B, 2 C, 2 D. Prepared by: Medical Control Point USCG Supply Center. Brooklyn: U.S. Coast Guard 1970.
65. Medical equipment on board Indian ships. The Gazette of India *42*, 1746–1812 (1966).
66. Medical first aid guide for use in accident involving dangerous goods. Chemical supplement to the International medical guide for ships (IMGS). Eds.: IMO, WHO, ILO. London: WHO 1982.
67. Medicinali, materiale sanitario ed istruzioni per il loro uso, di cui devono essere dotate le imbarcazioni e le zattere di salvataggio. Rome: Ministerio della Marina Mercantile 1965.
68. The merchant shipping (medical scales) regulations 1974. Statutory instruments. 1974, No. 1193 Merchant shipping: masters and seamen. London: Her Majesty's Stationery Office 1974.
69. Milcheva, Yem., M. Mikhaylov and T. Todorov: Za standartizirane ustroystvoto na korabnite aptechni shkafore i podrezhdaneto na lekarstvenite sredstva v tyakh. [Standardization of ship's medicine chest's design and the arrangement of medicaments therein]. Transp. med. Vesti *22*, 2, 44–51 (1977).
70. Nauticus. Encyclopédie pratique du bateau. 1. Médecine en mer sans médecin. 4. Guide pratique de la vie à bord. Ed.: G. Borg. Paris: Editions Maritimes et d'Outre-Mer 1977.
71. Nocht, B.: Vorlesungen für Schiffsärzte der Handelsmarine über Schiffshygiene, Schiffs- und Tropenkrankheiten. Leipzig: Thieme 1906.
72. Nomenclature du matériel médical et pharmaceutique à embarquer sur les navires de pêche (sans médecin à bord). Draft by an international group of physicians for E.C., 1978.
73. Nomenclature du matériel médical et pharmaceutique à embarquer. Paris: Journaux officiels 1971. (Navigation maritime No. 71–16)

74. Normal-Einrichtungen der Hospitäler und Operationsräume auf Schiffen - nach Angaben von H. Minning. Hamburg: Schulz & Zaage 1939.
75. Onnen, M.: Untersuchungen über die Versorgung der Schiffahrt mit Medikamenten, Verbandstoffen und Hilfsmitteln zur Krankenpflege. (Ein kritischer internationaler Vergleich). Dissertation, University of Hamburg 1975.
76. Pomorska medicina II [naučne rasprave]. Nautical Medicine II [Scientific reports]. Belgrad: Izdanje Mornaričkog glasnika 1979. (Pomorska biblioteka. Sveska 30)
77. Proceedings of the European nautical medical meeting, Hamburg, 1978. - Panel discussion of day to day problems. Ed.: H. Goethe.
78. Proceedings of the second European nautical medical officers meeting, West Sussex, 10–14 Sept. 1979.
79. Ram, J.: Maritime health services at sea. SAPANUT *6*, 2, 4–8 (1976).
80. Recommendation concerning the contents of medicine chests on board ship. Recommendation 105. Geneva: International Labour Conference 1958.
81. Sanitarnyie pravila dlya morskikh sudov SSSR. [Sanitary regulations for seagoing ships of the USSR]. Odessa: Moryak 1964.
82. Schadewaldt, H.: Bemerkungen zur Geschichte der Marinepharmazie. Veröff. int. Ges. Gesch. Pharm. *10*, 157–177 (1957).
83. Schadewaldt, H.: Geschichte der Schiffahrtsmedizin und Marinepharmazie. Wehrdienst Gesundheit *9*, 5–56 (1963).
84. Schadewaldt, H.: Lazarettschiffe und Marinelazarette. Ciba-Z. *7*, 2531–2533 (1955).
85. Schadewaldt, H.: Die Schiffsapotheke im Mittelalter. Sollemnia 700 annorum stationis aromaticae. Traguriensis de qua primitus memoria extat MCCLXXI. Zagreb 1973.
86. Schaefer, H.J.: Die medizinische Versorgung an Bord aus der Sicht des Schiffsoffiziers, unter besonderer Berücksichtigung der medizinischen Ausrüstung. Hamburg, Fachhochschule Hamburg, Department of Navigation 1980.
87. Schmidt, R. and A. Kludas: Die deutschen Lazarettschiffe im Zweiten Weltkrieg. Stuttgart: Motorbuch Verlag 1978.
88. Serdarević, S., O. Cupahin, V. Tonković et al.: Sastav brodske ljekarne. [Assortment of the ship's medicine chest]. In: Pomorska medicina. [Naučne rasprave]. Belgrad: Izdanje Mornaričkog glasnika 1975. pp. 99–105. (Pomorska biblioteka. Sveska 26)
89. Sherlock, P.: Recommended drug and equipment list. Manuscript 1969.
90. The ship's medicine chest. Department of Nautical Medicine, Hamburg 1977.
91. Ships' medicine chests. Boll. ann. C.I.R.M. pp. 10–11 (1971).
92. The ship's medicine chest and medical aid at sea. Ed.: U.S. Department of Health, Education, and Welfare, Public Health Service, Health Services Administration, Bureau of Medical Services. Washington: U.S. Government Printing Office 1978.
93. Sobol, Z. and K. Żurawiecki: Nowa wersja rozwiazania bloku szpitalnego na trawlerach-przetworniach. [New design of hospitals on manufacturing fish trawlers]. Bull. Inst. mar. Med. Gdańsk *14*, 3/4, 309–312 (1963).
94. Sobol, Z. and A. Krynicki: Design of hospital rooms and sickbays on ships. In: Human factors in the design and operation of ships. Proceedings of the First International Conference on Human Factors in the Design and Operation of Ships. Gothenburg, February 1977. Stockholm: Garmat Service 1978.
95. Socialstyrelsens Kungörelse om skeppsapotek. (4 Oct. 1968). Kungl. Sjöfartsstyrelsen Meddelanden *8*, 1–19 (1969).
96. Socialstyrelsens Kungörelse om skeppsapotek, 31 Oct. 1979. Socialstyrelsens författningssamling 25 (1979).
97. Staton, A.B.: Handbook of medicines and their use for the ship's medicine chest at sea. New Orleans: Lykes Lines 1980.
98. Stjepanović, R.: Priručnik o brodskim apotekama. [Handbook of ship's medicine chests]. Belgrad: Udruženje zdravstvenih radnika SR Crne Gore 1973.
99. Sudovye aptechki. [Ship's medicine chest]. In: Meditsinskoe posobie dlya kapitanov sudov. 2nd edn. Moscow: Reklambyuro 1970. pp. 202–233.
100. Tortori-Donati, B.: La attrezzatura ed il funzionamento del reparto sanitario di grandi transatlantici stranieri. Lav. e Med. *20*, 3, 105–118 (1977).
101. Ulrich, B.: Ärztliche Hilfe auf hoher See. Deutsches Forschungsschiff im Einsatz. Der schwimmende Operationssaal. General-Anzeiger d. Stadt Wuppertal, 20 April 1968. p. 29.
102. Urner, C.J. and A.B. Staton: The medicine chest at sea. New Orleans: Lykes Lines 1981.
103. Vinkovetski, A. Ya and Ye. P. Krivenda: Spravochnik po oborudovaniyu bytovykh i meditsinskikh pomeshcheni na morskikh sudakh. [Manual on the equipment of living rooms and medical centers on seagoing ships]. Leningrad: Izdatelstvo "Sudostroenie" 1968.
104. Volbehr, K.: Arzenei aus dem Meere vom 17. Jahrhundert bis heute. Bremerhaven: NW Ditzen.
105. Volbehr, K.: Gesundheit an Bord. Kleine Geschichte der Hygiene und Arzneimittelversorgung auf Schiffen. Bremerhaven: Deutsches

Schiffahrtsmuseum 1979. (Führer des Deutschen Schiffahrtsmuseums, No. 11)
106. Volkov, Yu. N.: Razvertyvanie rentgenologicheskogo otdeleniya na pasazhirskom teplokhode. [Establishment of an X-ray station on a passenger ship]. Voen.-med. Zh. *7,* 19–20 (1971).
107. White, P. C., jr.: A survey of medical care in the United States merchant marine. Milit. Med. *142,* 8, 613–616 (1977).
108. Zorn, E.: Einmalspritzen in der Krankenbehandlung an Bord. Hansa *106,* 3, 240–241 (1969).
109. Zorn, E.: Die Verwendung von Verbandpflastern an Bord von Schiffen. Hansa *105,* 1750 and 1760 (1968).

Addendum

110. Brochmann, J. H. H.: Førstehjelp ombord. [Oslo:] Grøndahl 1982.

1.4 Medical Care on Ships Without a Doctor – Radio Medical Advice

W. H. G. Goethe

1.4.1 Health Situation on Board

When considering the possibilities and the standard of health care on board and ashore, the following facts become evident:

In an emergency, people of industrial countries are used to prompt medical care in a clinic and/or a hospital. Even in developing countries medical services are generally available within several hours. On board ships the situation is quite different. Only a very few ships anywhere still carry a doctor; thus the crew members are dependent on the medical care of laymen with very limited medical qualifications. In others words, there is a discrepancy between the possibilities of medical care *ashore (high standard)* and *on board (low standard)*. This discrepancy increases from year to year, which might be explained by the fact that standards of health care ashore are constantly rising in most countries whereas, according to the experience of nautical medical experts, care on board has scarcely improved in recent years. It has to be emphasised that seamen on board represent a population at risk in respect of medical care in cases of accident and disease.

It is often assumed that in cases of accident or disease on board seagoing vessels only medical first aid is required. This is a complete misunderstanding as most seagoing vessels will be at sea for days or even weeks before they reach any port. Consequently not only first aid but also second and third aid have to be given.The crew member in charge of medical care (usually one of the officers) has a great responsibility to bear as he has to care for the health and well-being of the ship's crew. His judgement on the severity of an illness, on the need for radio medical advice and/or on whether to call at a port may, if faulty, put a life in danger.

The health standard of crew members on board often leaves much to be desired. In many shipping countries regular fitness check-ups are necessary as a preventive measure. If there are high examination standards the general state of health of crew members can be considered satisfactory, but irrespective of this fact intercurrent diseases or accidents still occur, requiring immediate medical treatment.

There are crew members on board many vessels of different countries who either have never had any medical fitness check-ups or only cursory inadequate examinations. The environment on board can exacerbate a pre-existing lesion which may in turn lead to life-endangering illness with no doctor on board.

In principle, the possibilities of improving the health care on board are rather restricted. There are only three ways of importance:

1. Training of personnel in charge of the health care on board;
2. Ship's medical kit (medical chest) including the ship's medical guide;
3. Radio medical advice.

The medical training of shipboard personnel is, without doubt, the most important factor in securing a satisfactory standard of health care on board. An adequate ship's medical kit must be complemented by an officer in charge who is competent in basic medical skills. Naturally, it is useless to have an excellent kit with unskilled personnel using it.

The standard of the medical outfit on board varies from country to country. Many seafaring countries do not have any regulations pertaining to the medical kit on board, whereas others are required by law to have excellent kits.

Industrial countries usually have their own medical guides (e.g. Great Britain: *The Ship Captain's Medical Guide* [46]; the United States: *The Ship's Medicine Chest and Medical Aid at Sea* [47]). The *International Medical Guide for Ships* (WHO/ILO/IMCO [20]) should be compulsory on board vessels of those nations not having national guides. Radio medical advice is in many cases a great help but its possibilities are still rather limited (see 1.4.4).

Only a very few publications are available concerning the general health situation on board. Most of them deal with specific health hazards only, excluding the general considerations. However, as long ago as 1968 Goethe [9] pointed to the general health situation on board and the necessity of improving the medical training of ship's officers. Turnbull [55] reviewed the different aspects of the seafarer's health in a study of European shipping countries and the USA. White [57], in his review, emphasises the need for strict health standards for ships' crews. Different authors report on the standard of health on board merchant vessels of their countries, expressing most varying opinions on the appropriate health care and/or relevant medical training: Ram [41]; Tenfjord [53]; Grewe [13]; Kharalanov et al. [27]; Goethe [10]; Ebert [3, 4, 5]; Turnbull [54]; Kraljević and Ditrih [28]; Mikhailova et al. [33]. Siem [48] reported specifically on self-care among seamen on Norwegian ships.

A questionnaire study was made on board 89 US merchant marine ships dealing with the training of personnel in charge of the medical care, sick-bay facilities, availability of medical references, inventory of medicines and supplies and immunisation procedures. White [58] found that midshipmen who received treatment aboard ship were not adequately treated. He recommended the following:

1. Improvement of the medical training, including better training standards;
2. Refresher courses for shipboard medical personnel;
3. The first aid requirements for first licences should exceed those of the basic first aid course of the American Red Cross;
4. Better and standardised medical content of the sick-bay and medicine chest aboard ship;
5. Improvement of immunisation schedules.

Another who reports on the necessity of improving the medical training of ships' officers is Vuksanović [56]. In his opinion the present medical tuition in maritime schools is restricted and quite inadequate. Consequently he urgently recommends extension of the medical tuition syllabus, with emphasis on how to render first aid until the ship reaches port and thus a hospital.

The WHO and the Joint ILO/WHO Committee on the Health of Seafarers in their various sessions dealt fully with the health care of seafarers and its resultant effects on the ship's operation. The Committee made a considerable number of recommendations which in many countries are still awaiting implementation [19, 22, 23, 24, 25, 26, 44].

Slutsker [50] and Gurvich and Styazhkina [16] report on the assignment of doctors and surgical assistants on board USSR vessels. Ships with more than 40 persons on board have to carry a doctor, 25–40 persons on board require a surgical assistant and if there are less than 25 one of the officers is usually entrusted with the medical care.

1.4.2 Who Performs Medical Treatment on Board?

In practically all seafaring nations the ship's captain has to bear the entire responsibility for the ship's operation, the crew members and the cargo. This naturally includes the health care of seafarers as well as medical aid in case of sickness and accident. Only in exceptional cases does he perform the medical care on board himself.

In general three occupational groups which may be assigned to the medical care of crew members and passengers on board can be distinguished:

1. The ship's doctor;
2. The paramedic (enfermero, feldscher, surgical assistant, marine physician assistant etc.);
3. Master, deck officer (chief steward on some English and Asian ships).

Nowadays very few doctors are employed at sea. In most countries only passenger vessels, fishery protection vessels, research vessels and large fish processing vessels still carry a doctor. There are a few exceptions in countries such as the USSR, Poland, the GDR, Bulgaria and Rumania, which provide a doctor on board vessels with a large number of crew members. It would seem that 95% of all seafarers are employed on board vessels without doctors.

The occupation of a so-called paramedic is recognised in only a few countries. Portuguese, Brasilian and other South American vessels carry an enfermero. This is usually a male or female who has had additional medical training for sea service. Besides their medical duties they are usually in charge of administrative tasks. USSR vessels with a medium number of crew members frequently carry a surgical assistant (feldscher) who is given a special medical training for several years, which, however, does not come up to a medical degree standard. The surgical assistant is responsible for the preventive and curative medical care on board. Ships sailing under the US flag may have a purser on board who has undergone the additional medical training of a marine physician assistant. This involves several years' paramedic training, which was introduced in the USA by the Staff Officers' Association. Of course, only a small number of US flag vessels carry a purser and thus a marine physician assistant. The training standards are rather high and consequently guarantee appropriate health care of the ship's crew [38].

On board most ships medical care is the duty of one of the deck officers who has been designated by the ship's captain. In many countries the first officer is entrusted with the task but in others it is the responsibility of the second or third officer. In the German Federal Republic it is traditional to delegate the duty to the second officer. In some countries, however, the most qualified officer is assigned, irrespective of rank.

The deck officer in charge usually gives the medical care in addition to his normal duty, e.g. watchkeeping. Normally there are no fixed consulting hours. The officer has to be present in case of sickness or accident. On some of the ships, however, fixed consulting hours have been instituted.

1.4.3 Medical Education of Shipboard Personnel

The extent of the medical training of the crew member in charge of health care on board is the decisive factor in successful treatment of sick or injured crew members. Incorrect diagnoses and/or careless handling of an accident may lead to severe physical disablement or even death. Cases have arisen where the disregard of certain symptoms and/or the failure to call at a port in emergency has had fatal results (e.g. high fever and no treatment in cases of malaria). The load of responsibility is rather heavy and can be made bearable only if adequate medical training has been given. The following possibilities and practices of basic medical training of ship's officers can be found world-wide:

No training at all;
"First Aid" course (Red Cross o.a.);
Theoretical medical lectures in nautical schools;
Theoretical medical lectures in nautical schools with short-term practical training in a hospital.

In some countries medical training is not compulsory. In these unfortunate circumstances, untrained laymen do what they can for sick or injured colleagues. A medical guide may or may not be available and the ship's medicine chest may be incomplete and inadequate. Instances have occurred where not even bandages and dressings have been available. The Joint ILO/WHO Committee on the Health of Seafarers urgently recommended in their resolution on the medical first aid training for ship's personnel: "More advanced medical training, based on the International Medical Guide for Ship's and/or similar national Guides" [44].

In many shipping countries the captain and the deck officers must complete a so-called first aid course by the Red Cross or another organisation prior to the issue of their certificate of competency. The syllabus naturally consists of immediate first aid such as control of haemorrhage and resuscitation, including the positioning of injured persons. The limited knowledge acquired on these courses is absolutely insufficient to make diagnoses and/or to take adequate therapeutic measures in cases of disease and accident on board. In some European and other countries, e.g. the USA, more extensive first aid courses including medical aid and cardiopulmonary resuscitation are held at various nautical schools.

Medical training in most of the nautical schools of the different shipping countries consists almost exclusively of lectures, with little or no practical training. Turnbull [55] published a review comparing the different aspects of seafarers' health problems and courses in medical aid in some European countries and the USA. It is evident that medical training is given preference within the normal lecture programme at nautical schools. The total training period differs considerably, ranging from 15 to 80 h. The lack of practical exercises, e.g. simple surgical procedures, application of bandages, making diagnoses, giving injections and dressing wounds, in many courses detracts from the usefulness of the training. Some shipping countries, however, have introduced short-term practical training courses in a hospital in addition to the normal medical course at nautical schools. This should help to overcome the lack of practical experience but will maintain the link with the general nautical and medical education of deck officers at schools. This type of education is given in some of the nautical schools of the German Federal Republic and the Netherlands.

In some countries there are theoretical training courses of one or even several weeks. In the UK there are courses of 12–13 h in first aid and of 20 h in medical aid (organised by the General Council of British Shipping in Liverpool) in addition to the basic first aid course of 12 h at the nautical schools. A similar course at the Dreadnought Seamen's Hospital in Greenwich lasts 20 h. The medical training of the German Democratic Republic also consists of several weeks' combined courses. In the meantime this branch of study has been subordinated to the "Ing. Hochschule für Seefahrt" as an independent teaching subject "transport medicine – navigation". The practical training will consist of assignments to clinical wards for several days and will include practical exercises, demonstrations etc. Ebert [2, 3]. Combined theoretical/practical medical training courses for officers in hospitals, lasting 4 weeks and more, are as yet practised only in Hamburg (FRG). The "Hamburg model" consists of a training programme of approx. 140 h. The courses are held at a special education centre for ships' officers attached to the Port Hospital of Hamburg (Goethe and Grewe [8]; Goethe [10, 12]).

The training programme of the 4-week course for licences AM and AG (senior officers and masters) is based on an agreement between the Free and Hanseatic City of Hamburg and the German Federal Ministry of Transport. The syllabus naturally alters slightly from time to time, but basically the content has remained unchanged in recent years. The theoretical lectures and demonstrations are given to the group as a whole, but for practical training, even bedside teaching, the 18 participants are split up into groups of three to achieve a better teaching impact. The course finishes with practical and theoretical examinations. In the practical examination the participants have to prove, inter alia, knowledge of physical examination techniques, emergency care, injection techniques and urine analyses. The theoretical examination is a written test according to the multiple choice system. The issue of licences is subject to the candidate passing the examinations.

For the AK licence (masters and mates in coastal trade) a 2-week course with a limited training programme was set up. The tutor has overall responsibility for planning the curriculum timetable and for co-ordinating the final examination. The success of the course depends to a great extent on his enthusiasm and ability to liaise with staff and students. Unless he can keep the course running smoothly and keep interest and morale at a high level, the results will suffer.

In planning the course, emphasis must be given to practical aspects as opposed to set lectures, which should be kept to a minimum requirement. Wherever possible, theoretical instruction should be interspersed with demonstrations, practical training and teaching in out-patient and in-patient wards of the Port Hospital. In addition, the participants should be given the opportunity to attend out-patient, night-time and weekend emergency duty services.

Refresher courses of 1 week on a voluntary basis are also offered for experienced mates and captains. Experience shows that good results have been achieved with participants sent by shipping companies. The seafaring officers and captains know the problems of medical treatment of sick or injured persons on board, so they are keen to become more proficient. The course consists of combined theoretical/practical lessons spanning roughly 35 h.

Similar refresher courses on a voluntary basis which, however, last 4 weeks are held at the Maritime Institute of Technology and Graduate Study (International Organization of Masters, Mates and Pilots) in Baltimore, USA. The training programme is quite intensive, predominantly involving practical exercises, but also including theoretical lectures and occasional assignments to in-patient wards in hospitals. The first part of the course ends with the award of a certificate of an Emergency Medical Technician [31].

1.4.4 Radio Medical Advice

Radio medical advice is the only possibility the ship's officer has of asking for medical help in the event of disease or accident when he is in difficulty [37]. The potential of radio medical advice is, however, often overestimated. Very often the opinion is heard that radio medical advice practically replaces the medical training of the shipboard personnel and makes a well-equipped medical chest superfluous. This is, in fact, a mistaken view. Radio medical advice from doctors can only succeed if there is a competent person on board with a basic knowledge of medicine. The crew member in charge must be able to describe the symptoms and must know what information is needed to make a diagnosis and to advise treatment. The risk of wrong diagnoses is very high when the inadequate basic medical knowledge of the shipboard personnel does not provide enough clear details of the history, signs and symptoms to enable a fairly safe diagnosis to be made. One should never forget that the advising doctor is not in a position to see and to examine the patient himself but that, on the contrary, he is dependent on the inexpert observations made by the shipboard personnel. He has to perform "teletherapy", a method of medical treatment which is not provided for in medical education at universities.

The following short history of radio medical advice was given by Goethe et al. [11]: Radio medical advice became possible with the introduction of radiotelegraphy by Marconi in 1897. With the introduction of radio equipment on ships and the construction of coastal radio stations it became possible for ships with or without a doctor on board to obtain medical advice by radiotelegraphy. There were, however, no national or international rules for this procedure. On November 18, 1920 a commercial radio license was issued to the Seamen's Church Institute of New York for the purpose of providing radio medical advice to ships. At that time the manpower losses of the world merchant fleet as a result of sickness and injury in the open sea averaged seven seamen daily. The station of the Seamen's Church Institute of New York, with a broadcasting range of 2500 miles, offered radio medical advice from a team of doctors. Information on the existence of radio medical advice was propagated on first - aid courses and in the *Manual on Ship Sanitation and First Aid for Merchant Seamen,* published by the medical team of the Seamen's Church Institute (Manning [32]).

International regulations in this field were not introduced before the 1927 Washington Conference, when a comprehensive medical section was added to the International Code of Signals with the support of the Office International d'Hygiène Publique. The medical part was intended to make radio medical consultation easier for the physicians. Radio medical services were set up in many maritime countries in the late 1920s and 1930s - namely Japan in 1928, the Netherlands in 1930, Germany in 1931, Yugoslavia in 1938 etc. Since 1932 the International Telecommunication Union (ITU) has published information on coastal radio stations which provide these services.

The International Radio medical Centre (CIRM) was founded in 1935 in Rome on the initiative of Professor Guida as the first institution for international cooperation on radio medical consultation. Over the years it became the main European centre for radio medical advice. After World War II the CIRM joined forces with the US Coast Guard and the Automated Mutual Assistance Vessel Rescue System (AMVER system), which has been providing invaluable help to shipping in the Atlantic since 1958 and the Pacific since 1966. The Coast Guard regularly issues information in the form of the AMVER Bulletin throughout the AMVER system.

The Joint ILO/WHO Committee on the Health of Seafarers at its second session in 1954 also discussed the matter of radio medical advice for ships at sea. After a number of meetings and conferences the following ILO Recommendation No. 106 [42] was adopted on 13 May 1958:

a) Medical advice by radio to ships at sea is available free of charge at any hour of the day or night;
b) The medical advice available includes, where necessary and practicable, specialist advice;
c) Adequate use is made of the radio advice facilities available, inter alia, by instruction of seagoing personnel and by medical guides which indicate clearly and concisely the type of information which will help the doctor in giving his advice, so that the person on board ship who seeks advice understands what sort of information is required by the advising doctor;
d) An up-to-date and complete list of radio stations from which medical advice can be obtained is carried on each ship equipped with radio installations, and kept in the custody of the officer or, in

the case of smaller vessels, of the person responsible for radio duties.

Today there are over 200 radio stations engaged in radio medical advice all over the world. Thus medical advice can quickly be obtained and proper measures taken in emergencies at sea.

There are very few international publications dealing with the problem of radio medical advice. Special attention has to be paid to the long-term in-depth studies of CIRM (Durante [1]; Guida [14, 15]). In the Netherlands, Steensma [52] was an early pioneer when he established the radio medical service which is attached to the telecommunication system of the coastal radio station Scheveningen. The study by Myhre [34] on the radio medical advice via radio Bergen became quite well known in Norway.

Goethe et al. [11] state in their review of the problems and the need for improvement of the radio medical service some essential points of qualified radiomedical advice:

1. Good quality of telecommunication;
2. Considerable improvement to be expected by means of satellite communication;
3. General medical and nautical medical skill of the advising physician;
4. Medical training of lay persons entrusted with medical care on board (ship's officer, paramedic etc.);
5. Medical guide with instructions on how to ask for medical advice;
6. Appropriate content of the ship's medicine chest (drugs and medical instruments), including directions for use.

Some authors report on the national facilities and practical experience of radio medical advice. Ohashi [35] published statistical data of the Japanese maritime radio stations. The evaluation of these data represents – beside the regular CIRM reports (Bollettino Annuale) – one of the very few available sources of any such information. The national experience of radio medical advice is also documented for the following countries: GDR, Paul [36]; Stanzeit and Ebert [51]; Ebert and Warncke [6]; USSR, Sinitsyn et al. [49]; Poland, Krynicki et al. [29], USA, Manning [32], Sweden, Hansson et al. [18] and the UK, Lamont [30]; Brayley [59]; Renfrew [43].

1.4.4.1 The Ship's Side – Medical Emergencies on Board

Radio medical advice is normally required on board vessels in emergencies only. The main reasons for medical consultations are as follows:

1. The medical skill of the ship's captain and/or officer or even the paramedic is insufficient for a proper diagnosis and the subsequent medical treatment.
2. The crew member in charge of the health care on board wants to share his sole responsibility by consulting a radio medical doctor. Legally the responsibility is then largely delegated to the consulting physician.
3. The medical kit/chest on board (instruments, remedies, other auxiliary material) is insufficient and the expert advice of a doctor is needed.
4. It may happen that in special cases the necessity for surgical procedures or special life-saving measures cannot be decided by those on board.

Häberle [17] interviewed 43 nautical officers and captains about their experiences with radio medical advice and found that the total number of radio medical consultations by German officers is low. Only 75 consultations took place during a total of 309 years of ship board service. In other words: approximately every 4 years a ship's officer asks for radio medical advice. Of the interviewed officers, 30% had never called for radio medical advice.

The radio medical advice call is normally instituted on board on agreement between the officer in charge and the ship's captain. An attempt at contact with a coastal radiostation of the home country is often made. Obviously the ship's officers have more faith in the doctors of the home country who on account of their knowledge of shipboard conditions and the language are expected to give the best advice. If this is not possible they try to reach a nearby coastal station or a particular station already known for high-quality advice, e.g. CIRM. On board USSR, GDR and other vessels an attempt is invariably made to reach their home countries.

Radio medical advice calls are made either by telegraphy or telephony. Both procedures have their advantages and disadvantages. The advantage of telegraphy is that the enquiry and the answer are transmitted in full text without any atmospheric interference. The scant information in a telegram however, provides insufficient information. The International Code of Signals provides a medical code. By using the code, language difficulties are easier to overcome, but the decoding is time consuming. In the *International Signal Book* [21] it is recommended that enquiries should be set out fully and that only in case of language difficulties should the code be used.

The advantage of telephone calls is that direct communication with the radio medical advice doctor ensues. Good communication is usually possible via UHF, but technical difficulties frequently occur and interfere with contacts via short wave or medium wave. The calls are occasionally completely disturbed through atmospheric interference. Satellite communication offers a considerable improvement of radiomedical advice facilities. It is, however, necessary to have the phone numbers of the radio medical advice institutions available on board. The use of coastal radio stations as intermediaries is not possible.

A precise diagnosis is a prerequisite for correct radio medical advice. The advising doctor is in a position to make a correct diagnosis only if the verbal information contains as many details as necessary to get a clear picture of the disease or accident in question. This requires adequate expertise from the officer in charge. Many countries developed questionnaires for use on board. The check-list form of these questionnaires differs, but they all basically rest on the criteria of collecting within a very short time all the necessary data on the medical history, the present state of the patient, the medical treatment already given, the medical facilities on board etc. Goethe et al. [11]. Unfortunately, radio medical check-lists are used to only a very limited extent world-wide. General use of this method would improve the quality of the advice given.

1.4.4.2 The Shoreside – Who Gives Radio Medical Advice?

More than 200 radio stations of countries world-wide transmit radio medical advice calls, mostly free of charge. With few exceptions the advice is given not only by the doctor attached to the radio station. A link is established with a nearby specialist, e.g. a port health officer or – as in most cases – a specialist in the nearest local hospital (Goethe et al. [11]). There are, of course, advantages and disadvantages to this method. It is very helpful to consult a hospital if a specialist is available at all times, but it may be that there is no specialist on duty. In that event there may be a relatively young, inexperienced doctor on duty, especially at night or at the weekend, which does not contribute to the effectiveness of the radio medical advice. Radio medical work differs in many ways from ordinary medical practice. The doctor is trained and required to examine the patient with the help of his own senses (eyes, ears, touch) and to establish a diagnosis on the basis of his own observations and additional laboratory, X-ray, ECG and other data. Establishing a diagnosis and proceeding with treatment without even seeing the patient (remote treatment, teletherapy) is not only unusual, but in several countries is also forbidden by law. In most civilised countries the treatment of the sick and injured is entrusted to qualified doctors only. Radio medical advice is an exception where both of the above-mentioned principles must be violated (an emergency where the law cannot be applied).

There are a few well-established radio medical advice systems with different structures:

Centro Internazionale Radio Medico (CIRM)

This system, which is linked with all Italian and also with numerous non-European radio stations, was founded in 1935 by Professor Guida in Rome. A nautical medical specialist is on duty at all times, thus ensuring high-quality advice. Additional specialist advice is available upon request.

Netherlands/Radio Scheveningen

This service always has one experienced nautical-medical specialist on duty. The doctor can be reached via a wireless receiver placed at his disposal by the Dutch Post Telephone–Telegraph Service (Semaphone Service similar to the Euro Signal System). Upon receiving the signal, the duty doctor calls Radio Scheveningen via telephone, receives telegrams or telephone messages and establishes a direct telephone link with the ship in trouble ([39]; [40]; Steensma [52]).

The Spanish Radio Medical Advice Centre in Madrid (Centro Radio Medico Español)

A doctor can be consulted day and night. The medical records of all Spanish seafarers are available.

Japan

The Seamen Relief Association set up radio medical advice facilities in 1928. Today 13 hospitals are linked with 10 coastal radio stations. Ten of these hospitals belong to the Japan Seamen Relief Organization, three to the Japanese Seamen Insurance Association.

1.4.4.3 Results of Radio Medical Advice

The number of consultations per year varies greatly from one country to another, ranging from a few cases to several thousand. The radio medical activities of different countries can be compared only to a certain degree. An idea of the incidence in some countries mentioned here can be seen in the following table (Goethe et al. [11]).

Average number of consultation cases per years

Up to	100 cases	Belgium, German Democratic Republic, Finland, Sweden
Up to	500 cases	Federal Republic of Germany, Great Britain, Israel, Yugoslavia, Norway, Poland
Up to	1 000 cases	Japan
More than	1 000 cases	Italy (CIRM), The Netherlands, USA

Unfortunately information on frequency rates of diagnoses in radio medical advice is scarce world-wide. Goethe et al. [11] gave a considerable number of further references, but it is impossible to compare these accurately because the diseases were classified in different ways. In no case was the International Classification of Diseases of the WHO referred to.

The most detailed documentation is available from Japan, Italy (CIRM) and the Netherlands. In addition, some of the data from Poland, the German Democratic Republic, Sweden and Yugoslavia could be evaluated.

The detailed statistical data from Japan show that the majority of diagnoses referred to diseases of the digestive system. It is evident from this analysis that the rate of diseases of the digestive system is higher on foreign (30.6%) than on Japanese vessels (27.9%). The statistics of CIRM also show a high percentage of diseases of the digestive system (19.6%). Nevertheless, in CIRM data the frequency rate of 21.2% for "symptoms, senility and morbid states not clearly defined" is even higher. This is a characteristic which does not appear in any other report. According to the data from the Netherlands, diagnoses of diseases of the digestive system present a rate of 18.8%, being considerably below that of accidents and intoxications (29.4%).

In the Swedish statistics, diseases of the digestive system (when putting together acute abdomen, gastritis and/or ulcers) are in third place, after infectious disease (place 1) and surgical cases and/or accidents and injuries (place 2). In the British statistics, diseases of the digestive system (24.5%) are followed by diseases of the urinary system (13.8%)and by accidents (13.1%). In Poland diseases of the digestive system (17.7%) are in second place, following infectious diseases (20.9%). It is not possible to compare the statistical data of the German Democratic Republic with the data of other countries. The frequency rate of internal diseases is the highest, followed by surgical cases.

It is peculiar that the frequency rates of accidents differ considerably. In Japan accidents (22%) range significantly behind diseases of the digestive system (28.1%). The same applies to the Polish data, where accidents and injuries come below infectious diseases and diseases of the digestive system. In the CIRM statistics accidents follows symptoms which are not clearly defined and diseases of the digestive system.

In Yugoslavia accidents rank third, below diseases of the digestive system and the genito-urinary system, whereas in the Netherlands accidents and injuries lead with 29.4%, followed by diseases of the digestive system and infectious diseases. In general the rate of infectious diseases remains average or towards the bottom of the scale. Strangely enough, the Polish and Swedish statistics are the only exceptions, these diseases being given at 20.9% (Poland) and 25% (Sweden).

CIRM data show a decrease in percentage rates of infectious diseases from 10.7 in 1971 to 0.8 in 1978.

Recently Schepers [45], in an analysis of the radio medical activity of the Federal Republic of Germany, found infectious and parasitic diseases (including VD) to be in first place with 22.4%, diseases of the digestive system (including dental problems, hernia and appendicitis) to be second (21.4%), and accidents (11.4%) and diseases of heart and circulatory system (10.3%) to be third and fourth.

An explanation for the significant differences in the diagnosis distribution statistics is difficult to find. Possibly they relate to the different structures of crews and the non-standardised medical training of ship officers and/or their motivation in seeking radio medical consultation. At any rate, it would be advisable to use the International Classification of Diseases world-wide when establishing diagnosis distribution statistics in future.

1.4.4.4 Conclusion

The quality of radio medical advice and its success depend on the following factors Goethe et al. [11]:

1. *The scope of telecommunication*. This can generally be accepted as good, but further improvement may be expected by means of satellite communication.
2. *General medical and nautical medical expert knowledge of the advising doctor*. Intensive training in emergency medicine and nautical medicine should be compulsory. Training on the job is necessary.
3. *Medical training of the lay person entrusted with medical care on board* (ship officer, purser etc.). The standard of medical training in different countries varies considerably and is very often insufficient. Combined theoretical–practical medical training courses should be brought up to an internationally uniform standard.
4. *Medical guides with instructions on how to ask for radio medical advice* (checklist). Many shipping countries have national guides. An international adaptation of the respective instructions is urgently necessary.

5. *Adequate provision of drugs and medical instrumentation.* Most countries enforce their national recommendations for the content of the medical chest. However, on many vessels the medical kit available is poor and/or obsolete so that treatment advised via radio medical advice may not be possible. International recommendations on the minimum requirements for the medical chest are indispensable.

References

1. Durante, F.: Servizio medico del C.I.R.M. e suoi riflessi nella condotta del comandante in occasione di malati a bordo. Atti del Centro di studi e ricerche per l'assistenza sanit. soc. dei marittimi C.I.R.M. 115–120 (1961).
2. Ebert, H.: Die Gewährleistung des Gesundheitsschutzes auf Seeschiffen ohne Arzt unter den Bedingungen und den sich abzeichnenden Entwicklungstendenzen im Zusammenhang mit dem wissenschaftlich-technischen Fortschritt in der Schiffahrt der DDR. Sci. Dissertation, University of Rostock 1979.
3. Ebert, H.: Die Gewährleistung des Gesundheitsschutzes auf Seeschiffen ohne Arzt unter den Bedingungen und den sich abzeichnenden Entwicklungstendenzen im Zusammenhang mit dem wissenschaftlich-technischen Fortschritt in der Schiffahrt der DDR. Verk.-Med. *27,* 3, 95–107 (1980).
4. Ebert, H.: Health care on modern ships. Arb. Hig. Rada *30,* suppl. 1597–1599 (1979).
5. Ebert, H.: Health protection on the GDR seagoing ships without medical personnel. Bull. Inst. mar. trop. Med. Gdynia *28,* 3/4, 125–128 (1977).
6. Ebert, H. and J. Warncke: Unterstützung der Gesundheitsoffiziere durch funkärztliche Beratung. In: V. Internationales Symposium über Schiffahrtsmedizin vom 19. bis 21. Okt. 1972 in Rostock. Vorträge. Ed.: Medizinischer Dienst des Verkehrswesens der DDR. Rostock [1973]. pp. 85–92.
7. First-aid and radio-medicine course. Boll. ann. C.I.R.M. 6–7 (1973).
8. Goethe H. and H.-E. Grewe: Gesundheitliche Betreuung und Notfallsituation auf See. In: Jahrestagung der Deutschen Gesellschaft für Verkehrsmedizin, Hamburg, 11.–13. April 1975, pp. 45–49.
9. Goethe, H.: Die medizinische Betreuung des Seemannes auf Schiffen ohne Arzt. [Lecture held at the meeting "Sektion Schiffahrtsmed." 3./4. April 1968]. Hansa *106,* 1, 27–29 (1969).
10. Goethe, H.: Probleme der medizinischen Betreuung an Bord von Schiffen ohne Arzt – Die Situation der Ausbildung in der Bundesrepublik Deutschland. In: V. Internationales Symposium über Schiffahrtsmedizin vom 19. bis 21. Oktober 1972 in Rostock. Vorträge. Ed.: Medizinischer Dienst des Verkehrswesens der DDR. Rostock [1973]. pp. 103–108.
11. Goethe H., E. Zorn and A. Azzuqa: The radio medical advice in seafaring. Problems and possibilities of improvement. Hamburg: Schiffahrts-Verlag "Hansa" 1981.
12. Goethe, H.: Sicknesses, injuries and health care on board – medical education of shipboard personnel. Lecture. International Workshop on Human Relationship on Board. Bremen, January 21–22, 1982.
13. Grewe, H.E.: Erste Hilfsmaßnahmen und Krankenbehandlung auf den Seeschiffen der Bundesrepublik Deutschland. Arbeitsmed. Sozialmed. Präventivmed. 7, 180–183 (1976).
14. Guida, G.: L'assistenza radio-medica. 1, 2. 2nd Ed. Roma: C.I.R.M. 1966.
15. Guida, G.: Le radio-communicazioni mediche del C.I.R.M. In: Atti del primo congresso int. sull'assistenza di malattia e la tutela infortunistica della gente del mare nei paesi della c.e.e. Vol. 2. Genova, 3–5 Ottobre 1960. pp. 487–491.
16. Gurvich, L.I. and W.I. Styazhkina: O rabote sudovykh feldsherov. [Work of ships' feldshers (physician assistants)]. Feldsh. Akush. 8, 41–42 (1981).
17. Häberle, W.: Die funkärztliche Beratung aus der Sicht des nautischen Offiziers – Fallstudie II. Hamburg, Abschlußarbeit Fachhochschule Hamburg 1982.
18. Hansson, L., S. Johannsen and G. Berglund: The Swedish Radio Medical Organization. J. roy. nav. med. Serv. *57,* 2, 95–97 (1971).
19. Health of seafarers: Study of the nature and extend of the health problems of seafarers and the health service available to them. Ed.: Executive board, 37th Session. Genf: WHO 1965.
20. International medical guide for ships. Ed.: ILO, IMCO, WHO. Geneva: WHO 1967.
21. Internationales Signalbuch. (I.S.B.) Amtl. dtsch. Ausg. Ed.: Dtsch. hydrograph. Inst. im Auftrage des Bundesministers f. Verkehr. Berlin: de Gruyter 1969.
22. Joint ILO/WHO committee on the hygiene of seafarers. Report on the first session. Geneva: WHO 1950. (Technical report series No. 20)
23. Joint ILO/WHO committee on the hygiene of seafarers. Second report. Geneva: WHO 1955. (Technical report series No. 92)
24. Joint ILO/WHO committee on the hygiene of seafarers. Third report. Geneva: WHO 1961. (Technical report series No. 244)
25. Joint ILO/WHO committee on the health of

seafarers. Fourth session. Geneva: ILO/WHO 1965.
26. Joint ILO/WHO committee on the health of seafarers. Sixth report. Geneva: ILO/WHO 1981.
27. Kharalanov, V., P. Polonov and I. Dimitrov: Mnenie moryakov otnositelno meditsinskovo obespecheniya na sudakh. [Medical treatment on board from the point of view of the sailors]. In: V. Internationales Symposium über Schifffahrtsmedizin vom 19. bis 21. Oktober 1972 in Rostock. Vorträge. Ed.: Medizinischer Dienst des Verkehrswesens der DDR. Rostock [1973]. pp. 59–62.
28. Kraljević, L. and Z. Ditrih: Hitna medicinska pomoć i hitne intervencije na brodu i u pomorstvu. [Medical first aid and emergency steps on board of ships.] In: Pomorska medicina. (Naučne rasprave). Beograd: Izdanje Mornaričkog glasnika 1975. pp. 415–420. (Pomorska biblioteka No. 26)
29. Krynicki, A., A. Dyzewski and L. Majewski: Radio-medical consultations in the years 1970–1972. Bull. Inst. mar. trop. Med. Gdynia *26,* 3/4, 249–260 (1975).
30. Lamont, D.: Medical aid to ships at sea by radio transmission. Community Hlth *2,* 3, 137–143 (1970).
31. Lesson plans for maritime module. Ed.: Maritime Institute of Technology & Graduate Studies. Linthicum Heights [abt. 1979].
32. Manning, R. D.: Radioed medical advice at sea. In: Atlantic International Air and Surface. Search and Rescue Seminar. New York, 22–25 April 1975. pp. 123–124.
33. Mikhailova, M. I., A. A. Dukhanina, V. Ya. Spesivtsev et al.: Zabolevaemost plavsostava bolshikh morozilnykh rybopromyslovykh traulerov: Prichiny i profilaktika. [Crew morbidity on big freezer trawlers (BMRT): Its causes and prophylaxis]. In: V. Internationales Symposium über Schiffahrtsmedizin vom 19.–21. Oktober 1972 in Rostock. Vorträge. Medizinischer Dienst des Verkehrswesens der DDR. Rostock [1973]. pp. 63–68.
34. Myhre, J. R.: Radiolegetjeneste for sjöfolk – evakuering av syke og skadete fra skip i sjöen. In: Sjöfartsmedisinsk forskning, Rapport fra nordisk symposium, Oslo 16.–17.6. 1975. Ed.: Nordiska raadet och Nordiska ministerraadets sekretariat i Oslo. Stockholm 1976: Gotab. pp. 15–18.
35. Ohashi, N.: Outline of medical aid to ships at sea in Japan. Personal Communication. Tokyo 1979.
36. Paul, W.: Erfahrungen der Universitäts-Augenklinik in Rostock mit der funkärztlichen Beratung von Seeschiffen. Verk.-Med. *17,* 10, 428–432 (1970).
37. Proceedings of the European nautical-medical meeting 1978. Panel discussion of day to day problems. [Including additional paper and appendices]. Ed.: H. Goethe. Hamburg 1978.
38. Purser marine physician assistant. Ed.: Staff Officers' Association of America Training Program. [New York] 1970.
39. Radio medische dienst voor de scheepvaart. Overzicht 1974–1976. [Scheveningen] 1975–1977. Manuscript.
40. Radio medische dienst van het Nederlandse Rode Kruis voor de scheepvaart, via het Rijkskuststation Scheveningen Radio (PCH). [Scheveningen 1978]. Manuscript.
41. Ram, J.: Maritime health services at sea. SAPANUT *6,* 2, 4–8 (1976).
42. Recommendation concerning medical advice by radio to ships at sea. Recommendation 106. Ed.: International Labour Conference. [Geneva] 1958.
43. Renfrew, R. R.: Medical advice by radio. Ed.: The Grimsby Fish Docks Medical Services. Grimsby [abt. 1978].
44. Report of the joint ILO/WHO committee on health of seafarers. [5th session]. Geneva: ILO/WHO 1973.
45. Schepers, B.-F.: Die funkärztliche Beratung von Seeschiffen am Stadtkrankenhaus Cuxhaven. Notfallmed. 7, 1146–1158 (1981).
46. The ship captain's medical guide. 21st ed. London: Her Majesty's Stationery Office 1983.
47. The ship's medicine chest and medical aid at sea. Ed.: U.S. Department of Health, Education and Welfare. Public Health Service. Health Services Administration. Bureau of Medical Services. Washington 1978: U.S. Government Printing Office.
48. Siem, H.: Health status and medical problems on Norwegian ships, as reported by the seafarers. Lecture. Symposium "Safety of life at sea", Oslo, 20.–21. Okt. 1980. Research program associated with The Royal Norwegian Council for Scientific and Industrial Research. System for Sikkert Skip. Manuscript.
49. Sinitsyn, S. A., M. P. Volchenko and A. S. Budanov: Meditsinskaya pomoshch moryakam v mirovom okeane. [Medical and aid for seafarers at sea all over the world]. Sovetsk. Zdravookhr. *30,* 2, 51–53 (1971).
50. Slutsker, D. S.: On the performance of shipboard medical staff. Bull. Inst. mar. trop. Med. Gdynia *25,* 2/3/4, 273–275 (1974).
51. Stanzeit, H. J. and H. Ebert: Zu den Ergebnissen funkärztlicher Beratungen und ihre Bedeutung für den Gesundheitsschutz auf DDR-Seeschiffen ohne Schiffsarzt. Verk.-Med. *26,* 4, 146–150 (1979).
52. Steensma, W.: De radio medische dienst van het Nederlandsche Roode Kruis voor de Scheepvaart. Dissertation, University of Amsterdam 1969.

53. Tenfjord, O.W.: Om behandling av sykdom og skadetilfelle ombord. Skip 6/7, 27–32 (1964).
54. Turnbull, T.A.: Problems associated with medical aid in the mercantile marine of the United Kingdom. J. roy. nav. med. Serv. *63,* 166–171 (1977).
55. Turnbull, T.A.: A review of medical and training facilities in the U.K. and other countries. Ed.: Merchant Navy and Airline Officers Association London 1979.
56. Vuksanović, P.: Medicinsko obrazovanje pomorskih officira. [Medical education of ship's officers]. Zbornik Više pomorske skole u Kotoru 1, 239–246 (1975).
57. White jr., P.C.: An evaluation of health standard and practices in the United States merchant marine. Milit. Med. *142,* 9, 706–709 (1977).
58. White, jr., P.C.: A survey of medical care in the United States merchant marine. Milit. Med. *142,* 8, 613–616 (1977).

Addendum

59. Brayley, N.F.: A review of three years experience of medical advice to seafarers by the Casualty Officer, Royalty Naval Hospital Plymouth, via Portishead Radio (W/T Medico Portishead). J. roy. nav. med. Serv. *66,* 2, 93–106 (1980).

2 The Seafarer's Environment

2.1 Work and Recreation at Sea

E. Zorn

Throughout the ages ships' crews have always had to adapt to the special circumstances of life at sea. Irrespective of the size and type of ship, the common factor in seafaring is the requirement to live and work in a restricted community under special environmental conditions. The hard life endured by seafarers in former years has been made much easier by revolutionary engineering progress and better ship design, but technical innovations always create new problems. The increasing trend towards automation on board has reduced considerably the physical work required, and the standard of safety at work has been correspondingly raised. This has naturally been accompanied by facilities for a healthier and generally improved way of life. While these changes are to be welcomed, there is still room for improvement. The change from traditional seafaring to a modern shipping industry, associated with fewer crew members and quicker ship turnround in ports has increased the mental strain and the isolation from social contacts ashore. Any research project on "the ship of the future" must take account of these aspects in addition to subjects such as the ship's operation and professional education of the seafarers.

2.1.1 Work Structure and Hazards of the Individual Shipping Branches

All the various shipping trades, whether foreign-going, coastal or fishing, have numerous hazards. These hazards vary according to the type of ship and the nature of the individual jobs, but common to them all is the unavoidable stress caused by the noise and vibration of the machinery, the motion of the sea and other macroclimate influences. The microclimate and possible chemical or radiation hazards at the individual work-place are additional dangers.

The work-load varies according to type of vessel, occupation and work-place. The work-load may be increased or decreased according to the environmental factors. Therefore, the data of work-load studies on board are not strictly comparable with each other. These very different results cannot be considered as representative data.

On board nearly all vessels world-wide, the crew is subdivided as follows:
Deck staff
Engine room staff
Catering staff

Attempts have been made in several shipping countries during recent years to integrate the deck and engine room personnel owing to the reduction of the ship's crew and the increasing rationalisation of the ship's operation. Modern merchant vessels have become larger in size and tonnage and are provided with greater propulsion power. Consequently, the average gross tonnage of German vessels increased from approximately 2000 gross tons in 1952 to approximately 10000 gross tons in 1970. Simultaneously, the ship's crew was reduced from, say, 70 in 1957 to 30 or even less in 1974. The duration of voyages and calls at ports were reduced to approximately half of the former time periods (Goethe et al. [10]). In the meantime, approximately 90% of German Federal vessels have been fully automated. This applies to nearly all highly developed shipping countries, whereas the situation of the countries of the so-called third world is frequently in conformity with the conditions of about 1950 in the industrial world.

The modern merchant fleet predominantly consists of motor vessels and only in small part of turbine-driven ships. The following groups of vessels are concerned:

Dry cargo vessels
Special cargo vessels (container vessels, LASH carriers, bulk carriers)
Tankers (crude oil tankers, chemical tankers, gas tankers etc.)
Multipurpose vessels
Passenger vessels

The peculiarities of the cargo to be transported by the above-mentioned types of vessels have a big influence on the workload and the hazards on board.

The fishery fleet, with its different types of vessels, naturally has its own particular problems.

The cargo vessels which make up the biggest part of the merchant fleet mostly serve as liners. They regularly visit a number of defined ports according to a timetable and then return to the home port.

There are no fixed shipping routes in tramping. Home ports are visited at extremely irregular intervals – maybe only every couple of years. Tramping means unfavourable work conditions because of greater mental stress.

If a vessel is chartered, it is assigned to a shipping company and/or agency for one or more voyages. This implies similar conditions for the crew as in tramping.

There are two types of cargo vessels: general cargo vessels and bulk carriers. General cargo consists of mixtures of cargo, e.g. engine parts, vehicles, technical articles, chemicals, wood and spices. The cargo has to be stowed safely. Therefore, stowing means very skilled and difficult work. Non-adherence to safety regulations and carelessness at work may lead to severe accidents. The number of general cargo vessels has been reduced considerably with the introduction of container vessels.

Bulk liners predominantly carry coal, ores, cereals and fertilizers. The severity of possible hazards depends on the peculiarities of the transported cargo. If, for example, the ventilation of the cargo tanks of a coal freighter is insufficient, this may cause a high concentration of carbon dioxide, methane and sometimes hydrogen sulphide in the air. When entering the tanks, crew members may consequently suffer toxic effects. Spontaneous combustion may sometimes occur. Although severe burns are the usual injury in this event, poisoning by carbon dioxide may also happen. The strict control of ventilation is essential to guarantee the safety of the ship's crew. Ore cargo carries the risk of inhaling high concentrations of dust in addition to gas produced by the ore. This may happen if the ore gets wet, forming toxic chemical combinations with hydrogen (e.g. hydrogen sulphide). Heavy ore cargo may shift with the ship's motion during rough seas, severely affecting the ship's stability. The transportation of cereals presents similar hazards. Wet cereals may also lead to spontaneous combustion and thus to a very high concentration of carbon dioxide. There is also the risk of cargo shifting. The same applies to other bulk cargoes, which, transported under the influences of high environmental temperatures and humidity, may form carbon dioxide and other kinds of toxic gas. This includes a large variety of cargoes normally considered absolutely harmless, e.g. vegetables, maize, rice, soya, potatoes and fruit. Fruit and vegetables which have been bruised and have rotted are a particular hazard.

Fruit carriers are special ships equipped with large cooling plants to prevent overripening. These cooling systems may leak coolants such as Freon, which may be dangerous because it displaces oxygen and can cause asphyxia. The regular inspection of cargo requires frequent lengthy visits to the cold stores. These temperature changes may precipitate minor ailments. There is the added danger that poisonous creatures may be present in the cargo (spiders, scorpions and sometimes snakes), especially when bananas are carried.

Container vessels are designed for the transportation of large cargo containers. The loading and unloading of the containers is very responsible work and thus involves a high mental load. This work is done by means of special "cargo computers" if larger vessels are concerned. LASH carriers (lighter aboard ships) are also special vessels carrying floating containers – the so-called barges – which go by inland waterways to the loading port and from there by ship to the final port of destination. The work procedures and the possible hazards are similar to those on board container ships.

Tankers are designed for the transportation of liquid bulk cargo (see Chap. 5.3). These vessels are equipped with special safety devices. Very strict regulations considerably reduce the potential hazards of explosions and burns. Gas and chemical tankers are special types of tankships. Liquid gas – mostly hydrocarbons – is pumped under pressure into the tanks of the ship from shoreside facilities. This implies a high risk of burns and explosions. Therefore the safety regulations are very strict. The tanker crew are subject to stress caused by the potential hazards and by certain personal restrictions (ban on smoking) and by the fact that the rapid loading and unloading mostly takes place in very unattractive and isolated port areas.

Passenger vessels have become less important during recent decades, when long voyage liners could not compete with air travel. There are still many passenger ferries in short coasting and intermediate trade, excursion steamers and, in foreign trade, the cruisers. The so-called combi-shipping, i. e. freight vessels with a limited number of passengers aboard, has also been considerably reduced.

On passenger vessels the catering staff is subject to the highest work-load (Israeli et al. [14]), which increases with every change of passengers. Frequently, the living quarters of the crew members on board passenger ships are fairly modest in comparison with those on cargo vessels, due to the limitation of available space and the preference given to passengers. There are no specific hazards from the occupational health point of view.

The fishery fleet has to be subdivided into (a) coastal fishery and (b) deep sea fishery. Both categories have various methods of fishing. Thus the work-load and the hazards differ considerably. Coastal fishing is done from small boats (cutters and others) at sea for only a fairly short time. These small boats are specifically exposed to the hazards of high wind and rough sea. Deep sea fishing is normally carried out by a fishing flotilla comprising one or more large processing ships besides smaller trawlers. Heavy physical work is required and the frequency rate of accidents is much higher than in seafaring as a whole (Goethe et al. [12]).

The fishermen have no regular working pattern with a restricted number of working hours. The fishing itself and fish processing represent unbalanced kinds of work in respect of intensity and duration. This, naturally, may lead to overstrain. As a consequence of the the very high work-load, living space and personal hygiene often leave much to be desired (see Chap. 5.4). Very often females do the fish processing on board. The employment of females does not seem advisable due to the unfavourable working atmosphere and the very high stress on the musculoskeletal system (Marschall and Kersten [16]). Fishery protection vessels are sent with the fishery fleets of several countries for the health care and technical support of the fishing boats within a special fishing area.

Some special kinds of ships have still to be mentioned, i. e. the buoy-layers and vessels serving as lightships. These vessels are to guarantee safe shipping lanes. All work required on board these special vessels has to be done irrespective of the prevailing weather and sea conditions. Thus the accident risk is rather high. Besides the monotony of shift-work (watchkeeping) it has to be emphasised that the crew is specially accident prone owing to the frequently very bad weather conditions. The same applies to work and life on board mooring and/or fastened offshore platforms. The risk of accidents on board salvage ships is very high because salvaging operations are usually carried out in severe weather conditions.

The function of the local sea pilot figures large as he is assigned to the ship's captain to operate the ship in dangerous sea and port areas (see Chap. 5.8). Sea pilots have a highly responsible and worrying job. The physical load is also fairly high because of the necessity to board vessels in open sea, which may be rather dangerous during rough weather (Zorn [32]).

2.1.2 Occupational Health Conditions of Individual Working Areas

Although there are typical working areas on board seagoing vessels, the working conditions themselves may differ considerably according to type of vessels, location and sea and weather conditions. So the work-load caused by one specific activity may differ considerably, ranging from low to extremely high. Therefore, the data of several occupational studies are hardly comparable.

The captain and his deck officers are responsible for navigating the ship in addition to their other duties. They share the watchkeeping duty on the bridge, which is by tradition divided into 4-h periods to ensure alertness and concentration. It is physically inactive work which, under normal conditions, does not have a high accident risk for the individual. On the other hand, it is very responsible work which is mentally tiring. During long voyages at sea it is much easier because, except for occasional chart work (calculating the ship's position and plotting the course) modern navigational aids have taken over a lot of the former tasks. Consequently, from time to time officers of the watch on these voyages suffer from monotony, lack of stimulation and a sense of isolation. This does not apply during voyages in dangerous shipping areas, in coastal trades and calls at ports when crowded shipping lanes, higher speeds and larger vessel size, put the navigators under considerable nervous strain. This strain is increased by the steady general trend to reduce the size of crews so that in emergencies, each individual on board is under extra strain (Hynitzsch [13]).

Watchkeeping at night is more difficult and darkness adds to the general strain of the job. High demands are made on the efficiency of vision and in particular on dark adaptation, as the density of light varies considerably during the individual tasks: observation of the sea route, radar control and chart work (Zorn [33]).

The deck officers also supervise loading and discharging of cargo. In this capacity they are naturally exposed to the same hazards as the deck ratings and port workers who carry out the work.

The physical load of the radio officer is insignificant whereas he has to endure a rather high mental load, especially from interference with the radio reception. Since the introduction of the ultra-short-wave radio-telephone, morse telegraphy is actually being used to only a small extent. Thus, the radio officer is under less strain. The vessels of the intercoastal trade nowadays carry a radio officer only occasionally. Wireless communications are then effected by the navigation officers.

In port, the deck personnel are occupied with loading or discharging cargo, with berthing the ship and with safety and maintenance work. However, in most ports, cargo handling is performed by special shore gangs and no longer by deck staff. Furthermore, the work-load has considerably decreased because of the increasing automation on ships, so that nowadays heavy manual work on deck is necessary only occasionally with the exception of rough weather at sea, when the work-load is usually increased. On board modern bulk and container vessels or LASH carriers, heavy physical work is required only in short bursts. Occasionally, the securing and strapping of containers or barges may be heavy physical work. In former times, cleaning and maintenance work (rust scraping, painting, washing of paintwork, rigging etc.) were compulsory. Nowadays, such work is performed at sea by the deck crew only to a limited extent due to the personnel reduction on board many vessels. At the same time, the volume of work on deck has been cut down considerably on board vessels manned by a so-called integrated or multipurpose crew. On board such fully automated vessels, requiring only little maintenance, the crew members do both deck and engine room work. In spite of the fact that the crew is rarely exposed to environmental weather conditions, climatic influences may, from time to time, have harmful effects. Making all secure on deck during heavy storm and bad weather may occasionally lead to severe injuries or even to being swept overboard. Severe contusions, fractures or injuries followed by amputation can be caused by broken steel wire ropes or cords. Adherence to the technical safety regulations (accident prevention regulations) largely eliminates these kinds of accidents. During maintenance work on board, e.g. rust scraping, injuries to the eyes are frequently caused by foreign bodies. Poisoning by inhalation may be caused by painting with spray devices in narrow rooms. Such accidents can be prevented by making it compulsory to wear individual protective equipment (eye protectors and breathing apparatus).

Engine room personnel are exposed to rather high noise and vibration levels and to unfavourable microclimatic influences in the engine rooms. With the introduction of high-speed propulsion engines (diesel engines), noise and vibration levels increased considerably. In addition to the main engine, the auxiliary engines (generators, converters, ventilators etc.) produce considerable noise. By the construction of sound-absorbing and temperature-regulated engine control rooms, these dangers can be considerably cut down. Furthermore, modern vessels are operated from the bridge, making the permanent manning of the engine room superfluous. This drastically shortens the periods of noise exposure of crew members. Also the work-load in the engine room has decreased considerably as an effect of the ship's automation. Engine room personnel are, however, still subject to a great physical load if repair work becomes necessary and this may even result in overstrain. The mental load of the engine room staff corresponds with the deck ratings, so the high-responsibility job of the chief engineer is accompanied by high mental stress. The chief engineer has to supervise the strict adherence to the ship's time schedule and the faultless functioning of the engine plant. His responsibility is shared by the engineer on watch, who works longer hours in the engine room than the chief engineer. Thus, he has to endure high mental stress too. The engine staff (mechanics, motormen, greasers, cleaners etc.) perform control functions, cleaning and repair work under the direction and supervision of the engineers. The physical load is much higher but the mental load is much lower than in the engineers.

Accidents also occur in the engine room, especially contusions during heavy seas. Burns and scalds, as well as electric burns, are rare on board modern vessels, as are toxic effects from the inhalation of smoke from loose exhaust pipes. Heat illness, formerly a frequent disorder in firemen (firemen's cramps), is exceptionally rare under normal conditions on board modern vessels. Engine crew members occasionally suffer from oil acne or allergic reactions of the skin to oil contact. Exposure to high noise levels [above 90 dB(A)] has frequently resulted in damage to the inner ear. Irreversible hearing damage was found in a large number of older engine room crew members by means of audiometric examinations (Goethe et al. [11]). Noise and vibration may explain why older crew members frequently complain of nervous exhaustion and neuroses. It has to be emphasised that the control of the complicated automatic engine plant – especially if there are any engine faults – produces a lot of mental stress which may be followed by exhaustion and neuroses in the older engineering staff.

The electrician is in charge of the whole electrical supply system and the many electrical devices on board, as well as being responsible for urgent repairs. By the introduction of numerous electrically operated devices in all areas – the navigation and engine area, on deck, in the galleys and the cold stores – his function became more important. The combined mental and physical stress can be regarded as from moderate to high. The pumpmen on board tankers have to supervise all activities associated with the liquid cargo. The hazards which may occur are poisoning from inhalation of gas fumes from the cargo, as well as injuries during work on deck during heavy seas.

The work of the catering personnel (pursers, male and female stewards) on board is harder than comparable duties ashore owing to the ship's motion and the environmental load factors (noise, vibrations, changes of the macroclimate). On board cargo vessels the work-load is fairly moderate, compared with passenger vessels, where it is quite high. Slight injuries may occur during work as well as dermatoses caused by the use of detergents. The ship's cook and his assistant personnel are exposed to high engine vibrations as the galleys are mostly lodged far abaft. Furthermore, the very unsatisfactory microclimate of the galleys may be even worse than that of the engine room. The large temperature drops in the cold stores, which have to be controlled by the crew members in charge several times per day, increase the load. Therefore, the physical load is high and, from time to time, even extremely high, especially for the ship's cook, who has a most responsible job. The galley crew as well as the catering personnel on board vessels of most shipping countries have to undergo regular medical examinations for infectious diseases.

2.1.3 Results of the Examinations of the Psycho-physical Load in Crew Members on Board Seagoing Vessels

Studies of the individual environmental load factors have been carried out frequently, whereas studies on the psychophysiclal load are rare. As the basis and the examination methods of these few studies differ, the data obtained are not comparable.

In 1963 Kersten [15] examined the workload of deep-sea fishermen by means of pulse and blood pressure recordings. He concluded that the work-load was extremely high during the fishing process itself and that the working capacity of young fishermen was reduced by the constant load.

In 1966 Sandratskaya [23] published examination results of working conditions on board fishery vessels during operation in cold climatic zones. Changes of the pulse and breathing rates as well as of the blood pressure were recorded which exceeded the physiological limit values.

Zorn [28] in 1966 reported on an extensive study of the environmental and workload of crew members on board different types of warships. Environmental factors such as macroclimate, noise and vibrations have a significant influence on board practically all navy vessels. The parameters were: records of pulse and blood pressure, body temperature, secretion of sweat as well as haematological and biochemical blood tests. Furthermore, psycho-technical tests were applied. It was found that the load was high, sometimes extremely high, owing to the special conditions on board navy vessels.

Biel and Vogeler [2] in 1967 made an ergonomical study of the work-places on board seagoing vessels, using empirical assessment. They found that efficiency depended on good motivation irrespective of the work-load.

A review was published by Israeli et al. [14] in 1967 on the work-load on board Israeli passenger vessels. They estimated the work-load by using work-place analyses and a graduated scheme developed by Maurer. They found that, generally, the expenditure of energy required by individual professional activities decreased, but the neuropsychic load continuously increased. In comparison with the engine room and deck staff, the catering personnel showed the highest expenditure of energy.

Dolatkowski et al. [6] in 1969 examined influences of climate on the psycho-physiological condition of seamen on board by means of psycho-technical tests. The "Tremo-test" demonstrated proneness to a delayed reaction and an increasing tendency towards making mistakes. An extraordinarily high load was found in the engine room staff.

Ohashi and Hirota [18] in 1969 published results of telemetric recordings of the heart rate of captains and sea pilots during the ship's operation when calling at ports. From time to time, considerable increases of the heart rate were found in heavy stress situations.

Marschall and Straube [17] in 1973 examined the physiological reactions due to the work-load on board by means of blood pressure monitoring. No clear results were achieved. Therefore the authors recommended telemetric control of the cardiovascular function.

Bondarev et al. [3] in 1973 dealt with energy consumption in the different climatic zones in order to set up standards for an optimal nutrition aboard.

Paslaru and Repta [19] in 1974 studied the stress problem. They recorded the changes of pulse and blood pressure which are also influenced by environmental load factors.

Some authors published examination results from 1974 to 1980 on work stress at sea. The heart rate and the level of urine catecholamine were recorded in crew members aboard merchant and fishery vessels. A higher physical load was found in the female catering staff. In extreme situations, e.g. when entering ports, the captain naturally showed the highest mental load (Rodahl et al. [20], Rodahl [21]).

Avot et al. [1] in 1977 reported on the estimated work-load of seamen. Also the socio-psychological conditions were considered, but the study does not contain any statement on the corresponding multifactorial influences on the work-load.

Within an extensive research project from 1972 to 1974, the so-called "Flensburger Studie", the environmental load factors, as well as the individual load during defined work procedures, were examined on board 24 modern seagoing vessels of different types [9]. The following parameters were applied: measurement of noise, vibrations, macro- and microclimate, lighting, high frequency radiation and chemical dangers. It was found that noise and vibrations are permanent dangers occurring at most of the work-places and in the recreational area too. The microclimatic load is also significantly reduced in the engine rooms by the remote steering control system, which makes long-term stays in the engine room unnecessary. The ship's motion and severe weather conditions may imply a heavy load. Insufficient lighting may be an additional load factor but is, however, less significant. High frequency radiation (radar beams) are of minor importance. Chemical dangers are practically excluded in the usual ship's operation (Goethe et al. [10]).

The individual load was recorded by means of telemetry during a total of 309 working cycles: heart rate and action (ECG), respiratory rate, skin temperature and internal body temperature and humidity of skin were noted.Self and observer assessment served as the basis of the graduated scheme (Zorn [30]). From the 309 recordings the following was evident: in 24 cases (7%) clear signs of mental load were found: 7 cases concerned the engine room, 17 the deck staff (including the bridge and the radio officer).

The mental load was follows:

Deck:	Very low to moderate	130 (42%)
	High	20 (6%)
	Very high	8 (3%)
Engine Room:	Very low to moderate	128 (41%)
	High	17 (6%)
	Very high	6 (2%)

No case of extreme physical load was found.

From these results the psycho-physical load may be assessed as follows: Normally the deck crew is under more strain in ports and the engine room staff more at sea. In the normal ship's operation the mental load was rather low, whereas it considerably increased in all cases under extreme conditions. It has to be pointed out that emergencies such as severe damage, shipwreck or fire were not experienced. The mental load is in conformity with the grade of responsibility of the respective crew member. Consequently, the ship's management is more stressed than the ordinary ratings. Normally the physical load is very low, but it may increase considerably with special repair work in the engine room or certain loading procedures on deck. The reduction of the ship's crew and the more and more applied practice of multipurpose manning, as well as the ship's automation, lead to more mental stress. The total individual load involving the psycho-physical load and the effects of the different environmental load factors may vary at any one defined work-place and any one special professional activity. Owing to the manifold mixtures of multifactorial effects, the work-load may be much higher than originally suspected for that work.

It goes without saying that the evaluated data may serve only as guide values owing to the lack of relevant criteria. The acceleration and deceleration caused by the ship's motion represent only a temporary and inconstant load, which affects, however, all ratings. Values between 1 and 3 m/s^2 were frequently registered; occassionally they increased to 7–9 m/s^2 which, besides kinetosis, have a harmful effect on crew members in any case, i.e. by the necessary compensatory activities of the muscles and the lowering of recuperative capacity.

The technical staff is more strained by noise and vibrations which particularly apply to some of the professional activities. At many work-places, vibration values above 4.0 K and noise levels even above 100 dB(A) were registered. Also, the values measured in the living quarters in any case imply a high load by interfering with the recreation of crew members. The climatic influences may be a constant load, predominantly for the ship's cook and the engine room personnel, and temporarily for the deck staff too. During voyages in tropical waters, the effective temperatures measured in the engine room and in the galley normally exceed not only the limit values, but in most cases also the limit of light permanent duty (above 30° effective temperature). Stenko [25] reported slight rises in body temperature and heart rate and a slight drop in blood pressure during tropical voyages. Ditrih and Celio Cega [5] found changes in the acid-base balance and the blood electrolytes.

Chemical dangers occur very infrequently in spite of the continuously increasing mixtures and quantities of dangerous cargo. This can apparently be attributed to strict safety regulations (Zorn et al. [34]). Nevertheless, a temporary load may occur for the deck officers and the engineering staff as well as for the ordinary crew. The levels of high-frequency radiations are generally below the limit values as the radiation intensity of the radar is fairly low. This hazard is, therefore, of no practical importance. Insufficient lighting may be an indirect load factor as the light intensity at many work-places is far below the required guide values. Frequently, the intensity of light in the different parts of the engine room differs considerably. In the bridge area, very often concern for the required dark adaptation of the personnel on duty leaves much to be desired. The insufficient lighting thus provided means an additional mental load.

Watchkeeping on board vessels is a load factor of great importance, but it is difficult to assess. The navigation officers are liable for watchkeeping. Only part of the deck staff is involved, and the engine room personnel only in exceptional cases and never on board automated vessels.

On most vessels the three-watch system is customary, i.e. 4 h duty, 6 h off duty. On board smaller vessels (mostly coastal vessels) the two-watch system is applied, i.e. 6 h duty, 6 h off duty or the so-called "English watch", i.e. 4 h duty, 4 h off duty and then 6 h duty and 6 h off duty, which means a continuous rotation (shifting) of working hours. This kind of shift work implies a permanent additional load which should not be underestimated. Colquhoun et al. [4] intensively studied the effects of the circadian rhythms, deprivation of sleep and fatigue on the watchkeeping crew member at night. The watch systems diminish the possibilities of private communication (social contacts). This is aggravated by the increasing proportion of watchkeeping crew members in relation to the total number of crew members on board. In any case, the permanently influencing psychological factors have, of course, to be included in the assessment of the individual total load, i.e. monotony during long sea voyages, mental isolation, reduced crews, seclusion from the family and related groups of people ashore, lack of spare time activities and possibilities of compensation and relaxation, unsatisfied sexual requirements and, finally, the potential hazards of seafaring (see Chap. 2.10).

2.1.4 Leisure Time – Hobbies and Games

Besides the lack of recreational possibilities, the unsatisfactory situation in respect of spare time activities has a harmful mental influence on crew members. Although the situation has considerably improved during recent years, it generally remains insufficient. The frequent lack of interest during long voyages may be related to the decrease of spontaneity caused by the monotony of life at sea. Repeated stimulation by reasonable hobbies or/intellectual activities may be adequate measures to ameliorate the situation (Zorn [29]).

In order to create a good psychological atmosphere on board, spare time activities are an essential prerequisite in addition to the collective working efficiency. These activities are necessary to guarantee satisfactory recreation. It is evident that passive behaviour during leisure time has a smaller recuperative effect than active participation in leisure interests (Stiewe [26]). It is very important to take into consideration the national and social peculiarities of the individual crew members on board when planning recreational activities. Individual crew members, and especially the ship's management, may have strong positive or negative influences. Unfavourable working conditions and the lack of any positive impulses often lead to abuses of stimulants, including tea and coffee but predominantly alcohol, as some kind of compensation. Especially on board deep-sea fishery vessels, enormous quantities of stimulants are consumed which at other work-places can scarcely be as high (Stiewe [26]). It has also to be emphasised that alcoholism on board only reflects the situation of the whole society. Therefore, national, social and religiuous differences figure largerly. The generally held idea that a "proper" seaman consumes a considerable quantity of alcohol has to be eradicated (Zorn [31]) (see Chap. 4.4).

Although a lot of attempts have been made during recent years to offer the possibility of spare time activity on most vessels, the situation differs substantially on board vessels of various nations. The facilities on board and the financial means are frequently insufficient to organise spare time activities. In other cases there may be a lack of stimulation towards any such activities in the ship's crew, especially towards educational work. It seems that the crew members on board vessels of the Eastern block countries show more interest, and that more possibilities of education are available, than crew members on board vessels of the Western shipping countries. On these vessels, all activities are normally left to the individual crew member. On board vessels of the Eastern block countries, special education programmes and planned spare time activities are offered.

Recreational requirements should already have been considered with the ship's design and equipment. On bigger vessels, special hobby rooms are provided for technical hobbies, wood-carving, painting, photographic works, preparation of sea animals etc. It is also possible to pursue sports. Besides physical exercises with dumb-bells, expanders and home athletic implements (like fixed ergometers or rowing devices), various ball games (like medicine ball) are possible. Table tennis is much favoured. A general enthusiasm for this easy form of sport can be observed when organising table tennis tournaments. Bigger vessels often have a swimming pool. During stays in port, occasionally, football matches can be organised, which may help to overcome passive attitudes and the deficiency of social contacts. Of course, this becomes very difficult with the increasingly shortened turn-round in ports. Visits to museums, theatres etc. should be included.

It is very important to have a library on board as many vessels as possible, provided that it is adapted to the on board conditions. It should contain books for general education as well as good literature and light reading. Audiovisual devices (radio, television, tape recorder, records, cine-projector) are available on most vessels. The screening of interesting films is very popular. So are parties and social meetings if there is a good working atmosphere on board. Of course, the desire for social contacts normally decreases during long voyages and from time to time there are increasingly petty misunderstandings as a result of monotony and the inclination to neuroses which afflicts seamen as a result of the special living conditions on board (Dolmierski [8]; Dolmierski et al. [7]).

In spite of the material improvements, the planning of spare time activities on board will become much more difficult in future owing to the busier life of seafarers caused by personnel reduction. In order to make reasonable spare time activity possible, the following facts have to be realised:

1. In the ship's design, sufficient space and /or rooms should have been provided for recreational activities (free deck areas, rooms for hobbies and sports etc.). Of course, they have to be equipped accordingly.
2. Improvement of possibilities of education via the library and audiovisual education appliances.
3. Delegation of a qualified crew member to organise spare time activities in a suitable way in order to oppose the passive attitude of the ship's crew.
4. Also, in nautical schools and training centres, attempts should be made to give guidelines for a proper planning of recreational activities on board.

2.1.5 Future Problems of Occupational Health and Physiology

The trend towards structural changes in seafaring with respect to the technical, economical and personnel situations continues. Consequently, classical seafaring will be replaced by a "shipping industry" which, besides the loss of romantic illusions, implies a very high mental load. The automation of the ship's operation (including working procedures on the bridge, in the engine rooms and in the loading area) will progress. The further reduction of crew members, resulting in a busier life on board, has to be considered in this connection. The activities of seamen will then largely consist of control and operational functions. This means a further reduction of physical work, the mental load increasing correspondingly. As the receptivity of human beings is restricted to a certain quantity of information, additional overstrain caused by a surplus of not absolutely essential information has to be excluded. This modern anthropotechnical system requires the best adaptation of on board facilities to the psycho-physiological factors of human beings. This predominantly refers to control functions and maintenance works (Schmidtke [24]).

The results for the ship's crew are as follows:

1. The future vessel will predominantly be at sea.
2. The turn-round time in ports will increasingly shorten. Thus leaves in ports will be reduced and the mental load will increase.
3. Total automation will lower creative activities in the daily work.
4. The frequent turn-over in crew members will largely prevent the development of camaraderie for people on board, which, in turn, will lead to a higher mental isolation.
5. Seafaring will no longer be considered as a lifelong profession.

The following conclusions have necessarily to be drawn:

1. Crew members should be relieved at regular intervals and should go on leave for longer periods (4 months per year).
2. The period of service should be shortened.
3. More facilities should be provided for individual leisure activitities on board. In spite of all difficulties, the well-being of people on board should be improved.
4. The professional training of seafarers should incorporate a possible change to a job ashore.
5. The still increasing mental load requires thorough fitness examination, including psychological tests (Rünger [22]).

References

1. Avot, Yu. K., V. V. Kanep, D. S. Slutsker et al.: Medico-sanitarnye voprosy truda moryakov. [Medical-sanitary problems of the seamen's work]. Riga: Swajgsne 1977.
2. Biel, H. H. and I. Vogeler: Ergonomische Betrachtungen über Arbeitsplätze in der Seeschifffahrt unter besonderer Berücksichtigung der psychophysiologischen Anforderungen. Arbeit und Leistung *21*, 8, 147–151 (1967).
3. Bondarev, G. I., O. A. Shovkoplyas, V. A. Petrovykh et al.: K otsenke tyazhesti truda ekipazhey promyslovykh sudov. [Wordload-estimation of ships' crews]. In: V. Internationales Symposium über Schiffahrtsmedizin, Rostock, 19–21 Oct. 1972. Rostock 1973. pp. 245–247.
4. Colquhoun, W. P., P. Hamilton and R. S. Edwards: Effects of circadian rhythm, sleep deprivation, and fatigue on watchkeeping performance during the night hours. In: Experimental Studies of shiftwork. Ed.: P. Colquhoun, S. Folkard, P. Knauth et al. Köln, Opladen: Westdeutscher Verlag 1975. pp. 20–28.
5. Ditrih, Z. and M. Celio Cega: Neka zapažanja o promjeni metabolizma vode i soli za vrijeme rada pri visokim temperaturama u zatvorenim brodskim prostorima. [Certain observations concerning the change of the water and salt metabolism during work at high temperatures in closed ship's rooms]. In: Pomorska medicina. (Naučne rasprave) Belgrad: Izadanje Mornaričkog glasnika 1975. pp. 317–321. (Pomorska biblioteka 26).
6. Dolatkowski, A., K. Dega and S. Klajman: The effect of working conditions at sea on the psy-

chophysiological state of seamen. In: III. International Symposium on Marine Medicine, Leningrad 1968. Moscow 1969. pp. 24–29.
7. Dolmierski, R., S. R. Kwiatkowski and J. Nitka: Neurotic disorders and the EEG picture in seamen. Bull. Inst. mar. trop. Med. Gdynia *25*, 2–3–4, 320–326 (1974).
8. Dolmierski, R.: Neurosen und Verhaltensstörungen bei Seeleuten. In: V. Internationales Symposium über Schiffahrtsmedizin, Rostock, 19–21 Oct. 1972. Rostock 1973, pp. 25–30.
9. "Flensburger Studie" Vol. 5 with Appendix: Untersuchungen über die psychischen und physischen Belastungen von Schiffsbesatzungen. Forschungsstelle für Schiffsbetriebstechnik. Forschungsauftrag "Schiffsbesetzungsordnung". Flensburg 1974.
10. Goethe, H., E. Zorn, R. Herrmann et al.: Die psycho-physische Belastung des Personals moderner Seeschiffe als aktuelles Problem der Schiffahrtsmedizin. Zbl. Bakt. Hyg., I. Abt. Orig. B *166*, 1, 1–36 (1978).
11. Goethe, H., E.-G. Schmidt, E. Zorn et al.: Lärmbelastung auf See- und Binnenschiffen, Untersuchungen zur effektiven Lärmbelastung der Besatzungen. Ed.: Bundesanstalt für Arbeitsschutz und Unfallforschung, Dortmund. Bremerhaven: Wirtschaftsverlag NW 1979. (Forschungsbericht 201).
12. Goethe, H., E. Zorn and J. Vrcelj: Unfälle an Bord von deutschen Seeschiffen und ihre Ursachen. Hansa *118*, 20, 1513–1517 (1981); Hansa *118*, 23, 1699–1700 (1981).
13. Hynitzsch, G.: Schiff der Zukunft – aus der Sicht des Praktikers. Eine kritische Betrachtung. Hansa *114*, 8, 743–744 (1977).
14. Israeli, R., M. Weinstein and D. Süssmann: Untersuchungen über die Arbeitsplatzanforderungen an Bord von Passagierschiffen. Neuzeitliche Gesichtspunkte bei Einstellungsuntersuchungen von Seeleuten. Arbeit und Leistung *21*, 8, 145–147 (1967).
15. Kersten, E.: Die Berufsbelastung der Hochseefischer. Bull. Inst. mar. Med. Gdańsk *24*, 1/2, 117–130 (1963).
16. Marschall, B. and E. Kersten: Arbeitshygienische Betrachtungen zum Strukturwandel in der Hochseefischerei unter dem besonderen Aspekt der Frauenarbeit an Bord. Verk.-Med. *18*, 11, 481–491 (1971).
17. Marschall, B. and E. Straube: Zur Erfassung physiologischer Reaktionen unter den Bedingungen der Berufstätigkeit auf See. In: V. Internationales Symposium über Schiffahrtsmedizin, Rostock, 19–21 Oct. 1972. Rostock 1973. pp. 45–51.
18. Ohashi, N. and Y. Hirota: The mental strain of a ship manoeuvrer. In: XVI International Congress on Occupational Health, Tokyo, 22–27 Sept. 1969. pp. 419–420.
19. Paslaru, V. and V. Repta: Data concerning sailor's activity and stress conditions in the Black Sea and the Mediterranean sea navigation. Bull. Inst. mar. trop. Med. Gdynia *25*, 2–3–4, 335–338 (1974).
20. Rodahl, K., Z. Vokac, P. Fugelli et al.: Circulatory strain estimated energy output and catecholamine excretion in Norwegian coastal fishermen. Ergonomics *17*, 5, 585–602 (1974).
21. Rodahl, K.: Arbeidsstress til sjös. Ed.: Arbeidsfysiologisk Institutt. Oslo 1980. (System for Sikkert Skip).
22. Rünger, H.: Individuale und soziale Probleme des Menschen auf dem zukünftigen Schiff. In: Bedingungen für den Betrieb zukünftiger Schiffe. Symposium, 26 Sept. 1980. Ed.: Fachhochschule Hamburg, Fachbereich Seefahrt.
23. Sandratskaya, S. E.: Izuchenie usloviy truda plavayushchego sostava na rybolovnykh sudakh tipa RT i BMRT. [Investigation on the crews' working conditions on trawlers and freezing trawlers]. Bull. Inst. mar. Med. Gdańsk *17*, 3, 231–234 (1966).
24. Schmidtke, H.: Mensch und Technik in Ortung und Navigation. Nationale Tagung "Mensch und Technik in Ortung u. Navigation", Dtsch. Ges. f. Ortung u. Navigation, Essen, 26, 27 Oct. 1971. Düsseldorf: Dtsch. Ges. f. Ortung u. Navigation 1971.
25. Stenko, Yu. M.: Usloviya truda i otdykha moryakov na sukhogruznykh sudakh pri plavanii v tropikakh. [Occupational and recreational conditions of seamen on dry cargo vessels in tropical zones]. Gig. i Sanit. *30*, 117–119 (1965).
26. Stiewe, M.: Die Freizeit der Seeleute an Bord in der Hochseefischerei. Verk.-Med. *18*, 8, 345–355 (1971).
27. Zade, G.: Simulatoren in der Ausbildung nautischer Schiffsoffiziere. Schiff und Hafen *28*, 11, 1116–1118 (1976).
28. Zorn, E.: Profesionale štetnosti na brodovima u ovisnosti od pogonskih uredjaja. [Occupational dangers on ships depending on ship-propulsion]. Dissertation, University of Zagreb 1966.
29. Zorn, E.: Freizeitgestaltung und Rekreation an Bord von Schiffen. In: V. Internationales Symposium über Schiffahrtsmedizin, Rostock, 19–21 Oct. 1972. Rostock 1973, pp. 355–361.
30. Zorn, E.: Umgebungs-und Arbeitsbelastungsstudien an Bord von Seeschiffen. In: Arbeitsmedizinische Probleme des Transport- und Verkehrswesens. Bericht über 14. Jahrestagung der Deutschen Gesellschaft für Arbeitsmedizin, Hamburg, 17–19 Oct. 1974. Ed.: G. Lehnert, D. Szadkowski and H. J. Weber. Stuttgart: Gentner 1975. pp. 125–135.
31. Zorn, E.: Alkoholkonsum an Bord. Beobachtungen aus der Praxis. In: Jahrestagung der Deutschen Gesellschaft für Verkehrsmedizin, Hamburg, 11–13 April 1975, pp. 7–16.

32. Zorn, E.: Beiträge zur Berufsbelastung und kardialen Mortalität der Seelotsen von 1945 bis 1973. Hamburg 1976.
33. Zorn, E.: Die Nachtfahrt und ihre sehphysiologische Problematik. Der Seewart *41*, 4, 157–162 (1980).
34. Zorn, E., B.-F. Schepers and H. Goethe: Gesundheitsgefährdung durch Chemikalien. Untersuchungen an Bord deutscher Seeschiffe unter besonderer Berücksichtigung gefährlicher Ladung. Hansa *116*, 6, 465–469 (1979).

Additional Reference

Goethe, H.: Arbeitshygiene in der Schiffahrt. In: Handbuch der gesamten Arbeitsmedizin. Vol. IV, Part 2. Ed.: H. Symanski. Berlin, Urban & Schwarzenberg 1963. pp. 597–648.

2.2 Ship Design – its Effects on the Seafarer's Physical and Mental Health

T. Ivergård

2.2.1 Introduction

Perhaps one of the worst of all working environments is that on board ship. Accident rates, sickness rates and death rates of seamen are several times higher than those among the equivalent age groups on land. At the beginning of this century, the frequency of marine accidents (ship losses) decreased drastically. In recent decades, however, the number of accidents involving ships has levelled out or even risen (Ivergård [14]; Otterland [17]). During the last decade several international conferences have also been devoted to the work environment aspect of ship design (e.g. the International Shipboard Environmental Design Conference in Maryland, 1974, and the First International Conference on Human Factors in the Design and Operation of Ships in Gothenburg, 1976).

The difficulties experienced by people at sea, the risks of collisions etc. are caused to a large extent by the lack of techniques that are available/used for adapting technological systems to man, his needs and his abilities.

The situation of mental and physical ill health among seamen is strongly influenced by bad environmental and working conditions which, in turn, are a result of unsuitable design of the ship system:

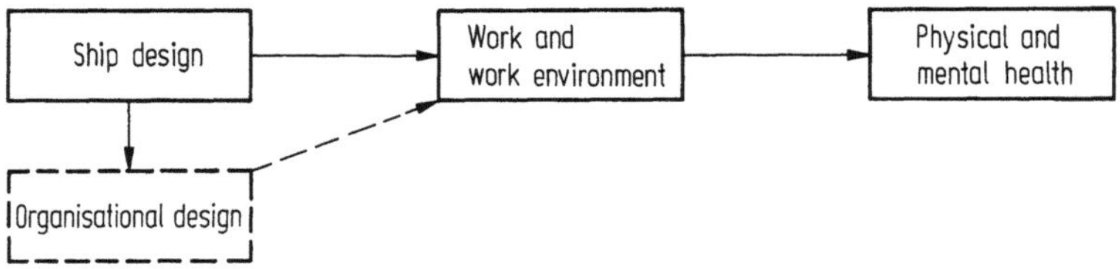

The first part of this chapter consists of a short description of typical work environmental problems on board ships and criteria to be used in ship design. The second part presents examples of solutions to the problems and a model for systematic design.

2.2.2 Work Environment Problems on Ships

This section describes the types of criteria which could be used in the assessment of different environments and also gives some examples of typical problems. The problems to be discussed are noise, vibration, lighting, thermal climate and some other environmental factors; the design of information equipment, controls and workplace layout are also discussed. Criteria applicable to the chemical environment will not be discussed in detail. In relation to the different environmental areas there is also a short commentary on the relevance of the different types of criteria to be used in the design process. A general criticism is that most of the existing types of environmental criteria are worked out mainly from land-based research. The criteria are often taken to be equally valid for maritime environments without any further knowledge. This is a great mistake, as the working conditions on board differ greatly from the conditions ashore. Exposure to the various environmental factors occurs in different ways from those on land; for instance, while on a voyage the crew is exposed to environmental conditions such as noise and vibration for 24 hours a day.

The large Swedish survey study *The Work Environment on Ships* (Ivergård [14]) and studies about ergonomics and reliability in ship handling (Istance and Ivergård [10]; Istance and Ivergård [11]) form the base for most of the results reported in this chapter.

2.2.2.1 Lighting (see also Chap. 2.5)

A ship is often likened to a miniature society. With regard to lighting this means that all the requirements made of lighting in society should also exist on board ship. This is indeed true when one considers that the ship contains work-places, homes (in the sense of individual living areas) and recreation areas. Considering that the work on board ranges from highly qualified navigational work to heavy lifting and moving objects on the deck, it can be said that every area on board has its own special lighting requirements. General lighting criteria have been published by the US Illuminating Engineering Society [20].

The ship can be divided into four areas, each with different lighting requirements:

1. Control rooms, i.e. the bridge, the radio station, the engine control rooms and, in certain cases, the cargo control room;
2. The engine room and other areas with technical equipment and apparatus;
3. The deck;
4. Living and recreation areas.

The problem of lighting is important in many steering and controlling jobs on board ships, and lighting is also important in the avoidance of accidents. The role of visual information is a crucial factor in the safe handling of the ship. Visual information comes from outside as well as inside the ship from: other ships, land contours, lighthouses, instruments, charts, weather maps and, not least, radar. Auditory information also plays an important role, but must be seen as subordinate to the visual. If the information is to be effective then the visual surroundings must be designed with consideration for the information transmitted and for man's needs.

Recommendations on lighting in ships are mainly concerned with the general lighting level. For example the Swedish Board for Shipping requires that the general lighting be at least 80 lux, and that occasional work-places have at least 40 lux. On gangways and platforms, at least 80 lux is needed. The authority also gives simple recommendations on comparative illumination, but there are no detailed descriptions of how lighting conditions should be arranged on the bridge in order to create optimal visual conditions. Night lighting on the bridge should be designed in such a way as to balance the need for dark adaptation of the eyes with the need to see with an acceptable degree of clarity. It is also important that the bridge lighting is suitable for daylight conditions. During daytime the illumination inside the bridge must be high, as this reduces the problem of glare from the bright external environment and also allows easier reading of instruments. Ivergård [12] has developed recommendations for bridge lighting.

The risk of reflections in instrument glass and windows is an obvious problem which can be solved by suitable positioning of lamp fittings and orientation of instruments and windows.

Lighting conditions on bridges are bad in most ships. The possibility of maintaining good dark adaptation is very slim. Work on the bridge is therefore normally done with only partly adapted eyes, which, of course, severely reduces visual ability. (The distance at which another ship can be detected on a clear night may be less than one-tenth of the detection distance for the fully dark-adapted eyes). The way in which information is presented on dials and instruments varies considerably. Sometimes they have white text on a black background, sometimes black on a white background and occasionally combinations of other colours. If the bridge is lit with standard red light at night then instruments with white text on red background can only be read with the help of a torch. Lighting in many other places in the ship is so bad that there are clear risks of accidents, particularly in stair areas and gangways.

Recommendations regarding illumination levels are normally given in lux. In ergonomics literature, one often finds discussions about the suitability of this type of criterion for lighting. It is, of course, the luminance and not the illumination which one experiences; but from a design point of view it is much easier to design a light fitting to fulfil certain illumination requirements than to fulfil certain luminance criteria. It should be possible to fulfil luminance criteria if the illumination engineer has detailed knowledge of the form of the room, the superstructure, the colour, the type of surface etc. This will probably be too complicated. Recommendations about suitable levels of luminance (cd/m^2) should therefore only be given for rooms with special requirements from a visual point of view. Instead, one has to combine the recommendations about illumination levels with recommendations about suitable values for reflection factors on walls, instruments etc. Maximum contrast differences for the surroundings should be recommended, using some type of suitable glare indices.

2.2.2.2 Noise (see also Chap. 2.6)

Noise is a factor causing substantial problems for work and recreation on board. In Chap. 2.6 limits are presented for noise levels in ships according to IMO [4]. General data about noise on ships are found in Berg [3].

Noise levels in the engine room can exceed 110 dB, but the fact that even in the living quarters noise is continuously about 60 dB means that recommendations about length of exposure are difficult to make. Noise masks sound signals and speech communications, making the use of the intercom system, phones, VHF radio etc. very difficult, and can cause considerable disturbance. Noise on ships often has a very large low frequency component; this is especially so on the bridge.

One must remember that noise not only affects man's hearing, but can also be disturbing and troublesome, and affect efficiency in other ways. Noise affects man's effectiveness and behaviour indirectly via the autonomic nervous system. It causes a "general stress reaction" in the body, which, at least temporarily, causes a higher level of alertness and tension. In the longer term, tiredness effects occur. Low frequency noise and infrasound cause risks of other psychological effects which can reduce man's ability to carry out monotonous work demanding a high level of vigilance.

The situation on the bridge is often worse due to extra infrasound arising from the funnel and also, being at a higher level on the ship, bears the greatest effect of amplification from low frequency vibrations in bulkheads etc. Infrasound can affect man in different ways, including slower reaction times.

As was mentioned previously, it is difficult to use normal hearing damage criteria, as men on board ships are exposed to the noise for 24 hours per day for many days. Probably the general stress criteria for noise exposure will be much more important. Before it is possible to define some general maximum exposure level for noise on board ships it is probably necessary to know a lot more about man's systemic reaction to noise. One could also question the value of general exposure levels as design criteria.

From a design point of view, ashore it is very useful to know the maximum sound power level from a certain machine unit. In industries it is often possible to compute sound pressure levels at different places from knowledge of sound power levels from different machine units. However, the ship's structure and the different machine units are so integrated that it becomes too complicated a procedure. Instead, one has to rely mainly upon knowledge of how noise from the main sources is distributed throughout the ship.

2.2.2.3 Vibrations (see also Chap. 2.6)

Vibration is an important environmental factor closely linked to noise. Its effects on man are either local or whole-body effects. The local effects are primarily those from handtools etc. and will not be dealt with here as these problems are the same as those on land. Of greater interest is whole body vibration to which in principle one is continuously exposed wherever one is on the ship.

The main resonant frequencies of the human body are between 3 and 7 Hz, and the impedance is considerably higher for people standing than for a relaxed, sitting person. Vibration can cause a feeling of discomfort and can become painful at higher amplitudes. Very low frequency vibration at high amplitude causes movements of the body and increased sweating and salivation, headache and nausea. At higher frequencies, headaches and fatigue occur.

Very powerful vibration over a long period can cause damage to the skeleton and inner organs, and visual ability is also reduced. It can also cause a general stress effect and increased metabolic rate. There are currently no recommendations on vibration, but there are some internationally agreed limits [7]. Chapter 2.6 presents some commonly used vibration criteria according to ISO recommendations. There is evidence which indicates that the levels in these recommendations ought to be lowered. As with noise, the values do not take into account that exposure exceeds 24 hours.

Vibration measurements on the deck at different positions in the ship have shown that vibration on the bridge floor is especially noticeable. Men are often standing still for long periods on the bridge (e.g. the helmsman). Subjective complaints of vibration, pain in the knees etc. have often been reported. Measurements have shown that the amplitudes exceed the ISO limit values for 24 hours' exposure, yet these measurements are taken only occasionally, which is surprising considering the number of complaints.

Use of damped chairs on board can be of great help in reducing the load on the body, and perhaps especially in legs and knees, which can eventually be injured by vibration. Skolnick [23] and Rumyantsev und Mekhelson [21] discuss the effect of vibration on seamen aboard.

2.2.2.4 Thermal Environment (see also Chap. 2.4)

The thermal environment is a very special problem on ships [5]. The main reason is that the ship moves through different climatic zones that can be either very hot and humid or extremely cold. Although passages through Arctic waters can cause severe problems for unprotected personnel, it is the hot climate that most often presents difficulties.

Most modern ships are equipped with air-conditioning in the control rooms and living quarters. In the engine room and cargo space it is not possible to control the thermal climate and this will result in an excessive heatload.

Work is being done in Sweden towards an international standard index for hot climates. The US limit values are based on the following formula, known as WBGT (wet bulb globe temperature index):

$$\mathrm{WBGT} = 0.7\,\mathrm{WB} + 0.3\,\mathrm{GT}$$

Out-of-doors, it is calculated thus:

$$\mathrm{WBGT} = 0.7\,\mathrm{WB} + 0.2\,\mathrm{GT} + 0.1\,\mathrm{DB}$$

where WB = wet bulb temperature
DB = dry bulb temperature
GT = globe temperature

The wet bulb temperature is measured with a thermometer which has a piece of

Table 1. Permissible US threshold limit values for exposure to heat (values are given in °C)[a]

Work-rest regimen	Work-load		
	Light	Moderate	Heavy
Continuous work	30.0	26.7	25.0
75% work 25% rest, each hour	30.6	28.0	25.9
50% work 50% rest, each hour	31.4	29.4	27.9
25% work 75% rest, each hour	32.2	31.1	39.0

[a] Higher heat exposures than those shown are permissible if the workers have been undergoing medical surveillance and it has been established that they are more tolerant to work in heat than the average worker. Workers should not be permitted to continue working when their deep body temperature exceeds 38.0 °C

wet gauze around the bulb, and the dry bulb temperature with an ordinary thermometer shielded from radiated heat. A globe temperature is read from a common thermometer placed in the centre of a 15-cm diameter black-painted copper globe.

Table 1 shows the allowed values for different working conditions and loads. These values are in fact experienced as fairly stressful, and heat stress is thus a serious risk which can cause special problems for the elderly and those with circulatory trouble. Studies show that many places on board show temperature levels above the recommended index values. In the engine room, conditions at times are such that the work/rest ratio should be 1:3.

In the galley the cook may experience thermal overload despite air conditioning, owing to heat radiation from the stove.

With respect to the thermal environment, the ship can be thought of as consisting of four principal areas:

1. Internal living and service areas (cabins, messes, the galley, offices etc.), which on most ships in world-wide services are equipped with air-conditioning.
2. The deck, where the external climate determines the thermal conditions.
3. The engine room, where the thermal environment is influenced by the external climate and the power output of the main engines.
4. The cargo holds and storage areas, where the climate is decided by the water temperature and the external climate.

2.2.2.5 Air Pollution

Air pollution on board is a problem that occurs in many different forms. Pollution can arise from the cargo, the engines and (most often) the work that is performed. Contrary to common belief, the air quality in the engine room is generally good. This is mainly because of the high air consumption of the combustion in the engines, which gives a high turnover of the air and dilutes air pollutants.

Air pollution is most serious while handling cargo. For instance, when loading a crude oil tanker a large amount of hydrocarbons is released on the deck and may spread to the living quarters (depending on the wind direction). On RoRo ships and ferries, the exhaust fumes from vehicles with internal combustion engines result in serious problems. Dust from bulk cargoes can also cause problems if open handling methods are used.

Local problems with air pollution arise while performing different kinds of jobs. Examples of this in the engine room are oil mist while working in the crankcase of large bore diesels a short time after stopping the engine and the handling of chemicals for boiler water treatment (hydroxine). Examples on the deck are rust removal and, of course, use of solvents while painting, especially in closed spaces with limited ventilation.

There are, in most countries, special threshold limit values or maximum allowed concentrations for air pollution exposure at work-places. Threshold limit values (TLV) are divided into time-weighted average (TWA), ceiling limits (CL) and short-term exposure limits (STEL). These limit values are of great importance in deciding if there are health risks from air pollution. However, in designing a ventilation system these threshold exposure limit values alone are of less value in avoiding excessive air pollution at work-places. Additional criteria have to be used. It has been suggested that consideration should be given to the maximum concentration of emitted air pollution from different machine units. One could for example specify that diesel engines should only be allowed to emit X mg SO_2 per hour. This value could then be used in combination with similar values from other machines to design a suitable ventilation system with local exhaust and general ventilation.

2.2.2.6 Accidents and General Work Problems

In investigating these problems, the types of task a particular crew member has to perform must be considered. Before deciding how a bridge, engine control room or cargo control room shall be designed, it is necessary to carry out a function and task analysis, and then to decide which functions will be performed by man and which by machine. When the various tasks to be done by man have been defined, they can be grouped into suitable jobs. From this one can decide upon the types of instruments and controls needed at a particular work-place. In a series of reports by Toni Ivergård and Howell Istance, published by the Swedish Ship Research Foundation, the problems of bridge design have been discussed and recommendations made [9, 10, 11, 12, 13].

The risk of *accidents* varies with the type of ship. In general, however, serious risks are present in mooring and certain forms of cargo handling (e.g. work with motor vehicles or with cargo hatch covers). Gangways and accommodation ladders are also serious areas of risk. The method of boarding large ships does not differ markedly from that of boarding small ships, in spite of the great differences, in, for example, the height from the dockside, and also the steep slope of the gangway, slippery steps and unsatisfactory or missing hand rails. The lighting is often very poor. Considerable risks exist in work at heights, and accidents due to slipping are very common.

Apart from the direct and obvious health risks, there are many problems of wear and tear and *fatigue*. On the bridge, these are often associated with standing and with constrained working positions. Changes of design of the equipment on the bridge should enable the conditions to be created for variation in sitting and standing work, for comfortable and effective working positions. Studies of work on the bridge have also revealed the occurrence of problems of vision, but the degree and seriousness of these could not be determined; neither has it been possible to show more exactly the reasons for these problems. It can be stated generally, however, that the lighting conditions on the bridge are often wholly unsatisfactory, and this in combination with specialised and difficult visual tasks (e.g. radar observations) could well be the cause.

Great problems of fatigue and a number of smaller injuries also occur in the engine room in connection with maintenance and service work. In all ships studied, even those which in other respects have been well designed, little thought has been given to the maintenance and repair of the ship. The main trouble, from an ergonomic point of view, arises from the very heavy work that is occasionally required and from a lack of working space, which leads to highly unsuitable working positions.

The galley is also the site of fatigue, owing to the bad working positions associated with standing work. In combination with these problems of fatigue, there is also a host of risks similar to those found in kitchens on land. The risks are, however, magnified considerably by the movement of the ship.

The notable factor about maritime conditions is that many problems often occur in combination. It is common for people to be exposed simultaneously to noise, the movement of the ship (both rolling and vibration), heat and mental stress. The psychological problems are often exacerbated by the feeling on board ship that one cannot get away from the problems, whether physical or psychological in origin.

As far as psychosocial problems on board are concerned, the following emerge as being of importance:

1. The "couldn't care less" feeling, i. e. apathy, passiveness and a general feeling of meaninglessness;
2. The hierarchy, imposing barriers which hinder conversation and free discussion between all the individuals on board;
3. High turnover of personnel, which leads to superficial relationships, lack of security etc.;
4. Resignation to feelings of homesickness and inability to change the present environment.

All these factors can have serious consequences for those on board.

In conclusion it can be said that the shipboard environment is an especially difficult one from the psychosocial point of view, placing particular demands on the officers and crew. The main aim must be to create conditions – through leadership development, education, training and organisational changes – to prevent psychological stress and to build up the ability of every man on board to handle in a constructive way those problems which will always occur.

Accidents and general work problems are discussed in [1]; Ivergård [13]; Laborit [15]; Otterland [17].

2.2.3 Design for Better Working Conditions

The first part of this section gives some examples of various recognised solutions to the aforementioned problems and also suggests some other solutions. In the second part, a model for systematic design and evaluation is discussed.

2.2.3.1 Examples of Measures

The physical loading and risk of accidents in the galley are often dependent upon the planning of communication routes. For example, the store rooms should be in close proximity to the main working area of the galley.

The risk of accidents in connection with mooring operations is often greater than necessary. The most important matter when mooring a ship is that the officer on deck is able to obtain an accurate picture of the developing operation. With this picture at hand and his experience of mooring operations, he is able to direct the actions performed on deck in such a way as to ensure satisfactory security for the ship and its crew. The following points are vital for this to be achieved:

1. The layout of the poop and forecastle must provide a safe position for the officer, with good visibility for observation of the ship's surroundings *and* for communication with the crew.
2. The layout must provide sufficient space for the crew to operate the equipment.
3. The noise level should be as low as possible, so as to permit verbal communication.
4. The lighting should be concentrated on the equipment and preferably be provided by a large number of low-voltage sources, rather than one or two large floodlights.

Vertical movement, both on board ship and when boarding, could also be made safer, for example by using lifts. Lift shafts with exits directly onto the dockside should be possible to arrange on many types of ship. It is also important to provide overhead cranes, lifts and traverses etc. in the engine room in order to make the handling and transport of engine parts easier.

To reduce the problems of noise on board the following points should be borne in mind when designing a ship:

1. The aft section of the underwater body and the propeller should be carefully de-

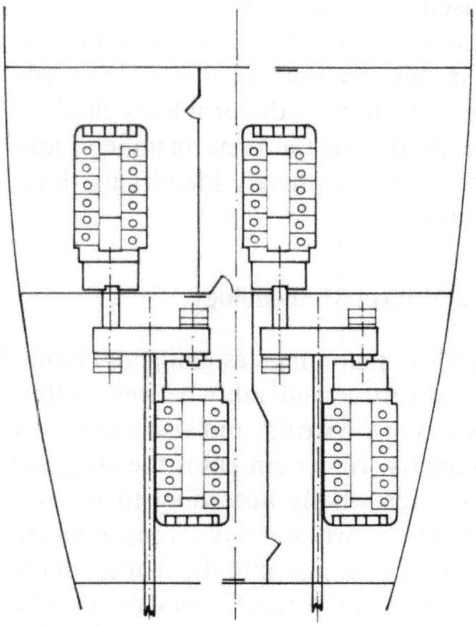

Fig. 1. Ideal design of engine room

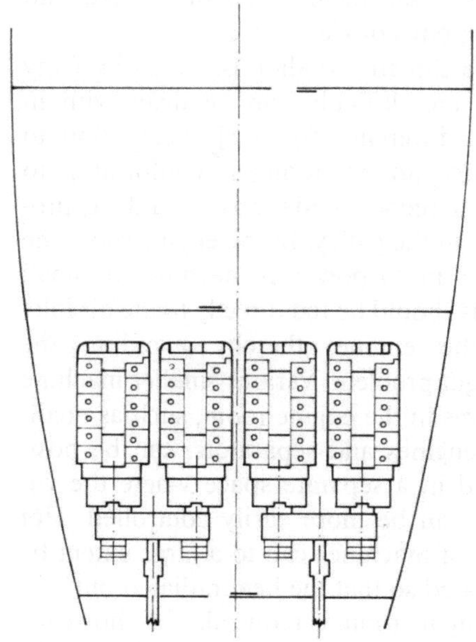

Fig. 2. Conventional arrangement of medium-speed engines between two watertight partitions

signed to avoid cavitation, which has a major influence in the noise level on board (Bark [2]; Söderqvist [24]).
2. The engine casing should, if possible, be separated from the superstructure;
3. Cabins and mess rooms should not be situated adjacent to spaces with high noise levels. Examples of noisy spaces are the engine room, fan rooms, the auxiliary engine room and pump rooms.
4. If possible, the decks should be constructed as "floating", which improves noise insulation and dampens vibrations (Hult [8]).
5. The cabins and all equipment within them should be carefully designed so that nothing will become loose and create rattling noises from vibrations in the hull. This kind of noise has been shown to have a great influence in terms of subjective disturbances.
6. Two access doors should be placed between housing and engine casing so as to prevent noise and other disturbances from spreading.
7. The engine room should, if possible, be designed as shown in Fig. 1. Figure 2 shows a conventional engine room with the same type of medium-speed engine. The partitioning of the engine room into small sections around each engine improves decisively both noise and temperature in the engine room.
8. The engine control room should be very carefully insulated from the noise and heat of the engine room in order to provide a place where the staff may talk in quieter and cooler surroundings and recover from the engine room noise.

There are also a number of unproven ideas for improvements, which would need to be investigated further before definite suggestions can be made. One such is the possibility of dividing the main engine room into several insulated parts whereever there is more than one main engine. Auxiliary engines should always be placed in special acoustically insulated rooms. When work is being carried out on one of the main or auxiliary engines, this work could then be done in conditions which are relatively satisfactory from the thermal and noise points of view.

The climatic conditions, which in many cases are difficult, can be dealt with in many different ways [18]: Ventilation to produce an environment conforming to current recommendations should be provided in the galley. In the engine room the intake air to powerful machines in small rooms should be fed directly to the air inlet on the engine, thereby avoiding the draught problem. Various smaller machine systems in the engine room, such as auxiliary engines and separators, can be positioned in a separate space where the climate can be more easily controlled. Hot parts of machines can to a large extent be insulated so that the heat radiated out into the engine room is reduced. This, however, must be investigated and planned carefully, so that maintenance is not made more difficult. Gardner and Coker [6] have presented occupational hygiene guidelines for ship construction. On deck at the bow and stern, observation places shielded from the wind can be provided, so that the waiting time involved in mooring and other activities in harbour can be spent in protected areas with good visibility. There are already examples of this, but the idea can be further developed.

As far as psychosocial factors are concerned, the only changes and improvements which can in the long term be of benefit for the officers and crew are those which are based on the willingness of the crew themselves. A move to tackle some of these problems involves, among other things:

The cooperation of the whole crew in the planning and sharing of the work,
Improved leadership training
The introduction of permanent crew members.

These measures can be expected to lead to considerable benefits – for example, increased interest and concern for one another, deeper relationships, fewer psychosocial problems, increased satisfaction with work, reduced turnover of personnel and increased safety on board.

Continued research and investigative work in this area must be directed towards finding solutions to the problems cited (in cooperation with the crew members) and not be limited to merely identifying those problems.

2.2.3.2 Project Methodology

Methods of planning, designing and building ships vary considerably between different places in the world, and also within any one country. In certain cases the shipyard builds ships wholly according to its own specifications, without any arranged buyer. The ship is then put onto the market in the same way as many other capital goods. The possibility for the purchasing shipping line to influence the working environment on board is almost non-existent in these cases. It is more common in Europe for the shipping line to put forward some form of general specification for the ship they require, and the yard which gets the order carries out a more detailed design. In these cases the shipping line has a good opportunity to influence the design and fitting-out of the ship with working conditions in mind.

In recent years some of the larger shipping lines in Europe have built up relatively large technical departments which actively participate in the design and construction of ships. This participation can occur in several ways. One way is to carry out a very detailed specification for the ship before offers from shipping lines are invited. Another is for a more general specification to be produced, the shippers then agreeing with the yard on cooperation in the design of certain parts of the ship. These two, and especially the latter project methodology, give the shippers an excellent opportunity to influence the future working conditions on board.

In discussing the possibilites for changing or influencing the working environment conditions in connection with ship design, three complementary methods can be used:

1. Expert cooperation, direct and indirect;
2. User influence in the planning process;
3. A systematic approach.

Expert Cooperation

This can take place in several ways. The first is by calling in experts from different fields concerned with the environment to take part in the planning process. This would apply in the production of specifications for which regulations or norms must be observed and in the design of ventilation, sound-absorbing equipment etc. It can also take the form of indirect cooperation, with the use of checklists, handbooks etc. which the working environment experts have produced. This latter method is difficult in practice, as there is little relevant knowledge which is accessible in such a form that it can be used easily by the non-expert. One is therefore dependent upon using experts directly in the planning work, and it is vital that they are called in early enough in the different planning phases. The basic environmental and ergonomic demands must be formulated at the specification stage. Care should be taken to include such general problems as the overall design, positioning of the whole superstructure, choice of the number and type of main engines, etc. It is also a matter of designing the specifications for the different environmental factors such as noise, vibration, lighting, thermal climate, accident risks and work factors.

Cooperation from Employees

In today's planning and construction stages of a ship there exist certain interest groups such as the future owner (shipping line), the shipyard, the constructors, the planners and the future crew members. It is the shipping line which holds the casting vote in making decisions. For those employed on land a law may exist which gives employees the right to take part in the planning of new industries and work-places. The thinking behind this is that they will have the chance to enrich the planning work with their own experience and knowledge. A proposal now being considered by the Swedish government will provide similar conditions for those employed on ships.

Planning should be carried out in such a way that the employees and/or their representatives are not merely given the function of examining drawings made in the traditional way. For those who are not familiar with reading a traditional drawing of, for example, a crew's mess, it is very difficult to understand and to get a clear picture of what this drawing will mean in terms of environmental conditions. A perspective drawing can give a considerably better understanding of how the environment will finally appear. For the participation of the employees to be fruitful, it is thus necessary to change the presentation methods of different construction suggestions so that it becomes easier for the employees to get a picture of what the different alternatives will entail.

One problem with the planning and design of a ship, which also occurs on land with the design of a completely new industry, is that when the planning begins there are no employees. Where the higher grades are concerned, this problem has recently begun to be solved by employing officers at a very early stage in the planning. This is good, and is used to the greatest possible extent. As regards the crew members, one could imagine representatives of the crews of similar ships taking part in the planning process. But it is perhaps even more important to try to build flexibility into the ship so that the employees themselves can take part in the design. This flexibility can be of several different types. In some instances it can be achieved by means of sliding partitions, adjustable lighting fixtures, or walls and partitions which can be taken down and re-installed elsewhere, although this may be difficult to reconcile with the requirements of ventilation, water and power systems etc.

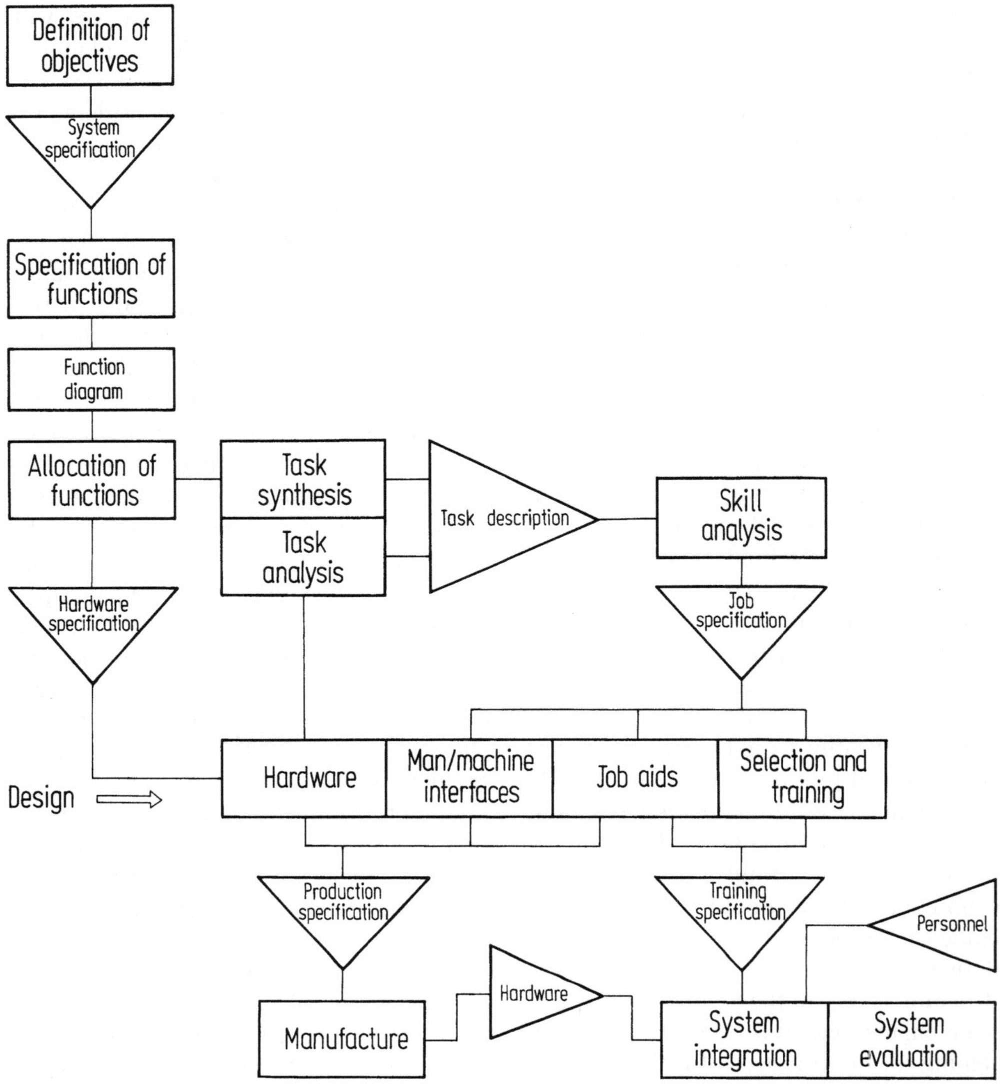

Fig. 3. Decisions in the systems design approach (Singleton [22])

A Systematic Approach

Various models exist for the design of complex man-machine systems. Singleton's model, shown in Fig. 3, is a well-known example. It starts with an analysis of the aims, followed by a function analysis, an allocation phase and then the various design phases. This form of systematic approach should also be applicable to the design of ship systems. It is not the intention that this approach in itself replaces cooperation from experts or from employees in the planning process; on the contrary, use of both methods is envisaged. In formulating the aims for a ship system, it is important to consider the main task of the ship and the limitations and assumptions which apply regarding, for example, speed and costs. There are soon found to be two main aims: the first concerns the manoeuvring and handling of the ship, and the second the maintenance and upkeep of the ship.

It lies outside the scope of this paper to

go into any function analyses for the different subsystems involved in the man-ship interface. It suffices to stress the importance of carrying out the function analysis with as few prejudices as possible, and of not deciding upon which technical solutions will be chosen for different applications during the function analysis phase. Neither should one decide in this phase whether a certain function should be performed by machine or man; this decision should be taken in the next phase of the work.

The allocation phase is, perhaps, in many ways the most important, because it is here that the degree of automation is chosen. It is therefore very important that the employees or their representatives are given the chance to participate. In discussing the degree of automation one must judge the effectiveness and abilities of man compared with machines; to do this one must have an understanding of the total work situation which the new system will involve. It is often easy, for example, to choose a technical solution for predicting collision risks (collision avoidance system) because it might be thought that the technical system is more effective. But in this case there is the risk of choosing the technical system without giving closer thought to what happens when it fails. One can discuss in this case how man's ability to handle the ship in the traditional way is affected by having worked for a long time with the automatic system, which may have led to a reduction in skill in controlling the system manually.

A badly designed automatic system used for too long can lead to impaired performance during normal work, and in abnormal situations (e.g. systems failures or other overloading) the crew member will have had insufficient training and consequently will function badly. This reasoning when choosing the degree of automation can be used in the discussion of both (a) bridge systems and machine control rooms and (b) maintenance and repair work.

It is important that design of the individual work-places does not follow directly upon the allocation phase. Starting with allocation, one should first analyse the tasks which the crew member has been given, and these tasks can then be divided into their separate components. In this way job descriptions are obtained. From these, work-places can then be built up which fulfil the needs of particular job. This is very important but very neglected in ships, where work-places are often put together without direct consideration of the work involved in the different jobs. This has resulted in there being only a few distinct work-places on board ship, which in turn leads to misunderstandings and a risk of mistakes.

2.2.3.3 Evaluation

In this section, only questions of evaluating work environment problems and man-machine systems will be discussed briefly. Special mention will be made of the need for a more continuous follow-up of the ships within one yard, or the merchant fleets of a whole country. It is obviously desirable to attempt to carry out different types of evaluation of those measures which one tried to introduce in the design of the ship. If, for example, one has attempted to comply with certain noise regulations or recommended pollution levels, it is desirable to measure how well the goal has been attained. But it is seldom that these follow-up studies are done later in the ship's life. It is often said by shipping management that they have a fairly good picture of the types of problems on their ships, the complaints received from the crew, and the repairs and service work needed to be done on board. Similarly, at the shipyard it is stated that one gets a good picture of how successful one has been in different ways through the complaints received and the work which has to be done under guarantee.

If ships are viewed from the purely technical point of view, it is possible to regard these present follow-up methods as sufficient. But when a ship is regarded as a man-machine system, the existing methods at company management and shipyard level are without doubt inadequate. Many of the ergonomic faults found on ships are not noticed in the same way as obvious technical faults or failings. Instruments unsuitably positioned on the bridge are perhaps felt by the bridge personnel to be somewhat irritating and troublesome, but they do not necessarily affect the work under normal conditions. On the other hand, an unsuitable instrument position or an unsuitable direction of movement of a control can be a serious fault in a critical situation where one must suddenly and quickly carry out a manoeuvre correctly. If no accident occurs, it is just a question of a common critical incident which is easily forgotten. The causes are not analysed in more detail and there is no feedback of this type of information concerning technical failings to the shipping company and shipyard. If an accident actually happens, it can be too late to report.

It can similarly be discussed whether one becomes accustomed to and does not notice many different types of failings in the man-machine system in a dangerous working environment, e.g. a machine room where one works many hours each day. Probably it is only when a really obvious accident occurs that the fault is noticed and there is a chance that it will be reported. In order to detect this form of failing it is necessary to have some sort of continuous follow-up of the ship under operational conditions. For example, one could conceive of some form of working group within a shipping company, consisting of officers and crew members working systematically, meeting regularly and discussing the faults in different parts of the ship which might endanger health or cause accidents or collisions at sea.

At the same time, in order to have a base for a broader national follow-up of new technical developments in shipping, these working groups within the shipping lines could also be incorporated in national, and perhaps also international associations which could follow-up the work of the groups and handle the statistics which could be produced by the groups. In this way, one should achieve a sufficiently wide statistical basis to be able to evaluate relatively quickly the effect of new technical developments on safety at sea. This form of evaluation system would also provide a basis for pinpointing areas where there is a need for technical research and development work.

Beside this form of evaluation of the direct man-machine interplay, there is also a need to follow-up individuals. There is, in Sweden today, a comprehensive system of industrial health care for employees on land, where they undergo health checks directed towards those problems, which exist at each employee's work-place. As yet, the shipping industry in Sweden has no similar system of health care. The creation of a similar system in the shipping industry, based (regarding choice of health screening, medical examinations etc.) on the type of health risks and working environment problems actually found on ships, would also be a valuable form of follow-up of the well-being of seamen.

References

1. Accident prevention on board ship at sea and in port. Geneva: ILO 1978. (ILO Codes of practice)
2. Bark, G.: Propellerkaviation som bullerkälla. Ed.: Statens Skeppsprovningsanstalt. Gothenburg 1978. (Allmän rapport No. 52).
3. Berg, P. Aa.: Noise abatement on ships. Machines and machinery. Measuring and presentation of noise data. Gothenburg 1972 and 1973. (SSF report No. 5309:12 E)
4. Code on noise levels in ships. Ed.: IMCO. London 1980.
5. Fläkten. Svenska Fläktfabriken *32*, 33 (1970).
6. Gardner, A. W. and D. Coker: Occupational hygiene guidelines for ship construction. Ed.: ESSO Petroleum Co. Ltd. Fawley/Abingdon 1977.

7. Guide for the evaluation of human exposure to wholebody vibration. 2nd ed. 1978-01-15. ISO 2631. 1978.
8. Hult, M.: Noise abatement on ships. Gothenburg 1976. (SSF report 118)
9. Istance, H.: Utformning av en manövermodul. Gothenburg 1978. (SSF report 178)
10. Istance, H. and T. Ivergård: Ergonomics and reliability in ship handling systems – Theories, models and methods. Gothenburg 1976. (SSF report 5311: 10)
11. Istance, H. and T. Ivergård: Ergonomics and reliability in ship handling system. Gothenburg 1978. (SSF report 157)
12. Ivergård, T.: Belysning på bryggan. Ed.: Sjöfartens Arbetarskyddsnämnd. Gothenburg 1977.
13. Ivergård, T.: Ergonomics and reliability in the handling of ships – A critical literature review. Gothenburg 1975. (SSF report 5311: 8)
14. Ivergård, T. (ed): Arbetsmiljö inom sjöfarten. Sjöfartens Arbetarskyddsnämnd. Gothenburg 1978.
15. Laborit, H.: Opinions concernant la fatigue et l'adaptation de l'homme a la chaleur. Résultats acquis et orientation actuelle des recherches dans la marine. Rev. Méd. nav. *14*, 3, 217–236 (1959).
16. Oborne, D. J.: Vibration and passenger comfort. Appl. Ergonomics *8*, 2, 97–101 (1977).
17. Otterland, A.: Accidents to Swedish Seafarers. International Transport Workers' Journal *23*, 5, 112–113 (1963).
18. Recommendation concerning air conditioning of crew accommodation and certain other spaces on board ship. Recommendation 140. Geneva: ILO 1970. pp. 32–33.
19. Recommendation concerning protection against hazards of poisoning arising from benzene. Recommendation No. 144. Geneva: ILO 1971.
20. Recommended practice for marine lighting, RP-12, of the Illuminating Engineering Society, USA, July 1974.
21. Rumyantsev, G. I. and D. A. Mekhelson: Vliyanie shumo-vibratsionnogo faktora v komplekse sudovykh uslovi na organism moryakov. [The effect of noise and vibration on seamen aboard oceangoing vessels]. Gig. i Sanit. *35*, 9, 25–27 (1971).
22. Singleton, W. T.: Current trends towards system design. London: Her Majesty's Stationery Office 1966. (Ergonomics for Industry)
23. Skolnick, A.: Crew performance requirements in the vibration environments of surface effect ships. In: Vibration and combined stresses in advanced systems. Aerospace Medical Panel Specialists' Meeting, Oslo, 22–23 April 1974. AGARD Conference Proceedings No 145, B3-1 – B3-9.
24. Söderqvist, S.: Propellerinducerat buller i fartyg. Gothenburg 1972. (SSF report No. 5309: 8)

2.3 The Effect of the Macroclimate

H. Ebert

2.3.1 External Climatic Conditions

Under *climate* we understand a group of permanent meteorological conditions that remain typical for a prolonged period. The term *weather,* in contrast, denotes only short-term meteorological changes lasting, say, for a day, a month, or even a season. The earth can be divided into four large climatic zones:

The *polar zone* is characterized by long, bitter and very foggy winters with considerable precipitation and cold summers with little sunshine.

The *temperate zone* characteristically has cool summers, moderately cold winters and frequent precipitation.

The *subtropical zone* is warm and sunny. Humidity is low, and there is little precipitation. The winters are short and mild.

The *tropics* are characterized by a hot, humid climate with intense sunlight (temperatures up to 36 °C with a mean humidity of 80%–90%).

The totality of meteorological and atmospheric conditions form the basis for the external climate (macroclimate) in a given part of the world. This external climate has a considerable influence on the climate within closed stationary or mobile spaces (microclimate) created by man as part of his living and working conditions. In general, working spaces and living spaces are not in the vicinity of each other. The conditions established in the living space permit, depending on the social situation, more or less complete recuperation of the productive capacity where working conditions are arduous. The situation in the shipping industry is different: the ship serves the seafarer as both living and working space simultaneously for considerable periods. It

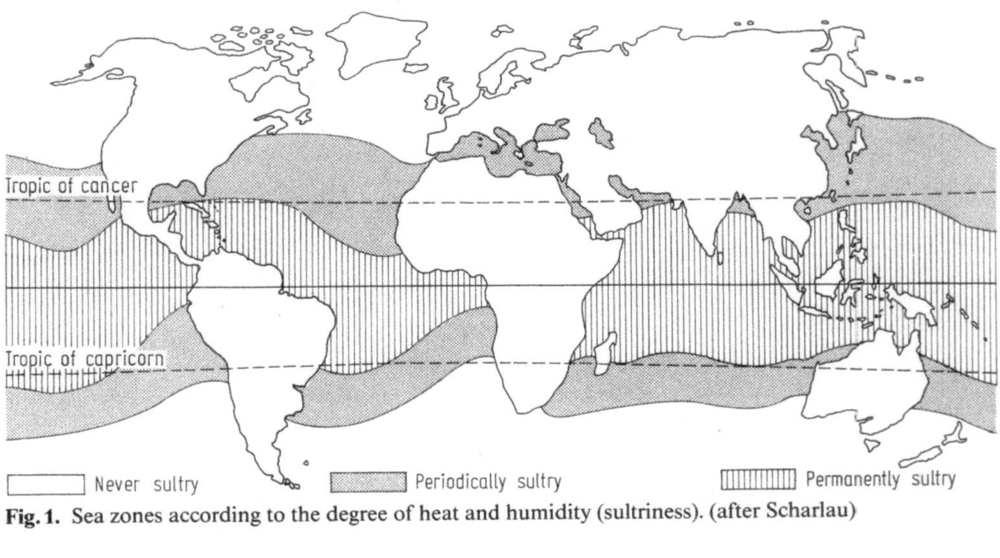

Fig. 1. Sea zones according to the degree of heat and humidity (sultriness). (after Scharlau)

is important that this be taken into account when assessing the requirements he must fulfil and the stresses he has to bear, including those imposed by the climate (Ebert [4]).

2.3.2 Effects of the Climate on Seafarers

Developments in science and technology have enabled modern ships to cover large distances in very short times. This results in rapid and frequent movement from one climatic zone to another and, consequently, substantial stresses on the human organism. Man is influenced by climatic effects and changes in atmospheric conditions (cyclones and anticyclones) which have a radical effect on his physical and mental reactions (loss of productive capacity, depressions, neuralgia etc. can occur). In view of this it is essential to take into account the variations in the performance capabilities of seafarers when exposed to different climates if harmful effects on their health and safety are to be avoided while at sea.

An analysis of the available literature reveals that the working capacity of people under different climatic conditions has been studied mainly at stationary workplaces or under simulated conditions in laboratories (climatic chambers). Such studies involve short-term loads and the results cannot be applied without further consideration of conditions on board. According to our present knowledge, the long-term effects of climate on well-being, physical and mental capability and health are expressed by two biochemical and physical reactions:

1. Increase of the basal metabolism from the normal 70 kcal/h (293 kJ/h) to about 100 kcal/h (419 kJ/h);
2. Constant regulation of the body temperature to a steady state of 36–37 °C.

The main load of these regulatory processes is carried by the heart and circulatory system because heat is exchanged between the organism and its environment via blood circulation and temperature. In warm climates this is manifested as increased circulation of blood through the skin, sweating and faster breathing. In cold climates, in contrast, blood circulation in the skin decreases and, to produce more heat, muscle tonicity increases until shivering sets in. Extreme overstressing of the circulatory sytem in either direction can lead to heart failure. From the standpoint of occupational medicine such stresses can be assessed by measuring changes in values such as body temperature, heart rate and sweat loss, which are measures of certain body functions.

According to Granz [16] the *acclimatization* of man takes place in two phases, each of which lasts about 60 days. The first phase is characterized by a reduction in overall capacity, i. e. a reduction in physical and mental concentration and the ability to react accompanied by diminishing oxygen consumption. In the second phase the above parameters increase again until they have returned to the original values. The heart rate is the most important criterion of physiological stress and it permits conclusions to be drawn regarding the adaptability of the organism. Under tropical conditions, physical work promotes acclimatization and has an additional training effect on the heart and circulatory system as shown by recent investigations published by Granz and Ziegler [17]. Factors which may delay adequate adaptation to a hot climate are obesity, lack of exercise, excessive adaptation to enclosed spaces, lack of sleep, tension, psychological instability and, finally, abuse of alcohol, nicotine and drugs. Under tropical conditions, sweating and, more important, evaporation of sweat, which depend on humidity, air temperature and air movement, are the most important phenomena that regulate the body temperature. Sweating starts at 30 °C and increases considerably with the temperature. Under conditions of extreme heat a liquid intake of 5–11 litres per day may be necessary (Granz and Ziegler [17]).

2.3.3 Prevention of Harmful Climatic Effects

Heat stroke and hyperpyrexia due to overloading of the temperature regulation system are possible harmful effects. These result from the accumulation of heat, hyperthermia and disturbances in the water and electrolyte balance, and cramps can lead to heat exhaustion and heat stroke (known commonly as "stoker heat-cramps" in steamship days). Rapid heat collapse and heat oedema may ensue if regulation of the circulatory system is not stable. Disturbances in the secretory activity of the sweat glands is another possible form of heat-induced damage and was the subject of extensive studies performed by Ejsmont et al. [6–12] in the ocean fishing and merchant shipping industries.

It is important to implement and maintain a certain system of liquid intake. It is advisable for those exposed to great heat to consume small amounts (about 0.25 litres) of a slightly acid tea several times a day. Ice-cold drinks should be avoided. It may also be necessary to restore excessive electrolyte losses by administering therapeutic doses of NaCl, and this should definitely be done prophylactically in the case of prolonged heat exposure. Appropriate clothing and a reasonable lay-out of the place of work can promote heat exchange and thus reduce the heat load. The clothing should consist of protection for the head, clothes that facilitate heat transfer but reflect heat radiation, and absorbent underwear. Appropriate arrangement of working hours and the inclusion of sweat breaks permit better adaptation to work in hot environments.

Persons suffering from disorders of the heart and circulatory system, whose pulmonary function is restricted, e.g. by pulmonary asthma, or who have suffered from myocardial infarct are unsuitable for work under hot conditions.

Acclimatization to cold generally requires no adaptation of the heat regulation system but merely modification of general habits. Minor physiological changes due to effects on the central nervous system, such as a slight reduction in subjective judgement of the degree of coldness, have been described (Noack and Schulz [26]). However, adaptation to cold climates is possible if appropriate clothing is worn, but high humidities and strong winds can cause heat losses that may impair intellectual and physical performance. The result may be poor concentration and loss of skill.

Disorders caused by excessive exposure to cold can appear during long periods of work in the open air, refrigerated spaces and cellars. In the shipping industry, such work would include, for instance, stowing operations in the holds of reefer vessels and vessels serving deep sea fishery (Ebert [5]). The principal form of damage resulting from the direct effects of cold is localized frostbite, but cold may also damage internal organs, causing renal anaemia and hyperaemia of the lungs. Susceptibility to illness is generally greater than normal. Owing to the specific nature of the seafarers trade, of course, cold effects on the body may also result from involuntary immersion in water (man-overboard and rescue operations etc.), but this will not be dealt with in this chapter.

Persons with disorders of the heart and circulation system, metabolic disturbances and great susceptibility to infection are unsuitable for work under cold conditions. Protection from cold is given by appropriate clothing with a high insulation effect and low water and wind permeability.

Summarizing, we see that the macroclimate can have a considerable effect on well-being and health. This must be taken into account when assessing the working and living conditions on board from the medical standpoint and when examining personnel with a view to their suitability for employment as seafarers.

References see Chap. 2.4

2.4 The Microclimate of the Ship

H. Ebert

2.4.1 The Components of Microclimate

Microclimate is defined here as the very localized climate existing within confined spaces – either working or living rooms. Although the sum of the microclimatic conditions is governed by external meteorological factors, the microclimate is not identical to the external climate, and may even differ from it very considerably. The microclimate can be characterized by four components:

1. The *air temperature*	(measured in °C)
2. The *relative humidity*	(measured as a percentage)
3. The *air flow*	(measured in $m \cdot s^{-1}$)
4. *Heat radiation*	(measured in $W \cdot cm^{-2}$)

Also, the strictly local climate immediately above the surface of the sea differs considerably from the meteorological conditions because heat radiation and the air temperature there are lower.

Special local climates are encountered on board on exposed decks. In summer the difference between external meteorological and microclimate conditions leads to a considerable rise in temperature when sunlight is intense. The deck and superstructures, which are heated by the sun, release heat to the air in their immediate environment, thereby raising its temperature by an average of 2 °C (Ebert [5]). This considerably increases the heat radiation to which crew members working on upper decks are exposed.

The microclimatic conditions inside the ship are subject to a variety of influences: they depend on meteorological conditions during the voyage, the presence and efficiency of heating and ventilation systems, the lay-out of the rooms on board, the proximity of heat emitting machinery or refrigerated spaces etc. [14; 19]. In overheated working spaces on board, such as the engine and boiler rooms, heat emitting engines, plants and appliances are generally major sources of convected and radiated heat. The microclimate of these spaces influences the human organism and imposes a major load on its heat regulation system (Goethe [15]). In the engine room, for instance, the body heat regulation system may be strained to the limits of its capacity during periods of great physical exertion such as may be encountered when repairing engines under emergency conditions (Blumenthal-Barby [1]).

The organism cannot be assumed to have adapted to a particular climate, i.e. acclimatization is not complete, until the person concerned has been active for at least 2 h a day under the new climate conditions for a period of 14 days. The organism in this way adjusts more effortlessly to the different components of the microclimate and becomes less susceptible. The effects of acclimatization are lost again if exposure is interrupted for long periods by, say, periods spent in another climate. Since modern ships pass from one climatic zone to another very quickly, complete adjustment in the form described above is impossible, unless, of course, the ship spends several weeks at anchor. The problem of acclimatization is particularly relevant nowadays, when seafarers frequently join ship by air travel. Often they are expected to take up their duties shortly after joining the ship, while suffering from jet-lag and before acclimatization has been possible. Granz [16] and Ejsmont et al. [6–12] have reported on the constantly changing loads to which seafarers are exposed due to acclimatization and their effects on performance.

2.4.2 Evaluation of Microclimatic Loads on Seafarers

Industrial hygiene values have been elaborated to permit assessment of the loads imposed on people by climatic conditions at their place of work and the microclimates existing in working spaces. However, these cannot be applied to work-places in the open air or in roofed structures which are only partly enclosed (Noack and Schulz [26]). It is necessary to distinguish between optimum and permissible microclimatic conditions:

1. *Optimum* microclimatic conditions are those which induce no change in the functional or general status of the human organism and do not load the thermoregulation of the body, even during prolonged exposure. They maintain a comfortable temperature and provide optimum conditions for work.
2. *Permissible* microclimatic conditions are those which no longer guarantee a comfortable temperature but, while imposing a major load on the temperature regulation system, do not exceed the limits of physical adaptability. They do not disturb or harm the health but, depending on the activity concerned and the values of the climatic components, are more or less detrimental to well-being and performance capacity.

When assessing these effects it is also appropriate to categorize the physical loads involved in different activities. Work categories are categories based on total metabolic activity into which activities are graded on the basis of the postures, motions and loads they typically involve. They do not, of course, take emergency situations into account. According to Noack and Schulz [26], work on board can be split into three work categories which can be used as a basis for deciding hours of work:

Category 1 contains activities that are performed standing or seated and in which the physical component of the work consists mainly of light handwork. The work of radio operators and deck officers, for instance, belongs in this category.

Category 2 contains activities that involve standing and walking, but not the movement of loads, and activities that are performed while seated and involve constant work with one and light work with two arms or heavy work with the hands. The work of the engine room personnel, for instance, belongs to this category.

Category 3 is characterized by the moving of light loads and activities performed mainly while standing or walking; activities involving constant heavy or moderately heavy work with both arms while seated also belong here. This category includes the work of the galley personnel, stewards and stewardesses and deck ratings.

In the shipping industry it will be impossible as a rule to obtain optimum microclimatic conditions on account of the constantly changing macroclimatic situation. It is therefore necessary to define permissible microclimatic conditions appropriate to the different seasons for the above work categories. Permissible values for the cold season are based on mean daily temperatures of 12 °C or below. The period when the daily mean temperatures are over 12 °C is referred to as the warm season. The permissible microclimatic conditions for the different work categories may be stipulated in national regulations for the various times of year.

2.4.3 Measuring the Microclimate

The different components of the microclimate can be measured separately or together to permit assessment of the climate within a space. The purpose of this is always to use the values thus obtained to assess the degree of comfort or compatibility of the microclimate with the human organism. In industrial hygiene it is usual to measure the components affecting the heat balance by means of appropriate measuring instruments. The standard instrument for measuring the *air temperature* and *humidity* is the Assmann psychrometer. This is well protected from radiation and shows the dry (air) and wet temperatures. These two values can be used to ascertain the vapour pressure and the relative humidity by means of psychrometer tables or a psychrometer nomogram (cf. Häublein et al. [18]). The black body radiation at the place of work is measured by means of a globe thermometer. After the instrument has been left to adjust to the ambient temperature for 20 min, the value is measured by means of a mercury thermometer, a thermo-element or a resistance-type thermometer at the centre of a dull black hollow sphere made of copper. The globe temperature is an integral value that includes the air temperature, heat radiation and air motion. The correct values can be calculated by extrapolation if the duration of the measurement is short. When assessing draughts in connection with the ventilation problem, the *motion of the air* is measured by means of a hot wire anemometer and the direction of the draught is identified by means of smoke cartridges. These traditional ways of measuring the microclimatic components have been supplemented in recent times by automatic and continuous recording apparatus [19]. These can remain in action for several hours at a time and not only for short periods like the instruments used for taking manual measurements. The latter have the drawback that they must be repeated at specified intervals in order to obtain a representative picture of the climate, e.g. throughout the course of a shift.

Automatic continuous data acquisition permits the construction of portable *microclimate measuring apparatus* for the simultaneous measurement of the following components:
Air temperature in room
Dew point in room
Globe temperature in room
External air temperature
External dew point

A modified anemometer can be connected to this apparatus so that the air current can also be measured. The apparatus measures the temperature by temperature-dependent electrical resistors and the dew point by means of a lithium chloride dew point sensor. The measured values are converted for practical use by means of a table. All sensors are connected to a calibrated pen recorder by appropriate leads so that readings are obtained for the whole time the apparatus is switched on. Additional information, such as the times of breaks, opening of doors and the like, can be noted at the appropriate times on the recording paper. All data required are thus available for the whole duration of the measurement and can be taken as discrete values from the diagram. This is a major advantage of this system over the more laborious manual method and makes it particularly suitable for scientific investigations into the microclimate and the assessment of performance under defined climatic conditions.

2.4.4 Air Conditioning on Board Ships

The microclimatic criteria to be met on board newly built or converted ships are specified in some national standards [14; 19] and are intended to ensure optimum working and living conditions. Table 1 summarizes the optimum microclimatic conditions.

The establishment of favourable microclimatic conditions, which, altogether, con-

Table 1. Optimum microclimatic conditions in ship spaces

Area	Air conditioning	Fresh air	Air conditioning	Room air	Relative humidity in the case of air conditioning	Air speed (draughts)
	Summer		Winter			
		Above outside temperature				
Accommodation, common rooms, etc. (cabins, messes, hospital, club rooms, radio and teleprinter room)	25 °C	≦5 °C	20°-23 °C	≧20 °C	50% ± 10%	≦0.2 m/s
Catering spaces (galleys, pantries)	28 °C	≦8 °C	20 °C	≧16 °C	50% ± 10%	≦0.3 m/s
Control centres (bridge, machinery control room)	28 °C	≦5 °C	22 °C	≧20 °C	50% ± 10%	≦0.4 m/s

stitute an important physical environmental factor on board, is a subject that must receive the unabating attention of the shipbuilding industry and of the health authorities concerned with the approval of facilities on ships. The works published by Frank [13], Reinders [27] and Vorobev [29] contain fundamental information in this respect and it seems advisable to use them to supplement the existing regulations.

Crew members entrusted with the control and operation of marine heating and ventilation systems must endeavour to use these systems as efficiently as possible to keep the load on the temperature regulation systems of their shipmates within tolerable limits.

References

1. Blumenthal-Barby, K.: Analyse der Arbeits- und Lebensbedingungen an Bord und Untersuchung zur Objektivierung des Einflusses wechselnder Klimate auf die körperliche Leistungsfähigkeit des Seemannes. Dissertation, University of Rostock 1964.
2. Costinescu, H. and M. Mihailescu: Das Mikroklima auf Schiffen. Rec. sanit. mil. Bucuresti *59*, 5, 869 (1963).
3. Dernov, A. I. and B. G. Zukerman: Mikroklimat na korablyakh v usloviyakh tropikov. [Microclimate on ships in tropical environment. (Based on data from foreign literature).] Voen. med. Zh. *8*, 58–62 (1965).
4. Ebert, H.: Die Arbeitsbedingungen auf einem Fang- und Verarbeitungsschiff unter den klimatischen Bedingungen an der Nordwestküste Afrikas. Rostock, unpublished 1967.
5. Ebert, H. (Ed.): Gesundheitsschutz an Bord. Berlin: Volk und Gesundheit. 1980.
6. Ejsmont, W., B. Lewalski, J. Waskiewicz et al.: The problem of acclimatization to hot-climate regions. Report I. Some physiological indicators in persons examined in the high temperature-chamber. Bull. Inst. mar. Med. Gdańsk *15*, 3/4, 185–192 (1964).
7. Ejsmont, W. and A. Went: The problem of acclimatization in the tropical zone. Report III. On some electrolites in organic fluids of men exposed to the action of high temperature. Bull. Inst. mar. Med. Gdańsk *17*, 1/2, 65–71 (1966).
8. Ejsmont, W. and J. Waskiewicz: The problem of acclimatization in the tropical zone. Report IV. Loss of body weight and increase of temperature-chamber. Bull. Inst. mar. Med. Gdańsk *17*, 4, 505–510 (1966).
9. Ejsmont, W., R. Dubrawski and Cz. Bartnicki: The problem of acclimatization in the tropical zone. Report V. Changes in the level of sodium, potassium and chlorides in organic fluids of man, under the influence of high temperature and humidity. Bull. Inst. mar. Med. Gdańsk *17*, 4, 511–519 (1966).
10. Ejsmont, W., Cz. Bartnicki and R. Dubrawski: The problem of acclimatization in the tropical zone. Report VI. Changes in the calcium and

phosphate levels in serum urine and sweat. Bull. Inst. mar. Med. Gdańsk *17*, 4, 521–528 (1966).

11. Ejsmont, W., Cz. Bartnicki, R. Dubrawski et al.: The problem of acclimatization in the tropical zone. Report VII. Dynamics of some physiological indexes in unadapted persons, under conditions of experimental humid heat. Bull. Inst. mar. Med. Gdańsk *19*, 1/2, 97–106 (1968).
12. Ejsmont, W., R. Dubrawski and Cz. Bartnicki: The problem of acclimatization in the tropical zone. Report VIII. Dynamics of sodium and potassium in urine of unadapted persons exposed to the effect of experimental high temperatures. Bull. Inst. mar. Med. Gdańsk *19*, 1/2, 107–115 (1968).
13. Frank, W.: Zum gegenwärtigen Stand der raumklimatischen Forschung. Gesundheits-Ingenieur *90*, 2, 40–46 (1969).
14. Gigienicheskoe osnovanie normirovaniya mikroklimata v sudovykh pomeshcheniyakh. [Hygiene guidelines for microclimatic standards for ship rooms]. In: Trudy nauchno-isledovatelskovo instituta gigieny vodnogo transporta. Eds.: E. P. Sergeev and G. I. Bondarev. Moscow 1968.
15. Goethe, H.: Klimabelastung in der Tropenfahrt. In: Fragen der Schiffahrtsmedizin. Internationales Symposium, Heiligendamm 28–31 March 1963. Medizinischer Dienst des Verkehrswesens, Special issue II, pp. 189–200.
16. Granz, W.: Untersuchungen über die Akklimatisation des Mitteleuropäers an natürliche tropische Klimabelastungen. Dissertation University of Leipzig 1980.
17. Granz, W. and K. Ziegler: Tropenkrankheiten. Leipzig: Johann Ambrosius Barth. 1976.
18. Häublein, H. G., G. Schulz et al.: Arbeitshygienische Normen und MAK-Werte. Berlin: Tribüne. 1974.
19. Hygienevorschrift für den Bau von Seeschiffen. Ed.: Medizinischer Dienst des Verkehrswesens der DDR. Rostock 1980.
20. Kersten, E.: Der Einfluß des Tropenklimas auf Arbeitsfähigkeit und Gesundheit der Seeleute. Bull. Inst. mar. Med. Gdańsk *17*, 3, 225–229 (1966).
21. Kersten, E.: Zur Beurteilung der Klimaverträglichkeit des seefahrenden Personals während der Tropenfahrt. Verk.-Med. *14*, 1, 29–36 (1967).
22. Knapik, A.: Microclimatic conditions on vessels. Bull. Inst. mar. Med. Gdańsk *17*, 3, 155–156 (1966).
23. Lehmann, G.: Die Arbeitsfähigkeit des Menschen im tropischen Klima. Köln, Opladen: Westdeutscher Verlag, 1968.
24. Lewalski, B. and W. Ejsmont: The problem of acclimatization to hot-climate regions. 2. Uropepsin contents in the urine from men staying in the chamber of high temperature. Bull. Inst. mar. Med. Gdańsk *15*, 3/4, 193–198 (1964).
25. Marine Air Conditioning. Shipbuilding International (London) *14*, 7, 2–12 (1971).
26. Noack, H. and G. Schulz: Klima am Arbeitsplatz. In: Arbeitshygienische Normen und MAK-Werte. Eds.: Häublein, H. G., G. Schulz et al. Berlin: Tribüne, 1974. pp. 43–90.
27. Reinders, H.: Mensch und Klima. Klima-Klimaphysiologie-Klimatechnik. Düsseldorf: VDI-Verlag. 1969.
28. Sadovskaya, N. N.: Ventilatsiya i otoplenie proisvodstvennykh i zhilykh pomeshchenii rybopromyslovykh sudov. [Ventilation and heating of working and living rooms on fishing vessels]. In: Gigiena truda i byta na promyslovykh sudakh v zapolyarye. Ed.: Ya. E. Neishtadt and L. Elpiner. Moscow: Pishchevaya promyshlennost 1967. pp. 52–63.
29. Vorobev, A. A.: Gigienicheskoe obosnovanie komfortnykh uslovii mikroklimata pomeshchenii sudov s uchetom akklimatisatsionnykh ismenenii u moryakov v reise. [Hygienic reasons for microclimatic comfort of ship's rooms in view of seafarers' acclimatization during voyage]. Gig. i Sanit 6, 24–28 (1976).

2.5 The Ship's Lighting

R. Herrmann

2.5.1 Introduction

In regard to receiving information, man is to be considered a "visual being". Approximately 70%–80% of all information received is registered by means of the sense of sight. In order for man to be able to process this information at an optimal level, great attention must be paid to adjusting the design of a lighting system to the peculiarities and requirements of the visual sense.

As well as exerting an influence on direct optical information, lighting also affects man's readiness to work. The sense of sight also affects the functioning (i. e. regulation) of the nervous system. Poor lighting can lead to errors in the regulation of the nervous system, resulting in fatigue, a change in oxygen requirement and unfortunate effects on the circulatory and digestive organs.

White light increases efficiency whereas red light leads to a decrease in efficiency.

An adequate lighting system on board should:

1. Guarantee ability and readiness to work productively;
2. Facilitate work;
3. Decrease the number of errors;
4. Aid the prevention of accidents;
5. Contribute to safety on board ship;
6. Increase the well-being and recuperative capacity of the crew.

2.5.2 Dimensions of Illumination Units

Luminous flux (Φ) is measured in lumen (lm) and is the total volume of radiated energy which emits from a luminous source and which is received by the eye over a given time period.

Luminous efficacy (η) is measured in lumen per watt. The efficacy of an illuminant (lm/w) is the ratio of luminous flux to electric input.

The luminous dose (Q, quantity of light) is calculated in lumen per hour (lm/h) and is the product of luminous flux and time period.

Luminous intensity (J) is measured in candela (cd). It is the existent visible radiation power in a certain direction and is mostly referred to in 1 000 lm and is relative to the dehedral (spatial) angle (ω).

Illumination (E) is measured in lux (lx). It is the ratio of luminous flux to the surface area in m^2. In rooms with lighting systems for general puposes it is measured horizontally at a height of 1 metre off the floor.

Luminance (L) is calculated in candela per m^2 (cd/m^2). This is the photometric dimension of a regarded object in relation to the impression of its luminous intensity. It is the ratio of luminous intensity to the surface area or of luminous flux to the dehedral angle.

2.5.3 Different Types of Light (Luminous) Source

The best known sources of light are thermal radiators (incandescent light sources).

They have a very low efficacy level and a large proportion of the available energy is emitted as heat. The light is produced by heating an incandescent filament. The colour of the light is determined by the temperature of the incandescent filament.

In the last few years luminescence and/or gas-discharge lights have found various new areas of use. Their light is produced through the electric discharge process in a gassy atmosphere. The efficacy of such a light is substantially superior to that of an electric light-bulb. The colour of the light produced is determined by the type of gas and the coating of the inner surface of the luminant. The use of semi-conductor light sources can be considered for special purposes. These are used almost exclusively for the illumination of scales and for warning lights.

2.5.4 Light Receptors in the Eye

There are about 6–7 million cones on the retina which convey impressions of colour and colour brightness to the brain. A luminance of 10 cd/m^2 is regarded as the outside limit for the efficacy of the cones. The maximum point of light sensitivity is reached at a wavelength of approximately 550 nm, i. e. in the yellow-green range, and decreases accordingly at shorter or longer wavelengths. Cones are to be found mainly on the central part of the retina. Towards the periphery their number decreases.

The approximately 100–125 million rods on the retina are needed for twilight vision (black/white vision). Pure rod vision begins at a luminance of 10^{-3} cd/m^2 or under. The rods and cones interact in a transition area found above this range, the rods gradually taking over vision when luminance decreases. The maximum wavelength at which the rods retain their sensitivity is to be found nearer the short wavelength range – at 507 nm.

The capacity to adjust to modifying luminance is called adaptation. The human eye can adapt to a change of intensity of the luminance level over a range of 10 decades.

The adaptation of the eye is brought about by alterations in the size of the pupil, by switching processes on the retina and by fluctuations in rod and cone sensitivity. The time needed for these processes depends upon the difference in luminance. The adaptation period is considerably longer in transition from light to dark than vice versa. A frequent need to re-adapt leads to signs of fatigue and impedes vision.

2.5.5 Special Points Regarding Illumination on Board Ship

Considerable problems arise in the fields of construction and evaluation of illumination in shipping. Cramped, narrow and windowless rooms are often to be found. The construction of lighting systems is made difficult because of the marked changes in luminance between the rooms themselves and between the rooms and the open deck. The danger of accidents is increased because of the limited visibility in the passageways due to construction requirements as well as the motion of the ship in rough seas. Areas of work which are interconnected or adjacent present problems because of the markedly different visual requirements involved.

It is usual practice that the type of illumination system to be found in inner, windowless rooms on a ship and its intensity are in accordance with the national standards in force. Examples of such rooms are: office rooms, control rooms, engine rooms, workshops, storerooms, provision stores and kitchens. The same applies to stairways and passageways.

Table 1 shows the approximate values of the luminous dose, illuminance and the required efficacy level and contains some general comments on the illumination of different areas and types of room on ships.

The illumination of the upper deck, cargo holds and engine rooms along with the

Table 1. Guideline values for illumination

Visual demands; examples of use	Illuminance (lx)	Incandescent lighting fixture W/m²	Fluorescent lighting fixture W/m²	Recommended light colour of fluorescent lgt. fixtures (L-Lp)[a]	General remarks	Points worthy of special attention
General orientation						
Adjoining rooms Upper deck Cargo holds	20–40 (exceptionally up to 60)	10	5	25	At low illuminances the source(s) of light must correspond to the type of visual demand, so enabling danger areas to be recognised, thus preventing accidents	Pay attention to anti-dazzling devices (nautical tasks) on the free deck. Greater illuminances on the upper deck, on fishery vessels, must be taken into consideration
Low visual demands						
Passageways Stairways Storerooms Magazines Cold Stores Toilets	50–75 (exceptionally up to 120)	20	10	25	The sources of light must be so arranged as to cast as few shadows as possible and produce no dazzling effects	The differences in brightness between inner and outer rooms must be considered when planning the lighting system
Medium demands						
Washrooms and bathrooms Sanitary accommodation Cabins (general)	100–150	30	15	25 or 32	In cabins and similar rooms where work-places are to be found, general illumination fixed at the work-places themselves should be used. Illumination at the work-places – at least 200 lux	With mirror illumination one should avoid dazzling caused by the light sources and the glaring reflection in the mirror itself
Medium demands: work illumination (permanent illumination)						
Operations, switch and pumprooms Air-conditioning centre	100–150 (exceptionally up to 250)	30	15	25	Principally general illumination is called for. Avoid reflection in the instruments	
Different demands (illumination in living-quarters)						
Messrooms Community rooms Music rooms	150–250	40	20	32	Mainly accentuated illumination is desirable	Lighting regulations must also be followed in regard to decorative lights

Table 1.

Visual demands; examples of use	Illuminance (lx)	Incandescent lighting fixture W/m²	Fluorescent lighting fixture W/m²	Recommended light colour of fluorescent lgt. fixtures (L-Lp)[a]	General remarks	Points worthy of special attention
Higher demands (permanent illumination)						
Operations rooms, e.g. engine and boiler rooms, control platforms and stations, technical and hobby rooms	150–250 (exceptionally up to 500)	40	20	25	If possible, general illumination. Illumination must be regular but not free of shadow. Exception: control platforms and stations. Unfavourable shadow effects, e.g. strongly cast shadows, to be avoided	Light sources must not dazzle. Use a screen/raster, lamina or optical medium
Illumination for special purposes						
Hospital area Examination rooms	200 and more (exceptionally up to 1000)	over 40	over 20	25 or 15 (19)	The standard of the general illumination must conform to the special illumination fixtures. (OP lights or other medical-technical apparatus)	Sick rooms, for example, must be designed in accordance with the experiences made with hospital illumination. When L-Lp is similar to daylight, at least 1000 lux is necessary
Illumination for special purposes (aggravating conditions)						
Bridges, chart rooms	100–150 (exceptionally up to 250)	30	15	25	General lighting is necessary for maintenance and care. In any other cases special illumination, e.g. the chart table (at least 500 lux adjustable to 0)	Variable workplace illumination, adjustable to the dark-adapted eye. Screening off of illuminated work-places (e.g. the chart table) with curtains

[a] (L-Lp): 25, universal white; 32, warm tone de-luxe; 15, daylight (6000 K); 19, daylight de-luxe (5000 K)

ancillary engine plants can present especially great difficulties. Substantially irregular illuminance levels sometimes appear here, forcing the eye to re-adapt itself continually. Adaptation from dark to light is accomplished relatively quickly, but for adaptation from light to dark a longer period is necessary which is not always allowed or foreseen. Therefore, with irregular lighting the danger of accidents is increased. For this reason regular lighting is desirable. Shadow-free illumination impedes orientation and should therefore not be used. Strong cast shadows should be avoided because adaptation problems arise within the area of the shadow. The problems of glare and dazzle should also be taken into account.

The transition areas between areas with artificial illumination and daylight (working passageways to the open deck) must be illuminated more brightly during the day and less brightly at night.

The transit area between the stairways and working passageways to the captain's bridge deserves particular attention. The bridge crew is adapted to the dark at night. Therefore when the entrance door is opened no light should fall from the working passageways onto the bridge. An adaptation zone must be created at the entrance to the bridge, necessarily adjusted to the room illumination level of the bridge.

General room illumination on the captain's bridge should contribute to keeping disturbances in the dark-adaptation of the crew to a minimum. The intensity of illumination must be variable, i.e. red light at a wavelength of 650–700 nm or filtered white light. By filtering the white light, the vital blue components are removed.

To this day illumination of the chart table has been accomplished with white light because the coloured signs and symbols would otherwise become totally illegible. The illumination of the chart table should be concentrated on the necessary chart section, the superfluous areas being covered by sector screens. The illuminated surface should therefore be kept as small as possible. The light must also be adjustable from 500 to 0 lx. The most favourable type of chart-table illumination device is the transillumination of the sea chart by means of a luminant table. This method of illumination has the advantage of less illuminance and fewer disturbances caused by surplus light. Instruments bearing signal lights or indicators must be illuminated with red light from 650 to 700 nm. The intensity must be infinitely variable. In order to confine the illuminated section to as small an area as possible, the scales, switches and other surfaces have to be darkly coloured. The pointers, figures, lines and lettering should be recognizable in white light during the day and at night be transilluminated in red.

In every observation room, such as the captain's bridge, the engine control room and the harbour operation centre, one should make sure that the lights for general illumination are placed so as to prevent reflections forming on instruments or shining surfaces, e.g. switches and windows at the customary place of operation.

Ruf [6] expounds on the basic principles of illumination on board ships. The author mentions the different sources of light, giving their application, the recommended efficacy and the type of light in table form. Special regulations are noted, whereby the requisites of waterproofing and precautionary measures against explosion are taken into account. Lastly the standard and quality of the lighting system in relation to the peculiarities of work on board are considered. The article defines the physiological and psychological demands on the artificial lighting on board. The illumination system should guarantee faultless orientation as well as optimal operational method. Attention should also be given to the maintenance of productivity levels and to the well-being of the crew members both in work and recuperation periods.

Adrian [1] describes the problem of illuminating the ship's bridge. In regard to the dark-adaptation capacity of the eye, a variety of unfavourably lit objects are to be found on board. Scales and low-voltage (weak) lamps etc. situated on the ship's bridge disturb considerably the dark adaptation of the personnel embarking on watch duty during the night or twilight periods because of their luminous intensity and colour composition. The author recommends red light for all indicators and lamps because the ability to adapt to darkness is then substantially increased.

Zorn [9] examines the ship's bridge from the viewpoint of ophthalmology and occupational medicine. He describes the working area on the bridge as an information centre and quotes the eye as being the most crucial receptor of the total information input. He goes on to describe short- and long-sightedness, colour differentiating ability, stereoscopic vision (tunnel vision), dazzlement and dark adaptation. Recommended or approved measurements often result in too high a luminance with unfavourable consequences for the dark adaption of the eye. It becomes clear from these data that the dark adaptation of seafarers is impaired because re-adaptation periods of 10–15 min. are necessary by currently prevailing luminances.

The article closes by making the following recommendations: painting of all components with a matt overcoat, avoidance of reflection through tilted windows, fitted doors to prevent infiltration of light, favourable positioning of light-source screening devices, avoidance of continuous indication when only intermittent supervision is called for, red light at a wave length of 660 nm and removal of the chart table from the general bridge area. The author suggests further experiments to determine more favourable illumination possibilities.

Schubert [7] deals with the problem of "red or white light on the ships' bridges". The author mentions previous claims in favour of red light for the ship's bridge but emphasises that this view is based only upon very theoretical principles. This aspect of dark adaptation was examined experimentally by Landolt-Rings. He describes experiments in which white light was used, the proportion (quantity) of blue components having been first filtered out. The brightness of the room illumination was 1–10 lx and the target contrast 113%.

The results show that the human operator is able to identify objects at practical night illumination levels within some seconds after having been exposed to brightness levels up to 3 lx. Red light has no advantage over filtered white light with regard to the identification time. The conclusions of these experiments are: it is not necessary to install red light with all its disadvantages in rooms like a ship's bridge. A "3-lx filtered white light" illumination will meet the requirements of shortest dark adaptation time for night vision. These experiments were conducted under marine conditions.

Lamoureux [5] says in the *Guide to Ship Sanitation* that illumination requirements are dependent on their purpose and the work being conducted and therefore they can vary greatly. Information on suitable illumination should be made available by the Health or Harbour Authorities – a requirement that is plagued with difficulties in practice.

In the technical regulations published by the government of the Federal Republic of Germany [8] with regard to the building and equipping of accommodation facilities on seagoing vessels, the illuminances for accommodation facilities on merchant ships are given in great detail.

An unpublished ergonomic checklist [2] drawn up by a committee on ergonomics of the Society of Naval Engineering gives various directives concerning the problem of lighting in habitability areas as well as a table (shown here as Table 1) with recommended illuminances for each area on a ship. DIN 5035 parts 1 and 2 (3, 4) contain valid guidelines for inner-room lighting with artificial light, including terms and general demands as well as critical values (approximate values) for work-places.

References

1. Adrian, W.: Die Beleuchtung auf Schiffsbrücken. Zbl. Arbeitsmed. *20,* 4, 101–110 (1970).
2. Ergonomische Checkliste. Ed.: Arbeitskreis Ergonomie der Schiffbautechnischen Gesellschaft. Hamburg 1974.
3. Innenraumbeleuchtung mit künstlichem Licht. Begriffe und allgemeine Anforderungen. DIN 5035. Part 1, Oct. 1979.
4. Innenraumbeleuchtung mit künstlichem Licht. Richtwerte für Arbeitsstätten. DIN 5035. Part 2, Oct. 1979.
5. Lamoureux, V. B.: Guide to ship sanitation. Geneva: WHO 1967.
6. Ruf, J.: Grundzüge der Beleuchtung an Bord von Schiffen. Schiff und Hafen *15,* 3, 260–268 (1963).
7. Schubert, E.: Red or white light on ship bridges? In: Proceedings of 5th Ship Control Systems Symposium, Annapolis, 1978. Ortung und Navigation 2, 301–317 (1978).
8. Technische Regeln für Bau und Ausrüstung von Unterkunftsräumen auf Seeschiffen. Bundesarbeitsbl. Fachbeilage Arbeitsschutz 1, 33–40 (1976).
9. Zorn, E.: Die Schiffsbrücke aus ergophthalmologischer Sicht. Schiff und Hafen *32,* 9, 327 (1980).

2.6 Noise and Vibration Aboard Ship

J. W. E. Pettersen

2.6.1 Shipboard Habitability

The quality of shipboard habitability is the integrated effect of all factors determining the behaviour, health and well-being of the seafarer under his specific conditions of service, comprising:

1. Physical environment: exposure to noise and vibration, climatic conditions, illumination, work and leisure considerations;
2. Working environment: man-machine interactions, ergonomic considerations;
3. Social environment: psychological interactions, sea service conditions.

Human factors in the design and operation of ships has been the subject of an international conference, the proceedings being edited by Anderson et al. [22].

Procedures for evaluating the integrated effect of simultaneous exposure to noise and vibration are not yet uniformly established, although Janssen [37] has put forward a proposal for a combined Annoyance Rating Scale for shipboard accommodation conditions. Present practice is, however, to evaluate separately the human reaction to noise and to vibration in guidelines applicable to shipboard conditions (national and/or international norms).

2.6.2 Appraisal of Effects of Exposure to Noise

2.6.2.1 Nomenclature

Some brief definitions should suffice:

- Sound pressure level, symbol L_p, unit dB $L_p = 20 \log p/p_o$ dB. reference pressure, $p_o = 20\,\mu Pa = 2 \cdot 10^{-5}\,N/m^2$
- Frequency (f), cycles per second in Hz
- A-weighted (frequency weighted) sound pressure level, symbol L_{pA}, unit dB
- A-weighted equivalent continuous sound pressure level, symbol L_{Aeq}, unit dB

These definitions follow recent ISO guidance on symbols, quantities and units of expression; see [26]. General practice has, however, been to quantify L_{pA} and L_{eq} in dB(A), which is the term used in present guidelines.

2.6.2.2 Risk of Damage to Hearing

Hearing. The sensitivity of the ear covers a wide range both in level and frequency, from the threshold curve of average minimum audible sound to a threshold of feeling at about 120 dB and a threshold of pain at about 140 dB. The middle frequency range (about 500–2000 Hz) is most significant for the understanding of everyday speech. ISO R266 [27] shows the equal loudness contours for pure tones, while ISO 1996 [28] contains an evaluation of noise rating (NR) curves for broad-band noise in octave bands. For typical shipboard noises the NR number is approximately 5 dB lower than the overall A-weighted sound pressure level, L_{pA}.

Steady-State Continuous Noise. Continuous exposure to excessive noise over a long period may cause irreversible hair cell damage and a permanent threshold shift, more commonly described as noise-induced hearing loss. Ear protectors should be worn during continuous exposure to noise from the ship's main propulsion machinery and auxiliaries where noise levels in the range of 90–110 dB(A) may be expected.

Impulse Sound. The ear is more vulnerable to damage from unheralded or unexpected impulse sounds, the extent depending on sound peak level and pulse rise time and duration. The sudden release of safety valves or the taking of indicator readings on diesel engines may expose engine crew to such impulse sounds.

Noise-Induced Hearing Impairment

The general effects of noise on hearing are discussed in Henderson et al. [10]. The reader should refer to ISO 1999 [29] with regard to risk of suffering a noise-induced threshold shift sufficient to impair the understanding of everyday speech.

Noise climates in ship engine rooms have been reviewed by Bailey [4] and Acton et al. [2], and the effect of noise on hearing among engine room personnel has been reported on by Quist-Hanssen [60], Harris [20], Nowak and Dahl [56], Kanda [42], Grewe and Rodegra [18] and Szczepanski et al. [67]. A comprehensive survey of the noise conditions in sea-going and inland waterway ships, focussing on the exposure of ship personnel to noise, is found in Goethe et al. [14].

The result of audiometric examinations is reported by Herrmann et al. [21]; they show that of engine room personnel, 21% suffered from significant threshold impairment. In addition, 12% of deck crew members showed hearing impairments (cause unknown), and threshold impairments were diagnosed in 40% of radio officers.

It may be noted that older ship personnel affected by presbycousis and possibly some noise-induced hearing loss in the upper frequency range may be handicapped in following the conversation in the dayrooms [about 65 dB(A) medium frequency dominated noise] compared with their younger colleagues, and are thus liable to loneliness, withdrawal and non-participation in leisure activities.

As a ship's engine room personnel may already have suffered some degree of permanent threshold shift during their training period in shore-based industries or during leisure activities, audiometric testing should be performed prior to entry into sea service. Regular audiometric screening tests during service would be useful in detecting personnel susceptible to noise-induced hearing loss. Screening tests should also cover higher frequencies (e.g. 4000, 6000, 8000 Hz).

2.6.2.3 Other Effects

A general survey on the behavioural and physiological effects of noise has been carried out by Lambert and Hafner [48] as background material for consideration of shipboard noise evaluation procedures.

The psycho-physical load on ship personnel under various environmental loads (incl. noise and vibration) is discussed by Goethe et al. [16].

Requirements for sleep, solving problems and speech communication in shipboard compartments are discussed by Lambert [47].

Interference with Speech and Aural Communication Signals

The speech interference level (SIL) is generally taken as the mean of levels of noise in the octave bands with centre frequencies of 500, 1000 and 2000 Hz (or the A-weighted ambient sound level). In some working situations the signals are limited to some well-established commands often accompanied by specific hand signals. Klumpp and Webster [45] showed that for shipboard noises (naval personnel) satisfactory signal comprehension occurred at a higher ambient A-weighted noise level than that corresponding to the general SIL level.

Discomfort and Annoyance

Noise is usually described as unwanted sound, and it is often taken that the louder the noise, the more likely it is to create annoyance. The noise composition is often, however, more important (irregular level/duration, high pitch, pure tones, impulse sounds).

Shipboard noise levels are reported by Conn [9], Godin [13], Lambert [46], Schmidt [62] and Goethe et al. [14]. In general the noise in the ship's accommodation spaces may be described as steady-state monotonous in character. Although the noise level [some 60–65 dB(A)] inherently is higher than in land-based dwellings, some noise may be beneficial to the ship's crew on open sea duty in relieving the feeling of voidness or in masking extraneous noise from adjacent cabins etc. Apart from complaints in cases of excessive noise levels, much of the nuisance experienced in ship accommodation spaces is due to rattling of components, doors, cupboard doors, mirrors etc.

The occurrence of sudden, loud and unfamiliar noise produces reactions following the natural instinct of self-preservation/emergency activation. The effects are transient and die away rapidly as the noise loses its "startling" character.

In some instances when a seafarer is situated in a precarious position or is handling delicate or dangerous objects, the involuntary muscle reaction to the startling noise can be hazardous.

Effect on Work Proficiency

Broadly it appears that:

1. Broadband steady noise rarely has any effect on proficiency when A-weighted noise levels are less than 90 dB.
2. Adverse effects are normally associated with complex, multi-component tasks, cognitive tasks and tasks with high information loads. Sound may improve the performance of simple, routine tasks by relieving boredom. Distracting noise components are likely to impair accuracy and efficiency of performance, and may adversely affect the quality of decision making.

It is to be emphasized that ship personnel, and especially the engine room crew, are subjected to additional environmental loads, such as the motion of the ship, vibration and climatic factors. The deck officers are exposed to considerable stress when manoeuvring in congested harbours and narrow restricted waters. The overall stress and fatigue loading is greater than that caused by exposure to noise alone.

Effect on Sleep

The awakening potential of noise is a function of the change in the level of noise components and of the prevailing steady-state ambient noise in relation to the stages of sleep (1–4 and REM). Motivation and habituation may be significant in the awakening process.

Loud and strange noises produce the more marked awakening response, while stimulation in response to familiar noise is to some extent filtered, awakening depending on the degree of 'harmful' meaning attached to the change in noise. Engine room personnel would wake on the sudden disappearance of noise, associated with the possible faulty operation of machinery.

Attention should particularly be paid to preventing combinations of noise with other (psychological) stress agents which might lead to prolonged deficiency of sleep, affecting general well-being and proficiency.

Infrasound Effects

Infrasound (e.g. pressure pulsation at frequencies below the audible range) has been considered in relation to possible risk of hearing loss, mechanical effects (middle ear), speech reception, work proficiency and discomfort (annoyance) [25].

Two samples from shipboard conditions:

1. Complaints of annoyance from infrasound at wheelhouse; infrasound excited by diesel engine exhaust pulsations and amplified by resonance effects in the light long-spanned ceiling;
2. Complaints of annoyance from infrasound at outboard positions in the aft passenger saloon in a passenger ferry; infrasound propeller excited and amplified by standing waves due to coincidence between excitation frequency half wavelength and distance between bulkheads.

2.6.3 Codes on Noise Levels in Ships

2.6.3.1 National Norms

Several countries have issued proposals for codes of practice involving recommendations for permissible noise levels in ships. Tables 1 and 2 give surveys of such guidelines. The data shown are mainly drawn from IMCO-DEXIX/WP7 [24]. In addition, Australia has also issued a code for ship noise.

For manned ship engine rooms the recommended limit is usually 90 dB(A), with the proviso of octave band levels not exceeding NR 85, and with a correction factor of 5 dB (stricter) for pronounced pure tone content. The noise level for present-day machinery exceeds this, thus entailing the installation of a separate control room, for which the recommended noise level limit is 75 dB(A). In some countries a limiting level of 85 dB(A) is set for the engine room workshops.

Noise levels for cabins and mess and dayrooms are generally set at 60 dB(A) and 65 dB(A) respectively.

Work has been in progress in several countries in updating ship noise level codes, and it should be ensured that the latest relevant edition is consulted for evaluation purposes.

2.6.3.2 International Code (IMCO)

Based on the national norms of the member countries, the Intergovernmental Mari-

Table 1. Noise requirements/recommendations in dB(A) from various countries (based on IMCO-DEXIX/WP7 [24]).

	USA	UK	WGerm.	Sweden	Norw.	Poland	Denm.	Finl.	Nethr.	Israel	Canada	Italy	France	USSR	DDR	Japan	IMCO
Engine room	110	110	110	105	110	–	110	–	110	90	–[e]	110	105[f]	95	–	–	110
Control room	75	75	75 + k[a]	70	75	75	75	–	80	75	–	75	70/75	70	80	75	75
Workshop	–	90	85	75	85	–	85	–	90	80	–	90	85	85	90	85	85
Wheel house	65	65	65	65	65	65	65	–	65	65	–	–	65	45	60	–	65
Radio room	65	60	60	55	65	60	65	–	65	65	–	65	60	45	60	–	60
Cabins	60	60	60	55	60 + k[c]	60	60	60 + k[c]	60	60	70	55	55/60	45	60	60 + k[g]	60
Hospital	60	60	60	55	55	55	–	–	60	–	–	60	–	45	55	–	60
Mess/recr. rm	65	65	65 + k[b]	65	65	65	65/70	60 + k[d]	65	70	74	65	65/70	45	60	60 + k[g]	65

[a] k = 0: BRT > 4000, k = 10: BRT < 4000
[b] k = 0: BRT > 8000, k = 5: BRT < 8000
[c] k = 0: BRT > 2000, k = 5: BRT < 2000
[d] k = 0: BRT > 10000, k = 5: BRT < 10000
[e] Can. tow-boat operators
[f] Turbine prop./eng. prop.
[g] k = 0: BRT > 65000, k = 0: BRT < 65000

Table 2. Sound insulation values (based on IMCO-DEXIX/WP7 [24]).

	IMCO[a]	Sweden[b]	Finland	Norway[a]	Denmark[a]
Cabin to cabin	30	35	30	30	30
Mess. recr. room to cabins	45	50	–	45	45
Cabin to corridor		30	30	30	30
Cabin to galley				45	
Accom. spaces to open deck					40

[a] Laboratory measured sound insulation index I_A
[b] Field measured sound insulation index I_A
(I_A – ISO R717. Rating of sound insulation of dwellings)

time Consultative Organization (IMCO) has more recently prepared a draft proposal for a code on noise levels in ships [IMCO-DEXXIII [23]]. The draft proposal deals with: general scope and purpose, measuring equipment, measurement conditions and procedures, noise exposure limits, noise exposure protection, acoustic insulation between accommodation spaces, ear protection and safeguards, instructions to crew and responsibilities, and format of noise survey reports; it also gives suggestions for methods of controlling noise exposure. Table 3 is reproduced from this code. This code should be consulted when finalized and ratified copies become available.

In addition IMO has issued *Recommendations on Methods of Measuring Noise Levels at Listening Posts* (IMCO Resolution A.343,IX), which recommends permissible noise levels at listening posts/bridge wing:
Maximum sound pressure levels in dB in octave bands at centre frequencies of

250 Hz – 68 dB
500 Hz – 63 dB

as measured at three-quarters of normal ship speed.

Noise levels relating to various types of ships are listed in Table 4, while Fig. 1 illustrates the ship types, and Table 5 outlines suggestions for noise control measures to meet IMO guidelines, taken from Brubakk [6].

Table 3. Limits for noise levels as specified in IMCO-DEXXIII [23, p. 20].

Work spaces	*dB(A)*
Machinery spaces (continuously manned)	90
Machinery spaces (not continuously manned)	110
Machinery control rooms	75
Workshops	85
Non-specified work spaces	90
Navigation spaces	*dB(A)*
Navigating bridge and chartrooms	65
Listening post, including navigating bridge[a], wings and windows	70
Radio rooms (with radio equipment operating but not producing audio signals)	60
Radar rooms	65
Accommodation and recreation spaces	*dB(A)*
Cabins and hospitals	60
Mess rooms	65
Recreation rooms	65
Open recreation areas	75
Service and office spaces	*dB(A)*
Galleys, without food processing equipment operating	75
Serveries and pantries	75
Offices	65
Normally unoccupied spaces	*dB(A)*
Spaces not specified	90

[a] Reference is made to resolution A.343(IX), which also applies

Table 4. Distribution of noise levels for various types of ship (Brubakk [6])

Ship groups		Positions: Engine room	Control room	A-(main-deck)	B-deck	C-deck	D-deck	E-deck	Wheel house	Radio room	Bridge wings	Open recr. area
Tank/OBO	A1 (turb.) L > 200 m	95–100	65–75	65	57	53	50	47	55	50	65	70
	A2 (diesel)	100–105	65–75	65	60	56	53	50	55	55	70	70
Tank	B1 (10–50000 tdw)	100–110	70–75	65	58	55	52	50	60	60	75	75
Bulk	B2 (5–10000 tdw)	105–110	75	70	62	58	56	54	65	65	75	75
LPG	B3 (1– 5000 tdw)	105–110	75–80	73	65	62	60	60	68	68	80	80
Cargo	B4 (< 1000 tdw)	105–110	80	75	68	65	63	63	70	70	85	80
Ro/Ro	C1 (aft/amid/fore)	100–110	70–80	75/55	65–45		60–43		55	50	60	75
Pass.	C2 (amid/fore)	100–110	70–80	60/45	55–43		50–43		55	50	60/70	70
Refrig. Cont.	D (L > 100 m)	100–110	70–75	65/70	60	57	55	53	60	55	70	75
Small Ro/Ro	E (L < 100 m)	105–110	75–80	60	55	50	–	–	55	55	65	70
Tug Supply	F (L < 100 m)	105–110	75–85	60	57	54	–	–	65/70	65	80	–

Table 5. Proposed measures to enable the various ship groups to meet the IMO code regarding noise (Brubakk [6])

	Ship groups / Noise reducing measures	Arrangement: Separate casing/accommodation	Arrangement: "Bufferzones"	Arrangement: Resiliently mounted deckhouse	Engine room: Elast. aux. eng.	Engine room: Noise red. contr. rm	Engine room: Elast. exh. syst.	Engine room: Exh. silencer	Prop.: Aft ship form	Prop.: Noise "weak" prop.	Accommodation: Floating accom. system	Accommodation: Damping layer	Accommodation: Absorb. ceiling	Accommodation: Elast. bow thrust
Tank/OBO	A1 (turbin) A2 (diesel) L > 200 m							×					×	
Tank/LPG/LNG/Bulk Cargo etc.	B1 (10–50000 tdw)		×		×		×	×	×			×	×	
	B2 (5–10000 tdw)	×	×		×	×	×	×	×	×	×		×	
	B3 (1– 5000 tdw)	×		×	×	×	×	×	×	×	×	×	×	
	B4 (< 1000 tdw)	×		×	×	×	×	×	×	×	×	×	×	
Ro-Ro/Ferries/Passeng.	C1 (aft/amid/fore)				×	×	×		×	×	×	×	×	×
	C2 (amid/fore)					×								×
Refrig./Cont.	D (L > 100 m)		×		×		×	×	×	×	×			
Small Ro-Ro	E (L < 100 m)					×							×	×
Tug/Supply	F (L < 100 m)		×			×	×	×			×	×		×

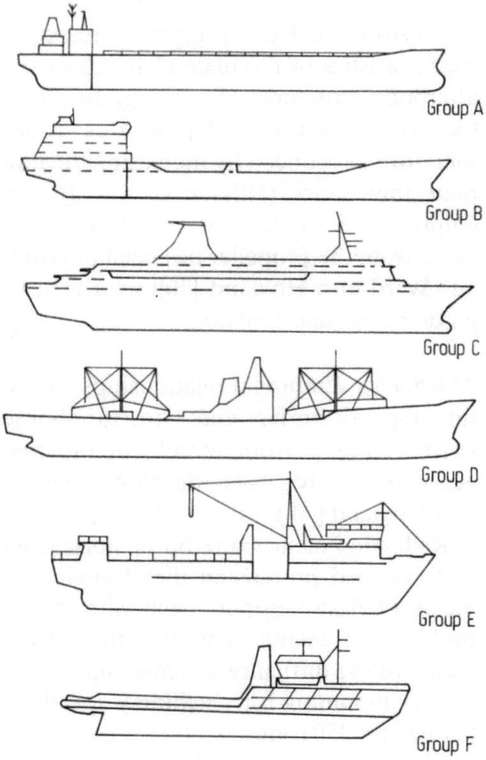

Fig. 1. Ship groups (Brubakk [6])

2.6.4 Noise Control in Ships

2.6.4.1 Acoustic Planning

The overall objective of the acoustic planning in ships should be to meet the specified noise level requirements by means of balanced, cost-effective design, due consideration being given to such factors as safety, habitability and comfort.

Preliminary and contract level consideration on noise control in ship design has been outlined by Maniar and Daidola [51], while the present state-of-the-art in ship noise control is surveyed by Noonan and Feldman [55] and ship trial noise measurements and evaluation are discussed by Pettersen [58]. Experiences with ship noise control are reported by Wragge [73].

The procedure for a systematic analysis of relevant factors involved in deriving a given noise climate is briefly outlined below:

1. Design objectives: Definition/specification of relevant noise requirements as given in national norms, international guidelines relating to work areas, accommodation spaces, navigating bridge etc.
2. Noise sources: Evaluation of the strength of the ship's main noise sources (air-borne and structure-borne sound) and of additional noise sources near occupied areas.
3. Arrangement plan: Where possible, accommodation spaces should be located remotely from main sound sources.
4. Noise prediction: Estimation of the expected noise level in relevant localities based on noise sources and arrangement plan (path of noise propagation). Comparison of results with design objectives.
5. Noise control measures: Evaluation of additional noise control measures necessary to reach the specified requirements in relation to noise reduction at the source, in the transmission path and at the occupied spaces. Consideration must be given to the weight, size and cost and ease of maintenance of acoustic devices applied to shipboard conditions.
6. Safety and reliability: Noise-reducing devices must comply with general requirements regarding fire resistance, strength/fatigue, moisture etc. as prescribed by national/international maritime authorities and classification societies.

2.6.4.2 Ship Noise Sources and Transmission Path

A brief outline is given below of important shipboard noise sources and major paths of propagation; noise control measures are covered in the following section.

Sources. The major noise sources on a ship are the propeller, the main propulsion diesel engine and auxiliary generating sets. Hydraulic systems often need particular attention to noise reduction measures. Contributory sources at the navigating bridge and wheelhouse are diesel exhaust noise and navigating equipment noise, while in deck recreation areas engine and cargo room air intake and outlet openings are probable offenders.

Transmission. The main path of transmission to the accommodation quarters, offices and living spaces is in the form of structural sonic vibration – structure-borne noise. The casing can be a source of radiation of air-borne noise into nearby cabins. Hydraulic noise may be transmitted through ducting system and supports, being radiated by supporting bulkheads. Noise from air conditioning in the accommodation quarters is primarily conducted through the ventilation piping, while excessive flow-induced noise may be generated and radiated at the ventilation outlet grille.

2.6.4.3 Elements of Noise Control in Ships

General principles of noise reduction are described in standard reference books. Noise control measures to be adopted aboard ship must, however, be evaluated in terms of the specific conditions applying to ship service environment.

Handbooks dealing directly with noise control in ships are available, e.g. [1]; [5]; [19]; Kluikin [44], Pettersen and Storm (Eds.) [59];

Reduction of Sound Sources

Propeller. Propeller cavitation leads to generation of high noise levels into the ship. Cavitation is caused by uneven wake distribution over the propeller plane, particularly the high wake peak behind the stern post. The most important noise reducing measures would be (a) designing the afterbody for minimal wake variations at the propeller plane and (b) optimal design of the propeller geometry for the given wake field, by appropriate choice of main parameters (rpm, diameter) to reduce propeller tip speed.

The transfer of acoustic energy into the ship's structure depends upon the response characteristics of the plate elements of the afterbody structure. The energy transmitted to the accommodation area could therefore be reduced by increasing the hull plate impedance (Nilsson et al. [54]). An empirical formula for structure-borne noise from the propeller has been developed (Ward and Hoyland [70]) as a general guide for noise estimation.

Machinery. Empirical relationships for estimating air-borne and structure-borne noise resulting from diesel engines and gear boxes have been developed (Ward and Hoyland [70]).

Reduction of structure-borne noise from a slow-speed propulsion diesel engine by means of elastic support meets with special problems of engine stability in the seaway owing to the difficulty in achieving a satisfactory mounting for machinery speeds of below, say, 350 rpm.

Structure-borne noise from auxiliary engines/generating sets may be of significant importance for the noise levels aboard ship. At the general rotational speed of generator sets, elastic mounting is quite feasible, although special precautions should be taken to ensure satisfactory operations under seaway conditions (Pettersen and Storm (Eds.) [59]).

Elastic mounting has today become a routine measure. The noise-reducing efficiency also depends upon the mass/stiffness distribution of the seating/foundation. Resiliently mounted engines on platforms tend to transmit higher structure-borne noise levels than those placed on ship's double bottoms.

Exhaust Systems. Exhaust systems should be fitted with suitable silencers. Reduction of structure-borne noise transmitted from exhaust piping is achieved by flexible mounting supported by adequately stiffened brackets.

Engine Room Acoustic Measures

The main requirement for noise control in the engine room space is a separately sound-insulated control room. To attain adequate noise reduction requires special high transmission loss bulkhead constructions, double leaf elastically fitted observation windows, preferably a double door arrangement and a floating floor to reduce structure-borne noise. Attention should be paid to reduction of noise in the control room air-conditioning system.

Engine room workshops are often separated from the engine room proper only by half-wall partition. Full partition would be beneficial to the personnel.

Noisy machinery components may be insulated by acoustic hoods, isolated from the foundation to avoid structure-borne emission. Adequate component ventilation, means of visual inspection and maintenance facilities should be incorporated in the design.

Design of the Ship's Superstructure

The global layout of deckhouses containing accommodation areas should be such as to facilitate the inclusion of suitable noise control measures.

Conventional Superstructure. The accommodation spaces are placed around the engine casing. The noise radiating from the casing may be reduced by placing stores, washrooms etc. close to the casing, thereby shielding cabins and mess rooms.

Separate Deckhouse and Casing/Funnel. In this construction cabins and mess rooms are placed in a superstructure freed from direct contact with the casing, thereby reducing the noise radiated by the casing into the accommodation areas.

These separate deckhouse arrangements may be prone to propeller-induced vibratory effects. Design calculations should be made to ensure avoidance of propeller-excited superstructure resonance at ship service speed, or adjudged from experience with similar ship structures.

Resiliently Supported Deckhouse. As the dominating noise in the accommodation area is structure-borne noise radiated from bulkheads, ceiling and deck (floor), noise attenuation in the transmission path may be introduced by mounting the complete superstructure on flexible mounts, whereby considerable noise reduction may be achieved (Falensky, [11]). Such a construction requires that great care be taken to ensure required structural strength and adequate dynamic behaviour under the load exposure from seaway forces.

Accommodation Areas. If the estimated noise level in cabins and mess rooms exceeds the design objectives after precautionary noise-reducing measures have been considered for the sources and for the general accommodation arrangement, then it becomes essential to incorporate noise control to protect the receiving areas from excessive noise. It would also be beneficial to prevent noise from propagating from one locality to another within the area and to keep the sound level generated inside any locality as low as possible (desired reverberation time).

Designing for low-noise ships is discussed by Ward and Hoyland [70], Kihlman and Plunt [43] and Nilsson [53] in the form of predicting noise levels at the ship design stage.

Floating accommodation systems provide the most effective way of reducing airborne and, particularly, structure-borne noise in accommodation quarters (Janssen and Buiten [38]; George [12]). In principle the system consists of a floating floor, inner partition walls and a suspended ceiling isolating the cabin from the steel structure of the ship. The efficiency of the floating floor depends upon the characteristics of the resilient interposed material and the radiation factor of the upper floor. The inner wall partition is resting on the floating floor and elastically supported at the steel bulkhead to prevent structure-borne noise transmission. Acoustic absorption material is fitted in the empty space to dampen acoustic standing waves. The suspended ceiling is mounted in a similar manner.

The facing of ceiling and walls may be fitted with acoustic absorption material to absorb noise generated in the room and to improve aural communication (adjusted reverberation time).

Instead of a floating accommodation system, visco-elastic damping layers (Asztely [3]; Burroughs et al. [7]) may be used to reduce the transmission of structure-borne sound in the steel structure.

The ventilation noise produced by the *air-conditioning system* often makes a noticeable contribution to the noise in cabins. The system should be fitted with silencers and absorption lining in the ducting. The air velocity at the outlets into the cabins should be kept low, and the outlet grilles should be designed for low noise generation.

The fan room containing the air-conditioning plant should be acoustically treated, and the plant itself and the air-flow ducting should be elastically supported.

Bridge/Deck Areas. A major component of noise from diesel propulsion at the bridge may be the exhaust noise. To maintain ease of listening, efficient silencers should be installed. Low frequency range attenuation is also desirable. Other sources of noise are air intakes and outlets from engine rooms fans and cargo room fans. The ducting should be fitted with acoustic absorption lining and special louvres at the air inlets and outlets. The air velocity should be kept as low as possible.

2.6.5 Appraisal of Effects of Exposure to Vibration

A comprehensive study of the load imposed on the ship's personnel by exposure to vibration aboard ship has been prepared by Goethe et al. [15], dealing with vibration measurements related to ISO 2631 [31]. Exposure of crew to disturbing vibration in work environment, leisure activities and periods of relaxation (sleep) is discussed.

2.6.5.1 Nomenclature

For sinusoidal vibration the following quantities apply:

- Vibration displacement, $x = A\sin\omega t$, numerical amplitude $= A$
- Vibration velocity, $dx/dt = \omega A\cos\omega t$, numerical amplitude $= \omega A$
- Vibration acceleration, $d^2x/dt^2 = -\omega^2 A\sin\omega t$, numerical amplitude $= \omega^2 A$
- Angular frequency, $\omega = 2\pi f$ in rad/s
- rms magnitude $= \left[\frac{1}{2\pi}\int_0^{2\pi} x^2\,dt\right]^{1/2}$
- Crest factor = ratio peak amplitude to rms value
- Mode of vibration: characteristic vibratory pattern related to number of nodes
- Node: positions of vibratory rest
- Natural frequency: a frequency of *free* vibration
- Resonance: state of coincidence between periodicity of excitation force and system natural frequency
- Critical speed: a speed (of machine, shafting etc.) at which resonance occurs

For further terminology see ISO 2041 [30].

2.6.5.2 Whole-Body Vibration Effects

Exposure of the human body to mechanical vibration results in relative displacement of adjacent tissue in various parts of the body. For small amplitudes these relative displacements may not be noticeable, but at higher amplitudes they can stimulate a variety of receptor organs, interfere with human perceptual and motor performance and cause discomfort, pain or, in extreme cases, injury.

Parameters affecting the evaluation of human response to vibration are:

1. Direction of applied vibratory motion with respect to the coordination of the human body;

2. Waveform of the vibratory input to the body;
3. Application of simultaneous multidirectional vibration;
4. Biodynamic response characteristics of the body;
5. Condition of the subject (physiological);
6. Psychological effects (motivation, habituation);
7. The activity of the individual;
8. Presence of additional environmental factors.

In dealing with shipboard vibration we are primarily concerned with two types of exposure to vibration:

1. Global vibration transmitted to the body through the feet of a standing person, through the buttocks of a sitting person, or through the supporting area of a reclining person. This type of exposure is termed *"whole-body vibration"*. It covers the frequency range of 1–80 Hz.

A proposal for evaluation of shipboard vibration has been put forward by Kanazawa [41]. A collection of Japanese shipboard vibration data evaluated from the point of view of habitability has been submitted to ISO/SC4 by the Japanese delegate [8]. Vibration load on ship personnel is discussed by Zaborski and Szczepanski [74] and Switaiski [66], while selection of measuring positions for vibration in occupied spaces is suggested by Wieg [72].

2. High displacement–low frequency vibration applied as wholebody vibration and related to motion sickness (kinetosis) and work proficiency effects. It covers the frequency range 0.1–1 Hz.

Measurements of ship motion effects have been carried out by Goto [17] on five training voyages for apprentices, using a motion sickness index (MSI):

Grade I Slightly uncomfortable.
Grade II Rather uncomfortable, feeling of nausea, difficulty in continuing ordinary tasks.
Grade III Very uncomfortable, vomiting, completely spiritless.

The measurements are related in frequency response to ISO 2631, addendum DAD/2 [32].

2.6.5.3 Evaluation of Human Whole-Body Vibration

For general-purpose evaluation, reference is made to ISO 2631 [31], which should be consulted for further study with respect to scope, field of application, method of measurement and evaluation procedures. Rectilinear vibration transmitted to man should be measured in the appropriate axis at the point of application to the human body. The frequency range covers 1–80 Hz.

The standard (i.e. ISO 2631) gives guidance as to the evaluation of exposure to various levels and durations of vibration. The evaluation concepts are:

1. Objective physical/physiological response (hazard) term: *"tolerance limit"*.
2. Efficiency of performing work (interference) term: *"decreased proficiency boundary"*.
3. Subjective (psycho-physiological) response (annoyance) term: *"reduced comfort boundary"*.

The standard is of a general nature, specific situations being covered by addenda.

One such addendum to ISO 2631 is in preparation as a draft proposal, ISO/TC108/SC4-N116 [33], concerned with evaluating exposure of crew to vibration. This addendum deals specifically with the vibratory input to the human body, so that information can be gathered for direct comparison purposes using the methods outlined in the parent document, ISO 2631 [31].

The rating curve for vibration in occupied spaces in this draft proposal is derived from the lower envolute of combining the requisite curves for vertical and horizontal vibration exposure from the parent document ISO 2631. This addendum [33] is presently under revision, and it may be altered so that the rating procedure follows the scale for evaluation of whole-body vibration described in ISO 2631.

Guidelines for evaluation of low frequency motion (0.1–1.0 Hz) are proposed by ISO draft addendum ISO 2631/DAD2 [32], which deals primarily with occasional travellers. Boundaries for risk of motion sickness (kinetosis) are given in relation to duration of exposure. Experienced seafarers, adapted to life at sea, may require a period of acclimatisation upon returning to ship after a prolonged stay onshore.

Further, an rms value of 1.75 m/s^2 (peak value of 0.25 g) has been suggested as the approximate disturbance level for writing and fine manual control (decreased proficiency).

2.6.6 Codes for Evaluating Shipboard Vibration

There are draft international codes for measurement and reporting of hull girder vibration (ISO DP4867 [34] and local vibration (ISO DP 4868 [35]). These codes apply to general vibration surveys, the main object being to verify the overall vibration response of the hull girder, superstructure and local spaces as well as selected positions for indication of vibratory force transmission. The test and ship operational conditions are outlined, and a format of reporting is given.

Special measurements, such as detailing exposure of personnel to whole-body vibration at all occupied areas, would require a comprehensive survey.

The codes do not deal with "troubleshooting" aimed at detecting causes and providing a basis for particular corrective measures – this would require more extensive investigations. Solumsmoen [64] and Ojak [57] describe service shipboard vibration problems.

ISO/TC108/SC2 has prepared a draft proposal: ISO DP6954 – *Overall Evaluation of Shipboard Vibration in Merchant Ships* [36]. This code is based on internationally collected data from shipboard conditions, the measurements being taken at relevant positions in the ship structure and

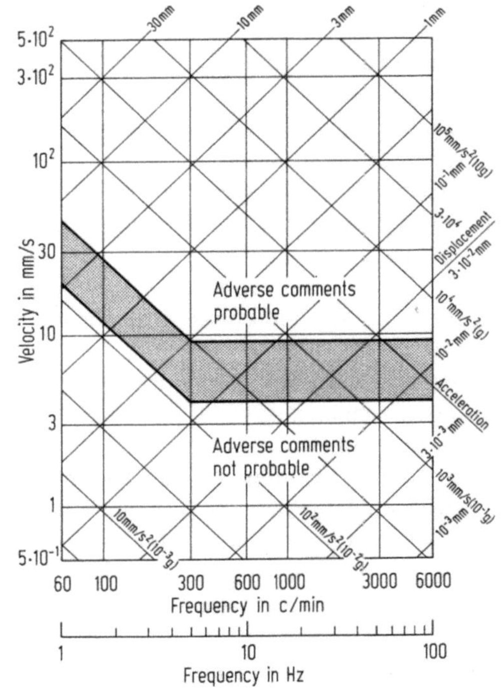

Fig. 2. Guidance for the overall evaluation of vertical and horizontal vibration in merchant ships (simplified). Quantities expressed in maximum repetitive magnitude (peak value) (ISO DP6954 [36])

primarily expressed in maximum repetitive magnitude (peak value). Through accumulated (semantic) data, cognizance of the human reaction to shipboard vibration is incorporated into ISO DP6954, the evaluation curves from which are reproduced in Fig. 2, the measurements being taken at deck structure. If a direct measurement of *whole-body vibration* is desired, this would, for a sitting person for instance, entail interposing a suitable measuring device between the buttocks and the seat cushion as outlined in ISO 2631 [31], and the addendum to it [33], which is currently being revised.

The rating curves in ISO DP6954 are based on information submitted to ISO/TC108/SC4-N116 [33] for sinusoidal vibration exposure, together with data submitted from other participant countries.

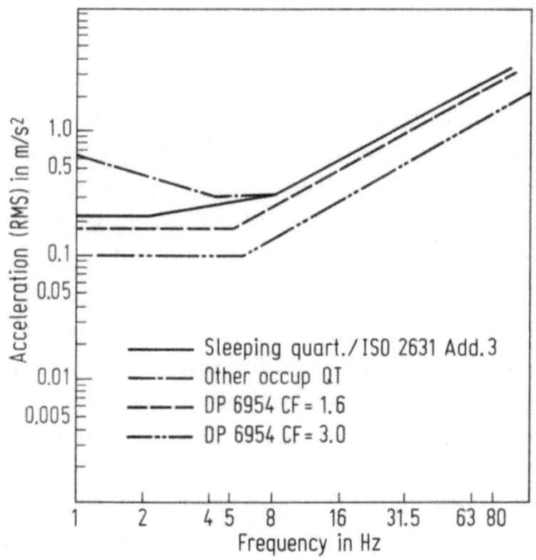

Fig. 3. Comparison between maximum repetitive values, including effect of crest factor (ISO DP6954 [36]) and rms value (ISO 2631 draft proposal addendum 3; working paper ISO/TC108/SC4-N116 [33]) From ISO DP6954 [36].

ISO DP6954 describes three categories, viz. a lower zone where adverse comments are not probable, a transition zone at which unfounded complaints may arise and an upper zone at which adverse comments are probable. Vibration levels exceeding the upper curve are to some extent met with in ship accommodation areas.

The rating curves of ISO DP6954 may be applied to shipboard vibration in both vertical and horizontal directions. This differs from the separate evaluation of vertical and horizontal whole-body vibration as outlined in ISO 2631. This difference in evaluation may be due to some additional effects in the complaints regarding exposure to horizontal vibration, e.g.:

1. Muscle tension due to relative motion of work surfaces rather than whole-body vibration
2. Discomfort induced by additional rotary motion
3. Nuisance increased by vibration 'beating' effects
4. Psychological effects (disturbance of leisure activities)

Note that ISO 2631 uses the rms value of acceleration as the descriptive quantity. For a comparison between ISO/TC108/SC4-N116 and ISO DP6954, Fig. 3 from the latter is included. For shipboard vibration, which may be characterized as narrow-band random in nature, crest factors (CF) of 1.6–3 are shown. Typical crest factors may be in the order of 2.0–2.5. From this diagram it follows that evaluation using DP6954 tends to be on the conservative side. With the present state-of-the-art in shipbuilding, good practice would be to aim in the design for the lower curve while applying corrective measures if vibration is found to exceed significantly the upper curve during trial trips.

2.6.7 Vibration Control in Ships

2.6.7.1 Design Planning

The overall objectives of vibration control in ships are to meet the requirements regarding structural strength and safety and to ensure a satisfactory level of exposure of the ship's personnel to vibration.

Preliminary contract considerations in ship design with regard to vibration are discussed by Maniar and Daidola [51], while the present state-of-the-art in ship vibration control is outlined by Noonan and Feldman [55]. Design stage measures to prevent harmful vibration are outlined by Leenaars and Forbes [49] and Johannessen and Skaar [39], while vibration measurement during a trial trip is discussed by Pettersen [58] and vibration problems are reported upon by Ojak [57].

Vibration in ships is conveniently categorized as (Noonan and Feldman, [55]):

1. Hull girder vibration
2. Vibration in major substructures
3. Local vibration (deck areas, bulkheads, accommodation areas)
4. Propeller, machinery and shafting vibration
5. Vibration in components, control panels and instrument on their supports

These items are all related to the dynamic structural behaviour and safety of the ship and to the safety and operational performance of machinery and equipment. The first three items are of particular concern with regard to the exposure of personnel to vibration.

The procedure for analysis of ship dynamic response follows the evaluation of:

1. *Design objective:* Clarify the requirements regarding ship and machinery performance and special requirements regarding levels of vibration exposure in relevant areas of occupation.
2. *Vibration sources:* Evaluate strength of ship's major vibration sources, propeller and machinery.
3. *Transmission:* Identify major paths of transmission to relevant structural configurations.
4. *Vibration prediction:* Estimate the dynamic response of major structural elements.
5. *Vibration evaluation:* Review expected levels of vibration to evaluate possible correction to attain a level of vibration satisfactory from the point of view of (a) the ship's safety and operational requirements and (b) exposure of personnel to vibration.

2.6.7.2 Sources of Vibration and Transmission Path

Sources. The propeller is the major source of vibration in ships. Some 90% of complaints about vibration in the accommodation spaces arise from propeller-induced local vibration (Solumsmoen, [64]). Secondary vibration effects, such as "rattling" and random movements of supported items, are frequent sources of annoyance to the crew. Free, unbalanced forces and moments in main propulsion diesel engines and in auxiliaries are potential sources of excitation of low-noded hull girder resonant vibration and/or vibration in platforms and other local structures.

Transmission Path. The excitation forces are transmitted from the major sources into the structure, setting the hull girder and major substructures (such as the deckhouse and engine room) into "global" modes of vibration. The global vibratory motion acts as input to local vibratory systems, deck areas, bulkheads and supported equipment. Owing to greater local flexibility and to mass distribution effects, local elements usually experience an increase in vibration level, in some cases magnified by local resonance effects. The major aim of the design is therefore to arrive at a satisfactory level of vibration in the hull girder and major substructures, as this would indicate adequacy in design as regards propeller source strength and dynamic behaviour of the ship as a whole. Additional refinements to ensure low-level vibration in local elements can then more readily be incorporated in the structure.

2.6.7.3 Elements of Vibration Control

Generally the evaluation of source strength and vibration response characteristics of a ship is comprehensive, requiring computerized prediction programs. Reviews based on accumulated data and experience, supported by preliminary estimates, may be applied at the early, conceptual stage.

The logistics of ship vibration control are outlined briefly below:

Propeller. The excitation from the propeller is propagated as (a) propeller-induced hull surface forces (pressure fluctuations) and (b) shaft-induced forces, transmitted to the hull through stern tube bearing and thrust bearing seating (Vorus [69]).

The optimal design of propellers for low excitation purposes requires testing of the ship aft-body lines (wakefield) in a model tank and cavitation testing of the propeller and/or calculations to arrive at an estimate of the expected range of propeller forces (Lindgren and Johnsson [50]; Rutherford [61]). The aim would be to optimize the propeller/aft end conditions for the extent of propeller cavitation, hull-induced pressure forces, shaft-induced forces and the total integrated propeller vibratory excitation forces.

The number of blades should be chosen on the basis of considerations of possible resonance effects in the hull and shafting system. Resonance for longitudinal vibration in the shaft system should not occur within the normal service speed range of the propulsion machinery in order to avoid magnified vibratory forces being transmitted to the hull structure. The propeller is the major cause of shipboard vibration (Skaar and Ræstad [63]).

Diesel Propulsion Engine. Free, unbalanced forces and moments may give rise to hull girder vibration, (Johnson and McClimont [40]; Volcy [68]). Resonance condition at ship service speeds should be avoided. Guide force moment may give rise to more localized vibration. The engine foundation is of importance, and staying the engine at its top ends limits transmission to the ship in case of resonant vibration.

Superstructure. The superstructure design should be evaluated for possible resonance effects, both in its "separate" modes and in coupled modes with the hull girder. The major considerations are to provide (a) adequate support aligned with the fore and aft transverse steel bulkheads, preferably continuously down to the double bottom, and (b) adequate shear stiffness in the sides (Noonan and Feldman [55]).

Attention should be paid to the taller deckhouse construction separated from the casing/funnel arrangement. Although beneficial from the point of view of noise, such taller structures will have a lower natural frequency due to greater flexibility, and thus be more prone to dynamic effects than the conventional continuous superstructure.

Local Areas. Vibration in local deck areas and bulkheads within the superstructure requires attention to beams, girders and panel stiffeners and to adequate supporting brackets. Long span deck areas may require supporting pillars to avoid resonance effects. Particular attention should be paid to ensure low vibration in control panels, instruments and items which would adversely affect the work environment. Also tables, beds and items affecting the relaxation and leisure activities of personnel should be checked for local vibration behaviour (Goethe et al. [15]). Measuring points for occupied areas are discussed by Wieg [72].

Propeller-induced hull structure vibration is discussed by Stiansen [65], while Ward and Willshare [71] give special reference to full-scale measurements. Mano et al. [52] give an outline of prevention and remedy of ship vibration.

Local vibration may be adequately controlled by selecting satisfactory mounting of the elements involved. Checks should be made on the trial trip.

References

1. Acoustic design manual for ships. Ed.: British Ship Research Assoc. Wallsend 1976.
2. Acton, W.I., R.R.A.Coles, R.P.Grime et al.: Noise in ships' engine rooms and machinery spaces. London, Clowes 1973 (B.S.R.A. Report NS.361)
3. Asztely, J.: The use of visco-elastic materials for noise reduction on ships. Noise Control, Vibration and Insulation p. 297 (1977).
4. Bailey, B.: Engine-room noise on board merchant ships. International Labour Review *88*, 3, 281–304 (1963).
5. Bauliche Maßnahmen gegen Schiffslärm. STG-Richtlinien 2201, March 1963.
6. Brubakk, E.: Consequences of IMCO's Code on noise levels. Paper. Det norske Veritas. Oslo 1981.
7. Burroughs, C.B., R.W.Fischer and F.L.Shiflet: Noise reduction for floating compartment and damped deck treatments in ship living spaces. ASA Meeting, Atlanta April, 1980.
8. Collection of Japanese shipboard vibration data from the habitability point of view. ISO/TC 108/SC 8/WG 2 (Japan-5) 18, April 1975.
9. Conn, R.B.: A survey of noise in merchant ships. Engineers and Shipbuilders *85*, 4, 61 (1969).
10. Effects of noise on hearing. Eds.: D.Hender-

son, R. P. Hamernik, D. S. Dosanjh et al. New York: Raven 1976.
11. Falensky, G.: Elastisch gelagerte Deckshäuser auf Seeschiffen. Schiff und Hafen *25*, 7 (1973).
12. George, A. W.: Shipboard airborne noise control. Ed.: SNAME. Philadelphia section 1980.
13. Godin, L. S.: Subjective ratings as a criterion in developing hygienic standards of noise and vibration on shipboard. Bull. Inst. mar. Med. Gdańsk *25*, 2/3/4, 372–374 (1974).
14. Goethe, H., E.-G. Schmidt, E. Zorn et al.: Lärmbelastung auf See- und Binnenschiffen, Untersuchungen zur effektiven Lärmbelastung der Besatzungen. Ed.: Bundesanstalt für Arbeitsschutz und Unfallforschung, Dortmund. Bremerhaven: Wirtschaftsverlag NW 1979 (Forschungsbericht 201).
15. Goethe, H., E.-G. Schmidt, H.-D. Bode et al.: Schwingungen an Bord von Seeschiffen. Ed.: Bundesanstalt für Arbeitsschutz und Unfallforschung, Dortmund. Bremerhaven: Wirtschaftsverlag NW 1981. (Forschungsbericht 262)
16. Goethe, H., E. Zorn, R. Herrmann et al.: Die psycho-physische Belastung des Personals moderner Seeschiffe als aktuelles Problem der Schiffahrtsmedizin. Zbl. Bakt., I. Abt. Orig. B. *166*, 1, 1–36 (1978).
17. Goto, D.: Evaluation of ship's vertical motion from point of view of motion sickness. Paper at U. K. Informal Group on Human Response to Vibration. Meeting of Herriot-Watt University, Edinburgh 1981.
18. Grewe, H. E. and H. Rodegra: Untersuchungen über die Lärmschwerhörigkeit des Maschinenpersonals. Hansa *112*, 21 (1975).
19. Handbook for shipboard airborne noise control. Ed.: U. S. Coast Guard Washington 1974. (Tech. Publ. 073–100)
20. Harris, J. D.: Hearing-loss trend curves and the damage-risk criterion in diesel-engine-room personnel. J. Acoust. Soc. Amer. *37*, 3 (1965).
21. Herrmann, R., H. Goethe, E.-G. Schmidt et al.: The noise load of crew members on board seagoing and inland waterway vessels of the Federal German Republic (Latest Results). In: VIII International symposium on marine medicine – Abstracts – 24–28 October 1978. Varna 1978. pp. 249–250.
22. Human factors in the design and operation of ships. Proceedings of the First International Conference on Human Factors in the Design and Operation of Ships. Ed.: D. Anderson, H. Istance and J. Spencer. Stockholm: Garmat Service 1978.
23. IMCO-DEXXIII (draft only). Code on Noise Levels in Ships, Intergovernmental Maritime Consultative Organization (IMCO), Sub-committee on Ship Design. London, 12 Dec. 1980.
24. IMCO-DEXIX/WP7 agenda item 9. Noise Levels in Ships (ad hoc group). London 1978.
25. Infrasound and low frequency vibration. Ed.: W. Tempest London: Academic 1976.
26. ISO gives guidance on symbols for quantities and units. J. acoust. Soc. Amer. *67*, 1, 360 (1980).
27. ISO R266 Normal Equal-loudness Contours for Pure Tones and Normal Threshold of Hearing under Free Field Listening Conditions. Geneva 1961.
28. ISO 1996 Assessment of Noise with Respect to Community Response. Geneva 1971.
29. ISO 1999 Acoustics – Assessment of Occupational Noise Exposure for Hearing Conservation Purposes. Geneva 1975.
30. ISO 2041 Vibration and Shock – Vocabulary. Geneva 1975.
31. ISO 2631. Guide for the Evaluation of Human Exposure to Whole-body Vibration. Geneva 1978.
32. ISO 2631, draft addendum ISO 2631/DAD2. Evaluation of Human Exposure to Whole-body Vibration in the Frequency Range 0.1 to 1.0 Hz. Geneva 1980.
33. ISO 2631, draft proposal addendum 3; working paper ISO/TC108/SC4-N116. Guide for the Evaluation of Crew Exposure to Vibration on Board Seagoing Ships. Geneva 1981.
34. ISO DP4867 (draft) Code for the Measurement and Reporting on Shipboard Vibration Data. Geneva 1980.
35. ISO DP4868 (draft) Code for the Measurement and Reporting of Shipboard Local Vibration Data. Geneva 1980.
36. ISO DP6954 (draft) Guidelines for the Overall Evaluation of Vibration in Merchant Ships. Geneva 1980.
37. Janssen, J. H.: Hypothesis on simultaneous noise-and-vibration annoyance rating in shipboard accommodation. Noise Control Engineering 16, p. 145 (1981).
38. Janssen, J. H. and J. Buiten: An acoustical design on naval architecture. Proc. Inter-Noise 73 (1973).
39. Johannessen, H. and K. T. Skaar: Guidelines for prevention of excessive ship vibration. Trans. SNAME *88*, p. 319 (1980).
40. Johnson, A. J. and W. McClimont: Machinery induced vibration. Trans I. M. E. *75*, 4, 121 (1963).
41. Kanazawa, T.: A proposal for the vibration limits of ships. Wissenschaftl. Z. Univ. Rostock *10*, 2/3, 313–321 (1961).
42. Kanda, H.: Present state of engine-room noise and crew's hearing impairment. Paper. The Marine Engineering Society in Japan, Tokyo, 12–15 November 1973.
43. Kihlman, T. and J. Plunt: Prediction of noise levels in ships. In: Proceedings of the International Symposium on Shipboard Acoustics. Amsterdam: Elsvier 1973.
44. Kluikin, I. I.: Control of noise and sonic vibration in ships. Transl. from the Russian lang. by the U. S. Dept. of Commerce, Office of Techni-

cal Services, Joint Publ. Res. Serv. Washington 1963.
45. Klumpp, R.G. and J.C. Webster: Physical measurements of equally speech-interfering navy noises. J. Acoust. Soc. Am. *35,* 1328–1338 (1963).
46. Lambert, D.R.: Airborne noise levels in merchant ships. Ed.: Naval Ocean System Center. San Diego 1979. (NOSC-TD 243)
47. Lambert, D.R.: Requirements for sleep, solving problems and speech communication in shipboard compartments. Ed.: Naval Ocean System Center. San Diego 1980. (NOSC-TR 559)
48. Lambert, D.R. and F.S. Hafner: Behavioral and physiological effects of noise on people. Ed.: Naval Ocean System Center. San Diego 1979. (NOSC-TD 267)
49. Leenaars, C.E.J. and P.E. Forbes: An approach to vibration problems at the design stage. RINA Symposium. London 1980.
50. Lindgren, H. and C.A. Johnsson: On the influence of cavitation on propeller-excited vibratory forces and some means of reducing its effects. Internat. Symposium, PRADS, SNAJ. Tokyo 1977. p.343.
51. Maniar, N.M. and J.C. Daidola: The considerations of vibrations and noise at the preliminary and contract levels of ship design. In: Ship Vibration Symposium, Arlington, 16–17 Oct. 1978. Ed.: The Society of Naval Architects and Marine Engineers, New York.
52. Mano, M., Y. Ochi and K. Fuji: Prevention and remedy of ship vibration. IHI Rev. *10,* 10 (1975).
53. Nilsson, A.C.: Noise prediction and prevention in ships. In: Ship Vibration Symposium, Arlington, 16–17 Oct. 1978. Ed.: The Society of Naval Architects and Marine Engineers, New York.
54. Nilsson, A.C., B. Persson and N.P. Tyvand: Propeller induced noise in ships. Paper. SNAME Propeller 81-Symposium. Virginia Beach 1981.
55. Noonan, E.F. and S. Feldman: State of the art for shipboard vibration and noise control. In: Ship Vibration Symposium, Arlington, 17 Oct. 1978. Ed.: The Society of Naval Architects and Marine Engineers, New York.
56. Nowak, R. and D. Dahl: Die Lärmschwerhörigkeit des Schiffsmaschinenpersonals. Z. ges. Hyg. *17,* 7, 488–492 (1971).
57. Ojak, W.: Vibration problems on modern ships due to propeller excitations. 4th Italian-Polish Seminar on Ship Structures and Hydrodynamics. Genoa, June 1979.
58. Pettersen, J.W.E.: On the philosophy of conducting and evaluating sea trials vibration and noise measurements. Ship Trials Symposium, Naval Architects Association. Zagreb 1980.
59. Pettersen, J.W.E. and J.F. Storm (Eds.): Handbook on noise control in ships. Oslo: Selvig 1975.
60. Quist-Hanssen, S.: Noise induced hearing loss amongst engine-room personnel on board Norwegian Merchant ships. Ed.: Det norske Veritas. Oslo 1964. (DnV Publication 44)
61. Rutherford, R.: Aft end shaping to limit vibration. Paper. NEC Inst. Eng. and Shpbldrs. General meeting, Newcastle, 26 March 1979.
62. Schmidt, D.R.: Noise levels and crew noise exposure aboard U.S. merchant vessels. Ed.: Naval Ocean System Center. San Diego, 1979. (NOSC-TR 405)
63. Skaar, K.T. and A.E. Ræstad: The relative importance of ship vibration excitation forces. RINA Symposium. London 1980.
64. Solumsmoen, O.H.: Ship vibration. Experience from service measurements. Ed.: Det norske Veritas. Oslo 1977. (DnV Publication 96)
65. Stiansen, S.G.: Propeller and wave induced hull structure vibrations. In: Ship Vibration Symposium. Arlington, 16–17 Oct. 1978. Ed.: The Society of Naval Architects and Marine Engineers, New York.
66. Switaiski, B.: Belastung des Menschen durch Schiffsvibrationen. Schiff und Hafen *31,* 11, 991–998 (1979).
67. Szczepanski, C., L. Zaborski and M. Taniewski: Acoustic and vibrational media aboard ship type B-516 and the state of hearing in the crew. Bull. Inst. mar. trop. Med. Gdynia *31,* 3/4, 165–175 (1980).
68. Volcy, G.G.: Interaction and compatibility between machinery and hull from a static and vibratory point of view. In: Ship Vibration Symposium. Arlington, 16–17 Oct. 1978. Ed.: The Society of Naval Architects and Marine Engineers, New York.
69. Vorus, W.S.: Calculation of propeller-induced vibratory hull forces, force distribution, and pressures, free surface effects. J. Ship. Res. *20,* 2, 107 (1976).
70. Ward, G. and A. Hoyland: Ship design and noise levels. Paper. Annual Meeting, March 1979. NEC Inst. Engrs. and Shpbldrs.
71. Ward, G. and T. Willshare: Propeller-excited vibration with particular reference to full scale measurements. Paper No. 4, RINA, Spring meeting 1975.
72. Wieg, P.: Orientierende Meßpunkte zur Einschätzung des Schwingungsniveaus der Aufenthaltsorte von Besatzungen auf Hochseeschiffen. Verk.-Med. *22,* 1, 11–17 (1975).
73. Wragge, F.: Erfahrungen bei der Lärmbekämpfung auf Seeschiffen. Hansa *113,* 2, 142–147 (1976).
74. Zaborski, L. and C. Szczepanski: A hygienic analysis of mechanical vibrations in a voyage aboard the semicontainer ship M/S "Kalinowski". Bull. Inst. mar. trop. Med. Gdynia *27,* 3/4, 279–288 (1976).

2.7 The Ship's Water Supply

Z. Sobol

2.7.1 Introduction

Technological progress in shipbuilding has solved the quantitative problems concerning a ship's fresh water supply, but the problem of ensuring that fresh water meets modern sanitary standards remains (Sobol and Szumilas [8]; Sobol and Elpiner [9]; Sobol and Wasilewska [10]; Sobol [11]). To obtain water meeting the standards, it is necessary to be conversant not only with the problems of the ship's water supply, but also, and primarily, with the structure and operation of the ship's water system. Little attention is paid to the problem of water systems since it is believed to have no direct connection with navigational safety. The crew keeps changing, and it is difficult for them to become fully acquainted with the water system. Thus the ship's doctor or officer charged with medical care on board is responsible for instructing the crew on the correct use of the water system and for supervising its operation (Sobol [11]; Zorn [12]).

2.7.2 Sources of the Ship's Fresh Water

Traditional ships may receive fresh water directly from the port's water system or from water boats (Goethe and Herrmann [2]). Since the 1950s seawater distillation plants have been reintroduced to enable fresh water supplies to be replenished. The choice of the ship's water supply, i.e. from shore sources or the ship's own distillation plant, is merely a question of economy on cargo liners since these ships frequently call at ports and since their stay at sea has been considerably reduced due to their increasing speeds (Elpiner [1]; Sobol and Wasilewska [10]; Sobol [11]). Another problem is that distilling plants often cannot be used because of short stays in the areas where sea water is fit for distillation. On the other hand, on specialised ships staying at sea for a prolonged period of time (fishing, hydrographic and research vessels, or even tramps), distilling plants may be the only source of unlimited fresh water.

The operation of seawater distilling plants results in additional responsibilities for the crew, i.e. checking the technical condition of distilling and purification equipment as well as turning off the desalination plants during the ship's stay in highly polluted zones. Generally, waters up to 12 miles off the coast, areas of mass outflow of oil products and fisheries with large numbers of fish processing vessels are reckoned to be polluted zones.

2.7.3 Quantitative Problems with the Ship's Water

Water consumption on a ship depends on a number of factors, i.e. the possibility of providing the required amounts of hot and cold water from the ship's water system, the standard of personal hygiene of the crew and the sanitary facilities in the living and working areas. Quantitative standards of water consumption defined in the 1950s affected the design of water systems on ships (Herrmann [5]; Lamoureux [6]; Mateev et al. [7]; Sobol and Elpiner [9]; Sobol and Wasilewska [10]). According to those

Table 1. Old and new standards for water consumption

Uses of water	Standards hitherto observed (litres per person per day)	Actual water consumption and the new sanitary standards (litres per person per day)
Morning wash	10	10
After-watch bath	35	70 (2 × 35)
Washing hands before meals	15 (5 × 3)	15
Preparing meals and dish-washing	30	30
Washing hands after visiting the toilet	10 (4 × 2.5)	10
Toilet flushing	–	35
Laundry	–	25
Cleaning in the living spaces	–	5
Total	100	200

standards, overboard water was used for toilet flushing and cleansing purposes, and the daily ration of water amounted to 100 litres per person.

In the 1970s, as a result of the increasing pollution of harbour and coastal waters, attempts were made to replace sea water with fresh water. Analysis of the actual water consumption on ships indicates that the standards for fresh water consumption are outdated and in practice considerably exceeded. Thus, it has become necessary to work out new sanitary standards based on actual needs (Table 1) (Lamoureux [6]; Sobol and Szumilas [8]; Sobol and Elpiner [9]; Sobol and Wasilewska [10]).

2.7.4 Quality of Fresh Water on Board Ship

The quality of potable water on board ship which has been obtained from shore sources depends on the quality of fresh water in ports as well as storage conditions and purification (Elpiner [1]; Goethe and Herrmann [2, 3]; Herrmann [5]; Sobol and Wasilewska [10]; Zorn [12]).

Water systems all over the world fulfil different requirements, depending on the number of users. The water systems at ports supplying fresh water for ships must have the highest standards. The standards of ships' water systems are usually somewhat lower. Since the quality of water obtained from different ports varies, it is difficult to control its mineral content. Therefore, the turbidity standards of the water stored in the ship's tanks for a few days or longer are not so strict (up to 5 mg/litre SiO_2). Very soft water is in some countries thought to have a harmful effect on the human organism. Therefore, the distillate used to supply fresh water should be mineralised to obtain a hardness of 5°–6° N (about 2 mval) and to provide a full complex of the micro-elements occurring in natural water.

In a number of countries, the value of the mineralised distillate is considered to be the same as or even higher than that of the water from shore sources but the sanitary standard of water may be inadequate in some ports. Irrespective of the bacteriological state of the water at the time when it is obtained from shore sources or purified aboard, the water should be disinfected directly before its distribution. Correct operation of disinfecting plants, now installed on all ships, makes it possible to meet the highest standards, i.e. not a single faecal coliform bacteria in 100 ml of water, while the coli index (or MPN in 100 ml) must not exceed l.

2.7.5 Water Systems on Ships

The ship's water system includes water storage tanks, pressure tanks, pumps, a purification plant and a distribution system (the piping) (Elpiner [1]; Goethe and Herrmann [2]; Lamoureux [6]; Sobol [11]).

To provide potable water for all purposes when using a single water system, independent tanks should be installed, that is, tanks having no parts in common with the ship's construction, but this is not the case in all seafaring countries. At present, it is possible to instal such tanks on all cargo ships. However, because of fewer crew members and the growing speed of ships, the size and number of storage tanks have been reduced. On special ships, such as fishing or research vessels, where the number of crew in relation to the capacity of the ship is high, it is necessary to store water in tanks which are not independent, e.g. double bottom, fore and aft peak tanks. In such cases, the potable water system must be separated from any non-potable water system. In dual systems, potable water should be supplied for culinary, dish washing, personal hygiene (wash basin, shower bath) and hospital purposes, as well as for cleaning refrigerated provision stores.

Storage tanks must either be constructed of corrosion-resistant materials or have protective coating of a type accepted by the health administration (Elpiner [1]; Goethe and Herrmann [2]; Sobol and Wasilewska [10]; Zorn [12]). Cement has been replaced by epoxide, and thus the durability of coatings has considerably increased. The water tank must be so designed that it can be completely drained and dried. The tank should be equipped with a manhole, located preferably on a side, a filling line leading to the open deck, equipped with a standardised fitting to connect the shore–water hoses, and a vent equipped with a backflow valve provided with an insect and ratproof screen (Lamoureux [6]).

Every tank should be equipped with a water-level gauge so constructed as to prevent water contamination. Thus, use of sounding rods is prohibited. The devices acceptable for determining the depth of water in the tanks include water-gauge glass, petcocks, float gauges, water-level indicators operated by air pressure or electricity and other gauges installed inside the tank, enabling remote control of the depth of water (see Fig. 1). To evaluate the technological condition of the water system, it may be useful to compare the readings of water consumption by means of a float water gauge installed in the distribution system, with the amount of storage in the tanks.

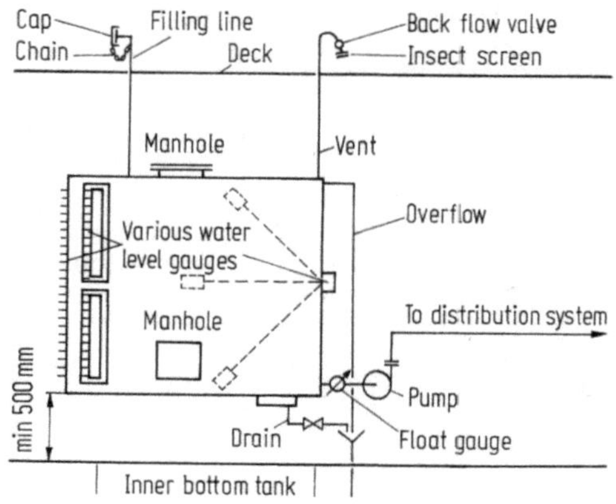

Fig. 1. Independent storage tank for potable water

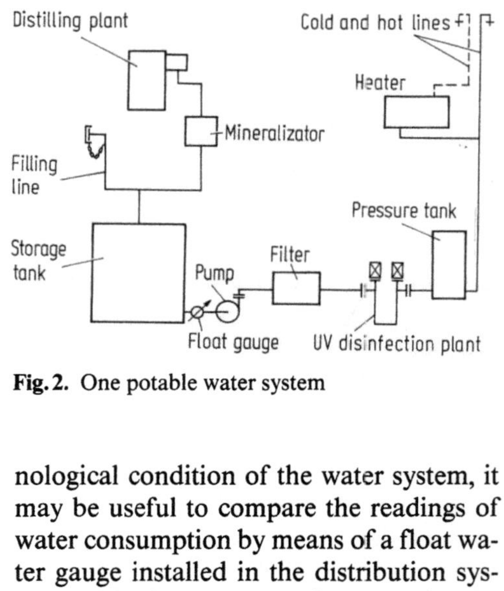

Fig. 2. One potable water system

When the potable water storage is supplied by water treated aboard, the size of the tanks may be decreased and a single potable water system may be used. A single potable water system is presented in Fig. 2.

The quality of the distributed water depends mainly on the technical condition of the water system and the materials used in its construction. Zinc-coated steel pipelines are acceptable when they are connected with zinc-coated fittings and can be dismantled. When the water system is damaged during the ship's voyage, welding of zinc-coated pipes often damages the protective coating. For this reason these sections must be repaired in the nearest port. Copper pipes can be used if they are accepted by the national health administration and do not contain harmful contaminants.

Technical systems should be connected with the drinking water system in case there is only one water system. This connection should be back-flow proof. Open-air gaps, vacuum breakers or pipe dividers are preferable. Non-return valves are not safe from the hygienic point of view.

Hot potable water (338–343 K, 65°–70 °C) should be piped to washbasins, showers and sinks, and to galley and pantry for scalding dishes and utensils (363–368 K, 90°–95 °C). Showers have to be fitted with automatic temperature limiting valves in order to avoid scalds.

2.7.6 Disinfection of Water

Water stored on ship for a long period may become contaminated and therefore should be disinfected (Elpiner [1]; Goethe and Herrmann [3]; Herrmann [4]; Sobol and Wasilewska [10]; Zorn [12]). The use of one of the disinfection methods restores the previous sanitary standard of the water. There is a need to improve the design of disinfection plants which will simplify the whole process of disinfecting and limit the participation required of the crew.

2.7.6.1 Chlorination

Until quite recently chlorination was the only method of disinfection (Goethe and Herrmann [3]; Sobol and Wasilewska [10]). Although effective, it has certain disadvantages. Firstly, the amount of chlorine needed to disinfect a given amount of water must be determined every time. When overchlorination occurs, the organoleptic properties of water change; therefore dechlorination must be achieved using activated charcoal. Secondly, chlorinating agents must be stored aboard, and their activity must be checked regularly. Chlorination can be applied only on a ship with a large crew where a particular crew member can be appointed to take care of the equipment. It is advisable to use the procedure after any kind of water system repairs, when the whole system must be disinfected.

2.7.6.2 Filtration

On ships with small crews (10–15 persons), filters with silver-impregnated ceramic candles are recommended (Sobold and Wasilewska [10]; Sobol [11]; Zorn [12]). The method consists of trapping all impurities on the filters. The filters are impregnated with silver ions, thereby preventing the growth of bacteria. In the 1950s and 1960s, this method was used on a number of ships, but recently some more effective methods have been introduced.

As impurities gather on the filter, effluent resistance increases and the filter's efficiency decreases. Therefore, filters must be cleaned when the resistance reaches a certain value. The filter can be regenerated 14 times, providing an average of 4000 litres of filtrate after each regeneration. Thus a total of 60000 litres of water can be gained from a single filtration candle. A serious disadvantage of this method is the labour-consuming regeneration of filters.

2.7.6.3 Disinfection with Ultraviolet Light

The bactericidal properties of ultraviolet radiation are also used to disinfect water. The method is simple to apply and the procedure can be automated. The most effective bactericidal action is observed at 2500–2800 Å. It is proportional to the radiation intensity and contact time (Elpiner [1]).

According to the manufacturer's data (General Electric), ultraviolet lamps transmit about 20% of the energy supplied. Further energy losses depend on the extent to which the water is polluted, since impurities absorb ultraviolet radiation. Suspensions of iron salts, acid carbonates, humus compounds and other substances reduce the transmission rate and gather on the protective quartz tubes separating the lamp from the water. Disinfection effectiveness depends on the following factors: lifetime of lamp (6000 h according to the manufacturer) measured by the lamp's work counter, cleanness of the quartz glass protecting the lamp and the degree of water pollution. The lamp's radiation intensity is measured by a photoelectric cell regulating the flow of water or warning of malfunctioning of the system. Impurities deposited on the lamp's quartz protections must be removed. The impurities can be reduced by filters installed before the unit. Because of the unit's simple construction it is easy to operate, uses little energy and seems to be the most suitable of all water disinfecting plants on the ship. Operating tests made aboard ship showed that a 100% bactericidal effect is observed at the exposure of 4 Wsec./litre, i.e. we can obtain 2 litres per sec. disinfected water with a lamp of 40 W. The organoleptic properties of water remain unchanged (Herrmann [4]; Sobol and Wasilewska [10]; Sobol [11]). Other disinfection procedures such as pasteurisation, ozonising and iodising are not generally used (Elpiner [1]; Goethe and Herrmann [2]; Zorn [12]).

2.7.7 Utilisation and Sanitary Supervision of Water Systems

To use a water system properly it is necessary to have complete working plans and operating instructions for all parts of the system. Good cooperation with the harbour medical service can be achieved when the doctor or officer charged with medical care on board is introduced to ship's hygiene and knows how to supply the ship with potable water and how to check the water's sanitary standard (Sobol [11]).

The following problems connected with using the ship's water system must be taken into account:

1. The method of taking water from the port system and especially the sanitary conditions of the watering equipment and hydrants, as well as the period of flushing the filling hoses (a minimum of 5 min).
2. The technical condition of the tanks and corrosion-resistant protective coatings; flushing the tanks before taking large supplies of water and draining the tank bottom as often as necessary to remove the sediment and impurities.
3. Disinfection of the tanks and water system after they have undergone any repairs.
4. Utilisation of spare pumps in the potable water system only when there is no possibility of them being used for liquids other than potable water.
5. To prevent water pollution, all connections and pump glands must be leakproof.
6. Measurement of water storage must be done by instruments not to be removed from the tank.
7. The method of seawater distillation, desalination and mineralisation of the distillate before the water is pumped to storage tanks.
8. Water-disinfecting equipment, its efficiency, following the operating instructions, periodical surveys and repairs.
9. Keeping records of all activities connected with the water-system equipment.

Water-system equipment is under sanitary control by the harbour medical service in the port of registry. Water samples, minimum of 100 ml each, for bacteriological tests are taken from all tanks and from nozzles of the water system. The frequency of sampling depends on ship traffic. The samples should be collected after each voyage lasting over 3 months, or in the case of shorter ones, after every fourth voyage. Water samples should be taken before filling the tanks, to find the hygienic standard of water from the last voyage. The harbour medical service is obliged to keep records of the sanitary inspection of the ship's water systems. Basic information concerning the water system, results of tests and recommendations after controls should be included. Physicochemical tests are also required by order of the harbour medical service. After all repairs or when the bacteriological condition of water has been found unsatisfactory, the ship's water system and equipment must be disinfected. Disinfection is done with 80 g of active chlorine per ton of water in the tanks and in the distribution system. After adding the chlorinating agent and filling the system with water, a 2-h contact period is required. To obtain an accurate disinfection of all equipment, the draw taps at the farthest section of the water system must be opened. Chlorinated water must flow through the entire system so that it will have the clear odour of chlorine. After 2 h, chlorinated water must be removed from the system, which is filled with clean water from the shore source.

2.7.8 Drinking Water on Lifeboats and Rafts

Lifeboats and rafts are equipped with a reserve of drinking water (Sobol [11]). The capacity of this reserve must at least be sufficient to replace the loss of body fluid for a completely occupied boat or raft. The outfit of lifeboats includes about 3 litres of drinking water per person, while in inflatable rafts there is a minimum of 1.5 litres per person. This reserve may be reduced to 2 litres per person on lifeboats and 1 litre in inflatable rafts provided with desalting equipment.

In lifeboats the drinking water is kept in at least two waterproof tanks of zinc-plated steel or other material resistant to corrosion and accepted by the sanitary authorities as being adequate for this purpose. The tanks should be provided with a dipper, a gauge and a cup fastened to a chain, serving for water rationing.

The crew members must change the water in the tanks at least once a month, and this operation has to be noted in the ship's log-book. To facilitate the exchange of the water in the lifeboats it is recommended that points taking potable water be installed on the boat's deck. During the exchange of water or other functions, the smallest of leakages of water from the tanks has to be immediately reported to the ship's captain and wherever possible these leakages must be eliminated. The traditional method of keeping water in lifeboats in tanks should be replaced by individual water rations in hermetically sealed tins made of material resistant to corrosion. On the tins the date of validity should be given. Drinking water in tins is used with success in inflatable rafts and retains an adequate quality providing that the principle of periodic replacement of the tins is observed. This duty to replace tins is often neglected on ships from various countries. The discharge of water from the tanks when a ship enters regions with temperatures below freezing-point is impossible. The water reserves on the lifeboats must be subjected to periodical control by the harbour medical services.

References

1. Elpiner, L. I.: Vodosnabzhenie morskikh sudov. [Water supply on seagoing ships]. Moscow: Izdatelstvo Transport 1975.
2. Goethe, H. and R. Herrmann: Hygienische Gesichtspunkte bei Konstruktion und Betrieb von Schiffswasserversorgungsanlagen. In: Jahrbuch der Schiffbautechnischen Gesellschaft, Vol. 63, 1969. Berlin, Heidelberg, New York: Springer 1970. pp. 293–302.
3. Goethe, H. and R. Herrmann: Zur Problematik der Trinkwasserdesinfektion an Bord von Seeschiffen. In: Desinfektion von Trinkwasser. Stuttgart: G. Fischer 1970. pp. 91–98. (Schriftenreihe d. Vereins f. Wasser-, Boden- und Lufthygiene No. 31)
4. Herrmann, R.: Die UV-Anlage an Bord von Schiffen. Hansa *116*, 2, 149–150 (1979).
5. Herrmann, R.: Wasserhygiene an Bord. Schiffs-Ing. J. *20*, 104, 10–14 (1973).
6. Lamoureux, V. B.: Guide to ship sanitation. Geneva: WHO 1967.
7. Mateev, I., V. Panteleev and G. Bumbalova:

Certain requirements to be observed in supplying ships with water. In: VII International symposium on marine medicine, Odessa, 23–30 Sept. 1976, USSR Ministry of Health, Moscow 1976. p. 310.

8. Sobol, Z. and T. Szumilas: Current trends of fresh water supply on ships. Bull. Inst. mar. trop. Med. Gdynia *30,* 2, 143–152 (1979).
9. Sobol, Z. and L. I. Elpiner: Elaboration of a uniform methodology of water supply investigation on ships. In: VII International symposium on marine medicine, Odessa, 23–30 Sept. 1976, USSR Ministry of Health, Moscow 1976. p. 305.
10. Sobol, Z. and H. B. Wasilewska: Supply of the sea going ships with fresh water. Budownictwo okretowe *26,* 5/6, 225 (1981).
11. Sobol, Z.: Zaopatrzenie statków w wode slodka. [Fresh water supply of ships]. In: Dolmierski, R. et al. (eds): Morski poradnik medyczny. [Medical guide for seafaring]. Warsaw: Państwowy Zaklad Wydawnictw Lekarskich 1981. pp. 341–356.
12. Zorn, E.: Wasserhygiene auf Schiffen. Mat. med. Nordm. *21,* 12, 708–713 (1969).

2.8 Waste and Waste-Water Disposal Aboard Ship

Z. Sobol

2.8.1 Introduction

To secure hygienic conditions for the crew and the passengers on board ship, it is essential to provide the ship with adequate sanitary equipment. This equipment has to discharge liquid human sewage, galley waste and waste from cleaning out the ship's holds. On ships, there may also be industrial waste requiring sanitary disposal (Buxton and Schormann [1]; Goethe [3]; Lamoureux [5]). At one time, the ocean was largely considered to be an unlimited dumping ground for many kinds of waste connected with human activities; it was not until the mass discharge of oil products began that the limitations of the sea in dealing with waste became apparent. This particularly concerns seas where the exchange of water with the ocean is limited – the Mediterranean Sea and the Baltic Sea. Up until the 1950s little attention was paid to the preservation of the natural marine environment. On the ships built up to this period, there were no restrictions on discharge of waste into the sea; the same was true for many ports all over the world.

The indiscriminate disposal of oil products from ships, either in the course of normal operations or as a result of damage, is more dangerous for the marine environment than the ordinary discharge of waste from vessels and shore. Nevertheless, when the international regulations for the prevention of pollution from ships were reviewed, attention was also paid to the less evident but likewise dangerous sanitary problem of pollution of the sea by non-oil waste from ship and shore. The International Convention for the Prevention of Pollution from Ships [so-called MAR(ITIME) POL(LUTION)], organised by the Intergovernmental Maritime Consultative Organization (IMCO) and held in London in 1973, was followed by local regulations concerning waste treatment. Since 1973, efforts have been made to achieve a technical solution to the problem of waste systems in the designs of ships, giving some consideration to the preservation of the natural marine environment. The international regulations should be regarded as the minimum requirements for protecting a narrow zone of coastal water from the waste discharged from ships. It is possible, however, that in future the sea as a source of food will be protected against pollution caused by the discharge of waste from ships into the sea. Hopefully, all oceans and seas as sources of food will in future be spared from devastation and pollution.

2.8.2 Types of Waste and Sewage Systems on Board Ship

Separate systems are traditionally used on ships for faecal and non-faecal sewage so as to prevent the backflow of faecal sewage from toilets into other areas in the event of a damaged outlet, freezing or considerable lurching. Ships are thus equipped with two sewage systems (Buxton and Schormann [1]; Sobol [10]): (a) a system receiving faecal sewage from toilets, urinals and toilet drains, called black sewage; (b) a system receiving non-faecal sewage from other sanitary facilities, such as washbasins, baths, showers, sinks and drains in places other than those in (a), called grey sewage.

Black sewage includes the waste from drains and toilets, the entire waste from the ship's hospital and the waste from holds where live animals are kept. Of the grey sewage, the most noxious components for the marine environment are galley and laundry waste since they contain the greatest amounts of impurities. Galley waste contains considerable amounts of food and grease, while laundry waste contains detergents. Waste from washbasins and showers is more diluted but contains the highest amount of bacterial impurities. Thus, in the event of contagious or infectious diseases on board ship, this waste must be disinfected along with the black sewage. They grey sewage contains only potable water, while the black sewage contains potable or sea water.

On ships built in the 1960s, i.e. ships that may still be in operation, overboard water is generally used for flushing toilets and urinals. Since the 1970s, single potable water systems have been used on cargo ships for all sanitary purposes, including toilet flushing and cleansing sanitary areas. The kind of water used for toilet flushing and cleansing sanitary areas is of particular importance to hygiene when a ship stays in a highly polluted harbour or coastal waters, especially in countries in which infectious and highly contagious diseases are endemic.

Black sewage makes up 20%–30% of the total amount of sewage, i.e. about 40–60 litres per person per 24 h. Its concentration depends on the sanitary habits of the crew and passengers, the frequency of toilet flushing and the technical condition of the flushing facilities. The amount of grey sewage on ships with individual sanitary facilities (washbasins and showers for all crew members) is 140–160 litres per person per 24 h (Sobol et al. [9]; Sobol [10]). With the dual sewage system, it is possible to isolate the sewage most noxious for the natural environment and treat it according to international regulations. The black and grey sewage systems are shown in Figs. 1 and 2.

2.8.3 Requirements of the International Conventions

The MAR POL IMCO Convention, London 1973, dealt with the prohibition of the discharge of black sewage into protected waters, i.e. harbour waters and a zone of coastal waters up to 12 nautical miles offshore. Black sewage discharge outside the protected areas is unrestricted. Discharge of grey sewage is unrestricted. According to the convention, ships must have holding tanks of adequate size proportional to the number of crew members and passengers aboard and the approximate duration of stay in protected waters. The sewage retained in the tanks may be discharged into the sea after leaving the protected areas or may be transferred to sewage-treatment plants ashore.

Crushed and disinfected waste may be discharged into the coastal waters 4–12 nautical miles offshore, provided the system comminuting and disinfecting the sewage intended for discharge fulfils the following effluent standards:

(a) Faecal coliform bacteria in the effluent should not exceed 1 000/100 ml; (b) the weight of the material retained on the filter screen (no. 12 with openings of 1.68 mm) after it has been dried to a constant weight in a oven a 103 °C/376 K must not exceed 10% of the total suspended solids.

To avoid the inconveniences resulting from having to retain sewage on protected waters, attempts have been made to work out effective methods of sewage treatment aboard ship. Treated sewage discharge is unrestricted, irrespective of the place, provided that the sewage treatment plant satisfies the following effluent standards: (a) the faecal coliform count does not exceed 250 faecal coliform bacteria per 100 ml; (b) the suspended solids do not exceed 50 mg/litre when the equipment is

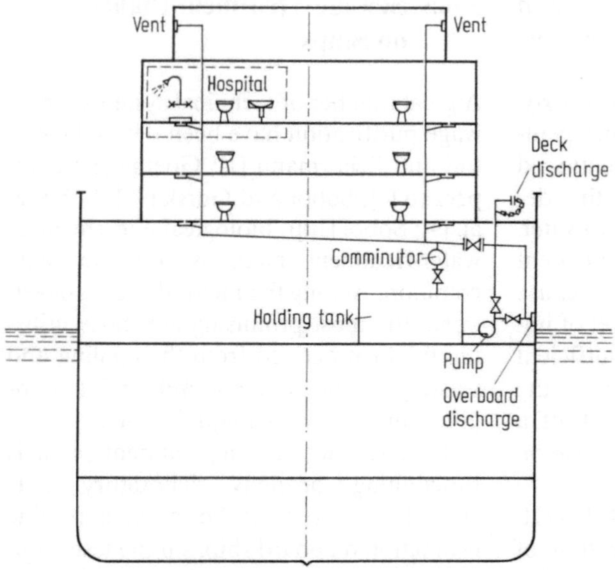

Fig. 1. Black sewage system

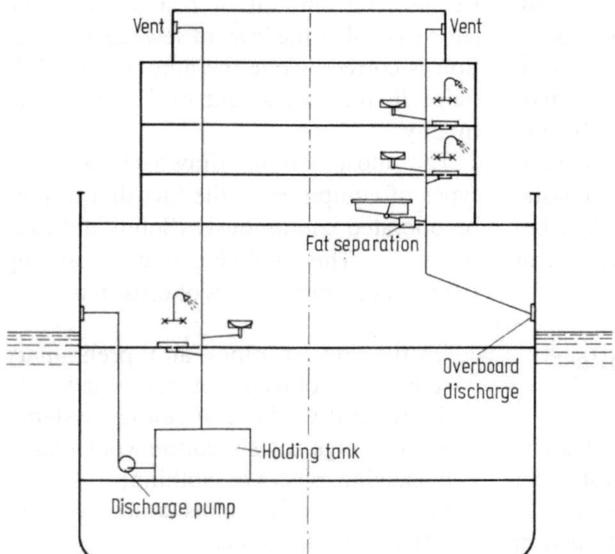

Fig. 2. Grey sewage system

tested on shore and are not 100 mg/litre above the suspended-solid content of the sea water used for flushing purposes when the equipment is tested aboard ship; (c) the residual level of chlorine in effluent does not exceed 5 mg/litre as free available chlorine. In addition to these conditions, the plant should be so designed that the geometric mean of the 5-day biochemical oxygen demand (BOD_5) of the effluent samples does not exceed 30 mg/litre (*International Conference on Marine Pollution* [4]). To meet the above standards is not easy and requires continuous operation of the plant by the crew. Care is absolutely essential – no objects or liquids that might interfere with the treatment process or even cause damage should be thrown into the toilets.

When operated and utilised properly, any of the sewage-treatment systems available are able to meet the above-mentioned requirements and contribute to the decrease in the level of impurities in seawater. All sewage-treatment systems, independent of the degree of sewage purification, cause a reduction of 70%–90% in the level of impurities in the effluent, which is sufficient to guarantee effective disinfection of the sewage in the event of an outbreak of a contagious or highly infectious disease on board.

As mentioned above, the MAR POL Convention dealt with the protection of harbour and coastal waters only. Waste discharge on the high seas by any ships, including fishing vessels, is unrestricted. Since, however, large numbers of vessels gather in the fishing zones and navigation routes intersect these zones, the problem of waste discharge into the seas of fishing zones must be solved. International regulations should protect not only the coastal waters but all other sea areas as well because of the great sanitary importance of this problem.

2.8.4 Sanitary Problems of Ballast Water

In view of the great speeds at which ships are now capable of travelling, ballast water may be carried over considerable distances in a short space of time and discharged in ports handling bulk cargo. Since the disinfection of such large amounts of water is practically impossible, ballast water taken up in countries in which infectious diseases are endemic should be replaced by clean seawater when the ship has left the coastal waters. This problem should be covered by international regulations.

2.8.5 Sewage-Treatment Plants on Ships

A great number of technical systems for sewage purification have been devised (Buxton and Schormann [1]; Goethe [3]; Perepeczko [6]; Sobol and Gorska [8]; Sobol et al. [9]; Sobol [10]); biological and chemical water-treatment methods are the most common. Among the methods being developed, the most promising are those utilising the heat derived from the cooling and waste gases of the main and auxiliary engines for evaporating liquid waste.

To assess whether a treatment plant is functioning properly, laboratory tests should be carried out. For a quick, routine estimation on board ship, simple tests indicating the amount of residual chlorine and sediment solids in the Imhoff tank are sufficient. The amount of residual chlorine shows whether the level of sewage disinfection is correct, while the amount of solids helps in the assessment of the treatment quality.

The most serious drawback with all types of equipment is the fact that it must be operated continuously (Sobol and Szumilas [7]). The following number among the most common causes of disturbance:

1. Obstruction of pipes and preliminary screens by objects not connected with the normal working of sewage systems, e.g. oily rags, towels, cotton wool, plastic packaging, pieces of clothing;
2. Leakage of oils, paints and chemicals into the sewage system;
3. Damage to equipment caused by changes in water salinity if overboard water is used for flushing toilets;
4. The decreased activity of chemical agents in the prolonged period of storage aboard;
5. Crew's reluctance to check and repair the sanitary equipment;
6. Poor knowledge of the servicing instructions and operating mechanism of the sanitary equipment.

It should be stated that systems properly used and operated can provide a degree of sewage purification in accordance with the international standards, if the sanitary requirements are strictly supervised by port or government authorities.

2.8.6 Sewage-Treatment Facilities in Ports

There are a great number of ships that have only holding tanks and thus the necessity arises that in all ports of the world there should be facilities for dealing with the sewage from such ships (Buxton and Schormann [1]; Environment Canada, Water Pollution Control Directorate, [2]; Sobol [10]). This is particularly important during long stays in ports when waiting on the roadstead or in the case of a ship being quarantined. In addition, ports are used by a great number of small fishing and auxiliary ships on which the installation of self-contained treatment plants would be impossible. Port authorities are, therefore, obliged to instal sewage-storage and purification facilities.

The transfer of the sewage to the municipal sewage plant is not possible because of the danger to public hygiene. Considering that in each port it is necessary to transfer the sewage from ships on the roadstead or direct from the wharf, ports must be equipped with floating sewage collecting and/or treatment units. These units may transfer the sewage to the reception facilities or treat it in their own plants, and afterwards discharge the treated sewage directly into the waters of the port or into the nearby coastal waters, without limit. The specialist crew on such ships guarantees the correct functioning of the treatment plants. An analysis of the transfer, handling and manoeuvring time indicates that one unit could deal with 10–15 ships in 24 h. The number of the sewage collecting and/or treatment units should be in accordance with the number of ships calling at the port within 24 h.

Table 1 Standard dimensions of flanges for discharge connections

Description	Dimension
Outside diameter	210 mm
Inner diameter	Dependent on pipe outside diameter
Bolt circle diameter	170 mm
Slots in flange	Four holes, 18 mm diameter, equidistantly placed on a bolt circle of the above diameter, slotted to the flange periphery. The slot width should be 18 mm
Flange thickness	16 mm
Bolts and nuts – quantity and diameter	Four, each 16 mm

In those ports in which the building of land-based sewage-treatment facilities is not expected in the near future, the sewage collecting and/or treatment unit ships are the only means of maintaining a sanitary barrier capable of protecting a country against the spread of infectious and contagious diseases. The transfer of sewage from ships to ports that do not have any sewage-purification installations is purposeless because the sewage will only be discharged untreated into the port or nearby waters.

To limit the contamination of the port waters by sewage during its transference from the ship to the port sewage-treatment facilities, both the transfer pipes of the treatment plant and those of the ship should be fitted with standard discharge connections in accordance with the dimensions presented in Table 1.

The flange is designed to accept pipes up to a maximum internal diameter of 100 mm and should be of steel or equivalent material having a flat surface. This flange together with a suitable gasket should be suitable for a service pressure of 6 kp/cm^2.

2.8.7 Holding Tanks

Holding tanks are especially used for sewage, i. e. faeces, urine and the associated

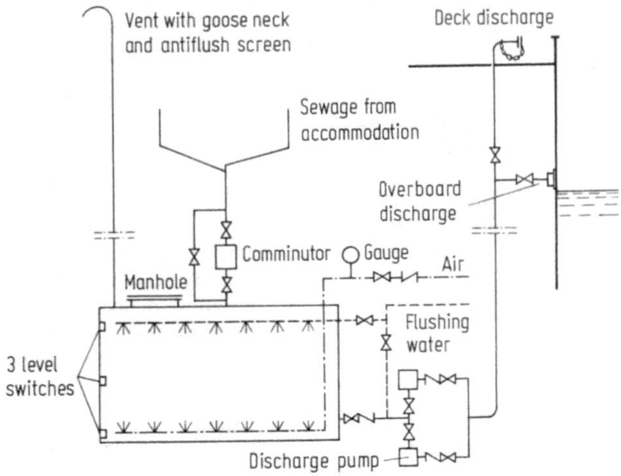

Fig. 3. Sewage system with holding tank

flush water. Raw sewage contains different solids, such as paper, rags, faeces and even garbage. To reduce the size of solids so that they can be more easily transported and pumped, holding tanks are equipped with a comminutor (*Environment Canada, Water Pollution Control Directorate,* [2]).

Fresh sewage contains an enormous number of aerobic and anaerobic bacteria. If the characteristics of the sewage favour aerobic bacterial respiration, then very little in the way of obnoxious odour will be present. For this reason, many designers prefer to aerate the sewage in the tanks.

If free air is in short supply in the sewage, then conditions become favourable for anaerobic bacteria and the presence of sulphur odour can be detected. If the contents of a holding tank are aerated so as to maintain a dissolved oxygen content in excess of 1.0 mg/litre, the sewage will be kept aerobic and the production of odours and dangerous gases should be minimised. The holding tank must have an outlet vent that should be located above the highest ship's deck to disperse any odours into the atmosphere. The vent pipe needs to be checked periodically to ensure that it is not blocked, especially during cold weather when the formation of ice in the vent can occur.

Each holding tank should be equipped with discharge pumps and it is recommended that two discharge pumps be fitted, one working and one standby. The pumps should be capable of handling heavy liquids and suspended solids of up to 5 mm. To facilitate cleaning of the tank, flush water should be supplied. Each holding tank should be equipped with a control system. The control system should consist of three level switches mounted in the tank and detecting the following levels – tank 90% full, tank 50% full and tank empty. The level switches activate alarms and lights according to the amount of sewage in the holding tank (Fig. 3). The capacity of the holding tank is dependent upon the flow rate in litres per man per day, the number of crew and passengers, and the sewage retention time in days.

2.8.8 Solid Waste on Ships

Solid waste accumulates on ships as a result of the preparation and consumption of food, the cleaning of the ship's holds and the professional work carried out on board (Lamoureux [5]; Sobol [10]). The solid waste comes (a) from the catering and accommodation areas – various kinds of wrappings and containers, food remains, old magazines and newpapers, old clothes; (b) from the working decks – old work materials, (e.g. paint containers, brushes, wire, ropes), old appliances no longer in use, loading and unloading waste; and (c) from the engine room – old engine parts, packing materials, discharged lubricants, old rags. The quantity of waste from the galley is estimated at 2 kg per person per 24 h on average and from all other areas 20–40 kg per 24 h.

The composition of the waste from ships is as follows: 40% paper, 14% metal, 20% food remains, 18% glass, 4% wood, 2% textiles and 2% plastic. On sanitary grounds, the greatest danger is caused by food remains and the wrappings from food products, as these can encourage insects and rodents. A danger to health can also exist in the residues from transported toxic materials. These residues are a constant problem during the loading and unloading of the ship. The other solid waste, e.g. kitchen waste, packing material (bottles, cans, boxes) and household waste, arises during the whole time the ship is being used.

Up to the time of the MAR POL 1973 [4] convention, solid waste from ships was (after leaving the port) usually dumped directly into the sea. In many countries, such a method of waste disposal is tolerated even now. As a result of the introduction of the MAR POL convention stipulations, solid waste disposal is now restricted not only in ports but also in coastal waters. Beyond a distance of 12 nautical miles from the coast, waste that sinks or that can be naturally broken down by the sea water can be jettisoned; beyond 25 nautical miles from the coast, wood and floating waste may be jettisoned (*International Conference on Marine Pollution*, [4]). The convention completely prohibits the disposal of plastic waste into the sea on most shipping routes (excluding the high seas).

On ships, therefore, the problem arises of finding a means of storing waste for a long period of time and making it as far as possible safe on board until it can be transferred to the sewage-treatment facilities. The difficulties connected with the storage of waste on ships and, in particular, the troublesome handling of it in ports, have led to the installation of waste combustion devices on ships, which continually burn away all kinds of waste. Although advantageous from the sanitary point of view, this solution does require great quantities of fuel and is very time consuming. Owing to the increased cost of fuel, the waste combustion device is often switched off in an effort to reduce expense. Irrespective of the methods of rendering the waste less harmful, there still exists the problem of storing it for a long or a short period of time on the ship. A good hygienic effect can be achieved by storing the waste in plastic bags, tightly closed after filling, in which form the waste can be taken to shore or disposed of in the combustion devices. The use of strong containers that can be tightly sealed prevents their being penetrated by insects and rodents. When the required quantity of plastic bags or suitable containers for waste is lacking, one observes on ships the increase of refuse on the open decks, which may present a sanitary danger not only for the ship itself but also for the environment (Sobol [10]).

With longer stays in ports or on roadstead, the sanitary state of the ship is dependent on the sanitation service of the port, which is responsible for accepting the waste from ships. Here, one observes certain deficiencies in many ports, and the keeping of rotting waste is a burdensome problem for both the ship and the port environment. It would be advisable for all countries to make the waste from ships as hygienic as possible in the port region so as to maintain a sanitary barrier. The delivery of waste to the communal dumping ground involves the possibility of spreading insects and rodents that normally do not occur in a given geographical zone, but could well be introduced by ships.

References

1. Buxton, G.V. and J.Schormann: Establishment of measures to control the discharge of vessels sewage. In: Proceedings of Symposium on prevention of pollution from ships. Acapulco 1976. VIII/2.
2. Economic and technical review report EPS 3-WP-76-3. Development of design guidelines for shipboard sewage holding tanks. Environment Canada. Water Pollution Control Directorate. March 1976.
3. Goethe, H.: Das Schiffsabwasserproblem - Die gesetzlichen Bestimmungen der USA und der UdSSR zur Vermeidung der Verunreinigung von Häfen, Flüssen und Seen durch Schiffe. Städtehyg. *22,* 9, 202–204 (1971).
4. International conference on marine pollution, 1973. Final act of the conference, with attachments, including international convention for the prevention of pollution from ships, 1973, and protocol relating to intervention on the high seas in cases of marine pollution by substances other than oil. London: IMCO 1974.
5. Lamoureux, V.B.: Guide to ship sanitation. Geneva: WHO 1967.
6. Perepeczko, A.: Okrętowe urzadzenia oczyszozające. [Clearance equipment on board of ships]. Gdańsk: Wydawnictwo Morskie 1976.
7. Sobol, Z. and T.Szumilas: Effect of pollution from vessels, on the sanitary state of coastal and port waters. In: VIII International symposium on Marine Medicine - Abstracts - 24–28 October, 1978. Varna 1978. p.297.
8. Sobol, Z. and T.Gorska: Hygienic estimation of the sewage treatment installation of ships. In: VII International symposium on marine medicine, Odessa, 23–30 Sept. 1976, USSR Ministry of Health, Moscow 1976. pp.315–316.
9. Sobol, Z., T. Szumilas and H.B.Wasilewska: The sanitary evolution of waste neutralization facilities on the Polish merchant ships. Bull. Inst. mar. trop. Med. Gdynia *32,* 314 (1981).
10. Sobol, Z.: Scieki i odpadki na statku. [Waste water and solid waste on board ships]. In: Dolmierski R. et al. (eds). Morski poradnik medyczny. [Medical guide for seafaring]. Warsaw: Panstwowy Zaklad Wydawnictw Lekarskich 1981. pp.357–366.

2.9 The Seafarer's Food

E. Zorn

In spite of the fact that undernutrition and avitaminoses have practically vanished nowadays, the standard of nutrition on board is in many ways deficient. The most frequent problems are:

Overnutrition
Malnutrition caused by an unbalanced diet
Monotony of meals
Unattractive and tasteless food
Poor hygiene in galleys

When dealing with the seafarer's food on board, the following points have to be considered:

1. The seafarer's nutrition on board is typical communal food, which rarely allows for any individual choice or extras.
2. Procuring provisions is practically impossible during voyages.
3. The energy consumption of seafarers differs according to type of vessel, occupation and shipping area. Generally energy consumption has shown a constant tendency to fall owing to continuously developing technology (increasing automation).
4. Changes of climate and the ship's motion may affect the appetite.
5. It may be difficult to prepare food on board small vessels during rough weather.
6. The psychological aspects of life on board during long voyages provoke a greater interest in food (Zorn [29]).

For the above reasons, nutrition on board is a delicate problem from a physiological and a hygienic point of view.

2.9.1 Nutritional Requirements on Board Vessels

In order to achieve high standards of nutrition on board, the following points should be observed:

1. Correspondence between the quantity of food and the average consumption of energy in order to achieve a balanced energy exchange
2. A mixed diet to provide the right amount of minerals and trace elements as well as vitamins
3. The prevention of microbiological and/or chemical contamination of food
4. The satisfactory timing of meals
5. Adaptation of type of food to the prevailing climatic conditions and the type of shipping trade
6. The aesthetic and tasteful preparation of food

2.9.2 The Energy Requirement

The physical load and, consequently, the consumption of energy have been constantly reduced by the developing standard of technology on board, i. e. the automation of the ship's operation. Heavy physical tasks like coal trimming, firing and handling of heavy hatches, which were still quite common not long ago have been reduced everywhere and the physical load is still decreasing. Most of the jobs consist of control and operational functions.

Studies on the work-load of crew members on board modern vessels have shown that members of the deck and the engine room staff are subject to a physical load of only medium level, but that occasionally they have to do heavier physical work (see Chap. 2.1). During the stay in ports the deck staff naturally work harder in the process of loading and unloading; the same is true of the ship's management. The engine room staff do extraordinarily heavy physical work during repairs and thus the consumption of energy is relatively high.

The physical work-load of crew members on board fishery vessels still represents an exception in seafaring. Although the physical work-load has generally been reduced, the tasks during the period of fishing must still be regarded as the heaviest physical work (Bühring [5]).

On passenger vessels the activities of the catering staff are defined as heavy physical work too (Israeli et al. [13]).

Unfavourable climatic and sea conditions mean additional load factors. Furthermore, factors like noise, vibrations and chemicals may affect the appetite and the metabolism of seamen. Finally, unfavourable psychological working conditions may influence the appetite and the energy exchange. On account of the many factors involved, evaluation of their individual effect is very difficult and the available data can serve only as a guide.

Balanced energy exchange (metabolism) is easily obtainable by exact measurement of the body weights of the individual crew members and the weight of the crew as a whole, as the body weights of healthy adults may indicate the differences between the storage and expenditure of energy. As the work-load on board modern vessels is fairly moderate, the average energy requirement is generally estimated at 12600–14700 kJ (3000–3500 kcal). Significant deviations may, however, occur as the load differs according to occupation. Additional deviations may be caused by work at sea or in ports. As the work-load of the catering personnel on board passenger vessels is rather high, the energy requirement is in general estimated at approx. 16800 kJ (4000 kcal).

The energy requirement of fishermen is considerably higher than the above figures: it is generally calculated at 16800–28400 kJ (4000–7000 kcal), although results reported by different authors vary considerably. Differences in type of vessel, equipment, weather and sea conditions in the fishing areas may figure prominently. For Polish deep sea fishermen average values of 16400–21000 kJ (4000–5000 kcal) per day are indicated by Kierst [14]. An even higher energy consumption was found in Soviet trawler fishermen, i.e. 17270–30400 kJ (4136–7238 kcal) (Bondarev et al. [3]). According to Weibelzahl [26], fishermen of the German Democratic Republic showed an approximate value of 23100 kJ (5500 kcal). Thorough investigations by analysis of breathing gas in Yugoslav seamen resulted in values from 14180 kJ to 18555 kJ (3376–4444 kcal) (Maver et al. [16]).

The high energy requirement and the high energy consumption of fishermen are exceptional in the merchant fleet. Consequently the food of fishermen has to be more nourishing, i.e. it has to supply more energy than that of crew members on board cargo vessels.

When comparing, very carefully and with restrictions, the average values of energy consumption of crew members of the merchant fleet with the values of the victualling bill and the calculated nutritive substances provided by allotments of provisions on board, it is evident that frequently the nutritive value of the consumed food is far higher than the value of energy consumption. The discrepancy between the supply of energy and the energy consumption may be related to the fact that physical work has decreased considerably on board modern vessels. The nutrition, however, has remained unchanged. The actual nourishment of crew members corresponds to the quantity of energy consumption several decades ago. Consequently the very substantial food intake involves the risk of overnutrition, whereas undernutrition occurs in very exceptional cases only.

The gross nutritive value of the food allotments of most maritime countries is above 16800 kJ (4000 kcal) (Wandel [25]; Bogetti [2]; Giannico et al. [8]; Øgrim [19]; Kierst [14]). The victualling bill of the German Federal Republic – which is not followed in practice – even contains a gross value of 25000 kJ (6000 kcal) (Zorn [29]). On an ocean-going oil tanker the average energy intake was 15070 kJ (3600 kcal) per man per day, of which 13230 kJ (3160 kcal) were derived from non-alcoholic sources (Eddy et al. [6]).

As stated above, weight measurements and medical examinations have proved that the mentioned nutritive values on board merchant vessels do not correspond with the actual energy consumption. Krynicki [15] found one-third of 1682 examined Polish seamen to be overweight, and several other authors have reported similar results (Goethe [10]; Roberts et al. [20]; Mitkova [17]). When calculating the total energy supply, alcohol should not be forgotten. On board West German vessels the average consumption is 4–5 bottles of beer per person per day (Zorn [28]).

The climatic influence on energy exchange should also be considered. As the rate of exchange decreases under high environmental temperatures and increases under low temperatures, the composition of food should be modified according to the conditions of the individual climatic zones to be crossed during long voyages. During voyages in the tropics the average energy requirement is approximately 10% lower than normal, whereas it is approximately 10% higher than normal during voyages in the polar zones. The changes in energy consumption caused by climatic influences may be even larger. The energy consumption is estimated at

- 12600 kJ (3000 kcal) in temperate zones
- 10500 kJ (2500 kcal) in the subtropics and the tropics
- 16800 kJ (4000 kcal) in polar zones (Giannico et al. [8])

The ship's motion and the resulting acceleration impulses affect the metabolism. It goes without saying that the gastrointestinal disorders caused by motion sickness lead to loss of nutriment and fluid. Slight cases of motion sickness involve a loss of appetite, and even in cases without the typical symptoms of nausea and vomiting the metabolism may be disturbed and glucose and ketone bodies are traceable in the urine (Goethe [9]). Consequently the energy exchange may be disturbed by acceleration impulses. Long-term motion sickness sometimes causes considerable loss of body weight.

2.9.3 Nutritive Substances

Adequate physiological nourishment consists firstly in the intake of well-balanced proportions of the main nutritive substances – proteins, fat and carbohydrates – as well as substances not providing energy: vitamins, minerals, bulk material and water. Consequently, the total value of nutritive substances is not the only important factor in optimal nutrition. A wisely balanced nourishment in respect of these substances is frequently unavailable on board. The proportions of the individual substances should be:

- Proteins, fat, carbohydrates 1:1:4
- In the tropics this should be 1:0.8:1 (Strothmann et al. [21])

Consequently, the following quantities are adequate:

- Proteins 100–110 g (in the tropics 80 g)
- Carbohydrates 400–440 g

relative to a total nutritive value of 12600–13440 kJ (3000–3200 kcal).

Calculations of the nutritive substances and the total nutritive value provided by the food allotments on board European vessels resulted in rather high values for lipids, which often exceeded 200 g. The proportion of fat frequently makes up 30%–40% of the total nutritive value, or even more, and thus is unreasonably high. According to the victualling bill of the German Federal Republic, the daily value of lipids amounts to 212 g per person, representing a rate of approx. 33%. On board Scandinavian and Polish vessels this value is even higher, i.e. 40% and more (Zorn [29]).

Overfeeding with lipids leads not only to adiposity, as already mentioned, but also to increased values of cholesterol and triglyceride in the blood. Kierst [14] stated that the average value of cholesterol in Polish seamen was 265.5 mg%; with a reduced supply of lipids the values became normal.

The proportion of proteins seems to be rather high in the seafarer's food on ships from the industrial countries. The average quantity is estimated at 130–160 g/person/day, sometimes even more. An evaluation of consumed food on board West German vessels showed the following results:
- Cargo liner 165 g/person/day
- Tanker 213 g/person/day (Zorn [29])

Giannico et al. [8] obtained similar results for the Italian merchant fleet, i.e. 165 g.

The required content of animal proteins in the usual seafarer's food are by far exceeded. A further increase should be avoided in order to exclude the risk of hyperuricaemia. A minimum of 30 g/person/day should be provided.

With respect to the important biological elements that are energy providers, the food should contain the following:

Mineral substances

Sodium	2–3 g
Chlorine	3–5 g
Calcium	800 mg
Potassium	2–3 g
Magnesium	260 mg
Phosphorus	800 mg
Iron	12 mg

Trace elements

Zinc	10 mg
Manganese	3–4 mg
Copper	2–5 mg
Fluoride	1 mg
Iodine	150 g
Cobalt	5–10 µg

Vitamins

A (axerophthol)	0.9 mg
B_1 (thiamine)	1.6 mg
B_2 (riboflavin)	2.0 mg
Niacin	15 mg
B_6 (pyridoxine)	1.8 mg
Folic acid	400 µg
Pantothenic acid	8 mg
B_{12}	5 µg
C (ascorbic acid)	75 mg
D (calcipherol)	2.5 µg
E (tocopherol)	12 mg

Finally, mention must be made of the bulk material, which consists of cellulose, the supporting substance of plants. This substance is not digested itself but stimulates the digestion and produces the subjective feeling of satiation.

Highly concentrated food with a high nutritive value is, mostly, poor in bulk material and therefore leads – particularly with hypokinesis – to chronic constipation, which is a frequent disorder in ships' crews.

The food on board ships of industrial countries, having rather high concentration of lipids and frequently proteins too, is sometimes poor in vitamins, mineral and trace substances. Additional factors that reduce the nutritive value are the small variety of foodstuffs and extended periods of storage. Although avitaminosis has practically disappeared, slight symptoms of deficiency are occasionally found. Especially during long voyages there may be a lack of fresh fruit and vegetables owing to difficulties in organising supplies or to economic factors. Furthermore, delicate food loses vitamins, particularly vitamin C, with long-term storage. Stutz and Reil [22] reported on a serious drop in the level of 1-ascorbic acid in the crew of a training vessel after a voyage of 4 weeks' duration. An examination of crew members after an 8-month voyage in the Antarctic showed a drop in vitamin C and B complex levels, and minor oral lesions were also diagnosed (Adams et al. [1]). Furthermore, it has to be remembered that vitamin levels are reduced considerably by the improper preparation of food and that the outer appearance and taste of fruit and vegetables alter with long-term storage, so that they are no longer liked. This may contribute to slight cases of avitaminosis, although satisfactory quantities of fruit and vegetable are available according to the victualling bill.

The level of different vitamins in the human body may be depressed by work in a hot environment and exposure to chemicals. Both these factors occur from time to time, or even regularly, during some special occupations on board (e.g. handling dangerous cargo). Additional environmental loads may affect the metabolism. According to the findings of the Nautical Medicine Institute in Moscow, vibrations may disturb the glycometabolism. The acceleration impulses (as mentioned already) and other factors may influence the crew members' appetite, digestion and assimilation of food (Bondarev et al. [4]).

The nutritive content and the timing of meals is mainly based on tradition and is subject to watch shifts and national habits. On board German vessels, breakfast is served from 7.30 to 8.30 a.m., lunch from 11.30 a.m. to 12.30 p.m., afternoon coffee from 3.00 to 3.15 p.m. and evening meal from 5.30 to 6.30 p.m. The timing of the meals largely corresponds with the rating on watch, i.e. shift work. It is, however, a great disadvantage that the interval from evening meal until breakfast in the morning is too long and therefore unfavourable for crew members doing shift work at night. This is, however, generally compensated for by making special kinds of food available in the refrigerator, e.g. sausage, cheese and sandwiches. The following distribution of nutritive value is recommended (Strothmann et al. [21]):

First breakfast	20%–25%
Second breakfast	5%–10%
Meal at noon	30%–35%
Afternoon coffee/tea	5%–10%
Evening meal	20%–30%

The above-mentioned percentage rates are based on a total requirement of approx. 14700 kJ (3500 kcal). The distribution over five meals has the advantage that sudden decreases in the blood sugar level, and thus excessive hunger, are prevented. Also, the load on the digestive system is reduced by several smaller quantities of food.

2.9.4 Scale of Ship's Provisions

It is necessary to develop a scale of provisions for all kinds of communal feeding and thus for the nutrition on board. The following items have to be considered (Wandel [25]):

1. Nutritive substances of foodstuffs and physiological aspects;
2. Provisions available and to be procured;
3. Seasonal, climatological and hygienic requirements;
4. Funds available;
5. Expenditure of work, equipment of galley and catering personnel available.

It goes without saying that the food should have a high concentration of biological elements and be nutritious, tasteful, budget priced and varied. The most important foodstuffs are meat and meat products, fish, potatoes, milk and milk products, rice, vegetables, pulses, farinaceous products, sugar, flaked oats and a lot of additional substances to achieve a greater variety of meals. When planning the weekly scale, one has to consider the special conditions of the shipping area, the kind of work on board, possible trends in the crew's taste etc. Of course, communal feeding cannot replace home meals and consequently cannot meet individual requirements fully. Advice on suitable diets should be part of general health education. It has to be emphasised that, in communal feeding, physiological and hygienic aspects are of major importance.

2.9.5 Procurement of Provisions

The procurement of provisions may be effected in three different ways:
1. By the shipowning company;
2. By the shipowning company together with crew members in charge of nutrition on board;
3. By the catering staff only.

Presumably the procurement of provisions by the shipping company only, is unfavourable for the ship's crew, as it is fairly difficult to meet the actual requirements of crew members.

Furthermore the following points are to be borne in mind (Wandel [25]):
1. Fruit and vegetables should be supplied when they are in season.
2. Only certain kinds of foodstuff can be prepared in the galley, given the available equipment and the numbers and knowledge of the catering staff.
3. Storage facilities aboard may limit the choice of food.

The cost of foodstuffs should not be the most important factor. Very often ready-made deep-frozen dishes, packed meat in individual portions, or fruit and vegetables of high quality seem to be more economical as there is less waste and the catering staff have less work to do (Troeder [23]; Wolf [27]).

Some further points are important:
1. Duration of voyage;
2. Climatic zone to be crossed;
3. Long periods at deep sea, when it is impossible to procure further provisions.

2.9.6 Storage of Provisions on Board

The preservation of foodstuffs is dependent on the storage facilities available. They should be highly effective to guarantee good, wholesome food which is greatly appreciated by the crew. It has to be pointed out that, owing to improper storage and inadequate preservation facilities, spoiled food formerly led to outbreaks of food poisoning during long voyages.

Naturally, different foodstuffs have to be stored in different ways:
1. In deep-freeze rooms,
2. In cold-stores,
3. In store-rooms with temperatures from +2 °C to +12 °C,
4. In store-rooms with living room temperatures.

The deep-freeze rooms should be kept at temperatures of −18 °C and below. A temperature of −30 °C is recommended for long-term storage, i.e. for more than three months. This prevents losses of vitamin C in foodstuffs. Premature thawing of deep-frozen foodstuffs must always be avoided. The food should be thawed only directly before use. Quick heating to +100 °C (by micro-waves) is most favourable. If there are temperatures higher than −15 °C, the refrigerating requirements of deep-frozen foods are no longer met, and they can no longer be stored. Temperatures of +2 °C to +4 °C guarantee preservation of perishable food for a few days only.

It is necessary to keep a cold-store absolutely clean. Meat, fish, vegetables and fruit should be stored in separate compartments. Preserved foodstuffs should be stored in well-ventilated rooms with temperatures of +4 °C to +12 °C. Dried foodstuffs in original packing can be stored at living room temperatures.

In order to preserve the taste and quality of the individual foodstuffs, they should be stored vacuum packed in foil or bags and be protected against damage by destructive insects. Mouldy foodstuffs should be destroyed because of their aflatoxin content.

The following kinds of store-room should be available on board larger vessels (Strothmann et al. [21]):
1. Deep-freeze room with temperatures of −20 °C to −30 °C for meat, meat products and fish;
2. Deep-freeze rooms with temperatures of

−18 °C to −30 °C for ready-made dishes, vegetables and ice cream;
3. Cold-store with temperatures of +2 °C to +4 °C for butter, margarine, eggs, cheese, milk products, prepared food, bread and confectionery;
4. Cold-stores with temperatures from +2 °C to +8 °C for fruit and vegetables;
5. Dry-store (approx. +15 °C) for preserved food, coffee, tea, flour, rice, potatoes, fresh and dried vegetables etc.

The store-rooms should be inspected regularly in order to avoid shortcomings. The following instructions should be observed:
1. Before starting the voyage: cleaning and disinfection of store-rooms; inspection of store-rooms; older provisions to be stored at the front of the rooms.
2. During the voyage: regulation and control of air temperatures and humidity; opening of rooms only once per day, especially deep-freeze rooms, to take out food-stuffs; older provisions and perishable food to be used first.
3. At the end of the voyage: old provisions to be marked and stored at the front of the rooms.

It goes without saying that if the ship carries a doctor, he is in charge of sanitary control, including inspection of store-rooms and the catering area.

2.9.7 The Qualification of the Ship's Cook

The qualification of the ship's cook is of utmost importance for the quality of nutrition on board and thus affects the well-being of crew members. A high-quality catering staff is a conditio sine qua non on board passenger vessels, whereas the qualification of cooks employed on cargo liners often leaves much to be desired. Three months' theoretical-practical training, as practised in the German Federal Republic at Travemünde and in the UK at Gravesend, should be compulsory. A ship's cook should be more creative than a conventional cook ashore, i.e. he should be able to offer a lot of different dishes from a restricted variety of foodstuffs in order to prevent monotony. Furthermore, he has to have and employ a basic knowledge of sanitary hygiene. Naturally, the shipowning company requires the ship's cook to make the best use of food and to victual economically in foreign ports (Herrmann [12]).

2.9.8 Further Problems of Nutrition on Board

1. The future vessel will predominantly be at sea.
2. The stay in ports will be shortened to a minimum.
3. The number of crew members will be reduced to the lowest possible level (see Chap. 2.1).

This will naturally complicate the procurement of provisions in foreign ports. The personnel reduction, of course, also involves the catering staff. It will then be necessary to deliver ready-prepared food to the ship and to adequately adapt the facilities of the galleys and store-rooms to the special requirements (Troeder [23]; Hein [11]). Semi-prepared foodstuffs (e.g. potato products, dry soups, cakes and ready mixed pastries) make preparatory work unnecessary. They require only brief cooking or baking. The same is true of dehydrated products (e.g. dried vegetables). Ready-made products (dishes, soups, puddings etc.) require only brief heating (Wolf [27]; Wachtel [24]). There are several advantages in using these products: minimum waste disposal, space-saving storage, no seasonal difficulties with the supply of fruit and vegetables, satisfactory level of hygiene and quick preparation for serving. Technical prerequisites for the storage and preparation of these products are sufficiently large deep-freeze rooms and galleys with quick-thawing devices (micro-waves etc.). Disadvantages are higher prices, organisational difficulties in procuring deep-frozen products in some ports and maintenance of the required temperature. A psychological aspect to be considered is the reduction in motivation of the ship's cook caused by the underuse of his professional skills. Finally, it has to be emphasised that on board the vessels of the future, the mental load of crew members will be rather high. Owing to the additional monotony of long voyages and in the absence of other stimulation, crew members will become unreasonably interested in food, and high-quality food is thus very important in maintaining morale.

In conclusion, it should be mentioned that some other problems on board may be related to nutrition, i.e. infectious diseases caused by contaminated food (see Chap. 4.3), water hygiene (see Chap. 2.7), drinking habits and consumption of alcohol (see Chap. 4.4) and the problem of sea survival rations (see Chap. 5.11).

References

1. Adams, R.J., R.S. Harding and W.R. Stanmeyer: Antarctic stress and vitamin requirements. J. dent. Med. *17*, 1, 36–42 (1962).
2. Bogetti, B.: Considerazioni sulla razione alimentare per gli equipaggi delle navi della marine mercantile italiana. Ann. Med. nav. *80*, 2, 191–218 (1975).
3. Bondarev, G.I., E.Sh. Zinovyev, Yu.A. Nepoklonov et al.: Energeticheskie zatraty i vitaminnaya obespechennost organizma promyslovykh rabochikh bolshikh morozilnykh rybolovnykh trawlerov pri lovle ryby v vodakh severnoy Atlantiki. [Energy expenditure and vitamin supply of workers engaged in big refrigerator fishing trawlers operating in waters of North Atlantic]. Vop. Pitan. *21*, 22–26 (1964).
4. Bondarev, G.I., E.N. Aronova, D.A. Mikhelson et al.: K voprosu o vliyanii obshchey vertikalnoy vibratsii i shuma na ryad pokazateley belkovogo, shirovogo i uglevodnogo obmena u teplokrovnykh schivotnykh. [Effects of vertical vibration and noise on the exchange of albumen, fat and carbohydrate of warm-blooded animals]. Gig. Tr. prof. Zabol. *12*, 10, 58–59 (1968).
5. Bühring, J.: Die Ernährung auf Hochseefischereifahrzeugen der Deutschen Bundesrepublik mit Berücksichtigung der Arbeits- und Klimasituation. Dissertation University of Hamburg 1971.
6. Eddy, T.P., A.L. Stock and E.F. Wheeler: Nutritional and environmental studies on an ocean-going oil tanker. 3. Energy balances and physique. Br. J. industr. Med. *28*, 330–341 (1971).
7. Empfehlungen für die Nährstoffzufuhr. Ed.: Deutsche Gesellschaft f. Ernährung. Frankfurt: Umschau Verlag 1975.
8. Giannico, L., B. Tortori-Donati and S. Biancone: L'alimentazione dei marittimi a bordo delle navi mercantili italiane. Considerazioni sugli aspetti igienico-sanitari. Ann. Sanità pubbl. *29*, 6, 1473–1490 (1968).
9. Goethe, H.: Kinetosen – Reisekrankheiten. In: Innere Medizin in Praxis und Klinik. Vol. 3. Ed.: H. Hornbostel, W. Kaufmann and W. Siegenthaler. 2nd edn. Stuttgart: Thieme 1977. pp. 1439–1445.
10. Goethe, H.: Personal information 1968.
11. Hein, G.: Die Verwendung von Tiefkühlkost in Gemeinschaftsverpflegungs-Einrichtungen an Bord. In: Referate d. Arbeitstagung über "Probleme d. Ernährung an Bord". Hamburg 1969. pp. 131–137.
12. Herrmann, H.: Probleme der Bordverpflegung aus der Sicht der Reederei. In: Referate d. Arbeitstagung über "Probleme d. Ernährung an Bord". Hamburg 1969. pp. 61–73.
13. Israeli, R., M. Weinstein and D. Süssmann: Untersuchungen über die Arbeitsplatzanforderungen an Bord von Passagierschiffen. Neuzeitliche Gesichtspunkte bei Einstellungsuntersuchungen von Seeleuten. Arbeit und Leistung *21*, 8, 145–147 (1967).
14. Kierst, W.: Ernährung der Fischer und Seeleute. In: Fragen der Schiffahrtsmedizin. Vorträge aus dem Int. Symp., Heiligendamm, 28–31 March 1963. Special issue Medizinischen Dienstes des Verkehrswesens II. pp. 244–251.
15. Krynicki, A.: Occurrence of overweight and obesity, and their influence on the health condition of crews of the Polish merchant marine and deep-sea fishing companies. (Summary of the doctor's degree dissertation). Bull. Inst. mar. Med. Gdańsk *24*, 1/2, 17–33 (1973).
16. Maver, H., M. Kovačević and Z. Grgić: Energetska potrošnja ribara. [Consumption of energy with fishermen]. In: Pomorska medicina. (Naučne rasprave). Belgrad: Izdanje Mornaričkog glasnika 1975. pp. 307–315. (Pomorska biblioteka 26)
17. Mitkova, N.: The scientific fundamentals of nutrition for seamen on tankers. In: III International Symposium on Marine Medicine, Leningrad 1968. Moscow 1969. pp. 136–138.
18. Mitkova, N.: About the problem of overfeeding and obesity of seamen. Bull. Inst. mar. trop. Med. Gdynia *25*, 2/3/4, 459–460 (1974).
19. Øgrim, M.E.: Kosthold til Sjøs. T. norske Laegeforen *84*, 18, 1257–1263 (1964).
20. Roberts, R.H., W.I. Morse, W. Josenhans et al.:

Studies in obesity among naval personnel. Med. Serv. J. Can. *19*, 8 604–630 (1963).

21. Strothmann, H., R. von Richthofen, E. Zorn et al.: Ernährung und Proviant an Bord von Seeschiffen. Ed.: Sozialwerk für Seeleute e. V. Lübeck 1978: LN-Druck. (up to date, Weiterbildung an Bord 14)
22. Stutz, E. and G. Reil: C-Vitaminspiegeluntersuchungen während der Westindienreise der Segelschulschiffe "Horst Wessel" und "Albert Leo Schlageter". Veröffentlichungen aus dem Gebiet des Marine-Sanitätswesens 30, 148–156 (1938).
23. Troeder, H. G.: Zukunftsprobleme der Bordernährung. In: Referate d. Arbeitstagung über "Probleme d. Ernährung an Bord". Hamburg 1969. pp. 96–108.
24. Wachtel, U.: Die Verwendung von vorgefertigten Produkten in Gemeinschaftsverpflegungseinrichtungen. In: Referate d. Arbeitstagung über "Probleme d. Ernährung an Bord". Hamburg 1969. pp. 119–130.
25. Wandel, A.: Die Ernährung in der Bundesmarine. In: Referate d. Arbeitstagung über "Probleme d. Ernährung an Bord". Hamburg 1969. pp. 42–60 a.
26. Weibelzahl, H.: Ernährung unter Bordbedingungen. Verk.-Med. *14*, 7, 239–250 (1967).
27. Wolf, W.: Dehydrokost im Dienste moderner Küchenpraxis. In: Referate d. Arbeitstagung über "Probleme d. Ernährung an Bord". Hamburg 1969. pp. 138–147.
28. Zorn, E.: Die Ernährung der Schiffsbesatzungen. Zbl. Arbeitsmed. *28*, 10, 280–283 (1978).
29. Zorn, E.: Die Ernährungssituation der Seeleute. In: Referate d. Arbeitstagung über "Probleme d. Ernährung an Bord". Hamburg 1969. pp. 19–30.

2.10 Psychological Problems in Seafaring

H. Böhm

2.10.1 Introduction

The common objective of nautical medicine and nautical psychology is to improve the working and living conditions in seafaring. Both disciplines use similar methods: *observation* to collect the multiple factors of a distinct phenomenon (behaviour); *diagnosis* to find and define the common denominator and the underlying structure; and *therapy* to contrive, develop and apply means to change (to "improve") the phenomenon.

There are two main differences between nautical medicine and nautical psychology:

1. Nautical medicine has a long history, whereas nautical psychology is in its infancy.
2. The reactions of the human body are less influenced by sociocultural factors than those of the psychological structure.

To understand the present state of nautical psychology (especially in connection with nautical medicine) and the form future cooperation between the disciplines may take, it is necessary to have a closer look at these differences.

ad 1:

Some facts prove the short history of nautical psychology:

a) There were but few publications in this special field before 1960.
b) Psychological selection (unlike medical selection) is not obligatory in nearly all countries.
c) The first step to improve human relationships on board internationally was taken in 1978 by the IMCO-resolution 22:

The conference
Having adopted the International Convention on Standards of Training, Certification and Watchkeeping for Seafarers 1978

Recognizing that not only safe operation of the ship and its equipment but also good human relationships between the seafarers on board would greatly enhance the safety of life at sea

Noting that the knowledge of personnel management, organization and training aboard ships is required for certification of supervisory personnel

Recommends that this knowledge includes knowledge of basic principles of human relationships and social responsibility

Invites all Governments:

a) to establish or encourage the establishment of training programmes aimed at safeguarding good human relationships on board ships;
b) to take adequate measures to minimize any element of loneliness and isolation for crew members on board ships;
c) to ensure that crew members are sufficiently rested before commencing their duties.

This resolution started a growing international cooperation; as yet the cooperation is not institutionalized, i.e. there are no common research projects, but this will in all probability change, within the next few years.

ad 2:

The "reactions" of the psychological structure are deeply influenced by sociocultural factors. The consequences of this psychological principle are obvious: *Even if the basic individual psychological structures and the factors of the environment are the same in a defined situation, two people will react differently according to their sociocultural "programme" if they are members of differ-*

ent groups. Applying this to seafaring leads to the observation that, although seafarers of different countries share similar problems, they react in different ways; in addition, since research is not internationally coordinated, its main emphasis lies on solving specific national problems – consequently the possibility of comparisons is very limited. There is another consequence: giving the results of national research can lead to bias in the psychological assessment and favour wrong decisions. Very often there is but one national result available and there is no scientific possibility of generalizing this result without further knowledge. General scientific statements presuppose general knowledge based on differentiated research and comparisons on the basis of a defined level of significance.

The present state of nautical psychology does not allow us to generalize *results* of psychological research but does permit us to describe *problems* in seafaring.

2.10.2 Main Psychological Problems and Factors

Nautical psychologists of different countries agree on the statement that seafarers share similar problems, but they differ in the proposed solutions. Since this handbook addresses doctors involved in the practice of various aspects of nautical medicine, it seems reasonable to describe the main psychological problems and factors in order to help the asking of pertinent questions and to provide background material.

The following features are selected according to their importance and their relation to the well-being and health of seafarers.

2.10.2.1 Mental Capacities and Selection

Men working on board need general and specific mental capacities:

Perception. The seaman should know the limits of his power of observation, the causes of hallucinations (formed by certain "outside" constellations of stimuli or "inside" structure of motivation) and the resultant errors and dangers.

Intelligence. Intellectual factors such as quick apprehension, flexibility, concentration, imagination, faculty to abstract and a retentive memory are of basic importance. Especially, the officers must be able to recognize inter-relationships in new situations, to find adequate solutions and to verbalize them. We do not yet know the effects of intelligence – whether a higher level produces fewer mistakes or an average one produces a better capacity for observing.

Knowledge. Professional knowledge is probably more effective as a result of experience.

Motivation. The structure of motivation influences the power of observation and decision.

Emotion. Emotions affect the capacity for work. Stability and well-balanced emotions are necessary to withstand different stress situations.

Will. The strength of will influences efficiency. Discipline, self-control and organization of work depend on the ability to prevail over factors such as tiredness and weakness. Decisions must be made in conflict situations and under stress.

Man–Machine Interface. The technical components of the ship demand special capabilities: technical knowledge and know-how, control of precise motions (to adjust instruments), quick reactions, carefulness, thoroughness etc. Next to these relatively constant factors are short-term circumstantial ones which alter efficiency, e.g. illness, overtiredness, alcohol and anger.

To find out which capacities really are needed, an exact psychological analysis of the working and living conditions on board is necessary. This requires the cooperation of psychologists and experts with nautical, ergonomic, medical, physical and technical knowledge and experienced operators, masters and pilots of ships. The differentiated picture of capacities and the order of priority could be shown by a flow-diagram. This would enable us to perform the important task of selection in the best (objective and efficient) manner possible. The different capabilities of persons could be made useful in different parts of the systems. Furthermore this would help us to observe and discover the effects of the system regarding men working in and depending on it and to control the changing of the system for the benefit of man.

"Selection" can also help the candidate to avoid a wrong decision and thus avoid an unhappy, unsuccessful life at sea, and would support the efforts to reduce accidents and improve safety at sea.

Nobody believes it to be a foolish waste of time to select according to defined standards of professional knowledge and skills. The value of health and body fitness as criteria in the selection of seamen is beyond all dispute, but many of the responsible people in the shipping industry hesitate to accept mental structure as a similar criterion. By contrast, in other industries the importance of psychological tests has been known for a long time and selection made obligatory.

It is not my intention to go into further details – all I want to do is, as a result of many discussions with colleagues from different countries, to promote the idea of selection and to ask all experts for help.

2.10.2.2 Function and Role

Working and living conditions normally can be separated into (a) place of work, (b) social field and (c) individual sphere. This is applicable to most conditions ashore, an exception being so-called total institutions (prisons, hospitals, military units etc.). The ship is a sort of total institution, because all three fields are nearly inseparable and unchanging. They form a unit in which each part influences the others constantly and to a high degree. There is almost no chance for the crew members to forget their function within the working system and play another role during their leisure time. An officer, for example, is an officer in all situations and during his entire presence on board. His role, i.e. his expected behaviour according to his position in the hierarchy, is like an armour which he cannot leave off. This can have advantages and disadvantages: advantages if he is a labile, unstable person who needs support, disadvantages if he is a "normal" (in the statistical sense), "average" person. Psychological theories agree on the fact that it is important for the mental hygiene and development to change roles. If a person is denied this chance the consequences can be frustration and rigidity.

Frustration leads to: aggression, regression, indifference and fixation. The ability to tolerate frustrating situations differs from person to person. Accidents, sicknesses, crimes and misdeeds, quarrels and fights, hard drinking etc. are significant symptoms of widespread frustration.

The fixed working hierarchy and schedule, the unvarying living conditions and quarters, and the ever-present and never-changing company of other crew members form a pressure which makes it understandable that rigid roles, with all their drawbacks, are chosen as a method of self-defence.

2.10.2.3 Watch System

A specific factor of the working conditions on board is the watch system. On most ships the watch of the deck officers is 4 hours twice a day in a never-changing pattern:

Officer A:	0.00– 4.00	12.00–16.00
Officer B:	4.00– 8.00	16.00–20.00
Officer C:	8.00–12.00	20.00–24.00

This system stresses the physical and mental capabilities of man. It is proven that working in shifts and during the night has a cumulative effect with the consequence of a higher rate of sicknesses. This situation cannot be totally changed as long as ships work for 24 hours a day. All that can be done is to test different watch systems and to minimize the harmful effects by medical and psychological compensations.

2.10.2.4 Social Climate

It is not an easy task to define what is called "social climate". It would be very satisfying to have an all-round definition but it is reasonable to confine the attempt to the more pragmatic side of the problem. Trying to analyse "social climate" leads to the conclusion that there are at least two categories of psychological and sociological factors which are used to define it:

1. The first category is based on scientific research and includes results of a wide range of experiments and observations. Some of these factors are: type of organization, information, communication, cooperation, interaction, group relations, role functions, participation, social adaptation, acceptation etc. Also part of this category are descriptions of the influence of working and living conditions on board and the knowledge that a "negative" social climate decreases productivity and activity and increases the number of accidents and sicknesses.
2. The second category contains factors which express more the direction in which "social climate" should be developed. The words used are more emotional and philosophical than rational and scientific. Some examples: good will, mutual help, responsibility for others, confidence, social mind, understanding, friendship, respect, care, compassion, peacableness and loyalty. In many fields the negative form is better known than the positive type. This is applicable to the social climate too. There are a number of well-known factors which create a "negative climate": envy, jealousy; tension, discordance; quarrel, struggle, conflicts; defamation; insecurity, uncertainty; compulsion, force, constraint, pressure; excessive strain, tediousness, dullness; lack of organization; dissatisfaction. It is one of the main tasks of all those responsible for the well-being of seafarers to reduce as many negative factors as possible.

2.10.2.5 "Natural" and "Artificial" Environment

Observing man and his environment leads to the general sentence that man lives – to state an extreme case – within two environments: the one is formed by "natural" conditions, the other by "artificial" ("technical", "man-made") conditions. The "borders" are not exactly defined, because there are overlappings and mixtures of every kind. But it seems to be important to show the psychological difference between those two environments.

In the natural environment, man reacts to conditions as if by instinct; in the artificial environment he lacks the pattern – which is replaced by the limitations of his intelligence. He must be guided, through ongoing conscious relearning of the laws and rules of procedure. Frequently automatic response replaces conscious effort as a result of training.

Present-day ships do not belong to the natural environment of man. Their specific problems can be solved in greater part only with the aid of additional instruments and methods. The naive transposing of natural patterns of behaviour into the technical world of seafaring leads to gross oversimplification and apparent solutions in many cases. The resultant feeling of security creates an additional danger; "additional" because we can expect more failures within the technical environment than within the natural one.

Specific laws and rules must be developed to master the technical world – rules which are adapted as much as possible to human nature. Rules which are not adaptable require rational learning, sometimes conflicting with natural patterns of behaviour. The quality of rules and remedies depends on the more or less successful approximation to natural behaviour and the more or less comprehensible, clear, simple and precise formulation and definition.

Consequently, we have to find out the borders between the natural and the artificial environments, to adapt technical remedies as closely as possible to human nature and to adapt man to the remainder by suitable means and methods.

2.10.2.6 Safety and Proneness to Accidents

It is known that a certain mental structure predestines a person to become involved in accidents, either actively as the "producer" or passively as the victim. If determinate characteristic attributes appear, it would be reasonable to check the candidate more closely in order to prevent safety risks. The long-term aim of the project is a contribution to aptitude tests for seafaring personnel. Some day it will probably become possible to select the "non-successful" even before he (or she) sets foot aboard a ship.

Below are set out the main theoretical considerations from which it could be concluded that the "safety attitude" and the "risk-taking attitude" form a stable mental set which does not change quickly under different influences.

1. It is common psychological knowledge that *patterns of behaviour* are stable and do not alter in similar situations. According to the behaviouristic learning theory, reactions are innate or learned. If they are innate, they appear at all times in the same or slightly modified course like instinctive behaviour. Whether reactions are learned or not depends on whether they are successful: Unsuccessful reactions more or less vanish – speaking of the normal and not of the psychopath – whereas successful reactions are repeatedly shown. Positive reinforcement leads to repetition until the individual is conditioned and the reactions follow a constant path. A certain stimulus (for example a certain traffic situation) produces a conditioned response.
2. Being prepared to take risks is – amongst other things – an expression of *self-confidence* and *self-evaluation*. This self-rating shows the subjectively perceived power to cope with the problems of life; and it is in just this part of the individual mental structure that a relative constancy of behaviour can be observed. Variations of behaviour connected with self-confidence in the direction of self-overrating or underrating point to mental disorder and a psychopathological personality.
3. In situations to which the individual is not (yet) adjusted, the subject tries immediately to acquire this adjustment by *self-regulation*. In order to master risky circumstances and to react effectively, a conscious or unconscious regulation is needed. This regulation of behaviour strives towards the long-term aims of the individual. It is part of the personality structure. Experiments have confirmed that this typical self-regulation lasts nearly continuously during the individual's lifetime.

Persons with a high accident rate do not adjust their behaviour to the rules and standards of their group easily and without problems. They tend to violate laws and regulations. Very often they grew up in families with various problems (economic distress, divorced parents, mental disorders and sicknesses). During their time in school they faced specific difficulties: reduced learning capacity and power of concentration, falling behind in their work, quarrels, first encounters with the police, actions contrary to an order, offering resistance, penalties etc.

These problems continue uninterrupted during their vocational career: interruption of apprenticeships, changing of companies, fights and quarrels with colleagues and officers, irregularity, unpunctuality, sicknesses etc. The devil's circle often closes with the same problems in their own family as were present in their parents' family.

2.10.2.7 Communication on Board

The existence of communication difficulties caused by language barriers on board many ships is a well-known fact, at least to those concerned. Outsiders, on the other hand, tend to handle these problems by "easy solutions". Usually their proposal is to make the language of the country of registry the compulsory means of communication. In reality, however, this is not always feasible. Multinational crews have become an accepted feature of seafaring and efforts to overcome language barriers connected with this trend must be made by all concerned.

Communication among crew members is not possible on all vessels to the same extent. Five typical situations may be distinguished:

1. All crew members come from the same country and speak the same language – their mother tongue. Communication problems do not arise, as long as all have a command of nautical terminology.
2. All crew members but one speak in their same mother tongue. There are bound to be few communication problems, as this linguistic outsider has to adapt quickly and will do so, in order to become integrated into his social surrounding.
3. On board ship there are members of different national groups with no common mother tongue. Even in this case no major problems are to be expected as all have to agree to the use of one common language. Experiences on tramp vessels have shown English to be this lingua franca.
4. Two or three national groups are encountered aboard ship, being employed in different departments, types of work etc. Generally an interpreter in a key function, e.g. as boatswain, will be a member of the crew. Thus communication causes few problems, at least in the operational field.
5. Members of two or three linguistic groups are on board and have to cooperate in all sectors. This is where the real problems do arise, since a common basis for communication has to be created.

From linguistic points of view, three different levels of linguistic performance can be distinguished:

1. Level of instructions and orders
2. Level of simplified conversation
3. Level of perfection

The differences between these levels are not only in the extent and complexity of grammar and vocabulary, but also in their main sectors of application.

Good communication is indispensable for:

1. *The safety of the crew and vessel.* Communication on board is not a personal matter for crewmen – it is above all necessary to ensure the safety of all.
2. *Smooth operation.* All crew members must possess a common basis for (verbal and non-verbal) communication if the ship is to operate smoothly.
3. *The social climate on board.* Communication with other people is necessary if individuals are to be balanced and efficient. Isolation results in mental alterations and abnormal behaviour which may have undesirable consequences.
4. *Individual satisfaction.* Beyond its immediate applicability as a means of communication, linguistic competence can be a medium to achieve a more complex personality and a broader approach to life.

All these aspects show communication and language to be a vital feature of life on board.

It will be difficult to reach a general agreement on the issue of *who* has to learn the other's language – if it should be (a) the foreigner, who has to master the ship's language, or (b) the officer, who must be able to employ the language of his foreign crew members in order to achieve perfectly functioning working conditions. As the safety of all crew members is at stake, every ship or possibly every shipping company must find their own solution.

2.10.2.8 Separation from Society and Family

One of the factors with the greatest consequences for the psychological situation of seafarers is the separation from their society, family and friends. The time of absence is sometimes 6–9 months or even longer. During this time, their connection with the groups they belong to is very loose, which can lead to significant changes and effects:

1. The complicated and differentiated norms and standards, rules, regulations and patterns of behaviour in (modern) societies are not constantly modifying behaviour and, as a result of less "training", are more or less regarded as unimportant and neglected.
2. Seafaring and, very often, each company and even each ship builds up a catalogue of norms and rules: the "style". Everyone on board has to adjust his behaviour to this demand; if somebody does not, his personal situation will become difficult and he has to live as an outsider with all the negative consequences.
3. The separation from the family not only influences the emotional relations between the partners but also causes problems in the family management and affairs and the bringing up of children. In many countries the patriarchal system is traditionally favoured. This changes, necessarily, to the matriarchal system during the absence of the seaman father. The mother has to solve the daily problems. The situation changes again during the (often long) vacations of the seaman.
4. Aboard a ship the seaman has to live together with other seamen whom he had no chance to select. He is forced to come to terms with the others whether he likes them or not. His real friends ashore are far away and the opportunities to talk to them rare. He misses – if he has no friends aboard – the favours and privileges of friendship: confidence, veracity, relaxation, empathy, common interests etc.

2.10.2.9 Information

Closely connected to the separation is the fact that seafarers very often live in a vacuum regarding information. In comparison to the ever-present information they receive ashore (press, radio, T.V.), the chances to receive information about the events in the "world" (especially "back home") are very limited. Theoretically there are some possibilities but in practice they are very often neglected. This can lead to a reduction in knowledge and to indifference.

There is another consequence: not being well-informed often implies not being able to look after one's own interests.

2.10.2.10 Image

Many, and in other aspects very different, countries face a common problem: the necessity to improve the image of the seafarer. This image, i.e. the picture of seamen held by non-seamen, has lost many of its positive details during recent years, negative items becoming dominant.

The image of the seafarer has a direct relation to the "climate" on board: If we succeed in improving the image, "better" people will be attracted and these will change the climate. This task is sometimes part of a wider project, but mostly it is handled by smaller units alone (for example shipping companies), often with insufficient resources. The best way to achieve greater success will be to combine efforts and to provide everyone who is willing and able to help with adequate information. And there are many persons and institutions who are able to help – in fact, everyone earning his money directly or indirectly from the sea.

2.10.2.11 Teaching and Training

There are more psychological problems in seafaring than this short survey, highlighting some examples, could show. To enable the reader to achieve a deeper insight and find possibilities to help as an expert in nautical medicine, it seems reasonable to give an overview of the world-wide state of teaching and training of personnel management and human relationships on board.

The following incomplete list of topics shows those subjects which are regarded as important in many countries: basic psychological and sociological knowledge; leadership; role functions; responsibility; information; communication; training and instruction; decision making; group dynamics; sensitivity training; interpersonal skills; assessment of co-workers; team work; negotiation skills; conducting meetings; motivation; management of conflicts, stress and emergencies; alcohol and drugs; introduction of a new worker; leisure time; basic ergonomic knowledge.

2.10.3 Future Aspects

Technical development alters the traditional and familiar environment of the sailor: ships become faster and larger, a few ship classes develop into numerous special ships, automation takes over in more and more areas of ship operation, lay-times become shorter, ports are built far from the next town etc. These changes influence seafarers and their mutual life on board. Some of the major consequences are:

1. Reduction of the crew – with more isolation and boredom on the one hand and rising stress and over-strain on the other;
2. Greater demands for theoretical learning and practical training;
3. Less leisure time and opportunities for sightseeing and making and meeting friends abroad;
4. Less time to compensate for the strain of a voyage.

The traditional hierarchical systems of leadership can no longer satisfactorily overcome the new problems; more and more new methods of leadership are replacing the old forms, paying more attention to the individual and relations in a group.

To overcome the negative effects of reduced manning, new models of living and leisure time and quarters are being developed.

The traditional connections and links between ship and company ashore are being revised.

World-wide, national and international institutes are trying to find practical and theoretical solutions to the problems of life on board ship. The factor "man" is finding increasing attention in scientific publications and the considerations of those working with seamen.

References

Publications

In view of the short history of nautical psychology as an entity, no complete integration of conclusions can be expected. In most cases psychological and sociological research has been done by individual scientists in limited circumstances. International co-operation and coordination – now initiated during some international meetings and slowly developing – has been restricted to personal communications and occasional discussions about common problems. The outcome of this situation is a widespread variety of publications. The future research should be better coordinated and more representative regarding the situation in seafaring.

The following list contains examples of publications from different countries and various aspects of nautical psychology connected in some way with nautical medicine.

Psychological Changes and Abnormalities, Psychopathology, Alcohol and Drugs, Suicides

Bevilacqua, C.: Le psiconevrosi dei marittimi come causa di inidoneità alla navigazione. Lav. e Med. *18,* 105–112 (1964).

Bokum, P.: Život i rad na brodu, mogući provokator paranoidnog reagiranja. (Life and work on board ships – possible provocators of paranoid behaviour.) In: Pomorska medicina II (Naučne rasprave). Belgrad: Izdanje Mornaričkog glasnika 1979. pp. 227–231 (Pomorska biblioteka. Sveska 30)

Brykin, I. S., V. M. Krivobokov and L. I. Klishchenko: Psikhoprofilaktika psikhoterapiya v dlitelnikh morskikh pokhodakh. (Psychoprophylaxis and psychotherapeutics during long sea voyages.) Voen.-med. Zh. 9, 53-54 (1974).

Dolatkowski, A., K. Dega and S. Klajman: The effect of working conditions at sea on the psychophysiological state of seamen. In: III. International Symposium on Marine Medicine, Leningrad, 1968. Moscow 1969. pp. 24-29.

Dolmierski, R. and J. Palubicki: Anxiety level in seamen during sea trip. Bull. Inst. mar. trop. Med. Gdynia *31*, 1/2, 15-20 (1980).

Dolmierski, R.: Neurosen und Verhaltensstörungen bei Seeleuten. In: V. Internationales Symposium über Schiffahrtsmedizin, 19-21 Oct. 1972. Rostock 1973. pp. 25-30.

Dolmierski, R. and K. J. de Walden: Ocena kliniczna przyczyn samobójstw u marynarzy. (Clinical evaluation of suicides by seamen.) Psychiat. Pol. *6*, 3, 255-258 (1972).

Ejsmont, W.: Higiena pracy na statkach a stan zdrowia marynarzy w Polskiej Marynarce Handlowej. (Occupational hygiene on ships and seaman's health state of the Polish Merchant Marine). Warsaw: Panstwowy Zaklad Wydawnictw Lekarskich 1966.

Engelhardt, H.: Seelische Faktoren bei der Seekrankheit. Ärztl. Prax. *10*, 33, 573-574 (1958).

Grimmer, G.: Probleme der psychophysischen Einwirkungen der Seefahrt. In: V. Internationales Symposium über Schiffahrtsmedizin, 19-21 Oct. 1972. Rostock 1973. pp. 11-17.

Haeberle, E. G.: Psychosomatische Erkrankungen bei Seeleuten. Empirische Untersuchung aus Versicherungsdaten und einer Feldstudie an Bord deutscher Schiffe auf See. Dissertation, University of Hamburg 1979.

Horbulewicz, J.: From studies on the influence of work on the personality of man in nautical environment. Bull. Inst. mar. Med. Gdansk *17*, 3, 379-381 (1966).

Nishibe, T.: Untersuchungen über Krankheiten und Schädigungen bei Seeleuten im Hinblick auf die Arbeitsbedingungen. Report 5: Arbeitsbelastung bei Seeleuten. (Summary in German from Japanese) J. Sci. Lab. *35*, 9, 656-663 (1959).

Reimer, F.: Suizide bei jugendlichen Seeleuten. Int. J. prophyl. Med. *6*, 1, 7-11 (1962).

Wodarg, W.: Psychische Krankheiten der Seeleute. Dissertation, University of Hamburg 1977.

Wodarg, W.: "... auf dem Pott wird unheimlich gesoffen". Seefahrt *2*, 12-15 (1978).

Zorn, E.: Zur mental-hygienischen Problematik bei Seeleuten. Arbeitsmed. Sozialmed. Präventivmed. *15*, 7, 166-168 (1980).

Zorn, E.: Alkoholkonsum an Bord. In: Verkehrsmedizin. Probleme in der See- und Binnenschifffahrt. Hamburg 11-13 April 1975, pp. 7-16.

General Situation on Board, Working and Living Conditions, Leisure-time

Aubert, V. and D. Arner: The ship as a social system. Oslo: Institute for Social Research 1962.

Backhaus, A.: Vom Leben an Bord. Physische und psychische Betreuung der Seeleute. In: Unfall- und Sicherheitsforschung Straßenverkehr. Kongreßbericht Jahrestagung 1981 der Dtsch. Ges. f. Verkehrsmed. gemeinsam m. d. Dtsch. Verkehrswacht. Hamburg, 7-9 May 1981. Ed.: Bundesanstalt f. Straßenwesen, Bereich Unfallforschung, Köln, i. Auftrage d. Bundesministers f. Verkehr. Braunschweig: Waisenhaus-Buchdruckerei 1981. pp. 107-114.

Campailla, G.: Indagini e metodi psicologici nel lavoro marittimo. In: Atti del primo congresso int. sull'assistenza di malattia e la tutela infortunistica della gente del mare nei paesi della c. e. e. Genoa, 3-5 Oct. 1960, Vol. 2, pp. 399-402.

Christiansen, H.: Neue Gesichtspunkte für die Unterbringung der Besatzung. In: Referate und Diskussionsbeiträge d. Sitzung des Fachausschusses "Schiffsentwurf und Schiffssicherheit" d. STG vom 15-17 Oct. 1975. Hamburg 1975. pp. 415-430.

Dean, L. M.: The effects of shipboard living conditions upon personnel. In: International shipboard environmental design conference, 21-25 April 1974. Maryland: Center of adult education. University of Maryland. Vol. II. pp. 9.

Jakobsen, G.: Mennesket i skipssamfunnet. In: Sjøfartsmedisinks forskning. Rapport fra nordisk symposium, Oslo, 16-17 June 1975. Ed.: Nordiska radet och Nordiska ministerradets sekretariat i Oslo. Stockholm: Gotab 1976. pp. 33-35.

Kiryakov, Kr., P. Polonov and Ts. Kardashev: Prouchvane varku nyakoi trudovo-meditsinksi i sotsialnopsikhologhicheski polozhenye na plavsastavite. (Investigations of occupational medical and socio-psychological situation of ships' crews.) Transp. med. Vesti *18*, 1, 1-5 (1973).

Rünger, H., W. Kleemann und E. Ingenhoven: Ergebnisse einer Befragung zur sozialen und beruflichen Situation des seemännischen Personals in der deutschen Seeschiffahrt. DAG-Schiffahrt *21*, 2, 2-9 (1968).

Schadewaldt, H.: Die psychische Situation des Menschen an Bord. Lecture. Nautischer Verein Lübeck 10.3. 1977.

Tenfjord, O. W.: The personal and family implication of being a seaman. Lecture. International Christian Maritime Assoc.

Tkachenko V. D. and S. T. Hramtsova: Questions of psychology and sociology in the commercial fleet. In: VII. International symposium on marine medicine, Odessa, 23-30 Sept. 1976. Moscow 1976. pp. 297-298.

Stiewe, M.: Die Freizeit der Seeleute an Bord in der

Hochseefischerei. Verk.-Med. *18*, 8, 345–355 (1971).

Zorn, E.: Rekreationsmöglichkeiten in der Seefahrt. Lecture. II. Internationales verkehrsmedizinisches Kolloquium. Hamburg 1971.

Zorn, E.: Freizeitgestaltung und Rekreation an Bord von Schiffen. In: V. Internationales Symposium über Schiffahrtsmedizin, 19–21 Oct. 1972. Rostock 1973. pp. 355–361.

Selection

Böhm, H.: Psychische Anforderungen an die Führung von Seeschiffen. Arbeitsgruppe "Psychische Probleme der Schiffsführung". d. Dtsch. Gesellsch. f. Ortung u. Navigation e.V. Sitzung, 9 Nov. 1973.

Boganelli, E.: Orientamento e selezione psicotecnica dei marittimi. In: Atti del Centro Studi e ricerche per l'assistenza sanitaria e sociale dei marittimi pp. 122–126 (1959).

Dolmierski, R. and J. Nitka: Analysis of the reasons for subjecting officers of the Polish merchant marine to psychophysiological examination. Bull. Inst. mar. trop. Med. Gdynia, *30*, 2, 123–125 (1979).

Zorn, E.: Das Problem der psychischen Eignung für den Seefahrtsberuf. Kehrwieder *21*, 8, 9–10 (1977).

Future Ships Reduced Manning/Automation

Bey, H.-P.: Gedanken zur menschlichen Isolation an Bord. ESSO-Reporter 2, 7–8 (1976).

Jensen, H.-J., H. Studt and W. Fink: Das zukünftige Schiff und seine Besatzung. Ed.: Verband Deutscher Reeder. Hamburg 1976.

Schepers, B.-F.: Auswirkung der Besatzungsreduktion auf die Belastungssituation des Seemannes, Aspekte auf das "Schiff der Zukunft" und seine Besatzung. In: Unfall- und Sicherheitsforschung Straßenverkehr, Kongreßbericht Jahrestagung 1981 der Dtsch. Ges. f. Verkehrsmed. gemeinsam m. d. Dtsch. Verkehrswacht. Hamburg, 7–9 May 1981. Ed.: Bundesanstalt f. Straßenwesen, Bereich Unfallforschung, Köln, i. Auftrage d. Bundesministers f. Verkehr. Braunschweig: Waisenhaus-Buchdruckerei 1981. pp. 37–41.

Schadewaldt, H.: Der Mensch an Bord. Schiffahrt international 6, 273–280 (1974).

Talkenberger, W.-D.: Probleme der Arbeitsorganisation und der Entwicklung der Arbeits- und Lebensbedingungen auf teilautomatisierten Schiffen des VEB Deutfracht/Seereederei. Verk.-Med. *22*, 8/9, 323–330 (1975).

Safety

Böhm, H.: Seafarers and safety – an experimental approach. Lecture. Meeting on "Marine traffic". Liverpool, April 1978.

Soerhaug, H.-Chr.: Social science and research on safety at sea. Lecture. Symposium "Safety of life at sea". Oslo, 20–21 Oct. 1980. Research program associated with The Royal Norwegian Council for Scientific and Industrial Research. (System for Sikkert Skip).

2.11 Psychological Aspects of Work-load on Board

N. Ohashi

2.11.1 Recent Studies on Board

Past research and studies into the psychological aspects of the work-load on board Japanese ships have mostly been carried out as supplements to other surveys. Some of them attempted to assess the correlation between practical work on board and the ensuing fatigue while others tried to measure various changes in psychological and/or biological functions during the voyage. The result was a considerable amount of knowledge and information about individual cases. However, it was very difficult to generalise and arrive at definitive figures for the work-load of seafarers because their working and living situations are quite complicated and often variable.

This experience was used aboard a container ship to carry out a research project which attempted to produce a non-quantitative description that would highlight the actual working and living situations of seafarers (Ohashi [3]; Ohashi and Aoki [4]). Twenty-six crew members worked and lived on board under a set, tight schedule for approximately 2 months, for the purpose of safe transportation of cargoes. To accomplish this purpose, seafarers expend considerable effort that is practically impossible to quantify but, nevertheless, should not be neglected. During the research project their actual work was observed precisely. Particular attention was paid to their conversations, expressions, actions, the flow of important information and the process of some important decision making. Everything was recorded as precisely as possible.

A profile was established of each crew member not merely as a workman on board but as an individual person working and living on a most technically advanced container ship. Furthermore, such a profile was not based on observations of their superficial behaviour or on simple interviews with them. It was this very personal role which could not be extrapolated from analysis of the crew's job descriptions. It was found that the essence of their work-load could not be measured by a fatigue survey, even though it was feasible on board. Several disparate factors had to be considered, e.g. their difficulties in establishing good human relationships based on new concepts that replaced those derived from longstanding custom and tradition, the professional difficulties of engineers facing rapidly advancing technological innovation, and the crew's warm concern toward their families thousands of miles away. These and numerous other factors persuaded the authors that it was a profile of seafarers which was impossible to quantify.

The authors were convinced that their concept of the seafarer not simply as *"a workman on board"* but as, *"an individual person living on board"* was correct, and every study and research project should be carried out and developed on the basis of this concept.

The work-load of seafarers is one of the most important aspects of this concept to be studied. There are, however, no established and effective methods available to evaluate work-load within the framework of the concept. Therefore, Ohashi and Hat-

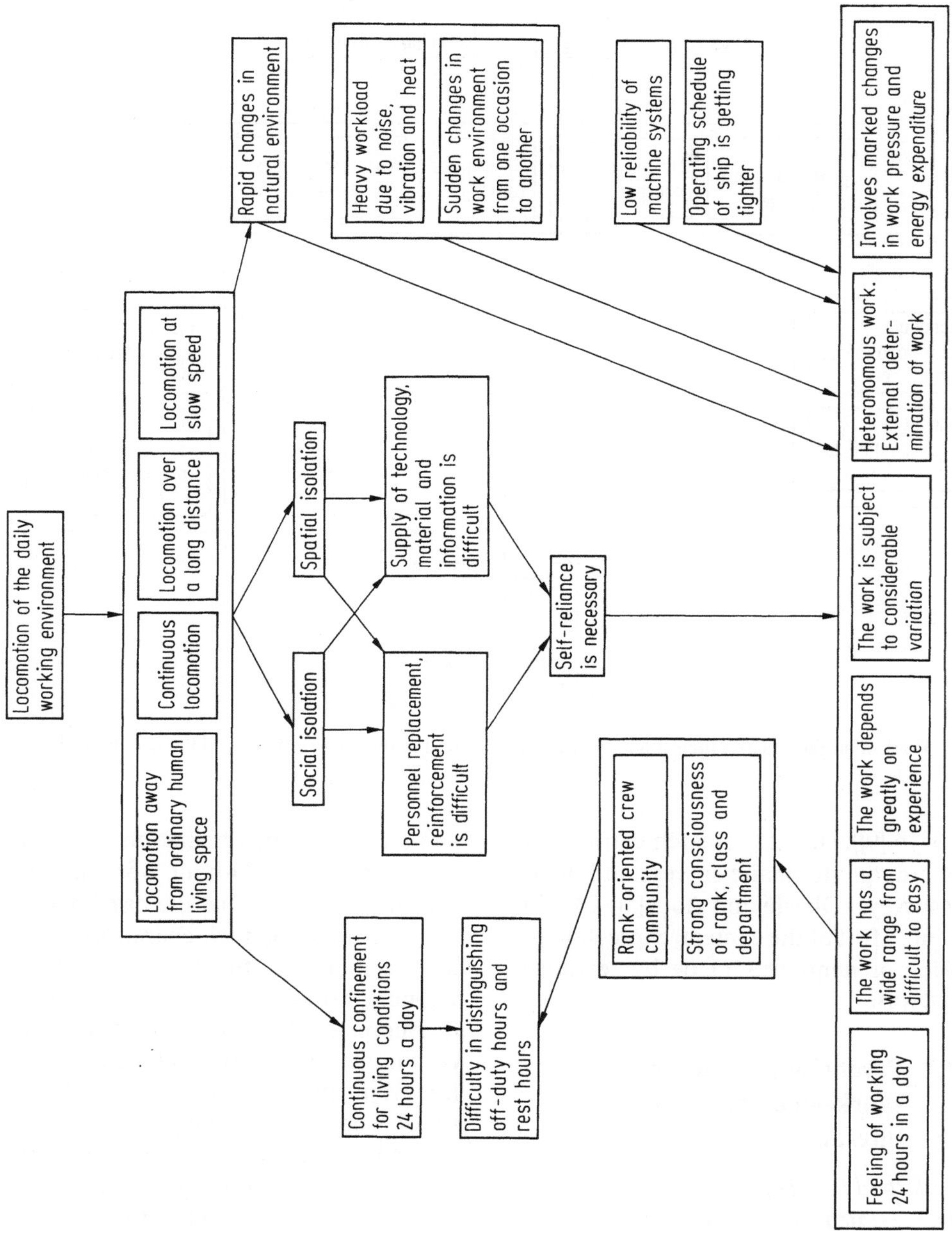

Fig. 1. **Work-load factors and their inter-relationships, related to the characteristics of the work on board**

tori [7] performed a trial study on psychological factors of the work-load of seafarers and their inter-relationships, analysing the results by means of the so-called K.J. method (Kawakita Jiro, problem solving method, [10]).

Approximately 400 cards (hereafter referred to as the Card Group) were used in this analysis. Each card had an item expressing seafarers' awareness, attitude, evaluation of work-life, career, occupational circumstances and so on. These items were adopted from the data which had been obtained and filed from the various past researches (Morikiyo et al. [1]; Ohashi [2]; Ohashi and Hirota [8]; Ohashi and

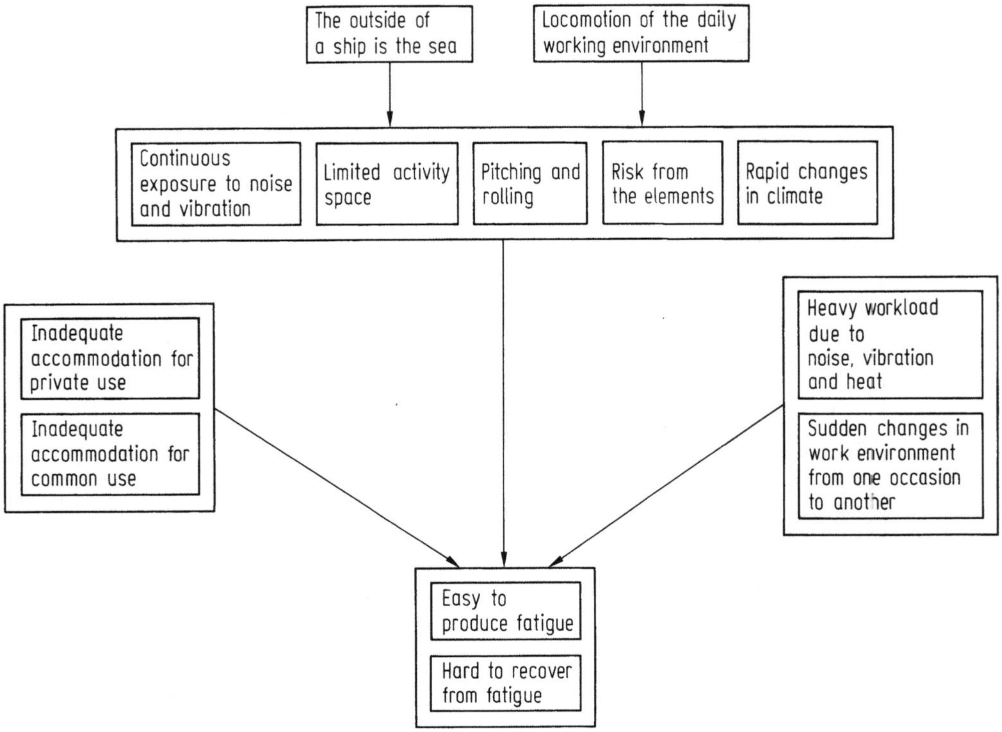

Fig. 2. Work-load factors and their inter-relationships, related to the environment and the accommodation

Morikiyo [9]), such as research carried out on board, questionnaire surveys and interview surveys (Ohashi and Aoki [5]; Ohashi et al. [6]). Most of the content, expression or wording of items was made by seafarers themselves.

2.11.2 Psychological Factors of Work-load and their Interaction

1. *Work-load factors and their inter-relationships, related to the characteristics of the work on board.* The result is shown in Fig. 1. However, items related to labour conditions in a narrow sense or to a particular shipping company have been excluded. As shown in the figure, seafarers' work ranges widely from difficult to easy, depends greatly on experience, is subject to considerable variation, involves marked changes in work pressure and energy expenditure, is heteronomous (external determination of work) and seems like a 24-hour working day. The authors found that the basic reason why the work has such characteristics is the locomotion of the daily working environment (movement of the ship). Furthermore, this locomotion is a slow and continuous process over a long time and far from the ordinary human living space ashore. This is the paramount factor which sets the pattern of seafarers' work. The items listed in Fig. 1 can be considered as work-load factors.
2. *Work-load factors and their inter-relationships, related to the environment and accommodation.* Items related to the environment and accommodation were withdrawn from the Card Group and sorted, with some slight generalization. The results are shown in Fig. 2. The study of the relationship between the items listed is not comprehensive and there may be some additional items that should have

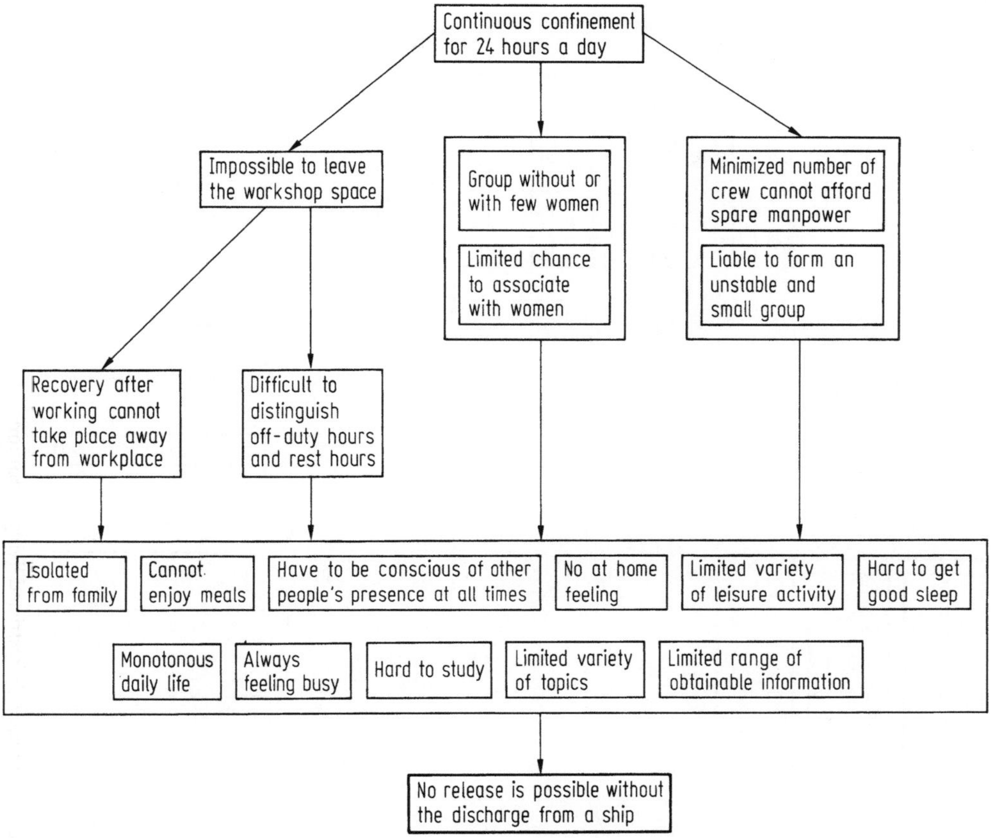

Fig. 3. Work-load factors and their inter-relationships, related to continuously restricted living conditions

been included. However, it is clearly indicated that a decisive factor is the locomotion of the daily working environment. Under such circumstances, when sufficient consideration has not necessarily been paid to accommodation, the work-load factors increase.

3. *Work-load factors and their inter-relationships, related to continuous restricted living conditions (confinement).* The result is shown in Fig. 3. The effect of 24 hours' confinement is not, of course, limited to the items shown in the figure and various other significant effects are also produced. If the generalization is possible, it can be concluded that confinement creates difficulties for seafarers in their social life. Also, the figures indicate that seafarers can have rest hours and off-duty hours in the genuine sense of the terms only when they are signed off from a ship. This indicates the importance and necessity of their paid leaves.

Figure 4 shows another result of analysis of the correlation between these factors. The item "Cannot enjoy meals" in Figs. 3 and 4 was further analysed to clarify the reasons for this condition, as shown in Fig. 5. Some elements with a probable bearing on the reason, however, such as environmental factors like "Rapid changes in climate", were not included. Nevertheless, it is clear that various factors affect adversely the enjoyment of meals. Another example is shown in Fig. 6. This gives a result of analysis on the item "Limited range of obtainable information". It is clear how various sorts

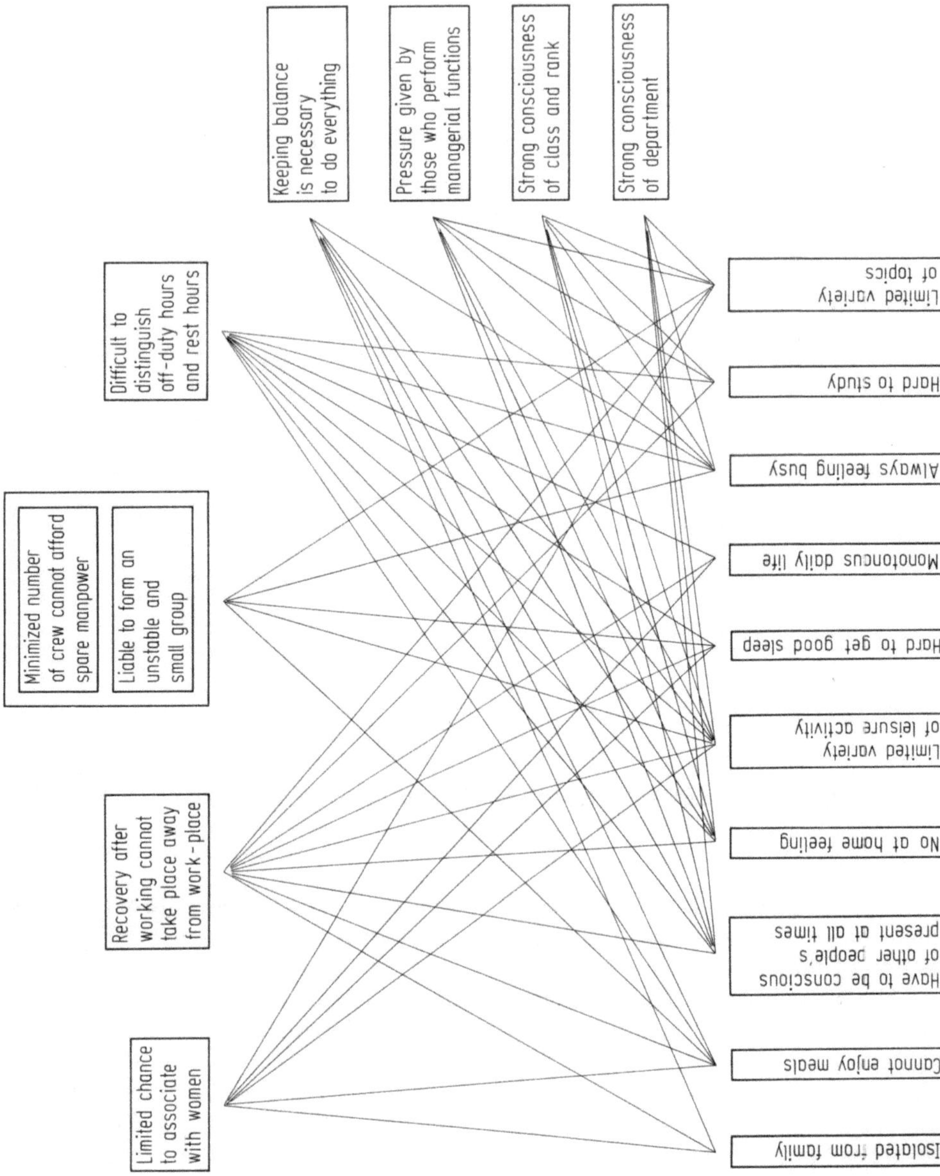

Fig. 4. Correlation between factors related to continuously restricted living conditions

of factors contribute to limiting the range of information obtainable, and this also creates more and different work-load factors.

4. *Other work-load factors, including the dissatisfaction of seafarers with their work and life.* As mentioned before, approximately 400 items concerning awareness and attitudes of seafarers to their work and lives were analysed. Some of these items have not been used in this article so far, but of course they may be useful for understanding the work-load of seafarers as related to a particular company or the society in general. As an example, Fig. 7 demonstrates work-load factors re-

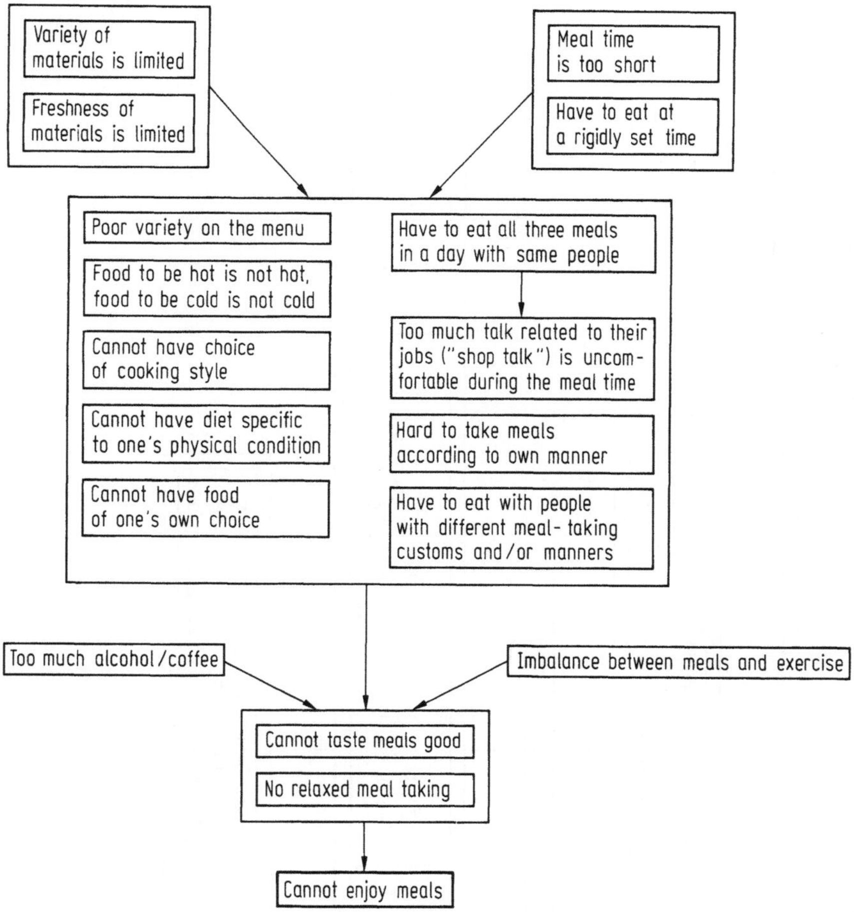

Fig. 5. Factors affecting seafarers' enjoyment of meals

lated to companies or the society, including dissatisfaction with the work and the life, using such remaining items. (Some items already used are shown again here.)

5. Figure 8 shows a summary of this article so far. Various complex interrelated factors can be seen as creating a situation where the seafarer's work easily produces fatigue from which it is difficult to recover. In view of the psychological aspects, it is possible currently to term them as work-load factors. In addition, there are other work-load factors to be analysed, e.g. the constitutional characteristics of shipping companies in general (lower left box in Fig. 8) and change according to shipping circumstances, i.e. increase of international competition or North–South problems in shipping. The diversification in the values of a society (represented in "Recent changes in various situations are very pronounced" at the lower right in Fig. 8) is also a work-load factor, because it also affects seafarers by creating awareness of, attitudes towards and evaluation of their occupation, sea-going life and occupational circumstances.

Therefore, further analyses of each item listed in Fig. 8 are needed. For example, "Cannot enjoy meals" and "Limited range of obtainable information" have been analysed and the results given, but

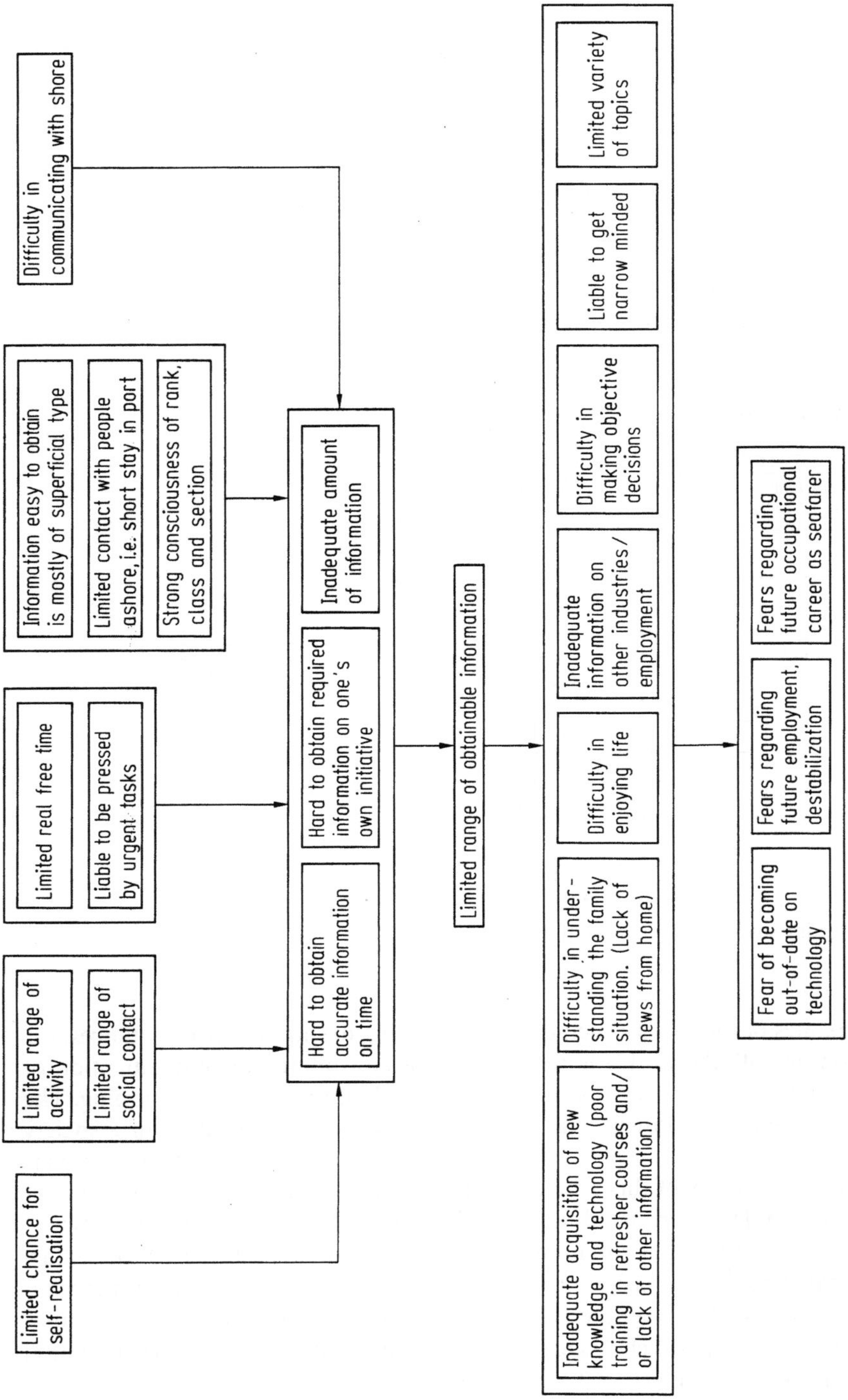

Fig. 6. Factors limiting the range of information obtainable

Fig. 7. Other work-load factors, including the dissatisfaction of seafarers with their work and lives ▶

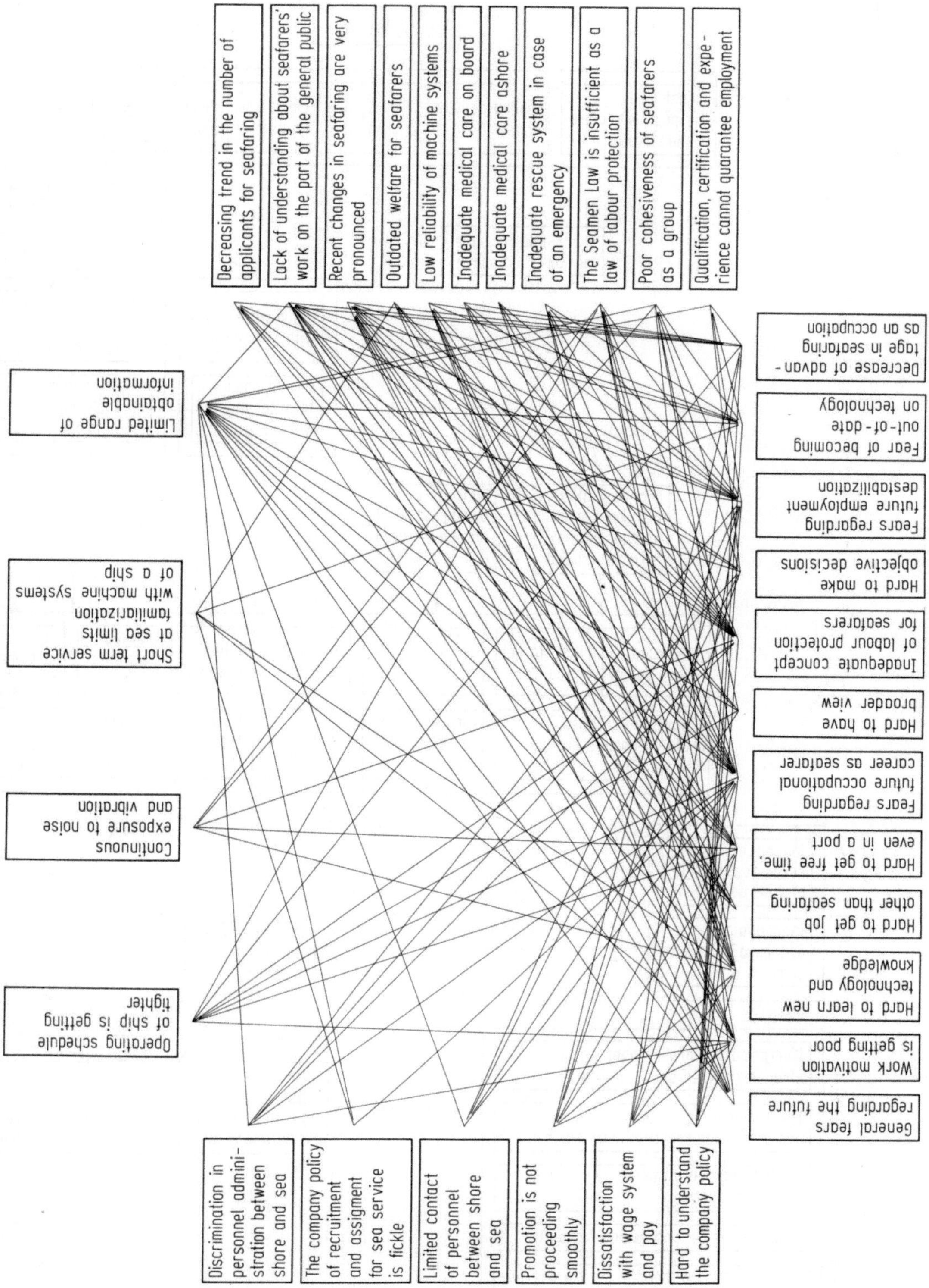
Decreasing trend in the number of applicants for seafaring
Lack of understanding about seafarers' work on the part of the general public
Recent changes in seafaring are very pronounced
Outdated welfare for seafarers
Low reliability of machine systems
Inadequate medical care on board
Inadequate medical care ashore
Inadequate rescue system in case of an emergency
The Seamen Law is insufficient as a law of labour protection
Poor cohesiveness of seafarers as a group
Qualification, certification and experience cannot guarantee employment
Limited range of obtainable information
Short term service at sea limits familiarization with machine systems of a ship
Continuous exposure to noise and vibration
Operating schedule of ship is getting tighter
Decrease of advantage in seafaring as an occupation
Fear of becoming out-of-date on technology
Fears regarding future employment destabilization
Hard to make objective decisions
Inadequate concept of labour protection for seafarers
Hard to have broader view
Fears regarding future occupational career as seafarer
Hard to get free time, even in a port
Hard to get job other than seafaring
Hard to learn new technology and knowledge
Work motivation is getting poor
General fears regarding the future
Discrimination in personnel administration between shore and sea
The company policy of recruitment and assigment for sea service is fickle
Limited contact of personnel between shore and sea
Promotion is not proceeding smoothly
Dissatisfaction with wage system and pay
Hard to understand the company policy

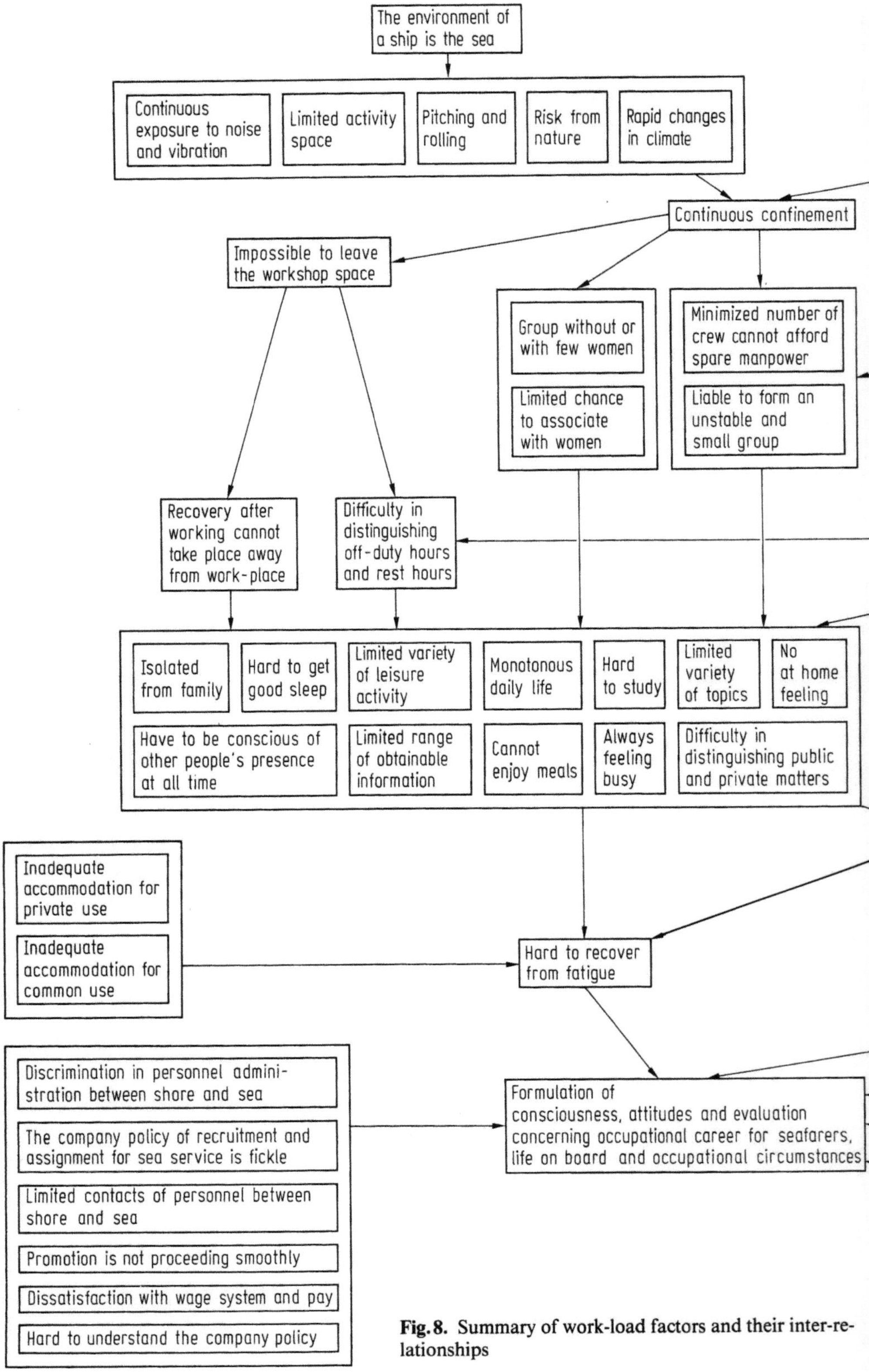

Fig. 8. Summary of work-load factors and their inter-relationships

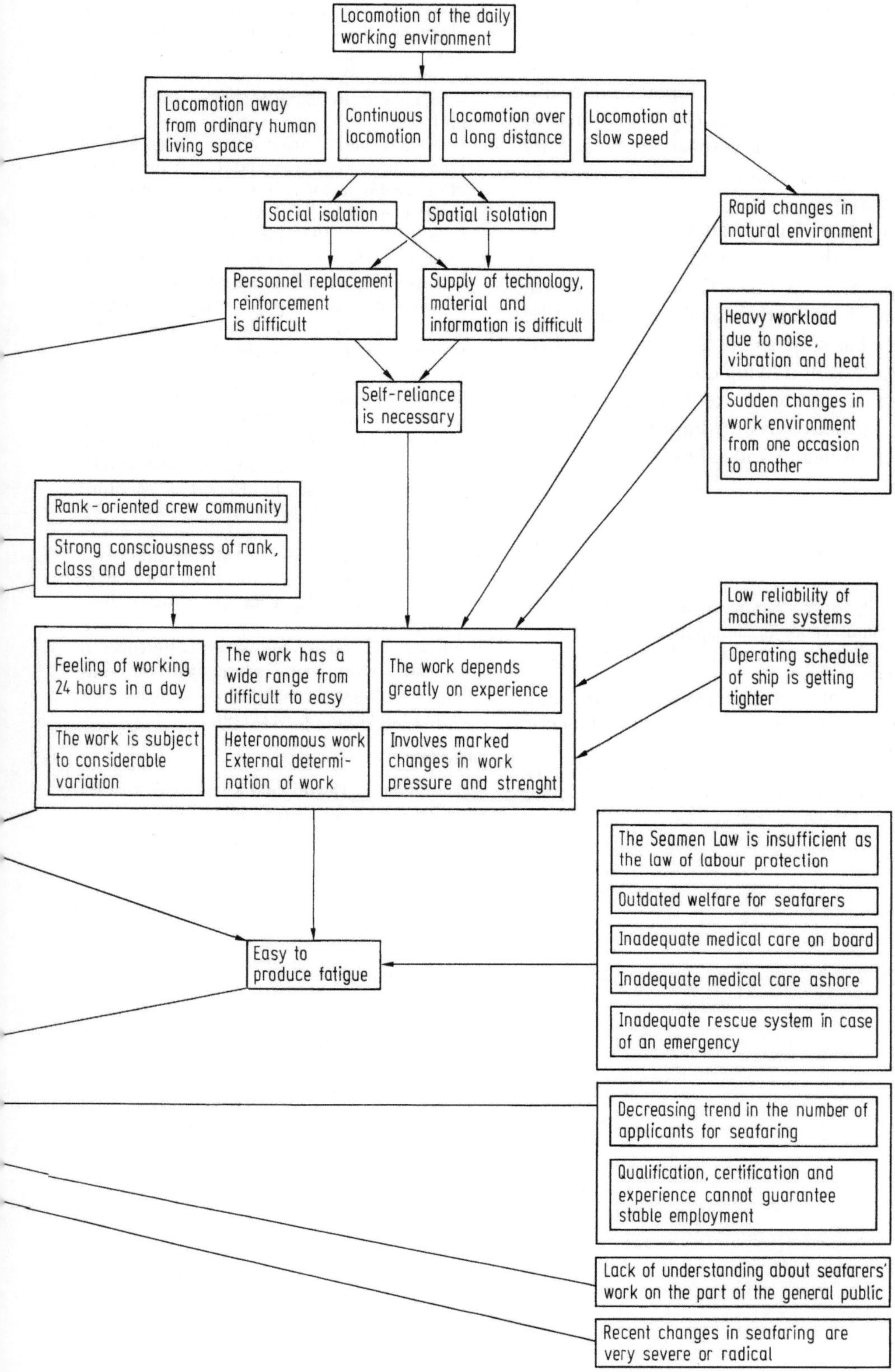
Locomotion of the daily working environment
Locomotion away from ordinary human living space
Continuous locomotion
Locomotion over a long distance
Locomotion at slow speed
Social isolation
Spatial isolation
Rapid changes in natural environment
Personnel replacement reinforcement is difficult
Supply of technology, material and information is difficult
Heavy workload due to noise, vibration and heat
Sudden changes in work environment from one occasion to another
Self-reliance is necessary
Rank-oriented crew community
Strong consciousness of rank, class and department
Low reliability of machine systems
Operating schedule of ship is getting tighter
Feeling of working 24 hours in a day
The work has a wide range from difficult to easy
The work depends greatly on experience
The work is subject to considerable variation
Heteronomous work External determination of work
Involves marked changes in work pressure and strenght
The Seamen Law is insufficient as the law of labour protection
Outdated welfare for seafarers
Inadequate medical care on board
Inadequate medical care ashore
Inadequate rescue system in case of an emergency
Easy to produce fatigue
Decreasing trend in the number of applicants for seafaring
Qualification, certification and experience cannot guarantee stable employment
Lack of understanding about seafarers' work on the part of the general public
Recent changes in seafaring are very severe or radical

the remaining items should also have been analysed further.

Analyses of work-load factors by this method should be developed and established as one of the effective methods of describing the work-load situations as fully as possible to ensure further progress in future studies.

Work-load factors on board are numerous and their interrelationship is quite complicated, as these figures have shown so far. These work-load factors should be reduced as soon as possible to provide better working and living conditions on board for seafarers, to make their occupation more attractive and to improve important aspects of health and safety.

References

1. Morikiyo, Y., N. Ohashi and H. Iida: Verbal communication in human information processing for ship manoeuvring. J. human Ergology *1*, 129–142 (1972).
2. Ohashi, N.: Designed and real working situations in machine systems operation. J. human Ergology *5*, 187–193 (1976).
3. Ohashi, N.: Life and work of seafarers on an ocean going container vessel. (Japanese) J. Jap. appl. Psych. *1*, 17–38 (1978).
4. Ohashi, N. and S. Aoki: Shinéi Kosokusen ni okeru Seikatsu to Shudankino no Kanren ni tsuite. (Work and life of seafarers on the most advanced ship). (Japanese) In: Report of Maritime Labour Research institute. Tokyo 1975. pp 1–82.
5. Ohashi, N. and S. Aoki: Nihon Yusen Sen' in Iken Chosa. (Attitude and consciousness of NYK seafarers to their work, life, and company). (Japanese). NYK Special Report. S. Mihara (ed) Tokyo 1976. pp 1–179.
6. Ohashi, N., S. Aoki and A. Hattori: Sen' in no Seikatsu Taiyo to Ishiki Chosa. (Attitude and consciousness of deep sea trade seafarers to their actual living and working conditions). (Japanese) Report of Nihon Kaigi Kyokai, Tokyo 1975. pp 1–218.
7. Ohashi, N. and A. Hattori: Kaijo Rodo no Tokushusei ni motozuku Rodo no Hyokaho ni kansuru Yobiteki Kenkyu. (A preliminary analysis of work-load factors and their mutual relationship). (Japanese) In: Report of Maritime Labour Research Institute. Tokyo 1982. pp 1–49.
8. Ohashi, N. and Y. Hirota: Mental strain of a ship manoeuvrer. In: Proc. 16th Int. Congr. Occup. Health. H. Kita (ed) Tokyo 1969. pp 419–420.
9. Ohashi, N. and Y. Morikiyo: Differences in human information processing for ship manoeuvring in the daytime and at night. J. human Ergology *3*, 29–43 (1974).

Addendum

10. Kawakita, J.: The original KJ method. Kawakita Research Institute (ed) Tokyo 1983.

3 The Pathology of the Seafarer

3.1 The Occurrence, Frequency and Aetiology of Diseases and Trauma Among Seamen

P. Vuksanović and W. H. G. Goethe

3.1.1 Factors Which May Affect the Health of Seamen

3.1.1.1 Macroclimate, Microclimate and Other Load Factors

Modern technology enables ships to sail at high speed and thus pass through different climatic zones within a very short time. The consequent rapid climatic changes may affect the physical and mental health of seamen considerably. Sudden temperature changes, combined with more or less high degrees of air humidity, wind, rain, fog, strong solar radiation and other macroclimatic factors, have a greater effect on board seagoing vessels than elsewhere. In spite of all the technical facilities, the macroclimate also has a big influence on the microclimate on board. Seamen work and live on board within a most restricted space and with an almost isolated environment. When there are extremely high exterior temperatures and humidity, the microclimate on board, particularly in the engine rooms of older ships, is adversely affected. Also, climatic conditions in the living quarters of those ships without (or with insufficient) air conditioning lead to a considerable reduction of the recuperative capacity of crew members. This may also happen on board modern ships with efficient air conditioning under extreme macroclimatic conditions.

Noise and, particularly, vibration may be stress factors not only in the engine rooms but also on the bridge and other workplaces and in the living quarters. These factors may increase the psycho-physical load, resulting in a considerable reduction of the recuperative capacity, particularly when they occur during the sleeping time.

Poor illumination, insufficient ventilation and, amongst other things, chemical fumes caused by work materials and dangerous cargo create a potentially adverse effect on the health of seamen.

The ship's movement is a special load factor. It not only causes motion sickness in sensitive persons but also represents a stress factor for crew members by reducing the depth of sleep because of the unavoidable muscular compensatory movements. It is considered that 95% of seafarers suffer once, or even several times, from motion sickness, if only when starting service on board, irrespective of the fact that motion sickness does not appear as a disease in the statistics of distribution of diagnoses.

3.1.1.2 Working Time

Crew members work partly under abnormal physiological conditions. On board modern ships, heavy work is rare but on many older vessels such duty is still unavoidable, especially in connection with repair work in the engine room. The recuperative capacity is, moreover, additionally reduced by multifactorial environmental loads, resulting in a total load which is much higher than the original workload.

A further stress factor for some crew members is watchkeeping, which, in practice, is the oldest form of shiftwork. The rotating three-watch system, with 4 h on duty and 8 h off, guarantees longer times of rest, whereas the two-watch system, with 12 h duty per 24 h is highly demanding with respect to health. This particularly affects older seafarers.

3.1.1.3 Socio-psychological Factors

According to former investigations the average seaman spends 20% of his working life at home with the family and 80% aboard his ship. This may still apply to many maritime countries. Only in the industrial maritime countries and some other shipping countries with a highly developed social system is the duty on board restricted in favour of more spare time ashore. Thus it is thought that seamen spend two-thirds of their working life on board and one-third ashore (including holidays and all other days off). In the United States this relationship is 1:1.

During his leisure time aboard, the seafarer is almost isolated from all social events ashore as nowadays the turnround time in ports is generally very short and is still being reduced in the so-called quick ports. Turnround times from 1 to 2 days down to only a few hours are, in fact, not exceptional. Because of their heavy work-load aboard, many crew members then have no time to go ashore.

The continuous modernisation in shipbuilding has altered the seafarer's life considerably. The ship's automation has released the crew members from heavy physical work, but has simultaneously increased the mental load. The additional standardisation of working procedures aboard has allowed a large reduction of crews. There is also a high personnel turn over which was formerly unknown. Instead of a permanent crew having some kind of family relationship, nowadays there is a heterogeneous crew in a multifactorial sense, resulting in an unfavourable sociological and psychological environment on board.

3.1.1.4 Nutrition

Formerly, partial or absolute malnutrition directly affected the health of seafarers. Undernutrition and avitaminosis then belonged to the most frequent diseases of seamen and scurvy and beriberi were terrifying diseases aboard ships.

The physical work-load, and thus the requirement for energy, have now been considerably reduced. Combined with overfeeding, this leads to health disorders, such as obesity, diabetes, arteriosclerosis and cardiovascular diseases. Additional disturbing and not exceptional factors are, unfortunately, abuses of alcohol, coffee, tea and tobacco and the consumption of too cold drinks, which has an adverse effect on the gastro-intestinal tract.

3.1.1.5 Other Factors

Doctors who, because of their specific medical education and motivation, are positively influencing general health standards on ships have become rare nowadays. In most maritime countries, only passenger vessels, some cargo ships with very large crews, fish processing and fishing protection ships and research or similar special vessels still carry a doctor.

Most seafarers world-wide are likely to be employed on vessels without a ship's doctor. Appropriate courses of medical instruction for nautical officers who are in charge of medical care on board, no doubt, contribute much towards better health standards on board. An officer with insufficient medical knowledge cannot render efficient help in emergency cases. In extreme cases this may be fatal. It has often been noticed that, particularly on board vessels of developing countries or those sailing under flags of convenience, this officer has very scant medical knowledge.

3.1.2 General Characteristics of Diseases in Seamen

Vuksanović, in his epidemiological study [26], analysed the diseases of approximately 8000 sick Yugoslav seamen within a period of 10 years. Port workers served as a control group. The study showed the following result: The average age of sick sea-

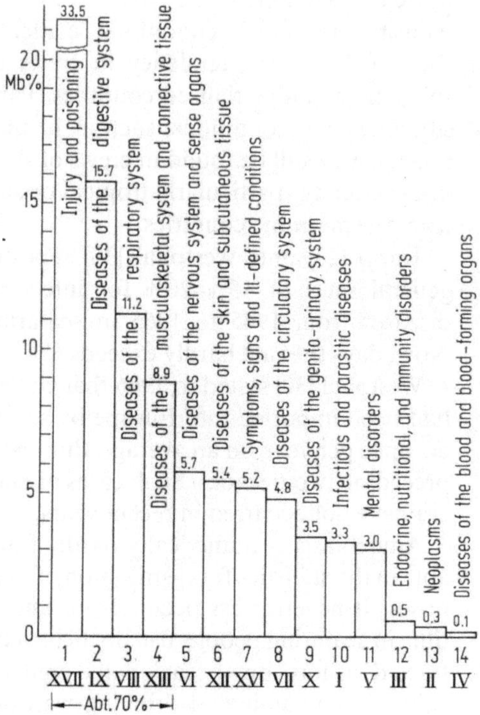

Fig. 1. Sequence of seamen's diseases from 7 countries, 1954–1979

farers was 31.2 years; that of the control group, 34.3 years. The average period of duty on board of the sick seafarers was 8.2 years; that of the control group ashore, 11.8 years. Seamen who had to do physical work fell ill after an average of 9.8 years, whereas the labourers of the control group showed an average of 11.5 years. The sickness days of seafarers amounted to an annual average of 20.1 days and those of the control group to an average of 11.7 days. The seasonal distribution showed a peak from June until September.

Statistical data on diseases of or accidents to seamen are scarce world-wide; data from very few countries are available, and they have been collected according to varying criteria. In 1981 Vuksanović and Goethe [27] compiled a survey of available data from seven shipping countries, covering the period from 1954 to 1979. This statistical evaluation was based on approximately 2 million sick or injured seamen. The diseases were classified according to the International Classification of Diseases (ICD) – main groups I to XVII. Figure 1 shows the frequency of the different diseases or accidents according to ICD, i.e. the morbidity rates. From this it is evident that accidents and injuries exceeded by far the other rates and thus ranked first in the sequence, followed by diseases of the gastro-intestinal tract in second place, diseases of the respiratory system in third place and diseases of the musculoskeletal system in fourth place. These four groups accounted for 70% of all disorders.

Oliver [21] stated that the accident incident rate, based on the total of reportable lost-time accidents related to the work force per 1000, is 45.8. This compares favourably with many shore industries; the rate for ship building and ship repairing is 66.2. Among 6630 diagnoses on board, 1559 accidents were reported.

3.1.3 Calculation of Morbidity Rates Among Seamen

For the calculation of standard morbidity rates on land the following factors should be considered:

1. Number of persons suffering from the defined disease within a given area;
2. Total number of inhabitants within that area;
3. Time period (generally 1 year).

The morbidity rate is calculated per 1000, 10000 or 100000 inhabitants. The formula is as follows:

$$\text{Mb}\,‰ = \frac{\text{number of sick persons} \times 1000}{\text{total number of inhabitants}}$$

This formula is not applicable to seamen as the total number of inhabitants is not available. The Soviet authors Komarov et al. [17] proposed the following formula to calculate the Mb of seamen:

$$\text{Mb}\ ‰ = \frac{E \times 1000 \times 365}{St \times 365}$$

E = number of sick seamen
St = number of seamen's days on board

This formula offers the advantage that it is possible to calculate the annual morbidity rate for an individual vessel, for several vessels of one shipping company or for the total national merchant fleet. It may be of great value in circumstances of high personnel fluctuations and thus continuously changing total numbers of employed seamen.

A very simple calculation method for the morbidity of seamen is the so-called structural index according to the formula

$$\text{Mb}\ \% = \frac{n}{N} \times 100$$

n = number of seamen suffering from a defined disease
N = total number of sick seamen

This method is frequently practised and recommended for routine work.

3.1.4 Genesis, Frequency and Aetiology of Some Diseases in Seamen (International Classification of Diseases I–XVII)

3.1.4.1 Infectious and Parasitic Diseases (I)

In recent decades, these diseases occurred only sporadically in seamen and very seldom epidemically. In the international statistics regarding distribution of diagnoses, infectious diseases, making up only 3.3%, are not very high in the numerical order (Vuksanović and Goethe [27]). Experience has also shown a decrease in alimentary bacterial and parasitic diseases. They occasionally still occur on board old ships, particularly vessels sailing under flags of convenience and with a low standard of hygiene. Salmonelloses, shigelloses and parasitic intestinal conditions evidently show a decreasing tendency in crews on ships of the industrialised countries. Parasitic intestinal conditions, such as helminthiases, may still be found in crews of ships of developing (particularly tropical or subtropical) maritime countries.

Trapp [23] and Westphal [30] reported general rates of 15%–20% for infectious diseases from 1945 to 1965 in seafaring. Nowadays the rate hardly exceeds 3%.

Westphal [30] stated in 1966 that cholera had been imported into Europe by seafarers once per year, on an average, during the preceding two decades. Such cases of cholera have not occurred in recent years.

Amoebiasis is numerically hardly traceable in the statistics for distribution of diagnoses. It nevertheless occurs from time to time in seafaring people, usually being contracted ashore but occasionally epidemically via contaminated drinking water on board. Chronic sub-clinical amoebiasis may well be underdiagnosed. A much feared complication of amoebiasis is liver abscess, which may be fatal. A similar danger is posed by malaria. Liver diseases do not play an important numerical role in the statistics regarding distribution of diagnoses. The industrial shipping countries try to protect crew members on board against malaria by more or less strict prophylaxis. The results are, however, unsatisfactory as experience has shown that the longer the seafarer's service at sea, the more unwilling he is to take tablets regularly. Severe complications of malaria have developed time and again because it was not recognised in its early stage. In the statistics regarding causes of death, which are available in only a few maritime countries, malaria plays a role not to be underestimated.

Tuberculosis was fairly widespread among seafarers for 10 years after the Second World War. Molfino [19] found that in Italian seamen tuberculosis accounted for 30% of all infectious diseases. The number of cases among seafarers from the industrial countries has decreased considerably during the past two decades. Strict preventive measures in most of the shipping countries, involving medical fitness and control examinations, may have made an essential contribution in this respect.

Tuberculosis is, however, time and again found in seafarers of those developing countries which have no regulations regarding prevention. According to investigations by Ejsmont [7] and Vuksanović [26], in most cases it is the deck personnel who are affected by tuberculosis.

Venereal diseases represent a continuing problem in seafaring. Mohar et al. [20] consider that 20% of seamen contract venereal infection at least once during their time at sea. In many maritime countries, venereal diseases are more frequent in seamen than in the population ashore. The frequency no doubt varies from country to country according to the structure of the crews and the geographical sailing areas.

Gonorrhoea is most frequent, making up approximately 90% of the VD diagnoses excluding non-specific urethritis. The remaining percentage covers all other venereal diseases. Because of a great many specific factors influencing their lives (such as separation from the family, monotony, insufficient sexual contacts and mass prostitution in ports) seamen are naturally prone to venereal diseases.

3.1.4.2 Neoplasms (II)

The statistical evaluation of data from seven maritime countries (Vuksanović and Goethe [27]) showed a slightly rising tendency for neoplasms in seamen, although they are in the last but one place in the morbidity structure (0.3%). Seafarers carrying out work on deck for long periods under tropical and subtropical climatic conditions obviously fall ill more often from skin carcinoma, which is probably due to increased ultraviolet radiation. Körbler [16] however states that seamen apparently suffer more frequently from neoplasms than the population ashore.

3.1.4.3 Endocrine, Nutritional and Metabolic Diseases (III)

Undernutrition and avitaminosis seem to be of minor importance in modern seafaring. It is a controversial question whether hypovitaminosis may occur from time to time owing to inefficient storage of provisions on board; in any case, a considerably larger number of crew members worldwide are confronted with problems of overeating and obesity than are affected by undernutrition. Diabetes mellitus is considered to be the most frequent disease within this group to be found in seamen, the so-called maturity onset diabetes forming 95% and diabetes of adolescents 5% of the total. The low percentage rate of diabetes of adolescents might be a result of the sometimes very strict selection of seamen (Jović-Paškvalin et al. [15]). Seafarers with diabetes under treatment, particularly those who need insulin injections, should not run the risk of going to sea. Diabetic coma is rarely treatable on board.

Metabolic and endocrine diseases are, with scarcely 0.5%, in the third from last place in the international morbidity structure (Vuksanović and Goethe [27]). Nevertheless, a slight rise in their incidence is noticeable.

3.1.4.4 Diseases of the Blood and Blood-Forming Organs (IV)

These diseases, with a rate of approximately 0.1%, take last place in the sequence (Vuksanović and Goethe [27]) and do not show a rising tendency.

Pathological blood pictures are only occasionally found. In crew members of tankships they are most probably the result of chronic intoxication caused by aromatic hydrocarbons. Tankship crews should be liable to regular medical checks including blood examinations.

3.1.4.5 Mental Disorders (V)

Mental disorders, with 3%, are fourth from last in the international morbidity rates

(Vuksanović and Goethe [27]). Most probably there is a large additional number of unrecognised mental disorders which are diagnosed and classified only according to their somatic symptoms. In an epidemiological study on Yugoslav seamen, Vuksanović [26] came to the conclusion that the rate of mental disorders was significantly higher than among the population ashore. Young seamen with no seafaring experience and insufficient adaptability to the environment on board are the most predisposed to psychoses and neuroses. There has been an increasing world-wide tendency to mental disorders during the past 20 years, the deck personnel showing higher rates than the engine room staff (Carev and Šokec [5]).

In this connection the problem of alcoholism is frequently considered. Naturally, alcohol consumption varies according to national and cultural habits, but Carev and Šokec [5] emphasise that seamen seem more inclined to alcohol abuse than the average population ashore. Last but not least the special situation of seafarers may be considered a reason for mental disorders.

3.1.4.6 Diseases of the Nervous System and the Sense Organs (VI)

In the international distribution of diagnoses, these diseases are represented with 5.7% (Vuksanović and Goethe [27]). It is very difficult to classify the individual diagnoses within this heterogeneous group (it includes diseases of the eyes and ears as well as the different diseases of the nervous system). Some of the cases of myalgia and/or lumbo-ischialgia may be classified either under this group or under group XIII (diseases of the musculoskeletal system and connective tissue). Lumbo-ischialgia and similar disorders of the nervous system are extremely frequent in seafaring. Heavy physical work under unfavourable conditions (motion of the sea, engine repairs in restricted space, work on deck under unfavourable climatic influences) leads to disorders of this kind. Other diseases of the nervous system are rare.

Diseases of the eyes are not specific in seafaring. Nevertheless, pterygium is sometimes diagnosed, particularly in seamen from Asia and in fishermen, although the total number of cases is not very high in the distribution of diagnoses. Many seamen complain of hearing disorders due to the high noise levels on board vessels. The engine room staff are specially affected. Impairment of hearing capacity is not exclusive to the engine personnel but is found in some deck workers and radio officers too (Goethe et al. [12]). Hearing disorders are not obvious from the statistical data as, presumably, they are in most cases not perceived or indicated as a disease. Hardness of hearing due to noise is an occupational disease subject to an award only in maritime countries with a highly developed social security system.

3.1.4.7 Diseases of the Circulatory System (VII)

These diseases are found in eighth place in the international statistics (4.8%) (Vuksanović and Goethe [27]). Myocardial infarction and other ischaemic cardiac diseases are predominantly diagnosed in older seafarers, especially in masters and ships' officers, who have a high load of responsibility, and, of course, in sea pilots. Zorn [32] found that myocardial infarction was responsible for 51% of the deaths among sea pilots in the age group 41–50 years in Hamburg between 1945 und 1973.

The death rate of sea pilots in this age group amounted to 2.66‰, whereas the rate of the comparable group of the male population in Hamburg was only 0.63‰. Ejsmont [7] reports similar findings. Fedele [9] came to the conclusion in his extensive study that more than 80% of ischaemic cardiac diseases occurred on the sea. Cardi and Puddu [4] also worked on the importance of cardiovascular diseases on board, and found that varicose veins are often a problem, particularly with the catering staff. Mundal et al. [33] and Rodahl [34] found that the risk of coronary heart disease among Norwegian ship captains and officers was considerably higher than in a comparable population ashore.

3.1.4.8 Diseases of the Respiratory System (VIII)

These diseases are in third place in the morbidity statistics, with 11.2% (Vuksanović and Goethe [27]). Predominantly the deck personnel are exposed to adverse macroclimatic conditions and so the sickness rate is higher than in the engine room staff.

3.1.4.9 Diseases of the Digestive System (IX)

Diseases of the digestive system (15.7%) are in second place in the morbidity statistics, behind accidents. Nearly all nautical medical experts throughout the world are aware of the fact that these diseases represent a considerable problem among seamen. Statistical morbidity data show that in some countries the rate even reaches 30% (Vuksanović [26]). It was found that gastritis and ulcers were chiefly represented.

Laba [18] and Gras and Parodi [14] found that young seamen fall ill more frequently from these diseases. Several authors came to the conclusion that gastric or duodenal ulcers are more often diagnosed in seamen than in the average population ashore. Watt [29] speaks of the "sailor's stomach".

The following aetiological factors are considered as perhaps significant here:

1. Kinetic load from the ship's motion (kinetosis, fatigue);
2. Noise and vibration as well as other load factors such as macro- and microclimate;
3. Work under abnormal physiological conditions and lack of recreation on board;
4. Mental stress;
5. Abuses of stimulants such as alcohol, coffee and tea, and consumption of too cold drinks in hot zones;
6. Monotony in nutrition;
7. Dental caries, particularly in the seamen of some countries;
8. Uncontrolled intake of medicaments.

Dental disorders naturally represent a big problem among seamen. According to Trunov et al. [24], 92.7% of examined seamen suffered from dental caries, while Zannini and Tortori-Donati [31] found a rate of 95%.

3.1.4.10 Diseases of the Genito-urinary System (X)

These diseases, with 3.5%, are in ninth place in the total morbidity of seamen (Vuksanović and Goethe [27]). They show a rising tendency. Deck staff are affected most frequently, possibly owing to the influence of macroclimatic factors.

In many cases, ureter and kidney stones are found. It is known that these diseases often appear in tropical zones because of insufficient fluid intake and this obviously applies to seamen as well. According to different authors (Chmielewski et al. [6]; Pellegrinelli [22]; Arduini and Rizzo [1]), typical stones account for up to 60% of all diseases within this group.

3.1.4.11 Diseases of the Skin and Subcutaneous Tissue (XII)

These diseases (5.4%) are in sixth place in the morbidity structure (Vuksanović and Goethe [27]). They show a slightly falling tendency, most probably owing to improved general and personal hygiene on board.

Contact dermatoses are very frequent skin diseases among seamen, presumably being caused by chemical work materials and additives in oil and lubricants as well as by detergents as used by the catering staff. Allergic reactions to detergents are also found in the deck staff.

Fishermen world-wide suffer from skin diseases caused by contact with salt water while working with nets during fish processing. On modern processing vessels, however, the number of cases of such diseases has been reduced considerably.

All over the world fishermen may also contract contact dermatitides, such as Dogger Bank itch and coral dermatitis, from sea animals. In addition a large number of seamen suffer from foot mycoses (athlete's foot), probably owing to a low standard of personal hygiene.

3.1.4.12 Diseases of the Musculoskeletal System (XIII)

These diseases, with 8.9%, are in fourth place in the morbidity statistics (Vuksanović and Goethe [27]), thus being relatively frequent. Conditions such as myopathy, arthropathy, lumbago of any kind and rheumatoid and rheumatic diseases mostly arise during voyages in cold and foggy sea areas, especially when moving from warm to cold zones. This has quite often been noticed in crews from tropical and subtropical countries and seamen's doctors in northern ports are often consulted by crew members of vessels from the tropics. Not only seamen doing heavy physical work on board are affected – others, too, suffer from these diseases.

3.1.4.13 Other Groups of Diseases (XIV, XV, XVI, XVII)

Group XIV refers to congenital diseases; group XVI contains certain symptoms and ill-defined conditions. The number of cases within this group is quite high as it is not always possible to diagnose precisely a disease on a ship without any further test facilities; lack of time may also be a factor. In many statistics concerning the distribution of diagnoses, the symptomatic and ill-defined conditions as per group XVI do not appear at all. In the international statistics they are in seventh place (Vuksanović and Goethe [27]).

Accidents, poisonings and violence (XVII) are dealt with in another chapter (i.e. 3.2 – "Accidents in Seafaring").

References

1. Arduini, M. and N. Rizzo: Etiologia e profilassi della calcolosi renale nei naviganti. Atti della "Sezione Studi" del C.I.R.M. 47–59 (1962).
2. Bogetti, B. and B. Tortori-Donati: Considerations about morbidity, diseases, sick leave and accidents among seamen according to the data concerning Italian seafarers. Folia med. *57*, 7/8/9, 130–138 (1974).
3. Burić, J., D. Jakac, N. Mohar et al.: Patološke manifestacije na koži pomoraca i ribara (Pathological manifestation on the skin of seamen and fishermen) In: Pomorska medicina (Naučne rasprave) Beograd: Izdanje Mornaričkog glasnika 1975. pp. 445–450 (Pomorska biblioteka 26).
4. Cardi, L. and V. Puddu: Le malattie cardiovascolari dei marittimi. Atti della "Sezione Studi" del C.I.R.M. 27–38 (1962).
5. Carev, V. and P. Šokec: Neki etiološki faktori alkoholizma na brodu. (Some aetiological factors regarding alcoholism on ships). In: Pomorska medicina II (Naučne rasprave) Beograd: Izdanje Mornaričkog glasnika 1979. pp. 315–320 (Pomorska biblioteka 30).
6. Chmielewski, J., R. Tomaszewski, W. Renke et al.: Urolithiasis in seamen. Bull. Inst. mar. trop Med. Gdynia *25*, 1, 228–232 (1974).
7. Ejsmont, W.: Stan zdrowia i zachorowalność marynarzy. (Health status and morbidity of seamen) In: Ejsmont, W.: Higiena pracy na statkach a stan zdrowia marynarzy w Polskiej Marynarce Handlowej. Warszawa: Panstwowy Zaklad Wydawnictw Lekarskich 1966. pp. 103–138.
8. Fedele, E.: Indagine sull'incidenza della gastrite, della duodenite e dell'ulcera gastrica e duodenale dei marittimi. Atti del Centro di studi e ricerche per l'assistenza sanit. e soc. dei marittimi C.I.R.M. 63–74 (1961).
9. Fedele, E.: Studio sulla frequenza dell'angina pectoris e dell'infarto miocardico nei lavoratori del mare. Atti del Centro di studi e ricerche per l'assistenza sanit. e soc. dei marittimi C.I.R.M. 105–113 (1961).
10. Goethe, H., R. Herrmann, R. Geister et al.: Die Frage der toxikologischen Beeinflussung der Besatzung von Tankschiffen. Eine vergleichende Pilotstudie über Tankschiff- und Nichttankschiffahrer. Arbeitsmed. Sozialmed. Präventivmed. *11*, 2, 46–51 (1976).
11. Goethe, H.: Gesundheitliche Probleme bei Tankschiffbesatzungen. Bull. Inst. mar. Med. Gdansk *17*, 3, 241–248 (1966).
12. Goethe, H., E.-G. Schmidt, E. Zorn et al.: Lärmbelastung auf See- und Binnenschiffen, Untersuchungen zur effektiven Lärmbelastung der Besatzungen. Ed.: Bundesanstalt für Arbeitsschutz und Unfallforschung, Dortmund.

Bremerhaven: Wirtschaftsverlag NW 1979. (Forschungsbericht 201).

13. Goethe, H., E. Zorn, R. Herrmann et al.: Die psycho-physische Belastung des Personals moderner Seeschiffe als aktuelles Problem der Schiffahrtsmedizin. Zbl. Bakt. I. Abt. Orig. B 166, 1, 1-36 (1978).
14. Gras, G. and V. Parodi: Relievi clinico-statistici sull'ulcera gastroduodenale nei marittimi. Lav. e Med. *5*, 1, 8 pp. (1951).
15. Jović-Paškvalin, L., V. Prpić and V. Furlan: Diabetes mellitus u pomoraca (Diabetes mellitus among sailors). In: Pomorska medicina II (Naučne rasprave) Beograd: Izdanje Mornaričkog glasnika 1979. pp. 311-314 (Pomorska biblioteka 30).
16. Körbler, J.: Bolest rak kod pomoraca (Cancer among sailors) In: Pomorska medicina (Naučne rasprave) Beograd: Izdanje Mornaričkog glasnika 1975. pp. 439-444. (Pomorska biblioteka 26).
17. Komarov, F. J., L. E. Poljakov and D. P. Zuikhin: The methods of studying the morbidity of sailors in navigations. In: VII Int. Symp. on Marine Medicine, 23-30 Sept. 1976 Odessa. Moscow 1976. p. 254.
18. Laba, L.: Some chronic diseases of the alimentary tract in sailors in the light of periodic health examinations. Bull. Inst. mar. Med. Gdansk *11*, 1/2, 21-27 (1960).
19. Molfino, F.: Le malattie della gente del mare. (Aspetti etiologici, clinici, preventivi ed assistenziali). Dagli atti del primo congresso intern. sull'assistenza di malattia e la tutela infortunistica della gente del mare nei paesi della c. e. e. Genova, Napoli, Trieste: Casse marittime per gli infortuni sul lavoro e la malattie 1960.
20. Mohar, N., F. Gruber and A. Wolf: Dijagnostika i liječenje spolnih bolesti u pomoraca. (Diagnosis and cure of venereal diseases of seamen). Pomorska medicina II (Naučne rasprave) Beograd: Izdanje Mornaričkog glasnika 1979. pp. 335-338. (Pomorska biblioteka 30).
21. Oliver, P. O.: A study of the causes of medical attendance aboard British Merchant ships. Publ. Hlth (Lond.) *95*, 74-81 (1981).
22. Pellegrinelli, G.: La medicina al servizio di chi lavora nei porti e sul mare. Lav. e Med. *16*, 31-35 (1962).
23. Trapp, E.: Die Morbidität in der Handelsschiffahrt. Verk.-Med. *13*, 4-5, 174-185 (1966).
24. Trunov, J. I., N. V. Pavlov, L. M. Shafran et al.: Analysis of stomatological morbidity among seamen and its prophylaxis. Bull. Inst. mar. trop. Med. Gdynia *25*, 236-240 (1974).
25. Vuksanović, P.: Najčešće bolesti pomoraca. (Most frequent illnesses of seamen) In: Pomorska medicina II (Naučne rasprave) Beograd: Izdanje Mornaričkog glasnika 1979. pp. 297-302. (Pomorska biblioteka 30).
26. Vuksanović, P.: Uticaj savremene plovidbe na strukturu morbiditeta jugoslovenskih pomoraca (epidemiološka studija) [Influence of modern seafaring on the morbidity structure of Yugoslavian seamen - (an epidemiological study)] Dissertation, University of Sarajevo 1981.
27. Vuksanović, P. and H. Goethe: Diseases and accidents among seamen - an international comparison of distribution of diagnoses. Bull. Inst. mar. trop. Med. Gdynia *33*, 1/2, 13-33 (1982).
28. Vuksanović, P.: Primjena epidemioloških metoda u pomorskoj medicini. (Application of epidemiologic investigations in nautical medicine). Pomorski zbornik 12, 593-599 (1974).
29. Watt, J.: The sailor's stomach. J. roy. nav. med. Serv. *58*, 1, 12-34 (1972).
30. Westphal, O. R.: Magenerkrankungen bei Seeleuten. Bull. Inst. mar. Med. Gdansk *17*, 3, 257-262 (1966).
31. Zannini, D. and B. Tortori-Donati: Rilievi sulla morbilità dei marittimi in navigazione. Lav. e Med. *14*, 5, 88-95 (1960).
32. Zorn, E.: Beiträge zur Berufsbelastung und kardialen Mortalität der Seelotsen von 1945-1973. Hamburg 1976.

Addendum

33. Mundal, R., J. Erikssen and K. Rodahl: Latent ischaemic heart disease in sea captains. Scand. J. Work environ. Hlth 8, 178-184 (1982).
34. Rodahl, K.: Arbeitsstress til sjös. Ed.: Norges Teknisk-Naturvitenskapelige Forskningsgråd. Oslo 1980. (System for Sikkert Skip).

3.2 Accidents in Seafaring

P. Vuksanović and W. H. G. Goethe

3.2.1 Frequency and Aetiology of Accidents

Occupational accidents were at the top of the list of morbidity rates in a recent international comparison (Vuksanović and Goethe [24]). Numerous authors have published statistical data on the frequency of accidents on ships and on their occurrence and aetiology during recent decades. Fleets belonging to different countries show accident rates from 10% to 30%, while in some maritime countries accidents reached 50% of all diagnoses in seamen. Fortunately accidents in seafaring have shown a tendency to decrease in number (Vuksanović and Goethe [24]).

Normally, seamen suffer less from accidents than do labourers ashore. Nevertheless, the mortality of injured seamen due to accidents is 5 to 7 times higher than that of the labourers ashore. Fishermen generally show a higher rate of accidents than other seafarers. A study over 7 years by Goethe and Vuksanović [6] concluded that the rate of accidents is twice as high among fishermen as among merchant seamen. Vrcelj [22] investigated very thoroughly the aetiology of accidents among seamen. According to his findings, the age of seamen and the type and size of vessels play an important role. The smaller and older a ship is, the more accidents are registered. Accidents are most frequent among young seamen beginning seagoing duties. Causative factors may be the ship's motion caused by rough sea, a deck made slippery by spilled cargo, ice or rain, snow, bad vision etc. The load caused by macroclimatic changes no doubt increases the hazards. Work in the engine room, particularly repair work and the handling of engine parts, sometimes during severe movement of the ship, is associated with a higher accident risk. A large number of accidents are caused by the handling of ropes, hoists and cargo-lifting equipment. Environmental factors such as noise, vibration, insufficient illumination and dust are additional risks.

The mental stress due to the monotony of life at sea and its physical manifestations is an important cause of accidents. No doubt, alcohol is involved in a large number of accidents, but it is difficult to trace any reliable data. The number of concealed cases may be rather high (Vrcelj [22]).

Poisoning caused by dangerous cargo and chemical work materials play a special role in the causation of accidents. It is rather surprising that the number of accidents caused by chemical work materials (such as acids, solvents and detergents) is considerably higher than that of the accidents caused by dangerous cargo (Schepers [19]).

3.2.2 Occupational Accidents in Seafaring According to Different Parameters

3.2.2.1 Age

Most of the injuries occur in young seamen up to 25 years of age (Vrcelj [22]). The accidents are obviously due to the as yet poor adaptation to the work and life on board. Furthermore, young people take more risks than older persons. However, according to

Dimitrov [2] seamen of advanced age groups are more accident prone than middle-aged seamen. In a study by Vuksanović [25] dealing with occupational accidents of seamen the average age of injured crew members is 30.5 years while that of the control group of injured labourers ashore is 32.5 years. The difference is statistically significant.

3.2.2.2 Period of Duty on Board

It can be shown that seamen are most frequently injured at the start of their seagoing life (Dimitrov [2]; Vuksanović [25]). There is a high correlation between the number of accidents and the length of service at sea. This should supply a motive to pay more attention to the prevention of accidents among younger seamen when organising the work on board.

3.2.2.3 Work-places

The majority of accidents happen on deck (approximately 43%), in the engine room (approximately 41%) and in the working area of the catering staff (approximately 16%).

Nearly 80% of the injured seamen do heavy physical work. The remaining 20% are crew members with light physical duty, e.g. the ship's officers. Within the group of officers the engineers are more frequently injured than the deck or catering officers (Vuksanović [25]; Dimitrov [2]; Vrcelj [22]).

The frequency of accidents also depends on the type of vessel. More accidents occur on the deck of cargo vessels than on tankships. On fishery vessels, accidents predominantly occur during handling of the deck machinery. The accident rate on vessels of an older design is generally higher than on modern vessels (Goethe and Vuksanović [6]; Vrcelj [22]).

With respect to the time of the accident before starting work or at work, Vrcelj [22] came to the amazing conclusion that most of the accidents happened in passage-ways when moving from one place to another on the ship. These are the so-called passageway accidents.

3.2.2.4 Injured Body Parts

In recent decades numerous authors have been concerned with the subject of which body parts were more frequently injured (Dolatkowski et al. [3]; Giannico and Tortori-Donati [5]; Puskeiler and Kersten [16]; Ejsmont and Filipek [4]; Moore [13]; Dimitrov [2]; Vrcelj [22]; Vuksanović [25]; Crovari [1]; Tortori-Donati [20]). Nearly all of them came to the conclusion that the upper extremities are affected most frequently (approximately 45%); naturally, the hands suffer most. The lower extremities follow with approximately 31%, the head with approximately 13% and the trunk in last place with 11%.

3.2.2.5 Kinds of Injury

The statistical data show the following sequence: 1) contusions 34%, 2) wounds (predominantly lacerations) 22%, 3) fractures (predominantly closed fractures) 19%, 4) strains (predominantly of the ankle) 17%. The remaining 8% includes burns, injuries involving foreign bodies, injuries to the eyes and internal injuries (Dolatkowski et al. [3]; Giannico and Tortori-Donati [5]; Dimitrov [2]; Vrcelj [22]; Vuksanović [25]; Trapp [21]). The above-mentioned sequence closely corresponds with the evaluation of the data regarding labourers ashore (Vuksanović [25]).

As, evidently, one-quarter of all accidents aboard cause open wounds, appropriate preventive measures should be initiated and the ship's medicine chests should be supplied accordingly.

3.2.2.6 Number of Sick Days

According to Vrcelj [22] the average number of sick days following an accident is 37.6; Vuksanović [25] gave 21.3 days and Dimitrov [2] 29.4 days. No other seamen's disease involves so many sick days. More than 50% of the accidents require 10–30 sick days. Of the total number of sick days on board, 22% are due to occupational accidents.

3.2.2.7 Aetiology

Many authors (Dolatkowski et al. [3]; Dimitrov [2]; Vrcelj [22]; Ejsmont and Filipek [4]; Otterland [15]; Vuksanović [25]; Guida [7]) have analysed occupational accidents on board and come to the following conclusions: The most important cause is the human factor. More than 40% of the occupational accidents are due to inattention, overfatigue, unfitness, carelessness, alcohol consumption and other factors predominantly correlating with the personality of the victim. Approximately 20% of occupational accidents are considered to have been caused by engine parts or other technical fitments on board. A further 20% may be associated with bad work organisation, including macro- and micro-climatic load factors. As mentioned above, the movement of the sea has a considerable influence on the occurrence of accidents. Very often, severe accidents are caused by heavy objects moving as a consequence of a storm. Considering the fact that the human factor is the chief cause of occupational accidents on ships, preventive measures should be put into force urgently. Without doubt it should be possible to avoid a large number of accidents by strict accident prevention measures, including an optimum work organisation.

3.2.2.8 Further Parameters

International comparison of accidents in seafaring over the past 20 years fortunately showed a tendency towards a constant slow fall, presumably because of improved accident prevention (Vuksanović and Goethe [24]).

A seasonal correlation of accidents could not be demonstrated (Vrcelj [22]), whereas the time of day seems to be a very important factor. Approximately 60% of accidents happen between 8 a.m. and 5 p.m. (Dimitrov [2]; Vrcelj [22]). This is to be expected as the greater part of the work is done during the day. An investigation of the eventual result of the injuries showed that approximately 90% of the injured persons recovered completely. Approximately 7% remained invalids life-long and retired from the sea. Approximately 1%–4% of the accidents were immediately fatal or the victims died subsequently from the effects of their injuries (Dimitrov [2]).

International comparison of the rates of accidents, classified according to the type of vessel, shows the fishery fleet to be top of the list. Apparently, tankship crews are not greatly prone to accidents. The figures for occupational accidents on board other types of vessel vary considerably. The frequency rates of accidents according to ship sizes show a negative correlation. The smaller the ship, the higher the rate of accidents. Most of the occupational accidents occur on smaller vessels of up to 10000 gross tonnes (Vrcelj [22]).

3.2.2.9 Death Due to Occupational Accidents on Board

Death by drowning (56%) ranks first in the order of frequency, followed by death caused by closed fractures, predominantly of the skull (17%). *These two causes account for 73% of all deaths;* the remaining 27% cover all other kinds of accident (Vrcelj [22]).

The results of accident aetiology research have shown that, in fatal accidents also, the human factor is of the utmost importance, followed by moving objects and work organisation (Kersten [8]; Puskeiler and Kersten [16]). In the international comparison ca. 1.2% of all casualties die as a result of accidents on board. This rate is 5–10 times higher than that for labourers ashore (Otterland [15]; Vrcelj [22]; Dimitrov [2]; Nolan [14]) used the "Standard Mortality Rate" (SMR) in order to compare the rates of seamen with those of the population ashore. He came to the conclusion that, generally, life is much more perilous at sea and that, as a consequence, the rate of fatal accidents to seamen at sea is higher than that to labourers ashore. His figures for seafarers, however, include barge and boatmen.

The casualty rates among deck and engine room personnel are nearly equal. The number of casualties among deck officers is slightly higher than that among engineers. Seamen are considered to be more suicidal than labourers ashore. To a certain extent the unsolved disappearances of seamen are explainable in terms of suicide. It seems that young, inexperienced seamen are more suicide-prone. No doubt, alcohol has an adverse effect on the mental condition of men at sea (Reimer [17]; Wodarg [26]).

3.2.3 Treatment of Accidents on Board

On land, injured people are generally transferred quickly to the care of the nearest doctor or Hospital. In contrast injured crew members on ships are dependent on the medical first aid of laymen, as only a very few vessels still carry a doctor. On long voyages, the injured person sometimes has to wait for hours or even days to get medical treatment by a doctor. Incorrect medical first aid and subsequent treatment may seriously reduce the chances of recovery and in some cases may result in irreparable damage. Severe injuries, particularly fractures, may cause great pain and increased shock owing to the ship's motion in rough seas, when satisfactory immobilisation is impossible.

In a medical emergency on board a ship without a doctor, a designated ship's officer is responsible for giving the essential quick medical first aid. However he may be involved in other duties or asleep and precious time may be lost before he collects his medical kit and attends the casualty. In many instances it falls to comrades present at the incident to give such lifesaving measures as control of bleeding, treatment of shock and/or resuscitation. It is imperative therefore that every seafarer should undergo at least one medical first aid course.

After first aid has been completed, any necessary further care and treatment of the casualty should be given by a ship's officer who has been trained for the purpose to a level higher than that of the usual first aid certificate. This further treatment is often necessary because it may be days before the ship can reach port or a doctor be brought aboard to a seriously injured seafarer (see also Chap. 1.4).

In the case of mass casualties caused by collisions, explosions or other major accidents, many patients have to be treated simultaneously. Such a situation necessitates very calculated action by the captain and/or ship's officers, but often they are unprepared or untrained for this kind of crisis. The training of ship's officers should include the handling of such events (triage).

Many maritime countries make available national medical guides (*Ship Captain's Medical Guide* or similar). They contain detailed instructions for the treatment of accidents and injuries. Where there is no national guide available, the *International Medical Guide for Ships* (WHO) should be compulsory on board.

3.2.4 Prevention of Accidents

The aetiology of occupational accidents is multifactorial. Analysis of shipboard accidents points to the following as chief causes:

1. The human being and the human factor;
2. The work organisation;
3. The work environment.

Preventive measures should consider the sequence of the above-mentioned factors. Accident prevention should be an integral part of the education of officers and seamen at the schools for ratings and at the nautical colleges. It should be emphasised even more during the practical training.

Careful occupational selection of seamen is a precondition of successful accident prevention on board. Besides purely medical fitness, the psycho-social aptitude is of great importance. The psycho-physical selection, i. e. the medical fitness examinations, should include vision, hearing and psycho-motor function, and should attest the mental stability of the applicant. Under no circumstances should accident-prone people be employed on board vessels. Re-examinations should be performed at regular intervals.

During the actual operation of the ship, management should take special care of the mental condition of crew members. The social and political structure of some of the maritime countries certainly makes this possible, but often there is not much chance of doing so. Nevertheless, everything possible should be done to ameliorate the situation. Naturally, there is the problem of excess alcohol consumption on board, which, no doubt, leads to numerous accidents. Prevention of alcohol abuse results in the prevention of accidents.

A further important point is the work organisation. Overfatigue and/or insufficient vigilance are important factors. Overfatigue is caused by watch periods being too long and by overtime work being required too often. A higher accident risk is understandable under such conditions. Overfatigue can be eliminated by an optimum work organisation. It may be that the two-watch system (12 h watch), which is practised on small vessels, particularly coastal vessels, results in higher accident rates.

The work environment on board seems to increase any tendency towards accidents. Ship designers should pay particular attention to optimal design of engines, fitments, ladders, stairways and passages to ensure personal safety. Regretfully, anthropotechnics are, so far, applied too rarely in the design of ships. Movement of the ship is practically unavoidable at sea. As 13% of the occupational accidents are directly or indirectly caused by rough seas (Vrcelj [22]), only urgent repair work should be carried out under these circumstances.

Environmental factors such as high and low temperatures, noise and vibration are controllable only to a certain extent. Everything possible should be tried in the ship's design to keep noise and vibration levels below the permitted limit values (see also Chap. 2.6). Special attention should be paid to accident prevention under unfavourable macro- and microclimatic conditions.

Work clothes, as well as the use of protective methods, are a special field of accident prevention. It has frequently been observed that working seamen wear insufficient protective clothing. Very often they do not use safety ropes nor do they wear gloves or safety boots. Generally, they seem to be rather careless. Regular accident and safety education for crew members is required and certainly creates a higher consciousness of accidents. Psychological training in accident prevention can never be overdone. The effectiveness understandably varies from country to country and from company to company. It has been possible to eliminate a large number of accidents on the vessels of some shipping companies by intensive psychological and technical methods of accident prevention but, of course, this necessitates continuous educational efforts. Good behavioural patterns by captains, deck officers and engineers contribute a lot towards general acceptance of good safety practice, and awards or rewards for accident-free work can be a stimulating means of accident prevention. The aim of accident prevention on board ships must be "Education for Self-protection" as any accident to anyone on board threatens the health of the seaman himself.

References

1. Crovari, P.: Malattie dei marittimi e condizioni di vita a bordo delle navi nei loro aspetti igienico-sociali. Ed.: Istituto Italiano di medicina sociale. Roma 1962. (Collana di studi sui problemi medico-sociali).

2. Dimitrov, I. V.: Proisvodstvniyat travmatizam vsred balgarskite morjatsi [Occupational traumatism among Bulgarian seamen]. Autoreferendum medical dissertation. Varna 1975.
3. Dolatkowski, A., J. Burka and K. Dega: Unfälle auf Schiffen im Zeitraum von 1960–1962. In: Fragen der Schiffahrtsmedizin. Vorträge aus dem Intern. Symp. vom 28.–31. 3. 1963 in Heiligendamm. Sonderheft des Medizinischen Dienstes des Verkehrswesens II. pp. 93–105.
4. Ejsmont, W. and B. Filipek: Traumas, accidents and fatal cases in the Polish merchant marine. Bull. Inst. mar. Med. Gdańsk *17*, 3, 343–349 (1966).
5. Giannico, L. and B. Tortori-Donati: L'incidenza di infortuni a bordo di navi da passageri e considerazioni sulla relativa azione a caratere preventivo. Lav. e Med. *12*, 2 (1974).
6. Goethe, H. and P. Vuksanović: Distribution of diagnoses, diseases, unfitness for duty and accidents among seamen and fishermen. Bull. Inst. mar. trop. Med. Gdynia *26*, 2, 133–158 (1975).
7. Guida, G.: The pathology of the seaman (Report on the activity of the C. I. R. M. "Studies Section": 1959–1967). Atti della "Sezione Studi" del C. I. R. M. 19–23 (1967).
8. Kersten, E.: Erkrankungen der Seeleute – Eine Analyse des Lehrstuhls für Arbeitshygiene. In: Fragen der Schiffahrtsmedizin. Vorträge aus dem Intern. Symp. vom 28.–31. 3. 1963 in Heiligendamm. Sonderheft des Medizinischen Dienstes des Verkehrswesens II. pp. 23–32.
9. Kraemer-Hansen, H.: Diagnosenverteilung bei Seeleuten. Auswertung der Erkrankungsbögen der Abteilung für Schiffahrtsmedizin am Bernhard-Nocht-Institut für Schiffs- und Tropenkrankheiten in Hamburg aus den Jahren von 1966 bis 1975. Dissertation, University of Hamburg 1977.
10. Kraljević, L. and Z. Ditrih: Hitna medicinska pomoć i hitne intervencije na brodu i u pomorstvu. [First medical aid and urgent medical interventions on board]. In: Pomorska medicina (Naučne rasprave). Beograd: Izdanje Mornaričkog glasnika 1975. pp. 415–420. (Pomorska biblioteka 26).
11. Lungarotti, R. and A. Picciocchi: Alcune considerazioni sugli infortuni a bordo. (Osservazioni sul personale navigante di un transatlantico). Atti della "Sezione Studi" del C. I. R. M. 155–159 (1965).
12. Matthiensen, R. P.: Diagnoseverteilung bei Erkrankungen in der Schiffahrt. Auswertung von Schiffskrankentagebüchern und ein Vergleich mit dem statistischen Material der SBG sowie der Ortskrankenkassen. Dissertation, University of Hamburg [1969].
13. Moore, S. R. W.: The occupation of trawl fishing and the medical aid available to the Grimsby deep sea fisherman. Brit. J. industr. Med. *26*, 1, 1–24 (1969).
14. Nolan, B.: Triple doses: a view of seamen's health. Marit. Pol. Managemt. *6*, 2, 119–127 (1979).
15. Otterland, A.: Unfälle bei Seeleuten der Handelsmarine. Abbottempo *2*, 20–25 (1970).
16. Puskeiler, T. and E. Kersten: Tödliche Unfälle in der Seefahrt. Verk.-Med. *12*, 2, 69–75 (1965).
17. Reimer, F.: Alkohol und Selbstmord bei Seeleuten. Akt. Probl. Verk.-Med. 2, 190–193 (1965).
18. Reimer, F.: Suizide bei jugendlichen Seeleuten. Int. J. prophyl. Med. *6*, 1, 7–11 (1962).
19. Schepers, B.-F.: Gesundheitsgefährdung durch Chemikalien an Bord deutscher Seeschiffe unter besonderer Berücksichtigung gefährlicher Ladung. Dissertation, University of Hamburg 1978.
20. Tortori-Donati, B.: Considerations about morbidity, diseases, sick leave and accidents among seamen according to the data concerning Italian seafarers. Bull. Inst. mar. trop. Med. Gdynia *26*, 2, 159–164 (1975).
21. Trapp, E.: Die Morbidität in der Handelsschifffahrt. Verk.-Med. *13*, 4/5, 174–185 (1966).
22. Vrcelj, J.: Die Unfälle an Bord von deutschen Seeschiffen und ihre Ätiologie von 1974–1976. Auswertung des Materials der See-Berufsgenossenschaft – Hamburg. Dissertation, University of Hamburg 1981.
23. Vuksanović, P.: Najčešće bolesti pomoraca. [Most frequent illnesses of seamen]. In: Pomorska medicina II (Naučne rasprave). Beograd: Izdanje Mornaričkog glasnika 1979. pp. 297–302. (Pomorska biblioteka. Sveska 30).
24. Vuksanović, P. and H. Goethe: Die Morbiditätsstruktur der Seeleute – ein internationaler Vergleich. In: Unfall- und Sicherheitsforschung Straßenverkehr. Kongreßbericht Jahrestagung 1981 der Dtsch. Ges. f. Verkehrsmed. gemeinsam m. d. Dtsch. Verkehrswacht. Hamburg, 7.–9. 5. 1981. Ed.: Bundesanstalt für Straßenwesen im Auftrage des Bundesministers f. Verkehr. Braunschweig 1981: Waisenhaus-Buchdruckerei u. Verl. pp. 57–66.
25. Vuksanović, P.: Uticaj savremene plovidbe na strukturu morbiditeta jugoslovenskih pomoraca (epidemiološka studija). [Influence of modern seafaring on the morbidity structure of Yugoslavian seamen (an epidemiological study).] Dissertation, University of Sarajevo 1981.
26. Wodarg, W.: Psychische Krankheiten der Seeleute. Untersuchung über Selbsttötung, Alkoholismus und andere wichtige psychiatrische Erkrankungen anhand von 236 von der See-Berufsgenossenschaft gesammelten Seeamtsverhandlungen aus den Jahren 1960 bis 1973. Dissertation, University of Hamburg 1977.

3.3 Gastro-Intestinal Diseases

G.J. Milton-Thompson and J.G. Williams

3.3.1 Introduction

Gastro-intestinal disorders are common at sea. They comprise the largest group of problems requiring radiomedical advice at sea, a disorder of the digestive system being the cause in 24.5% of calls to the Royal Naval Hospital, Plymouth, England (Brayley [7]). Such disorders were also responsible for the highest percentage (7.8) of all landed cases. Upper gastro-intestinal conditions predominated and there is little doubt that smoking and alcohol contribute to this (Krasner [18]). During 100 consecutive operational patrols by British submarines with a mean duration of 50 days submerged, 30% of acute problems were abdominal. In addition to appendicitis, these included peptic ulcer, pancreatitis, jaundice and inflammatory bowel disease (Glover and Taylor [14]). Infective diarrhoea, tropical disorders and infestations are not uncommon in ships visiting foreign ports.

3.3.2 Oesophageal Disorders

Life on board modern ships limits exercise and encourages obesity and over-indulgence in alcohol and tobacco. Chronic alcohol abuse is associated with acute and chronic oesophagitis (Van Thiel et al. [33]). Alcohol is probably directly toxic to the oesophagus, but also reduces lower oesophageal sphincter pressure (Kaufman and Kaye [17]) and interferes with acid clearing mechanisms (Winship et al. [37]). Reflux oesophagitis is therefore a common condition among seamen, causing considerable but minor morbidity. Diagnosis depends on the history of epigastric pain and heartburn occurring after meals and related to positional change and the drinking of hot liquids or spirits. The pain may wake the patient at night, but is relieved by assuming the erect posture. Such waking is commonly associated with a late and heavy meal with which alcohol has been taken. Symptoms of oesophageal reflux may be associated with, or independent of, a hiatus hernia. Weight reduction is essential, together with moderation in smoking and alcohol intake; these measures must precede the use of antacids, alginates, metoclopramide and cimetidine, the latter two of which are usually most effective at night. It should be remembered that hyoscine, often used for motion sickness, may exacerbate the symptoms of oesophageal reflux. Referral for surgery should be considered when the symptoms are incapacitating and resistant to conservative measures.

Spontaneous rupture of the oesophagus is rare but may occur after vomiting as a result of motion sickness or an alcoholic binge; indeed, the majority of patients give a history of vomiting (Abbott [1]). Pain is usually severe at onset, epigastric and retrosternal, although if the cervical oesophagus ruptures, pain may be referred to the anterior triangle of the neck (Brayley and Wilkes [8]). Pain is soon associated with the signs of an acute abdomen, together with dyspnoea, cyanosis and rapid deterioration. Surgical emphysema may be a late sign and may be missed. When X-ray facilities are available, a straight radiograph of the chest may show surgical emphysema and a little fluid in one costophrenic angle, while the abdominal X-ray shows no air under the diaphragm. Mucosal tears without perforation of the oesophagus may occur in similar situations, when they often cause bleeding – the Mallory-Weiss syndrome (see "Gastro-intestinal Bleeding").

Although dysphagia may be associated with oesophageal reflux and other benign conditions, it should always be taken seriously and investigated as soon as possible.

3.3.3 Gastritis, Gastric Ulcer and Gastric Carcinoma

Acute gastritis is common in seamen, for it is associated with dietary indiscretion, alcoholic excess and staphylococcal enterotoxin in pre-prepared meals. This gastritis may be associated with acute gastric erosions which are likely to bleed. Chronic gastric ulcer and gastric carcinoma do not show any unusual characteristics in seamen.

3.3.4 Duodenal Ulcer

Although the incidence is changing, duodenal ulcer remains a common condition affecting males rather than females and most prevalent between the ages of 20 and 60. It has been suggested that it is more common in seamen than in a matched group ashore (Watt [34]). But such comparisons of incidence are complicated by constitutional, genetic and geographical differences and firm conclusions cannot be drawn.

The clinical picture is less clear-cut than traditionally believed, but periodic symptoms relieved by food and antacids and waking the patient at night are characteristic. It has been observed that seamen developing duodenal ulceration may notice an increase in the severity of motion sickness (Cliff [10]). The condition frequently occurs in association with reflux oesophagitis. At sea the condition may reasonably be diagnosed on the history and physical signs; this is supported by the response to treatment with H_2-receptor antagonists, but referral for specialist investigation in due course will confirm the diagnosis. It is accepted by the British Royal Navy that uncomplicated duodenal ulcer does not constitute a bar to men returning to sea since drugs are available that are highly effective both in the acute attack and in reducing the rate of relapse, but caution should be exercised with regard to those who have a history of bleeding. Men at sea with a history of duodenal ulcer should be treated at once when their symptoms recur with cimetidine or another H_2-receptor antagonist in full dosage for at least 4 weeks (Burland et al. [9]), but the need for maintenance therapy is controversial and it is probably as effective to treat attacks as they occur (Bardhan [5]). Seamen who develop pyloric stenosis or other significant complications of duodenal ulcer should have surgery. This general view is not shared by the majority of doctors looking after merchant seamen. Cases of peptic ulceration are often referred for full investigation and treatment ashore and, in some countries, H_2-receptor antagonists are not allowed to be carried on board.

3.3.5 Gastro-intestinal Bleeding

Upper gastro-intestinal bleeding has numerous causes, but the commonest amongst seafarers are alcohol, Mallory-Weiss tears and peptic ulcer disease. The effects of alcohol on the gastro-intestinal tract have been reviewed recently (Van Thiel et al. [33]). Vomiting induced by acute or chronic alcohol ingestion may cause linear tears at the lower end of the oesophagus (Mallory and Weiss [22]) or in the upper fundus (Axon and Clarke [3]). These lesions are also seen in relation to severe seasickness. Other lesions related to excessive alcohol ingestion which give rise to bleeding include oesophageal varices secondary to portal hypertension and liver disease (Baker et al. [4]) and Barrett's oesophagus with or without ulceration, secondary to chronic oesophagitis (Martini and Weinback [24]).

In the stomach, acute superficial erosions and acute haemorrhagic gastritis are common problems following an acute alcoholic binge (Gottfried et al. [16]), particularly when there has been concomitant aspirin ingestion. Both alcohol and aspirin cause rapid turnover and loss of gastric cells (Krasner [18]; Croft [11]) and disruption of the gastric mucosal barrier (Smith et al. [29]. Alcohol appears to be directly toxic to the gastric mucosa. It also causes acute haemorrhagic lesions in the duodenum and jejunum but these are of doubtful clinical significance (Gottfried et al. [16]).

Peptic ulcer disease in seafarers has already been discussed. Peptic ulcers are responsible for some 50% of bleeding episodes requiring admission to hospital in the United Kingdom (Dronfield et al. [12]), and although the proportion is probably smaller among seamen because of the higher incidence of Mallory-Weiss lesions and acute alcoholic gastritis, peptic ulcer remains a significant cause of bleeding. A pre-morbid history is suggestive of peptic ulcer disease, although dyspepsia is common in seamen in the absence of peptic ulceration.

Management of upper gastro-intestinal bleeding will be dictated by the facilities available on board and by the proximity of medical care ashore. Fortunately, both acute alcoholic gastritis and Mallory-Weiss tears tend to be self-limiting conditions with a good prognosis. Bleeding from peptic ulcer is more dangerous but only 20% do not stop bleeding spontaneously and this is related to age (Young [38]). In the absence of skilled medical care in hospital, resuscitation with intravenous fluids and preferably blood is still possible and should be carried out when there is evidence of considerable blood loss, hypotension and anaemia. However, transfusion of blood will not be possible on board merchant vessels and intravenous fluids are not always carried. Drugs do not reduce the likelihood of further haemorrhage, except for cimetidine in acute erosive gastritis (Welch et al. [35]). Although cimetidine has not been shown to lessen the possibility of bleeding from peptic ulcers, it will accelerate the healing of such lesions, both gastric and duodenal (Burland et al. [9]), and should therefore be given routinely if possible following a gastro-intestinal bleed.

Lower gastro-intestinal bleeding tends to be less dramatic than haematemesis. Although patients may present with an acute severe bleed, most will complain of chronic intermittent bleeding. The causes tend to vary with age, so that in young adults inflammatory bowel disease and adenomatous polyps are the most common, in middle aged patients carcinoma, diverticular disease and ischaemia predominate. Local anal conditions such as fissures and haemorrhoids are common in all age groups. Finally, the possibility that apparent lower gastro-intestinal bleeding may have an upper intestinal source should be borne in mind.

Dysenteric infections may be difficult to differentiate from other inflammatory bowel disease. Suggestive features will be the particularly acute onset of dysentery associated with systemic symptoms and the clustering of a number of cases. If there is doubt, such cases should be isolated. *Campylobacter enteritis,* usually caught from contact with animals (especially live or dressed chickens and other contaminated food) and transmitted by the faecal–oral route, may mimic inflammatory bowel disease very closely in its presentation. Fortunately it is a self-limiting illness that does not usually require antibiotic treatment.

Valuable pointers to the level of bleeding from the gastro-intestinal tract are the patient's age, sex and medical history. Bright red rectal bleeding is usually from the rectum or sigmoid colon. Dark red blood usually comes from the more proximal colon, or infrequently from brisk bleeding higher in the gut. Melaena usually reflects upper gastro-intestinal bleeding, but may also be associated with lesions in the terminal ileum or caecum where there is stasis of blood in the right colon. Associated alteration of bowel habit or weight may suggest neoplasia, while diarrhoea may suggest inflammatory bowel disease and dysentery. Abdominal pain, its site, radiation and relationship to food intake or defaecation may be highly significant, particularly if a new symptom.

Treatment must be conservative if on board ship, but should include isolation unless a dysenteric cause has been definitely excluded. Most cases will settle spontaneously and bleeding will not be severe enough to warrant resuscitation with blood, although iron may be necessary. All cases of rectal bleeding require full medical assessment when appropriate, as most cases will have a cause that can be successfully treated.

3.3.6 Diarrhoea

Diarrhoea is, surprisingly, a relatively uncommon complaint in seamen, unlike travellers overland. Infective causes of diarrhoea will be encountered at ports of call. Most common among such will be the simple change in bowel flora producing a self-limiting 24–72 h diarrhoea (Nye [26]). But other more florid infections, such as with *Salmonella* and *Shigella, Campylobacter* and *Giardia* may be encountered. The closed environment of a ship makes infection with dysenteric organisms liable to achieve epidemic proportions with great ease. It is therefore of great importance that sufferers from diarrhoea, particularly where an infective cause is suspected, should be isolated and instructed to be scrupulous in their personal hygiene. In most cases of infective diarrhoea, antibiotics are not indicated since they do not hasten the resolution of the symptoms and are more likely to promote a carrier state [32]. The same considerations apply to the prophylactic use of antimicrobials, which may have adverse effects on the bowel flora both in the short and long term, with an increased risk of superinfection, masking of more serious infections and difficulties in making a bacteriological diagnosis. The incidence of both symptomatic and asymptomatic *Salmonella* infections is higher in those taking regular oxyquinoline prophylaxis than in those who take no prophylactic medication.

Other causes of diarrhoea include parasitic infections, colitis, malabsorption and the irritable bowel syndrome. With the exception of malabsorption due to pancreatic insufficiency in the longstanding alcoholic, these diseases are no more likely to be encountered at sea than ashore.

Management of diarrhoea on board ship requires assessment to establish the cause and isolation until an infective cause has been confidently excluded. Assessment should include a dietary and a drug history. Control of diarrhoea, if severe, is best achieved by a fluid diet [27] with codeine phosphate by mouth each time there is a fluid bowel action. Antibiotics are not indicated unless a specific dysenteric infection has been diagnosed (Lambert [20]).

3.3.7 Constipation

Although the causes of constipation in seamen are those of any other social group, reduction of transit time and less frequent passage of stool tends to occur with variations in diet and the reduction in the crude fibre content of the diet that commonly occurs during voyages. The irritable bowel syndrome, manifested by constipation or constipation alternating with diarrhoea, with spasmodic abdominal pain often relieved by the passage of flatus, is a diagnosis of exclusion. Such patients should be referred for full investigation when time allows. It should not be forgotten that a change in bowel habit in the older patient must be regarded with suspicion.

3.3.8 Jaundice

The commonest causes of jaundice presenting in seamen are alcohol-induced conditions and viral liver disease, obstructive jaundice due to biliary disease, and malaria.

Alcohol damages the liver both as hepatotoxin (Lieber and Rubin [21]) and as a result of malnutrition. Histologically, three categories of alcoholic liver disease can be defined: fatty liver, hepatitis and cirrhosis [2]. All of these may present as jaundice. Fatty liver is a reversible response to subacute alcohol ingestion which does not necessarily progress to chronic liver disease. Alcoholic hepatitis is a more severe form of injury, with a mortality ranging from 10% to 30%. It is possible that alcohol, by damaging the liver, predisposes to the development of chronic active hepatitis whether this be auto-immune or hepatitis-B mediated. Cirrhosis is a severe irreversible form of alcohol-induced injury.

Alcoholic fatty liver typically affects the patient who has been drinking heavily for some weeks to months. There is loss of appetite, weight loss, upper abdominal pain, nausea and vomiting and the patient is usually mildly jaundiced. Hepatomegaly is common and the liver is usually tender. Occasionally patients with alcoholic fatty liver present with an illness suggestive of obstructive jaundice.

Alcoholic hepatitis presents as jaundice, abdominal discomfort, fever and, on examination, usually some evidence of chronic liver disease.

Cirrhosis is often detected as an incidental finding and the patient does not have an acute illness as tends to occur in acute fatty liver and hepatitis. The stigmata of chronic liver disease may also be detected.

In alcohol-induced liver disease the severity of the histological lesion correlates poorly with the history of alcohol consumption, both in relation to duration of drinking and the amount consumed. This is partly because the history in such cases is notoriously unreliable. The diagnosis will ultimately rest on liver biopsy and all such patients will require hospital assessment and treatment which must include psychiatric advice. The mainstay of treatment of alcohol-induced liver disease is complete abstinence from alcohol. Nutrition should be restored and this must include vitamin supplements.

Viral hepatitis (A, B, non-A and non-B) is common among seafarers because of the closed community life which hastens the transmission of hepatitis A and the prevalence of homosexuality and tattooing, risk factors for hepatitis B and the non-A and non-B viruses (Zuckerman [39]).

Hepatitis A is endemic throughout the world but the exact incidence is unknown because of asymptomatic and anicteric infections, and differences in surveillance and patterns of disease. It is spread by the faecal–oral route and is particularly common in conditions of poor sanitation and overcrowding. The virus is shed in the faeces during incubation of the illness (28 days). The clinical illness resolved, there is no evidence of persistence of infection nor of progression to chronic liver damage.

Management should be symptomatic with attention to personal hygiene and, if necessary, a low fat diet. Human immunoglobulin given early in the incubation period will prevent or attenuate a clinical illness, but not necessarily the excretion of the virus. For these reasons, prophylaxis with immunoglobulin is recommended only for those without hepatitis A antibody who are visiting highly endemic areas. Hepatitis B causes a more sinister infection. Hepatitis B surface antigen can be detected between 2 and 8 weeks before the appearance of biochemical evidence of liver damage or onset of jaundice. The antigen persists during the acute illness and is usually cleared from the circulation during convalescence. Hepatitis B is not spread exclusively by blood and blood products and transmission may occur by intimate contact and by the sexual route. The sexually promiscuous, particularly male homosexuals, are at high risk. Hepatitis B surface antigen has been found in blood and various body fluids such as saliva, menstrual and vaginal discharges, seminal fluid, breast milk and exudates, and these have all been implicated in transmission of infection. The infection may also be transmitted by accidental inoculation of minute amounts of blood or fluids contaminated with blood such as may occur during medical, surgical and dental procedures, intravenous and percutaneous drug abuse, tattooing, ear piercing and acupuncture.

As for hepatitis A, management will be symptomatic with scrupulous attention to personal hygiene, while nursing staff should protect themselves from contact with blood and secretions. Hepatitis B immunoglobulin should be administered if there has been a single acute exposure to hepatitis B virus, such as occurs with inoculation from a known contaminated source.

Non-A, non-B hepatitis shares a number of features with hepatitis B. It is most commonly recognised as a complication of blood transfusion but may account for 10%–25% of adults with presumed viral A hepatitis. The illness is usually mild, often subclinical or anicteric, but may be severe and can cause fulminating hepatitis. Like hepatitis B, it may be followed by a persistent carrier state.

The carrier state associated with hepatitis B (and non-A and non-B) is defined as persistence of the B surface antigen in the circulation for more than 6 months. The carrier state may be lifelong and may be associated with varying degrees of liver damage. Several risk factors have been identified: it is more common in males, more likely to follow infection acquired in childhood and more likely to occur in patients with natural or acquired immune deficiencies. A carrier state becomes established in 5%–10% of infected adults. All patients with persisting hepatitis B antigenaemia require full clinical assessment, including liver biopsy, and will need long-term follow-up (36).

3.3.9 Other Infections Causing Liver Disease

A viral hepatitis may be caused by infectious mononucleosis. The association of lymphadenopathy, sore throat and palatal petechiae are helpful clues. Tropical causes include amoebiasis, schistosomiasis, hydatid disease, Lassa fever and yellow fever. These have recently been reviewed by Fakunle [13].

3.3.10 Biliary Disease

The spectrum of disease attributable to gallstones will be no different among seamen than among those ashore. Presentation will be with flatulent dyspepsia, biliary colic, acute cholecystitis or jaundice, all of which require appropriate management and, in due course, hospital assessment.

3.3.11 Pancreatitis

Alcohol-induced pancreatitis is the commonest form to be encountered among seamen, although the acute variety may also be associated with gallstones, certain drugs and other rarer factors which should be borne in mind (Trapnell and Duncan [31]).

Pancreatitis induced by alcohol tends to assume the chronic form although the mechanism is unknown. It occurs not only in alcoholics, but in the heavy social drinker, affecting the young or middle-aged male after years of over-indulgence (Benjamin [6]). Acute episodes tend to come on 12–48 h after a drinking bout, pain during the 'afternoon after the night before' being typical. Such attacks of varying severity last 3–7 days, with intervals of months or years. Later (but rarely before episodes of pain) evidence of pancreatic insufficiency, particularly diabetes, develops. Less common is the fulminating attack, in which the patient may become gravely ill with severe abdominal pain, distension, guarding, ileus and shock. A diagnostic laparotomy may be necessary.

The acute fulminating attack should be treated as a surgical emergency, with continuous gastric aspiration, parenteral nutrition and maintenance of fluid and electrolyte balance. Pethidine, rather than morphine, should be used for analgesia and surgery avoided unless to make the diagnosis (Trapnell [30]). The subject of alcohol-induced pancreatitis has been well reviewed by Marks [23].

Chronic alcohol-induced pancreatitis must be treated by total abstinence from alcohol, for no other regimen will abolish the episodes of pain. Other treatment must aim to improve the nutritional state and alleviate diabetes and steatorrhoea. In most countries a merchant seafarer suffering from chronic pancreatitis would be barred from further seafaring because of the possibility of (a) needing treatment that cannot be provided owing to the lack of medical facilities on board and (b) reduced working capacity.

3.3.12 Nutrition

Over the centuries nutritional problems have played a major part in the life of seamen (Milton-Thompson [25]). Modern methods of food preservation have combined with a greater understanding of nutritional requirements virtually to abolish these problems. Alcoholism remains a contributory factor to poor nutrition in individual seamen, and nutritional problems and vitamin deficiencies are still encountered in wartime (Schadewaldt [28]).

References

1. Abbot, O.A., K.A. Mansour, W.D. Logan jr. et al.: A traumatic so-called "spontaneous" rupture of the oesophagus: a review of 47 personal eases with comments on a new method of surgical therapy. J. thorac. cardiovasc. Surg. *59*, 67–82 (1970).
2. Alcoholic liver disease: morphologic manifestations. – Occasional survey –. Lancet *1*, 707–711 (1981).
3. Axon, A.T.R. and A.Clarke: Haematesis: A new syndrome? Brit. med. J. *1*, 491–492 (1975).
4. Baker, L., C.Smith and G.Lieberman: The natural history of esophageal varices. Amer. J. Med. *26*, 228–231 (1959).
5. Bardhan, K.D.: Intermittent treatment of duodenal ulcer with Cimetidine. Brit. med. J. *281*, 20–22 (1980).
6. Benjamin, I.S.: Alcoholism: New knowledge and new responses. Ed.: M.Grant. London: Croom Helm 1977.
7. Brayley, N.F.: A review of three years experience of medical advice to seafarers by the casualty officer, Royal Naval Hospital Plymouth, via Portishead Radio (WIT Medico Portishead). J. roy. nav. med. Serv. *66*, 2, 93–106 (1980).
8. Brayley, N.F. and F.R.Wilkes: A case of spontaneous rupture of the cervical oesophagus: a reminder. J. roy. nav. med. Serv. *68*, 1, 30–33 (1982).
9. Burland, W.L., R.H.Hunt, J.G.Mills and G.J.Milton-Thompson: Cimetidine. J. Pharmacotherapy *2*, 24–40 (1979).
10. Cliff, J.M.: Personal communication 1969.
11. Croft, D.N.: Aspirin and the exfoliation of gastric epithelial cells. Cytological and biochemical observations. Brit. med. J. *2*, 897–901 (1963).
12. Dronfield, M.W., M.J.S.Atkinson, T.W.Bell et al.: Outcome of endoscopy and barium radiography for acute upper gastrointestinal bleeding: controlled trial in 1037 patients. Brit. med. J. *2*, 897–901 (1963).
13. Fakunle, Y.M.: Tropical liver disease. Medicine *18*, 932–934 (1979).
14. Glover, S.D. and E.W.Taylor: Surgical problems presenting at sea during 100 British Polaris submarine patrols. J. roy. nav. med. Serv. *67*, 1, 65–69 (1981).
15. Gottfried, E.B., M.A.Korsten and C.S.Lieber: Gastritis and duodenitis induced by alcohol: an endoscopic and histologic assessment. Gastroenterology *70*, 890 (1976).
16. Gottfried, E.B., M.A.Korsten and C.S.Lieber: Alcohol induced gastric and duodenal lesions in man. Amer. J. Gastroent. *70*, 587–592 (1978).
17. Kaufman, S.E. and M.D.Kaye: Induction of gastro-oesophageal reflux by alcohol. Gut *19*, 336–338 (1978).
18. Krasner, N.: Alcohol and the gastrointestinal tract. J. roy. Coll. Phycns Lond. *12*, 15–20 (1977).
19. Krasner, N., T.J.Thomson, G.Crean et al.: Gastric epithelial cell turnover after acute and chronic alcohol ingestion. Gut *15*, 336 (1974).
20. Lambert, H.D.: Antimicrobial agents in diarrhoeal disease. Clin. Gastroent. *8*, 827–833 (1979).

21. Lieber, C.S. and E.Rubin: Alcoholic fatty liver in man on a high protein and low fat diet. Amer. J. Med. *44,* 200–206 (1968).
22. Mallory, G.K. and S.Weiss: Hemorrhages from lacerations of the cardiac orifice of the stomach due to vomiting. Amer. J. med. Sci. *178,* 506–515 (1929).
23. Marks, I.N.: Alcohol induced pancreatitis. In: Topics in gastroenterology 7. Ed.: S.C.Truelove and C.P.Willoughby. Oxford: Blackwell Scientific 1979.
24. Martini, G.A. and M.Weinback: Begünstigt Alkohol die Entstehung eines Barret-Syndroms (Endobrachyesophagus)? Dtsch. med. Wschr. *10,* 434–439 (1974).
25. Milton-Thompson, G.J.: Two hundred years of the sailors' diet. In: Starving Sailors. Ed.: J.Watt, E.J.Freeman and W.F.Bynum. Greenwich: National Maritime Museum 1981.
26. Nye, F.J.: Traveller's diarrhoea. Clin. Gastroent. *8,* 767–781 (1979).
27. Oral therapy for acute diarrhoea – leading article – Lancet *1,* 615–617 (1981).
28. Schadewaldt, H.: Nutritional deficiencies in the crews of German raiders in two world wars. In: Starving Sailors. Ed.: J.Watt, E.J.Freeman and W.F.Bynum. Greenwich: National Maritime Museum 1981.
29. Smith, B.M., J.J.Skillman and B.G.Edwards: Permeability of the human gastric mucosa: alteration by acetylsalicylic acid and ethanol. New Engl. J. Med. *285,* 716–721 (1971).
30. Trapnell, J.E.: The natural history and prognosis of acute pancreatitis. Ann. roy. Coll. Surg. Engl. *38,* 265–287 (1966).
31. Trapnell, J.E. and E.H.L.Duncan: Patterns of incidence in acute pancreatitis. Brit. med. J. *2,* 179–183 (1975).
32. Traveller's diarrhoea – leading article – Lancet *1,* 777–778 (1982).
33. Van Thiel, D.H., H.D.Lipschitz, L.E.Porter et al.: Gastrointestinal and hepatic manifestations of chronic alcoholism. Gastroenterology *81,* 594–615 (1981).
34. Watt, J.: The sailor's stomach. J. roy. nav. med. Serv. *58,* 12–34 (1972).
35. Welch, R.W., H.L.Bentch and S.C.Harris: Reduction of aspirin induced gastrointestinal bleeding with cimetidine. Gastroenterology *74,* 459–463 (1978).
36. What shall we do with the HBAg carrier? – leading article – Brit. med. J. *4,* 427–428 (1974).
37. Winship, D.H., R.Carlton and F.Calflesa: Deterioration of oesophageal peristalsis in patients with alcoholic neuropathy. Gastroenterology *55,* 173–178 (1968).
38. Young, A.E.: Stopping the haemorrhage from peptic ulcer. Brit. med. J. *284,* 530 (1982).
39. Zuckerman, A.J.: Acute viral hepatitis. J. roy. Coll. Phycns Lond. *15,* 88–94 (1981).

3.4 Respiratory Diseases

W. H. G. Goethe and T. Ball

3.4.1 Morbidity

Diseases of the respiratory system are as common at sea as they are on land. Statistical analysis of morbidity patterns among the seamen of seven seagoing nations according to the International Classification of Diseases [12] shows that respiratory diseases lie in third place after accidents and gastro-intestinal diseases (Vuksanović and Goethe [24]). Pons' statistics [17] put diseases of the respiratory system in second place, behind diseases of the digestive system. In the statistics of the *Centro Internazionale Radio-Medico,* cited by Tromp [20], respiratory diseases, at 4.9%, stood in fifth place among all diagnoses (excluding accidents) during the period 1935–1963. In these figures influenza appears under "infectious diseases", but if it is counted under "respiratory diseases", as in most classifications, then respiratory diseases again come second behind gastro-intestinal diseases. The international mean for respiratory diseases is 11.2% (Vuksanović and Goethe [24]), which corresponds to the figures given by the medical service of the *Deutsche Seeberufsgenossenschaft* (German Seamen's Cooperative Association).

The reasons for the leading position of respiratory diseases in morbidity among seamen certainly lie partly in exposure to the weather, but general meteorological factors, such as frequent changes of weather inside one climatic zone and rapid transitions between various zones within a short time, also take their toll.

Kraemer-Hansen [11] found in her material from an out-patient clinic for seamen that deck crew were on average affected more often than engine-room crew, although the difference was not statistically significant. It is undoubtedly true to say that working conditions play a decisive role. The engine-room crew often experience a marked and sudden change in temperature and humidity on leaving the working area, which could contribute to a general development of resistance. Crew members working on deck, however, are exposed to headwinds and simultaneous low temperatures and thorough soaking, particularly on voyages in cold sea areas. This undoubtedly makes them much more susceptible to common cold infections (Durante [2]; Ejsmont et al. [5]; Uselis et al. [22, 23]; Zannini and Tortori-Donati [26]). Uselis et al. [22] found parallel increases in diseases of the respiratory tract and of the cardiovascular system in higher age-groups. Kraemer-Hansen [11] found that officers became ill significantly more often than deck and engine-room ratings.

On the new high-technology ships, exposure to the weather has been substantially reduced. Time will tell whether this leads to any reduction in the incidence of diseases of the respiratory system.

No statistical data are available on the distribution of illnesses within the "respiratory diseases" category, but the experience of ship's doctors in general is that infections of the nose–throat area and the bronchi (common cold, pharyngitis, bronchitis, influenza) constitute an overwhelming proportion of the total.

3.4.2 Common Cold, Influenza

The relatively confined living quarters on board ship provide a particularly favourable environment for the spread of infectious diseases, especially those which are airborne. In past centuries the problem often reached epidemic proportions owing to the large numbers of people living together in crowded conditions. On most of the world's merchant vessels the seamen are still accommodated in shared cabins; it is only on the more modern ships from the industrially developed nations that the crew have individual cabins.

The crew of a ship is isolated from the normal continuous battle between a community ashore and the ever-changing infecting organisms ubiquitous in that community. The immunity of the crew may thus decline during a long voyage and render the members more prone to infections as soon as they start to mix with landsmen even at home. Colds and similar illnesses often spread like wildfire after the infection of one or more crew members by the locally current common cold or influenza virus in port. A few days after the ship has put to sea it is not uncommon for most or all of the crew to have become infected. Depending on the pathogen, there may be only slight symptoms or many crew members may suffer from fever and prolonged illness, which can in some cases cause significant problems in running the ship.

Abrupt changes in climate are obviously an important causative factor. Ejsmont et al. [4] found that acute diseases of the respiratory tract occurred chiefly on sudden changes of temperature in the macroclimate.

This problem is worsened on modern ships by the powerful air-conditioning systems, which impose an artificial microclimate and sometimes cause very strong draughts in the crew quarters. Naeve [15] attributed the very frequent common colds and the severe pharyngitis that he observed on board to rapid changes in temperature and in particular to the effect of the air-conditioning. Iwanoff [8] and Iwanoff et al. [9], in a study of the occurrence of common cold infections on board ship based on size of crew and duration of voyage (man-days), found a significantly higher incidence on air-conditioned ships than on non-air-conditioned vessels.

The seamen working on deck and in the superstructure on air-conditioned ships have a rate of diseases of the airways twice as high as that among those on vessels without air-conditioning, and on voyages in tropical regions the difference is particularly great. The authors draw the conclusion that air-conditioning on board ship must conform to outside temperatures, not to subjective comfort. For example, conditions of 25 °C and 50% relative humidity on board are probably too cold in the hot, humid tropics and too warm in winter in northern latitudes.

The type of air-conditioning can in certain circumstances be one of the contributory factors in the spread of infectious diseases. The air-conditioning system frequently cannot cope with unfavourable external macroclimatic conditions such as high temperature and humidity, and the ship's engineers then often drive it partly or totally as a simple air-circulating unit, i.e. the cool, dry air is circulated without any admixture from outside. In this way the whole crew can naturally very quickly become infected by any bacteria or viruses present in the air.

In a study of respiratory diseases in the United States Navy and Marine Corps, Hoeffler [7] found evidence to suggest that the use of suitably constituted adenovirus vaccines lessens the frequency and severity of respiratory illness in naval recruit populations. In merchant shipping, mass inoculations against influenza are not often carried out because of the difficulties in organisation.

3.4.3 Other Communicable Diseases

The literature contains only scanty material on other diseases. There are a few observations on bronchitis (sometimes chronic), pneumonia and tuberculosis. Sawyer and Sommerville [19] reported on an outbreak of *Mycoplasma pneumoniae* on board a nuclear submarine. The conditions on such a craft are, of course, not to be compared with those on a merchant vessel, but nevertheless similar epidemics could occur on a merchant ship through the functioning of the air-conditioning system.

Contact with cargo or with fuel in the engine room can lead to aspiration pneumonia; Wojdat and Winnicki [25] reported aspiration pneumonia from crude oil, where among other toxic effects there was liver and kidney damage.

3.4.4 Asthma and Others

Lung disorders such as asthma may be caused by allergens arising from the cargo or by substances the crew is working with. Bronchial asthma normally leads to unfitness for duty at sea at entry examination. But despite this, formerly undetected asthma may occur or asthma may be newly acquired due to allergens in the ship's environment. Allergens are frequent in cargo e.g. grain, castor beans and other seeds, animal products such as hairs, furs etc. Di Nardo [27] mentions among a considerable list of allergic disorders of seamen caused by environmental allergens on board only a few cases of asthma.

Ferraris [6], in 1960, studied the differential diagnosis in haemoptysis among seamen. He found that tuberculosis was the major cause, followed by tumours and tracheobronchitis.

In an investigation of smoking and respiratory disease in navy recruits, Pollard et al. [16] found that chronic respiratory symptoms were more frequent among heavy smokers than in light or non-smokers.

3.4.5 Tuberculosis

The once dreaded disease of tuberculosis no longer bears the significance it had in past decades. In a 1914 review of tuberculosis among seafarers, Sannemann [18] recorded that in the period 1896–1901, excluding accidents and suicide, 38.3% of all deaths were from tuberculosis, and in 1901–1910 the figure was still 31.7%. The highest mortality was in deck and engine-room ratings, officers and engineers being much less affected. Similar figures come from the records of the Dreadnought Seamen's Hospital in Greenwich, London, where 24.4% of all deaths in the years 1890–1910 were from tuberculosis.

The drop in the incidence of tuberculosis at sea, as on land, is attributable to better hygiene and to the widespread introduction of X-ray screening (obligatory for seamen). Durante [3] reported a considerable number of cases among Italian seamen as late as 1949–1954; the sufferers were identified in the course of mass radiography and treated. Molfino and Gennaro [13] recorded that tuberculosis accounted for 0.15% of the morbidity among all insured seamen and 0.60% of all illness. A classic example of the fall in tuberculosis in deep-sea fishing as a result of thorough screening is given by Kersten [10]; between 1957 and 1961 the annual incidence in the whole fishing fleet of the German Democratic Republic fell from eight to zero.

The statistics of the Marine Index Bureau of the USA merchant shipping fleet [1] show a similar clear fall from 0.10% in 1976 to 0.02% in 1980. Despite this welcome development, vigilance is essential, since in many countries, particularly in the developing nations, tuberculosis is still the most prevalent disease at all levels of society. Even in the highly developed industrialised nations a tendency to increase can be recognised.

Every seaman at the start of his career should undergo a medical examination, including a lung X-ray, before he signs on for a voyage. The experience of seamen's outpatient clinics in many parts of the world shows that failure to observe this basic rule, and especially the lack of regular repeat investigations, leads again and again to tuberculosis on board ship. Furthermore, in a case of open tuberculosis, the cramped living conditions make infection of other crew members very likely. If one of the crew is found to have tuberculosis, all the other members should be radiologically investigated.

References

1. Augenti, B.J. (Ed.): Statistical analysis No.79, Marine Index Bureau. New York 1981.
2. Durante, E.: Contributo allo studio della fisiopatologia dell'apparato respiratorio nei marittimi (Contribution for the study of physiopathology of the respiratory apparatus among seamen). Atti della "Sezione studi" del C.I.R.M. 211–220 (1968).
3. Durante, F.: Importanza dell'indagine schermografica ed umorale per la diagnosi precoce di T.B.C. nei marittimi. (The importance of humoral examination and screening for early diagnosis of tuberculosis among seamen). Atti del Centro Studi e ricerche per l'assistenza sanitaria e sociale dei marittimi 84–90 (1959).
4. Ejsmont, W., A. Knapik and E. Korytowski: Microclimatic conditions on vessels and morbidity among seamen. Bull. Inst. mar. Med. Gdansk *16,* 3/4, 201–203 (1965).
5. Ejsmont, W., J. Kruminis-Losowski, A. Krynicki et al.: Otsenka periodicheskikh profilakticheskikh isledovanii v polskom torgovom flote [Evaluation of periodical prophylactic examination in the Polish merchant marine]. In: V Internationales Symposium über Schiffahrtsmedizin, Rostock 19–21 October 1972. Rostock 1973, pp 173–189.
6. Ferraris, A.: Problemi diagnostici e terapeutici delle emoraggie tracheobronchiali nei marittimi (Diagnostic and therapeutic problems of tracheal and bronchial catarrh among seamen). In: Atti del primo congresso int. sull'assistenza di malattia e la tutela infortunistica della gente del mare nei paesi della c.e.e., Genoa: Casse marittime per gli infortuni sul lavoro e le malattie 1960. Vol. 2, pp. 451–457.
7. Hoeffler, D.F.: Current patterns of acute respiratory disease in the United States Navy and Marine Corps. Yale J. Biol. Med. *48,* 3, 171–178 (1975).
8. Iwanoff, I.: Klimaanlagen und Erkältungskrankheiten. Untersuchungen an Besatzungen von Frachtschiffen auf Tropenreisen. Dissertation, University of Hamburg 1975.
9. Iwanoff, I., H. Jungmann and P. Probst: Klimaanlagen und Erkältungskrankheiten. Arbeitsmed. Sozialmed. Präventivmed. *10,* 4, 78–81 (1975).
10. Kersten, E.: Zur Frage berufsbedingter Einflüsse auf die Morbidität in der Hochseefischerei. Verk. Med. *9,* 12, 551–574 (1962).
11. Kraemer-Hansen, H.: Diagnosenverteilung bei Seeleuten. Auswertung der Erkrankungsbögen der Abteilung für Schiffahrtsmedizin am Bernhard-Nocht-Institut für Schiffs- und Tropenkrankheiten in Hamburg aus den Jahren von 1966 bis 1975. Dissertation, University of Hamburg 1977.
12. Manual of the International statistical classification of diseases, injuries, and causes of death. Vol. 1 and 2. Based on the recommendations of the Ninth Revision Conference, 1975, and adopted by the 29th WHO Assembly. Geneva: WHO 1977 and 1978.
13. Molfino, F. and T. Gennaro: Rilievi ed osservazioni sulla tubercolosi polmonare nella gente di mare (Investigations and survey of pulmonary tuberculosis among seamen). Lav. e Med. *13,* 3, 41–43 (1959).
14. Montalto, G.: Sui casi di Pnx osservati negli ultimi dieci anni di attività della Marinferm Augusta: etiopatogenesi, terapia e rapporti del Pnx spontaneo con la Tbc; discussione di un caso di Pnx di etiologia incerta: secondaria o iatrogena (Cases of pneumothorax during the last 10 years of the activity of Marinferm Augusta: Etiopathogenesis, treatment and reports on spontaneous pneumothorax with tubercolosis). Ann. Med. nav. *82,* 3, 421–458 (1977).
15. Naeve, W.: Schiff ohne Schiffsarzt. Erkrankungen und Verletzungen der Besatzung eines Frachtschiffes im Liniendienst Europa-Südamerika. Münch. med. Wschr. *113,* 24, 909–913 (1971).
16. Pollard, R., L.J. Melton III, D.F. Hoeffler et al.: Smoking and respiratory illness in military recruits. Arch. environ. Hlth *30,* 11, 533–537 (1975).
17. Pons, R.: La pathologie du marin et sa prévention. Rev. int. Serv. Santé Armées *49,* 7/8, 579–586 (1974).
18. Sannemann, K.: Zur Frage der Tuberkulose unter den Seeleuten. Arch. Schiffs- u. Tropenhyg. *18,* 348–358, Beiheft 5, 192–202 (1914).
19. Sawyer, R. and R.G. Sommerville: An outbreak of mycoplasma pneumoniae infection in a nuclear submarine. J. Amer. med. Ass. *195,* 11, 958–959 (1966).
20. Tromp, S.W.: Some aspects of nautical biometeorology. Atti della "Sezione studi" del C.I.R.M., 23–39 (1965).

21. Tuberkulose wieder auf dem Vormarsch. Münch. med. Wschr. *125,* 8, 10 (1983).
22. Uselis, J., W. Ejsmont, L. Laba et al.: Gesundheitszustand der Seeleute in der polnischen Handelsmarine. In: Fragen der Schiffahrtsmedizin. Internationales Symposium, Heiligendamm, 28–31 March 1963. pp 252–254.
23. Uselis, J., A. Krynicki and S. Tomaszunas: Health condition of seamen examined at the outpatient's division for occupational diseases of the Institute of Marine Medicine in Gdansk (1961–1963). Bull. Inst. mar. Med. Gdansk *15,* 213–218 (1964).
24. Vuksanović, P. and H. Goethe: Diseases and accidents among seamen – An international comparison of distribution of diagnoses. Bull. Inst. mar. trop. Med. Gdynia *33,* 1/2, 13–33 (1982).
25. Wojdat, W. and St. Winnicki: Przypadek aspiracyjnego odoskrzelowego zapalenia pluc po zachlysnieciu sie ropa naftowa (A case of bronchial aspiration pneumonia due to a choke with crude oil). Bull. Inst. mar. Med. Gdansk *15,* 1/2, 83–85 (1964).
26. Zannini, D. and B. Tortori-Donati: Rilievi sulla morbilità dei marittimi in navigazione. In: Atti del primo congresso internazionale sull'assistenza di malattia e la tutela infortunistica della gente del mare nei paesi della c. e. e. Genoa: Casse marittime per gli infortuni sul lavoro e le malattie 1960. Vol. 2, pp 672–691.

Addendum

27. Di Nardo, U.: Su di alcuni aspetti particulari delle allergopatie nei marittimi. Atti della "Sezione studi" del C. I. R. M., 75–81 (1963).

3.5 Musculoskeletal Diseases

O. A. Jamall

The Dreadnought Seamen's Hospital in the Greenwich district of London is the main centre in the United Kingdom for the treatment of seafarers of all nationalities. The orthopaedic department plays an important part in the hospital function and it offers an ideal opportunity to study the pattern of orthopaedic diseases which affect seafarers. In this respect the hospital work is augmented by receiving orthopaedic patients who cannot spend time on the waiting list at other hospitals or who have been repatriated following illness or injury abroad.

This chapter is based on an analysis of the 1409 orthopaedic operations carried out at the hospital during the 5-year period 1977–1981 (Table 1). It does not attempt to classify a breakdown of the total attendances at the orthopaedic out-patient sessions. Nor does it distinguish the differing seafaring occupations. Included in the total number of patients operated upon are fishermen, entrants to seafaring, retired seafarers and an insignificant number of civilians. It is felt that despite the small dilution by these other groups, the figures given represent a clear indication of the orthopaedic disease pattern affecting merchant seafarers. A large majority of the patients were serving merchant seafarers, either British or of other nationality. It should be noted that Goethe and Vuksanović [3] found that accidents are more common in fishermen than in merchant seamen (see Chap. 3.2).

3.5.1 General Pattern

The series of operations at the Dreadnought Seamen's Hospital over the 5-year period shows virtually the same morbidity rate as that reported by the Naval Regional Medical Centre, Illinois (Konkel et al. [1]); of all operations, 66.8% were on the lower extremities, 25.9% on the upper limbs and 3.8% on the trunk.

3.5.2 The Knee Joint

In a study of musculoskeletal disorders needing surgical treatment over the period 1977–1981, disorders of the knee joint accounted for 479 cases, whereas the number of spinal problems needing surgery was only 53 – roughly nine times as infrequent.

In a survey of orthopaedic disease analysed in an article on *Orthopedic Diseases Treated in the Israel Merchant Marine Seamen's Clinic* by Sevilia and Shafrir [2], the incidence of spinal disorders was 252 as compared with 38 cases of disorders of the knee – a finding in reverse proportion to the statistical findings in London. However, the two surveys are not strictly comparable; the former deals with cases needing surgical care and the latter with the total number of cases seen in one orthopaedic clinic.

Many of the disorders of the musculoskeletal system in seamen are linked to their occupation and form an occupational hazard, though a large proportion of these cases come to light following relatively minor trauma on board ship. A predisposing instability of the locomotor system is often

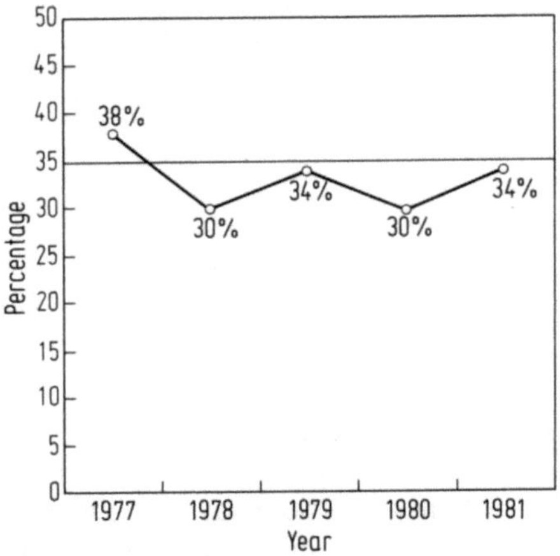

Fig. 1. Operations performed on the knees as a percentage of the total number of orthopaedic operations performed at the Dreadnought Seamen's Hospital per annum

present, having occurred after injuries sustained on a previous occasion.

Analysis of patients with surgical problems in the knee presenting for exploration of the knee joint during the three years 1977, 1978 and 1979 shows that derangement of the menisci accounted for 72 of 107 cases (67%) in 1977, 62 of 88 (70%) in 1978 and 77 of 105 (73%) in 1979. These figures represent a remarkable consistency.

The vast majority of cases presenting for surgery had a history of sporting injuries to the knee, mainly caused by playing football, in earlier years. Further exacerbation resulted from seafaring activities. Knees certainly form the major bulk of the problems needing urgent surgical intervention. This was born out in the Profile of Orthopaedic Surgical Practice reported from the Naval Regional Medical Centre, Illinois (Konkel et al. [1]).

Infra- and pre-patellar bursae or enlarged semi-membranous bursae are infrequently seen – only six cases needed surgery during 1977, 1978 and 1979, out of a total number of 300 knees, i.e. 2%.

The knee joint was explored for conditions other than derangement of the menisci in 9 of 105 cases in 1979, i.e. 8.5%, in 12 of 77 cases (15.5%) in 1980 and 17 of 102 cases (16.6%) in 1981.

Degenerative joint disease treated with osteotomy (upper tibial or combined upper tibial and femoral osteotomy) was infrequent: 3 of 105 knees treated in 1979, 6 of 77 knees treated in 1980 and 5 of 102 knees treated in 1981. It accounted for 4.9% of the total number of knee disorders requiring surgery over these three years.

3.5.3 The Hip Joint

Most of the patients needing hip replacements were non-seamen or seamen retired from active service. For example, of 39 patients who underwent total hip replacement in 1980, only seven of the patients were below the age of 50, the youngest being a 26-year-old male. However, over the 5-year period ten seafarers were able to return to work, albeit restricted to coastal duties.

3.5.4 The Upper Limbs

Disorders of the hands (Dupuytren's contracture, tenosynovitis, ganglion) also accounted for a significant percentage of the musculoskeletal disorders needing surgical care:

1977 42/281 – 14.9%
1978 37/293 – 12.6%
1979 61/306 – 19.9%
1980 52/258 – 20.2%
1981 44/271 – 16.2%

Recurrent dislocation of the shoulder is a common clinical problem seen at the Dreadnought Seamen's Hospital, and over the above 5-year period shoulder problems accounted for the following percentages of clinical cases needing surgical care:

1977 7/281 – 2.5%
1978 5/293 – 1.7%
1979 9/306 – 2.9%
1980 7/258 – 2.7%
1981 4/271 – 1.5%

In terms of morbidity, diseases of the elbow formed a group similar to that with shoulder-related conditions needing surgery.

The morbidity for the upper limbs in this series over a 5-year period was 25.9%. In a comparable series at the Naval Regional Medical Center, Great Lakes, Illinois, the upper limbs accounted for 20% of all cases of musculoskeletal disease (Konkel et al. [1]).

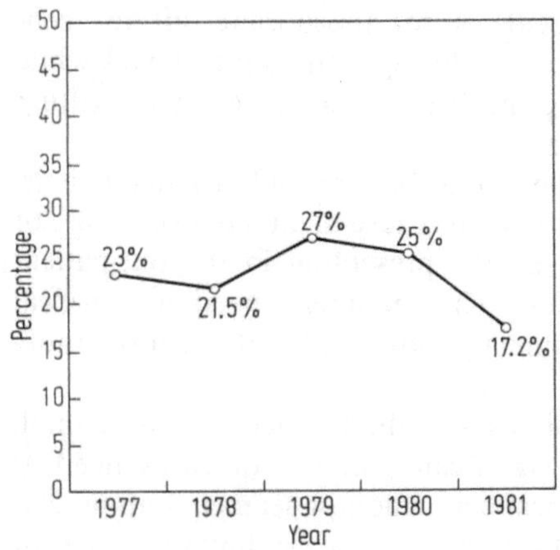

Fig. 2. Operations performed on the elbows and hands as a percentage of the total number of orthopaedic operations performed at the Dreadnought Seamen's Hospital per annum

3.5.5 The Trunk

Diseases of the trunk requiring laminectomy or spinal fusion were confined to male seamen.

Laminectomy	4/258 in 1980	1.5%
Fusion	1/258 in 1980	0.4%
Laminectomy	7/271 in 1981	2.6%
Fusion	3/271 in 1981	1.1%

These figures include only the small number of cases of back pain needing surgical care, and at first glance offer what appears to be a surprisingly low incidence of back problems treated. However, though an exact figure has not been compiled, the incidence of trunk problems in the form of recurring episodes of back pain and sciatica probably closely matches the figures quoted in Konkel et al. [1], where the incidence of diseases affecting the axial skeleton was 16.1% of the total attendances.

3.5.6 Discussion

In a study of the disease pattern in seamen from seven countries, diseases of the musculoskeletal system were fourth most frequent, with a morbidity rate of 8.9% (Vuksanović and Goethe [3]). Disorders of the knee joints produced the highest morbidity rate in our experience, accounting for 34% of all cases needing surgical care. Most of these give a history of earlier injuries to the knee joints made worse by trauma on board ship, caused through accidents on the deck or in the engine room. It was not possible to associate any particular task or type of work in either ship department with the occurrence of knee injury. The incidence of knee disorders over a 5-year period of study appears to be constant (Fig. 1).

Table 1. Orthopaedic operations performed at the Dreadnought Seamen's Hospital, London, between 1977 and 1981

Classification	Hips	Spines	Shoulders	Knees	Feet	Miscell.	Elbows and hands	Total no. of cases
1977	19	8	8	107	53	22	64	281
1978	29	12	6	88	81	14	63	293
1979	28	14	9	105	62	5	83	306
1980	44	8	11	77	49	4	65	258
1981	36	11	5	102	62	4	51	271
5-year total	156	53	39	479	307	49	326	1409

Disorders related to the elbows and hands accounted for 23% of all cases needing surgical care over the 5-year period. An interesting feature was the decline seen in 1981 (Fig. 2). It is possible to foresee a declining incidence of hand injuries with the changing techniques of handling cargo on board and with modernisation of the equipment in common use.

Recurrent dislocation of the shoulder is a small but interesting and continually recurring problem amongst seamen both on deck and in the engine room. Shoulder problems account for only about 2% of the cases needing surgical care.

The morbidity of recurring back problems has been adequately studied; facts have been collated in different studies amongst seamen and have tended to indicate that back disorders account for about one in ten cases presenting at out-patient clinics [Konkel et al. 1]. This figure agrees closely with the pattern observed at the Dreadnought Seamen's Hospital in Greenwich. Findings by Sevilia and Shafrir [2] in a Seaman's Outpatient Clinic of the Israel Merchant Marine show considerable differences. The majority of the patients (77.7%) consulted the clinic for back pains and among them 57% because of spondylosis.

Konkel et al. [1] also report a low incidence of spinal disorders needing surgery. They state that axial skeleton operations account for only 0.92% of all cases involving orthopaedic surgery. In the Dreadnought Seamen's Hospital over the 5-year period between 1977 and 1981, of the 1409 patients who underwent surgery, only 53 had spinal disorders, i.e. less than 3.7%.

In summing up, orthopaedic diseases form a high proportion of morbidity amongst seamen and in a relatively young and active group disorders of the knee joints provide most of the cases needing surgical care. It seems unlikely that this incidence of knee disorders will change significantly in the coming years.

Back pain will continue to be a significant disorder amongst seamen. Lifting of heavy weights on board will be necessary even in the seafaring of the future. The stress factor "lifting" will be increased by the ship's motions (rolling, pitching, slamming). Wrong techniques in lifting and carrying heavy weights with a bent vertebral column will lead to an increased risk of spinal disorders. The seaman should be instructed as to appropriate lifting techniques, i.e. lifting with a straight back while using the leg muscles to exert the lifting force.

Tendonitis, bursitis and degenerative arthritis are the cause of attendance in 30% of the seamen presenting in the out-patient clinics. The numbers needing surgical treatment, however, are considerably smaller.

Diseases of the hip account for a small but significant number of cases needing surgical care amongst seamen – about 2%.

Disorders of the upper limbs account for one-quarter of the surgical care needed in seamen, and as such their importance must be recognised.

References

1. Konkel, K.F., H.L. Spencer and R.C. Elliott: Profile of orthopaedic surgical practice at a non-teaching naval regional medical centre. Milit. Med. *143*, 8, 575–577 (1978)
2. Sevilia, J. and A. Shafrir: Orthopedic diseases treated in the Israel merchant marine seamen's clinic. Atti della "Sezione Studi" del C.I.R.M., 249–253 (1968)
3. Vuksanović, P. and H. Goethe: Diseases and accidents among seamen – an international comparison of distribution of diagnosis. Bull. Inst. mar. trop. Med. Gdynia *33*, 1/2, 13–33 (1982).

3.6 Venereal Diseases ("Sexually Transmitted Diseases": STD)

J. Huisman

3.6.1 Introduction

In the recent past, venereal disease has been most commonly associated with poverty and war; now its high incidence is associated with growing prosperity and relative peace (Morton [11]). Technical progress, rapid industrialization and urbanization have brought about an increase in production, while important industrial growth has also taken place in developing countries. This has resulted in intensive contact between ports via shipping. As in the old days, merchant seamen, deep-sea fishermen and navy personnel have a much higher incidence rate than people ashore; seamen must still be considered a high-risk group for acquiring STD (e.g. Eng and Jensen [5], Tomaszunas [18]). A seaman does not usually contract venereal disease at sea but on land and in a port which is not his home. The essential factor in the dissemination of STD, without doubt, is promiscuous sexual relations. Loose sexual behaviour is, of course, the essence of prostitution, but prostitution would not flourish if it were not for the traveller, and often he is encouraged by alcohol (Hawks [9]). One of the travellers *par excellence* is the (merchant) seaman and, by reason of his calling, he is more exposed to STD than those of many other occupations (Fergusson Ross [6]). For many years it had been felt that all attempts at STD control among seafarers would be in vain unless international agreement were reached for standardizing control methods in ports, irrespective of the nationality of the patient. An early move in this direction was the Copenhagen legislation of 1802 covering the free treatment of foreign sailors. By the time the Brussels Agreement came into force in 1924, Denmark had already had 125 years' experience in this field (Schokking [13]). In the Brussels Agreement the contracting countries undertook to establish, in each of their principal sea or river ports, services for the treatment of venereal diseases, free of charge and open to all merchant seamen regardless of nationality.

According to the Brussels Agreement, each patient receives a personal booklet ("carnet"), on which he is designated by number only. On the card the diagnosis and the treatment given are entered [1]. The World Health Organization publishes periodically a list of STD treatment centres – the World Directory of Venereal Disease Treatment Centres at Ports [17]; this gives the addresses of treatment centres and should be available in the ship's medicine chest and at all port medical offices. The Brussels Agreement also lays down the minimum requirements for equipment and supplies to be kept on board for the treatment of patients with venereal disease. They are also listed in the World Directory. In practice, however, the Agreement does not function optimally. For instance, not all countries are party to the Brussels Agreement; some behave as if they were, others bound by the Agreement do not fulfil their obligations. The treatment given is not always free of charge, designated clinics are not always easily accessible and consulting hours are not always convenient for seamen. In summary, the Agreement functions only partially and many seamen are treated by private physicians and not by the officially designated "free" clinics.

Besides the provision of treatment, free of charge, to seamen ashore and of treatment on board by doctors or (trained) laymen, the importance of health education as a preventive measure cannot be stressed enough. It should be directed at stimulating the seaman to seek medical advice after exposure and at enabling him to recognize the symptoms of STD, and should be offered in a way that is acceptable to modern seamen. It goes without saying that the positive effects of social welfare, education and recreation activities on board also play an important part in the prevention of STD in seamen.

A few words about personal preventive measures. The simplest of these, washing with soap and water, has been widely advocated, but the effect of this technique is, in fact, to date undocumented. So-called "prokits" were used by troops and naval personnel in World War II. The exact make-up of these kits varied but basically included a solution for urethral irrigation containing silver, mercury or permanganate and an ointment to be applied to the penis following intercourse.

Although carefully controlled studies were not carried out, infection rates in personnel using kits were generally lower than in non-users (Darrow and Wiesner [4]). Condoms have been in use for more than 400 years and when used properly appear to be highly effective in preventing the transmission of genitally located STD. However, the value of the condom as an STD prophylactic has been limited by improper and infrequent use. Barlow [3] showed that, when correctly and invariably used, the condom can be associated with decreased incidence of gonorrhoea in particular. Washing with soap and water and using condoms are advocated as preventive measures in the International Medical Guide for Ships [10], as is supplementary washing with 1:1000 mercuric chloride solution (Wandel [15]).

It should be accepted that there are differences of opinion on the treatment of venereal diseases at sea by laymen, especially syphilis and gonorrhoea. These differences are conditioned not only by the opinions of shipping doctors and specialists working in venereal disease clinics but also by government regulations concerning treatment on board and the content of the ship's medicine chest. The following guidance must, therefore, be regarded as the opinion of the author.

3.6.2 Gonorrhoea

Gonococcal infection causes purulent discharge from the anterior urethra with dysuria in men 2–7 days after infection. Some men, however, have no symptoms or symptoms so slight that there is no discomfort. Rectal infection, common among homosexual males, is at times also asymptomatic but may cause pruritis, tenesmus and discharge. It is evident that, in general, medical advice will be sought only in the case of symptoms. It is of prime importance that two or three urethral smears should be taken from all patients with suspected gonorrhoea. On board ship, it may not be possible for such a smear to be examined at once, but the glass slides, when dry, should be sealed in an envelope, dated, marked with the patient's initials and taken by him for examination by the specialist when he visits the clinic at the next port of call. Typical Gram-negative intracellular diplococci can be considered diagnostic in male urethral smears. Bacterial culture on special media confirms the diagnosis. Treatment of gonorrhoea with inadequate doses of antibiotics leads to resistant chromosomal mutants of *Neisseria gonorrhoeae*. The percentage of strains less sensitive to penicillin is considerably higher in countries where drug control laws are not strictly enforced – the rate increased by 30% within 5 years in Ethiopia and by almost 13% in 3 years in Singapore (Antal [2]).

In January 1977, *N. gonorrhoeae* strains producing β-lactamase appeared almost simultaneously in various parts of the world (*p*enicillinase-*p*roducing *N. gonorrhoeae* = PPNG) (Perine et al. [12]). It has been shown that PPNG strains contain a separate plasmid which codes for β-lactamase production. It is assumed that this plasmid has been transferred from enteric bacteria under a selective ampicillin (or penicillin) pressure. It is generally agreed that, unless penicillin treatment failure becomes a serious problem, penicillin (plus probenicid) should remain the drug of choice for initial use in uncomplicated gonococcal infection because of its efficacy, low cost and ability to abort incubating syphilis (Antal [2]).

In cases of uncomplicated urogenital/rectal gonorrhoea, the Centers for Disease Control in the USA [8] advise (a) aqueous procaine penicillin G 4.8 mega-units injected intramuscularly at two sites with 1 g of probenicid by mouth, or (b) tetracycline hydrochloride 0.5 g (taken 1 h before or 2 h after meals) by mouth four times a day for 5 days (total dosage 10 g), or (c) ampicillin 3.5 g or amoxycillin 3 g, both with 1 g probenicid by mouth. Evidence suggests that the two regimens listed under (c) are slightly less effective than the other recommended regimens. Treatment with tetracycline results in fewer cases of post-gonococcal urethritis in men and tetracycline may eliminate coexisting chlamydia infections. Patients incubating syphilis (seronegative, without clinical signs of syphilis) are likely to be cured by any of the regimens mentioned. Patients with uncomplicated PPNG infection should be treated with spectinomycin sulphate, 3.2 g intramuscularly (1.6 g injected at two sites) (Goethe and Backhaus [7]). Spectinomycin-resistant PPNGs may be treated with cefuroxime 1.5 g (750 mg injected at two sites) with probenicid 1 g by mouth. Considering all the evidence, treatment on board by laymen (captains, first mates or other responsible ships' officers) could probably be most effective with tetracycline, ampicillin or amoxycillin orally (the latter two with probenicid). At the first appropriate port of call a visit to the venereal disease clinic is necessary. Here the case will be assessed (involving, among other things, a bacteriological check for a cure and serological tests for syphilis) by a specialist who will also arrange for subsequent surveillance as required.

3.6.3 Non-gonococcal Urethritis (NGU)

Non-gonococcal urethritis (diagnosed by failure to demonstrate *N. gonorrhoeae* by smear and culture) is an STD that is diagnosed in the USA and the UK twice as frequently as gonococcal urethritis; its incidence in the general population is increasing more rapidly than that of gonorrhoea. In 40%–50% of cases, *Chlamydia trachomatis* is identified as the cause of NGU. Other causes are *Ureaplasma urealyticum*, herpesvirus hominis type II and *Trichomonas vaginalis*. In ±10%–20% no microbial cause can be found. Because of the difficult laboratory diagnosis of genital chlamydial infections, all cases of NGU are best treated as though they were chlamydial in origin, especially since many chlamydia-negative cases respond to the antibiotic therapy. The treatment of choice is tetracycline hydrochloride 2 g daily orally (in four doses) for 7–10 days which has been shown to be effective; erythromycin is an alternative. On board, treatment of gonorrhoea with tetracycline will also be effective for most chlamydial infections. As with gonorrhoea, a visit to a venereal disease clinic in the first port of call is necessary.

3.6.4 Syphilis

Clinical syphilis occurs in several stages. The primary and secondary stages usually end 6 months to 1 year after the infection with *Treponema pallidum* has been acquired. During these symptomatic stages, syphilis is highly infective and easily spread by sexual contact. After this "early syphilis" the disease enters a state of latency during which the disease can be detected only by serological tests. Latency may last many years but still be followed in some patients by the development of late lesions. For our purpose we will deal only with early syphilis. The first steps are to make an accurate diagnosis of syphilis, to establish the stage of the disease and then to consider it in relation to the patient's wife, family, fiancée or other sexual consort (male or female). For a disease with the consequences of syphilis, with a long period of observation following treatment, an accurate diagnosis is essential.

After an incubation period of 10 days to 10 weeks (usually 3 weeks) a primary lesion appears, usually as a single papule at the site of initial invasion; after erosion it presents a variety of forms, the most distinctive (but not the most frequent) being an indurated, hard, painless chancre. Invasion of the bloodstream precedes the initial lesion, and a firm, non-fluctuant, painless satellite bubo commonly follows. After 4–6 weeks, even without specific treatment, the chancre begins to heal and a generalized secondary eruption may appear. Syphilitic exanthema, generalized lymphadenopathy and condylomata lata or "plaques muceuses" are often accompanied by mild constitutional symptoms (malaise, fever, headache, soreness of the throat, arthralgia and skeletal pains). The saliva and discharges from sores in the (untreated) secondary syphilitic patient are highly infectious, but indirect transmission by contaminated articles must be considered rare. Primary and secondary syphilis are confirmed by dark-field (or phase-contrast) examination of exudates of lesions or aspirates from lymph nodes (if no antibiotic has been administered) and by serological tests of blood. Positive tests with *non*-treponemal antigens should be confirmed by tests employing treponemal antigens (i.e. fluorescent antibody or treponemal haemagglutination) to aid in excluding biological false-positive reactions. A dark-field examination is indicated in *all* suspected cases of primary or secondary syphilis and is indispensable in early seronegative primary syphilis.

Penicillin continues to be the drug of choice for all stages of syphilis. Whenever there is a history of penicillin allergy, every effort should be made to confirm the specific allergic state before choosing other antibiotics, because these antibiotics have been studied less extensively than penicillin. Treatment of early syphilis (primary, secondary or latent syphilis of less than 1 year's duration) should be with a long-acting benzylpenicillin (benzathine penicillin) 2.4 mega-units total by intramuscular injection at a single session. Benzathine penicillin is the drug of choice because it provides effective treatment at a single visit [14]. This is of prime importance for the treatment of seamen.

Patients who are allergic to penicillin may be given tetracycline hydrochloride 500 mg four times a day by mouth for 15 days or erythromycin (stearate, ethylsuccinate or base) 500 mg four times a day by mouth for 15 days. In-patient treatment for early syphilis is almost never indicated (except in patients with very extensive lesions of secondary syphilis). All patients with early syphilis should be encouraged to return for repeat quantitative, non-treponemal tests 3, 6 and 12 months after treatment. Careful follow-up serological testing is particularly important in patients treated with antibiotics other than penicillin. Examination of the cerebrospinal fluid should be planned as part of the follow-up visit after treatment with alternative antibiotics. Some prefer examination of CSF 2 years after treatment with penicillin. Generally no penicillin should be administered on board ship by laymen to patients with undiagnosed genital or other sores of possible venereal origin, and it must be explained to the patient that it is better to wait till the next port of call. A course of sulphonamides (e.g. sulphadiazine) may be considered as many non-syphilitic genital conditions will be cured by this, while not preventing syphilis being diagnosed later. Only if it takes more than 3 weeks to reach the next port of call and the symptoms are very suspicious, may penicillin treatment as described be given. It is always best to seek radio medical advice in such cases. Patients should be advised to visit a venereal disease clinic at the first port of call and at the home port the previous treatment must be assessed by a specialist. If the treatment is considered incomplete it might be advisable to start again.

3.6.5 Ulcus Molle

Chancroid or ulcus molle (soft sore) is an acute infectious disease of the genital tract caused by *Haemophilus ducreyi.* Most often, the diagnosis of chancroid is made through the exclusion of syphilis, granuloma inguinale and lymphogranuloma venereum. It is seen more often in the (sub-) tropics, especially in underprivileged promiscuous groups with poor body hygiene.

In temperate zones ulcus molle is seen in seamen and prostitutes in the big ports, where the incidence may be even higher than that of syphilis. The most important aspect of its treatment is the exclusion of syphilis. Any genital sore, whatever its appearance, should be suspected of being syphilitic until proven otherwise. At least three (daily) negative dark-field tests should be performed and negative serum tests for syphilis should be obtained over a period of 3 months before syphilis can definitively be excluded (Willcox [16]). The treatment of choice is sulphonamides (no masking effect on syphilis), but more and more sulphonamide-resistant ulcera mollia are observed. Sulphadiazine is given in an initial dose of 2–4 g orally, followed by a maintenance dose of 1 g every 6 h for 7–14 days. The sore should be washed with physiological saline, or a burn or wound dressing without local antibiotic may be applied. The latter should not be used when a seaman presents his lesion only a few days before arriving in port, as it may prejudice the dark-field examinations. Depending on the number of days before a port is reached and the clinical picture (risk of suppurating buboes), radiomedical advice should be considered. Any case or suspected case of chancroid must be referred to a venereal disease clinic at the first port of call so that the diagnosis can be confirmed and syphilis excluded.

3.6.6 Lymphogranuloma Inguinale (Venereum)

Tropical bubo or Nicolas-Favre's disease is caused by *Chlamydia trachomatis* and is mostly seen in the (sub-)tropics. In temperate zones it is rare and mainly observed in seamen as inguinal lymphadenopathy. The disease begins with a small painless erosion, papule or nodule, frequently unnoticed. The first signs and symptoms are, therefore, often the painful swellings, of the inguinal lymph nodes (mostly unilateral). The swollen lymph nodes become adherent to the skin and may undergo suppuration, fluctuation and sinus formation. General symptoms are fever, pain in the back and headache. Laboratory diagnosis is by demonstration of inclusion bodies in leucocytes of the bubo aspirate, by culture or by specific micro-immunofluorescence test.

The complement-fixation test is positive earlier than the intradermal test with Frei antigen. Treatment with tetracycline hydrochloride is effective in all stages. Dosage: 500 mg four times a day orally for at least 10 days or longer as indicated by clinical response (4–6 weeks). Bed-rest is necessary. Sulphonamides can be used when tetracycline is contra-indicated. Buboes should not be incised but, if necessary, be drained by aspiration. In the next port of call the venereal disease clinic should be visited so that tests for syphilis and confirmatory skin tests (Frei antigen) for lymphogranuloma inguinale can be performed. It should be realised that in 20% of patients with lymphogranuloma inguinale the non-treponemal tests for syphilis are falsely positive. In the home port, specialist assessment should be obtained.

3.6.7 Granuloma Inguinale (Donovanosis)

Donovanosis is a chronic, non-fatal, mildly communicable bacterial disease of the external genitalia and inguinal areas of the body. The disease begins with a papule in the genital area. This becomes a slowly spreading serpiginous, granulomatous lesion, which is frequently painless. Usually the patient has no fever and does not feel unwell. *Calymmatobacterium granulomatis* (or Donovan body) is the aetiologic agent. The diagnosis is based on demonstrating the intracytoplasmatic Donovan bodies in Giemsa-stained smears of granulation or biopsy material. Tetracycline hydrochloride (500 mg four times a day orally for 10–20 days) is the specific drug for the treatment of donovanosis. As granuloma inguinale develops rather slowly, there is no urgent need to start treatment on board. The condition requires examination by a specialist at a properly equipped clinic ashore. Treatment on board should be directed to the prevention of secondary infection. In many cases, hospital admission will be recommended.

References

1. The agreement of Brussels 1924. Geneva: WHO 1958. (Technical Report Series 150)
2. Antal, G.M.: The world situation on sexually transmitted diseases and its new aspects. Postgrad. Course on STD. Amsterdam 1977.
3. Barlow, D.: The condom and gonorrhoea. Lancet II, 811–812 (1977).
4. Darrow, W.W. and P.J. Wiesner: Personal prophylaxis for venereal diseases. J. Amer. med. Ass. *244*, 444–448 (1975).
5. Eng, J. and A. Jensen: Serologiske erfaringen ved rutinemessig undersøkelse av morske sjøfolk med Treponema Pallidum Immobilization Test (TPI). Nord. Med. 64, 2–8 (1960).
6. Fergusson Ross, A.O.: The different aspects of maritime venereal-disease control. In: Maritime Venereal-Disease Control, Selected Lectures Rotterdam 1953–1954, WHO, Reg. Office for Europe. Geneva 1956.
7. Goethe, H. and A. Backhaus: Die Gonorrhoe-Behandlung in der Schiffahrtsmedizin. Z. Hautkr. *52*, 1, 43–49 (1977).
8. Gonorrhea, CDC recommended treatment schedules. J. Infect. Dis. *139*, 496–501 (1979).
9. Hawks, D.: Getting the prostitutes off the ships: or health education as a design problem. Publ. Hlth Lond. *90*, 5, 247–250 (1974).
10. International Medical Guide for Ships. Ed.: ILO, IMCO, WHO Geneva: WHO 1967.
11. Morton, R.S.: Sexual freedom and venereal disease. London: Peter Owen 1971. p. 48.
12. Perine, P.L., R.S. Morton, P. Piot et al.: Epidemiology and treatment of penicillinase-producing Neisseria gonorrheae. Geneva 1979. (WHO Document WHO/VDT/79. 419)
13. Schokking, C.Ph.: The Brussels Agreement in retrospect. In: Maritime Venereal-Disease Control, Selected Lectures Rotterdam 1953–1954, WHO, Reg. Office for Europe. Geneva 1956.
14. Syphilis, CDC recommended treatment schedules. Morb. Mort. Wkly Rep. *25*, 101–107 (1976).
15. Wandel, A.: Elementare Prophylaxe der Geschlechtskrankheiten. Münch. med. Wschr. *114*, 452–459 (1972).
16. Willcox, R.R.: The therapy of venereal diseases in seamen. In: Maritime Venereal-Disease Control, Selected Lectures Rotterdam 1953–1954, WHO, Reg. Office for Europe. Geneva 1956.
17. World directory of venereal diseases treatment centres at ports. Geneva: WHO 1972.
18. Tomaszunas, S.: Venereal diseases among merchant seamen. Bull. Inst. mar. Med. Gdansk *13*, 1/2, 47–58 (1962).

3.7 Skin Diseases

Dorothy I. Vollum

Seamen are affected by a wide range of skin diseases which differ slightly in type and frequency from those found in the population ashore. Conditions due to sun exposure, irritant and contact dermatitis of the hands and fungal infections in the groins and feet are common but the more usual chronic diseases such as psoriasis, atopic eczema and severe acne are not seen so often because shipping medical standards may not allow employment of men known to suffer from them.

Zorn [20] and Shaposhnikov [15], discussing skin disease in seafaring, have stated that fungal infections, dermatitis, oil acne and solar dermatitis are frequent. Büchner [3] reported that 17% of 38000 seamen had skin disease, the common conditions being skin infection, irritant skin disease, contact dermatitis and fungal infection. It should be noted that the diagnoses were not made by medical staff.

Ambrosius [2] found that a clinical diagnosis of fungal infection was made in 63 members of a crew of 102 on board a nuclear-powered merchant vessel and the diagnosis was confirmed by microscopy or culture in 31; the author emphasised that mycoses occur frequently in seamen.

Goethe [7] suggested that fungal infections in the hands and feet were common in seamen, especially in tropical sea areas. He blamed low standards of hygiene and communal baths and showers.

3.7.1 Solar Changes

Ultraviolet radiation in the wavelength 290–320 nm (UVB) causes sunburn, elastosis and eventually skin cancer in the fair skinned. As the effects of UVB are enhanced by wind and potentiated by reflection from the sea, seamen are particularly at risk from them. Even in cloudy weather enough UVB penetrates to cause sunburn. Sunburn can be intense and severe even in the dark skin. The erythema comes within hours of exposure and may be associated with oedema and blistering. There may be a high fever with shivering, headache and vomiting. UVB stimulates epidermal thickening and for some days after exposure increased melanin formation and tanning, which are protective. Treatment is to avoid further exposure until the erythema has settled. The patient should be questioned to make sure that he is not taking any drugs which may make him light-sensitive; sulphonamides, tetracycline and phenothiazines, to name a few. Mild burns will be soothed by frequent applications of calamine lotion or cream and more severe ones respond to topical steroids with non-adherent dressings.

Elastosis or changes due to degeneration in the dermal collagen ("sailor's skin") as a result of ultraviolet exposure are common in fair skinned seamen in early middle age. The facial skin is thinned and markedly wrinkled while that on the back of the neck may be deeply furrowed and thickened. The skin, particularly over the forehead and temples, may have a yellowish hue and the facial pigment may be irregular in distribution. In the older patient the changes around the eyes are particularly marked and there are multiple comedones. The V of the neck, the forearms and backs of the hands, areas which are always exposed, are similarly affected.

Solar keratoses often present in all these light-exposed areas but particularly on the bald scalp, forehead, cheeks, backs of the hands and forearms. They are yellow-brown scaly lesions up to a centimetre across with a well-demarcated scale. The scale is adherent and removal leaves a roughened surface with bleeding points. The lesions are premalignant and any with an enlarging or indurated base should be biopsied. About 20% of patients with multiple keratoses are said to develop squamous cell carcinoma in one lesion, but the incidence of metastases in carcinoma arising from these keratoses is low, probably less than 1% (Lund [11]).

Seccia et al. [16], in their study of cutaneous tumours in sailors, found that 90% appeared on the exposed skin.

Multiple keratoses can be treated with curettage and cautery, or a topical cytotoxic cream such as 5-fluorouracil applied daily for about a month. Hydrocortisone cream can be used as well in an attempt to reduce the resulting inflammation. Cryotherapy with liquid nitrogen is also effective.

Rodent ulcers are not uncommon in the same light-exposed areas, particularly on the face in older seamen. Nodules with a pearly surface and dilated capillaries or superficial ulcers which fail to heal and have a beaded pearly edge are classical. However, any crusted or indurated lesion which persists should be regarded with suspicion and biopsy or cytology should be used to confirm the diagnosis. Adequate surgical excision is the treatment of choice but curettage and cautery can be used for smaller lesions and cryotherapy is an alternative (Zacarian [19]).

Malignant melanomata also occur but are less common than keratoses and rodent ulcers.

Prevention of the damaging effect of ultraviolet light is important, and susceptible fair-skinned seamen should be advised always to wear covering clothing – shirts with long sleeves and long trousers. The tightness of the weave of the cloth is more important than the thickness or colour in protection against light (Welsh and Diffey [18]). A sunscreen should be used on the exposed areas at least once a day. Preparations containing mexenone or para-aminobenzoic acid and its esters are suitable.

3.7.2 Urticaria

Urticarial attacks occur in 10% of the population so it is a fairly frequent cause of a generalised skin eruption in the fit seafarer. Urticarial weals are raised and red and soon appear white centrally. They have a well-demarcated edge and vary in size considerably. Each one lasts from 4 to 48 h. Irritation may be intense. Angio-oedema is a variant of urticaria with deep subcutaneous swellings. The eyelids and lips are often affected and in a severe attack there may be swelling of the tongue, laryngeal oedema and asthma. The weals are due to dermal or subcutaneous oedema from localised increased vascular permeability, and histamine is just one of the vaso-active mediators released from mast cells and basophils which may produce it (Munroe [13]).

Acute urticaria may sometimes be due to an immediate type I hypersensitivity reaction to foods such as nuts, fish and eggs or to penicillin. The allergen links with IgE on the mast cell and histamine is released. Other foods and drugs may produce urticaria by non-immunogenic means but usually no cause is found and the condition resolves within a few weeks.

Chronic urticaria, which is arbitrarily defined as an attack lasting more than 6 weeks, may sometimes be due to preservatives and dyes in foods – benzoic acid, salicylates and tartrazines. Occasional cases clear after treatment of intestinal parasitic infestations. Many drugs may prolong or provoke an attack by histamine release or other means; morphine, codeine, aspirin and indomethacin should all be avoided in the patient with urticaria (Akers and Naverson [1]). In cholinergic urticaria small weals appear in association with sweating after exercise or emotion. Cold and pressure may also cause urticaria (Warin and Champion [17]).

A history may suggest a cause and a general examination should rule out an underlying systemic disorder, such as an early infective hepatitis. If a routine blood count, ESR and stool examination are normal, antihistamines should be tried to suppress the condition. Hydroxyzine (Atarax) 10 mg t.d.s. and triprolidine (Pro-Actidil) 10 mg nocte may be helpful when promethazine hydrochloride (Phenergan) and tartrazine-free chlorpheniramine maleate (Piriton) have failed. Keeping a food diary may reveal an unsuspected cause and eventually challenge tests with dyes and preservatives in foods may be helpful. A diet free of preservatives and dyes may also be useful in the chronic case. Severe angio-oedema may require treatment with adrenaline 0.5–1 mg subcutaneously or intramuscularly. A chronic recurrent urticarial reaction on the trunk and arms in the crew of a tanker on the Orinoco river was eventually found to be due to the anal hair tufts of the female butterfly *Hylesia canitia* Stoll. The hairs were blown throughout the ship in the ventilation system (Goethe et al. [6]).

The differential diagnosis includes insect bite reactions which depend on the type of insect and the host's response to the injected irritant. There may be no reaction at all, a transient macule or weal, or after 24 h a papule which persists for several days and often has a central punctum where the insect proboscis has penetrated. The bites are usually grouped. Some, particularly mosquito bites, may cause large solitary blisters.

Jellyfish stings cause urticarial reactions at the site of the sting which often become necrotic and haemorrhagic (Halstead [8]). They may be associated with nausea, vomiting and sudden collapse. The weal is due to the toxic substances introduced by the nematocysts in the sting cells. The cause of the weal is usually obvious as it comes out more or less immediately after exposure and may be relieved by calamine lotion or topical steroids; supportive measures for the systemic side-effects may be necessary. Patients with scabies may have occasional weals and dermographism.

3.7.3 Miliaria

Miliaria rubra or prickly heat occurs as a result of obstruction to the sweat ducts. It is common in hot humid conditions in the tropics, particularly in men working in the kitchens or engine room. Minute erythematous papules in large numbers occur especially in the flexures and in areas of friction from clothing. There is an unpleasant sensation of prickling irritation. The only relief is to stay in air-conditioned surroundings and wear loose cotton clothing for a few days. The anhidrosis persists for at least 3 weeks after an attack. As a result of the anhidrosis, hyperpyrexia may develop.

3.7.4 Hand Eczema

Hand eczema is a fairly common disorder in seamen and may threaten their employment. It is therefore important to identify primary irritant and contact dermatitis as avoidance of the irritant or allergen may achieve cure.

The eczema may be acute with vesicles and erythema or more chronic with erythema, scaling and fissuring. There are many patterns of constitutional eczema but in most the palms of the hands and the sides of the fingers are affected, whereas in contact and irritant dermatitis it is the backs of the hands and fingers and frequently the ulnar borders of the forearms which are involved. Constitutional eczema tends to relapse and recur. Irritant and contact dermatitis may complicate it or occur alone. Anyone exposed to an irritant substance for long enough in a high enough concentration will eventually develop the irritant dermatitis. It is frequently seen in washing-up boys who do not wear protective gloves and do not dilute the detergent according to instruction and also in engineers exposed to oils and solvents.

Contact dermatitis is an allergic reaction and as well as an acute eczema on the backs of the hands and fingers, the face and genitalia may be involved. Frequently it is due to chemicals in rubber gloves, usually the accelerators, in which case the sharp cut-off line at the level of the top of the glove is obvious (Cronin [5]). A seaman with endogenous eczema may wear rubber gloves for protection and then become sensitised. Most shipping companies now recommend PVC gloves. Every case of hand eczema which persists after the standard treatment of avoiding water as much as possible, using emulsifying ointment instead of soap and applying a topical steroid ointment should be referred for patch testing.

3.7.5 Skin Problems on the Feet

Seamen often wear heavy protective boots in tropical heat and the subsequent sweating and maceration exacerbate any skin conditions on the feet. Endogenous eczema on the feet may be associated with palmar eczema or occur alone. The insteps and toe flexures tend to be involved symmetrically and the eruption is frequently vesicular or bullous and later erythematous, fissured and scaly. Contact dermatitis on the feet can be due to sensitisation to boots and shoes. The plantar weight-bearing surface is involved when it is due to the soles and the dorsum of the foot when it is due to the uppers – usually the dichromate used for tanning the leather or the dye.

Tinea pedis or athlete's foot is a dermatophyte infection of the horny layers of the epidermis. *Trichophyton rubrum, Trichophyton mentagrophytes* and *Epidermophyton floccosum* are the usual ones. All three may present as a soggy intertrigo with fissuring or as a vesicular eruption in the lateral toe webs. The nails are often infected and dystrophic. Asymmetrical vesicular and bullous lesions on the insteps are usually due to *Trichophyton mentagrophytes,* while the erythema and dry scaling in a slipper distribution is usually a *Trichophyton rubrum* infection. An acute tinea pedis will sometimes produce a secondary vesicular eruption on the palms. The diagnosis of the foot infection should be confirmed by microscopic examination of the skin scales for fungus or by a positive mycological culture. A topical antifungal application such as 2% miconazole cream or econazole lotion or powder is suitable for treating toe web infections. More extensive lesions should in addition have a course of griseofulvin 500 mg daily until the skin is clear, which usually requires several weeks. Treating nail infections with griseofulvin takes many months and is often unsuccessful.

A yellow-brown scaling of the toe web spaces may be due to erythrasma, a propionibacterial infection. Examination under Wood's light shows a brilliant coral red fluorescence, and 2% miconazole cream is a useful application. In very sweaty feet there may be superficial erosions of the horny layer of the epidermis and multiple pits on the weight-bearing surfaces. This is a condition known as "pitted keratolysis" and is thought to be due to a propionibacterial infection. It usually responds to treatment for the hyperhidrosis.

Groin rashes and irritation are common in seamen. Tinea cruris due to a dermatophyte causes erythema with a well-demarcated scaly border and is readily recognised. Mycological examination should be used to confirm the diagnosis and the treatment is as for tinea pedis. In eczema of the groins there is usually a history of spontaneous clearance and recurrence. There may be eczema elsewhere. The eczematous lesions often lack the clearly demarcated border of tinea. Here hydrocortisone or a weak topical steroid applied once or twice a day is useful. Erythrasma gives a macular hyperpigmentation with a well-demarcated border which is often symptomless. Wood's light examination shows the typical coral red fluorescence and treatment is with systemic erythromycin 250 mg three times a day for 21 days and topical miconazole. Flexural psoriasis may present as well-demarcated erythematous scaly intertriginous plaques in this area. Typical lesions of psoriasis may be seen elsewhere on the body or in the scalp.

Tinea versicolor is a yeast infection fairly common in seamen working in hot humid conditions. It is due to *Pityrosporum orbiculare*. It causes a macular rash on the trunk and upper arms with dark brown, light brown or depigmented and slightly scaly lesions. After sunbathing, the affected areas remain pale so that the eruption is fairly unsightly. The diagnosis can be confirmed microscopically. Treatment with econazole lotion or 10% sodium thiosulphate solution daily for a month is usually effective but the condition tends to recur. Recently ketoconazole in a dosage of 200 mg daily for 28 days has proved successful in the difficult case but liver-function must be monitored (Jolliffe and Ngai [10]).

3.7.6 Some Problems Due to Parasites

Scabies is a common cause of generalised irritation. It is due to infestation with the mite *Sarcoptes scabiei*. This burrows into the horny layer of the epidermis, laying eggs as it travels. The burrows are about 3 mm long and are seen as grey thread-like lines. They are found mostly between the fingers and on the flexor aspects of the wrists. There is a characteristic generalised papular excoriated rash. There may be some weals and dermographism is often a feature. Persistent papules are common on the scrotum and penis. The infestation is always transmitted by close bodily contact and in the adult is usually acquired sexually. In treatment it is important that the patient and his close contacts are treated at the same time to prevent re-infestation. After a bath 1% γ-benzene hexachloride cream is applied from the neck down to and including the soles of the feet, covering all areas of the skin. Another application is used 24 h later, and 24 h after that the patient has a bath, puts on clean underclothes and uses clean sheets. Alternatively benzyl benzoate emulsion 25% can be used.

Lice are small, grey bloodsucking insects which crawl among the body hairs. Different types infest the scalp, body and genital region – pediculosis capitis, corporis and pubis. They are difficult to see as they are almost translucent except after a meal of blood. The head louse lays about ten eggs a day which are cemented onto the base of the scalp hairs. The eggs hatch out after a week to 10 days and as the hair grows the now empty egg cases or nits grow out with it. Irritation from the lice causes excoriation and secondary sepsis with occipital lymphadenopathy. Scalp sepsis should always suggest a search for nits, which are frequently found in the area just above the ears. Treatment is with malathion 0.5% or carbaryl 0.5% lotion allowed to dry on the hair and left on for 24 h (Maunder [12]). This will kill the lice but not the egg, so the application should be repeated after 10 days when these have hatched. All close contacts should also be treated, and combs and hair brushes which cannot be properly cleaned should be destroyed.

Body lice cause a generalised irritation with a macular erythematous eruption, papules and many excoriations. The eggs are found mainly in the seams of the clothing and occasionally on body hairs. It is easiest to destroy the clothing and bed clothes if they are heavily infested or to put them dry into a hot tumbler dryer. The patient can be treated with applications of benzyl benzoate or γ-benzene hexachloride cream 1%.

Pubic lice are usually acquired by sexual contact and other forms of venereal disease may have been transmitted at the same time. Treatment is either by shaving or as for head lice.

Ulceration may be caused by contact with some corals. The trauma from the silica and the retained nematocyst barbs and the pharmacologically active substances it introduces are said to be the cause. The ulcers may take many months to heal but the chances are improved if the wound is cleaned and any traces of silica are removed initially and systemic antibiotics are given.

Dogger itch is an acute dermatitis on the face and hands caused by exposure to curly weed found in the North Sea (Newhouse [14]). This is a marine bryozoan *Alcyonidium gelatinosum*. The responsible hapten has recently been isolated (Carlé et al. [4]).

3.7.7 Tattoos

Tattoos are popular among seamen. A detailed report on the medical aspects of tattooing in seamen is contained in the thesis of Heron [9]. Pigment is introduced into the dermis with the needle so that early complications are usually localised infections such as impetigo or cellulitis, and occasionally infective hepatitis or even syphilis are introduced by this means. Late complications include allergic reactions to the pigments so that one colour in the area becomes swollen and painful. The red pigment is often mercuric sulphide (cinnabar), the green is usually chromic oxide and the light blue cobalt. Sometimes the yellow areas (cadmium sulphide) are photosensitive. Excision of the affected coloured areas is essential to remove the chemical particles causing the reaction. Some skin disease may present in the tattoos – psoriasis, lichen planus sarcoid and lupus erythematosus may be localised in the tattoo site. Removal of the larger tattoo presents many problems and nearly always a not very good cosmetic result. Plastic surgery, dermabrasion and laser treatment are usually not entirely successful.

3.7.8 Oil Folliculitis and Acne

Oil folliculitis is an irritant effect of petroleum oil. Oil acne is usually due to cutting oil and heavy lubricating oil. The primary lesions are comedones and there may also be papules and pustules. The backs of the hands, forearms, thighs, face, neck and waist are affected. The condition occurs when heavy oil-soaked clothes are worn for long periods and there is poor personal hygiene. It may take many months to clear even when exposure to the oil has ceased. Treatment with topical retinoid gels may be useful as they clear the comedones (Cronin [5]).

References

1. Akers, W.A. and D.N. Naverson: Diagnosis of chronic urticaria. Int. J. Dermatol. *20,* 32–40 (1978).
2. Ambrosius, G.: Mykosen bei Seeleuten aus der Sicht des Schiffsarztes. Mykologische Reihenuntersuchung bei 102 Besatzungsmitgliedern des Kernenergie-Forschungsschiffes NS "Otto Hahn". Dissertation, University of Hamburg 1971.
3. Büchner, E.: Hauterkrankungen bei Seeleuten. Dissertation, University of Hamburg 1976.
4. Carlé, J.S., M.Thybo and C.Christophersen: Dogger Bank Itch 3. Isolation structure determination and synthesis of a hapten. Contact dermatitis. Contact dermatitis *8,* 43–47 (1982).
5. Cronin, E.: Contact dermatitis. Edinburgh: Churchill Livingstone 1980. Oils 16, 839–850. Rubber 14, 714–70.
6. Goethe, H., R. Brett and H. Weidner: "Butterfly Itch", eine Schmetterlingsdermatose an Bord eines Tankers. Z. Tropenmed. Parasit. *18,* 1, 5–16 (1967).
7. Goethe, H.: Pilzerkrankungen in der Seefahrt. Hansa *96,* 10/11, 557–559 (1959).
8. Halstead, B.W.: Jellyfish stings and their medical management. U.S. armed Forces med. J. *8,* 1587–1602 (1957).
9. Heron, D.M.J.P.: Tatouages et gens de mer. Dissertation, University of Nantes 1972–73.
10. Jolliffe, D.S. and Y.L. Ngai: Systemic treatment of tinea versicolor with Ketoconazole in forty-four patients. Clin. Exp. Dermatol. *6,* 625–628 (1981).
11. Lund, H.S.: How often does squamous cell carcinoma of the skin metastasize? Arch. Dermatol. *92,* 625 (1965).

12. Maunder, J.W.: Clinical and laboratory trials employing Carbaryl against the human head louse. Clin. Exp. Dermatol. *6,* 605–612 (1981).
13. Munroe, E.W.: Urticaria. Int. J. Dermatol. *20,* 32–40 (1981).
14. Newhouse, M.L.: Dogger Bank Itch: Survey of trawlermen. Brit. med. J. *1,* 1142–1145 (1966).
15. Shaposhnikov, O.K.: Profilaktika dermatitov u mory akov. [Dermatitis prohylaxis among seafarers]. Voen.-med. Zh. *7,* 77–79 (1973).
16. Seccia, A., R. Bracaglia and E. Farallo: La cute del marinaio e gli epiteliomi; Problemi di fisiopatologia cutanea. Terapia e prevenzione. Atti della "Sezione Studi" del C.I.R.M. 14 pp. (1978).
17. Warin, R.P. and R.M. Champion: Urticaria. Philadelphia: Saunders 1974.
18. Welsh, C. and B. Diffey: The protection against solar actinic radiation afforded by common clothing fabrics. Clin. Exp. Dermatol. *6,* 577–582 (1981).
19. Zacarian, S.A.: Cryosurgical advances in dermatology and tumours of the head and neck. Urbana: Thomas 1977.
20. Zorn, E.: Die Bedeutung der Hauterkrankungen bei Seeleuten. Berufsdermatosen *16,* 215–227 (1968).

Addendum

Rook, A., D.S. Wilkinson and F.J.G. Ebling: Textbook of dermatology, 3rd ed. London: Blackwell 1979.

3.8 Cardiovascular System Diseases

W. H. G. Goethe, T. Ball

3.8.1 Morbidity, Mortality

The increase of cardiovascular diseases (CVDs), especially hypertension, arteriosclerosis, myocardial infarction, arterial occlusive diseases, arrhythmias and circulation disturbances, have been attributed to certain harmful aspects of the environment and our way of life.

In the statistical breakdown of diseases at sea, cardiac and circulatory disorders are not so common as among comparable populations on land, especially among those of developed industrial countries. This is definitely attributable to the more favourable age structure among seamen and to the selection procedures.

Applicants with cardiac and circulatory system diseases are eliminated at the preliminary and periodic examinations for fitness for duty at sea. If such diseases occur during a voyage the seaman affected will in most cases become unfit for seafaring duty very quickly and will appear in the statistics only once. As he is no longer a seaman, no relapse or new incidence will reappear in the medical statistics of seamen. When comparing the statistical data of the morbidity pattern of seamen from seven seafaring countries according to the International Classification of Diseases [15], Vuksanović and Goethe [29] found that cardiac and circulatory system diseases (group VII of the ICD) occupied eighth place with 4.8%.

There are, however, considerable differences in the rates of the nations included, varying between 2.1% (Denmark) and 7.4% (Fed. Rep. of Germany). In an analysis of diseases in the Italian navy, Pons [21] found that cardiovascular diseases took third place with 11.4%. A comparison of the conditions of merchant shipping and the navy is, however, possible only to a limited extent. In an analysis of the diagnostic statistics in an outpatient clinic for seamen, Kraemer-Hansen [14] found 4.6% in ICD group VII. In a thorough review of the literature published on this subject, she points out that most authors found disease rates between 1.6% and 8.8%. Rates over 10% are very rare in the literature and are probably caused in most cases by different assumptions and formulation of questions, as well as by the difficulty of classification. Furthermore, the often too specialised selection and the restriction to certain shipping areas or certain types of activities may be reasons for the range of variation.

Leaving aside their frequency, cardiovascular diseases exhibit a few particular characteristics with regard to nautical medicine. Their possibly dramatic sudden occurrence at sea and the associated problems of diagnosis and therapy put these diseases in a special position.

Unfortunately, there are only a very few statistical data available on the reason for the death of seamen during their career. According to Otterland [19] the most common medical cause of death among Swedish seafarers proved to be "heart disease". In the sequence of the distribution of causes of death, accidents and violence led with 42%, followed by drowning with 22% and diseases of the circulatory system with 10% (in third place). Unfortunately, this latter term was not further differentiated (coronary heart disease?, cerebral stroke?). The Danish Shipowner's Association has published yearly reports of the mortality among Danish seafarers [1]. In a summary of the years 1971–1981 there were 513 deaths. The most frequent reason was accidents (135 cases), followed by death of uncertain cause (122 cases). Third in the sequence were CVDs with 116 deaths, followed by carcinoma with 36. According to British Department of Trade statistics on the mortality of seamen whilst on articles at sea, it was repeatedly found that 60%–70% of all deaths from disease at sea are caused by cerebral strokes and heart attacks including CHD (Watson [31]). In contrast to the morbidity statistics, the mortality data of several seafaring countries demonstrate that some of the cardiovascular diseases may be of high risk to seafarers – higher than all other diseases.

3.8.2 Risk Factors

The main risk factors, such as smoking, hypertension, obesity, arteriosclerosis and psychological stress factors, are basically the same at sea and ashore. Some authors, however, point out specific aspects pertaining to sea travel. Pons [21] mentions disorders of the cardiovascular system brought about by the influence of the ship's movements on the neurovegetative system and by vasomotor strain during voyages in the tropics. This strain is said to cause cardiovascular diseases indirectly through general arteriosclerosis. Muzyka and Levina [18] report on shipboard examinations showing a severe demand and stress on the cardiovascular system during sudden changes of climate.

Jungmann [12] arrives at similar conclusions, pointing out that adaptation of the cardiovascular system to climatic changes will be achieved only after several weeks, especially on tropical voyages. Apanasenko [3] and Apanasenko and Gura [4] report on the increase of mean arterial blood pressure caused by sea voyages in rather high air temperatures and humidity. This indicates a semi-pathological condition.

Vasilev [26] considers possible an ischaemic change of the myocardium through the alteration of the coagulation potential of the blood which he observed during long sea voyages. A number of authors carried out selected electrocardiographic examinations on board ship. Di Nardo [9] found frequently occurring extrasystoles of different types and in some cases P-wave changes. Together with the changes in blood pressure which he observed, he attributes these findings to the climatic changes during voyages.

Wittwer [33], in conducting selected electrocardiographic investigations and determining cholesterol levels of seamen on automated ships, also found ECG changes, which he interpreted as signs of stimulation of the autonomic nervous system in the precordial lead. No definite correlation with the degree of automation of the vessel could be established. Waskiewicz and Banaszkiewicz [30] made exhaustive investigations into the state of the cardiovascular systems of Polish Ocean Lines seamen who were over 40 years of age. Among 307 officers investigated in accordance with the accepted principles of classification of the Minnesota code, 69.38% of ECGs were normal and 30.62% abnormal. The number of abnormal ECGs among the officers investigated considerably exceeded the figures from studies of industrial populations in Poland. Q-wave, ST-segment and T-wave disorders were considerably more frequent than similar abnormalities reported in the literature concerning the industrial population in the same age group.

3.8.3 Hypertension

Several authors mention blood pressure changes and the tendency to hypertension. Rizzo and Tumbiolo [22] examined 1175 seamen who were considered to be healthy. Hypertension was present in 16.9% of those over 50 years of age. Hypotension was found in 15% of the same age group and in 20% of those aged 25 years or under. Among 8000 long-serving seamen of the Russian merchant marine, Vinnikova and Matsevich [28] found 5.9% with arterial hypertension.

Barnatskii et al. [6, 7] report on hypertension, which is common in seamen and is thought to be in direct correlation with increased salt consumption. They consider successful prophylaxis with sodium hydrogen carbonate to be possible. Wolf [34] found a temporary increase in blood pressure in about 40% of the crew members of ships travelling in or through the tropics and a temporary decrease in about 50%. At the end of the voyage 53% of the crew members showed an increased blood pressure, which persisted even after disembarkation. In an examination of Polish seamen Filikowski [10] reports on the well-known correlation between obesity and hypertension.

A number of very different diseases are to be found classified in group VII of the ICD cardiac and circulatory system diseases. In his statistics concerning frequency, Pons [21] gives the following sequence:

Circulatory system disorders	64.3%
Angina pectoris	19.7%
Myocardial infarction	11.6%
Phlebitis	2.2%
Varicosity	2.2%

Kraemer-Hansen [14] reports that the frequency distribution of diagnosis in the material she worked on is as follows:

Cardiac disorders, including hypotension	55.11%
Haemorrhoids (piles)	36.36%
Varicosity, varicose ulceration, phlebitis	9.53%

Without giving exact data, Guida [11] expresses the opinion that diseases of the cardiocirculatory system are more frequent among seamen than among other workers. Among the CVS illnesses found on board ship the most frequent are the acute forms, such as collapse, hypotension and congestive heart failure. The higher incidence of cardiocirculatory diseases is found among engine-room personnel and among the "general staff", with those worst afflicted being ships' captains.

3.8.4 Angina pectoris, Myocardial Infarction

It is surprising that only a very few authors deal with the occurrence of angina pectoris or myocardial infarction (coronary heart disease – CHD) in seamen, which due to the frequently dramatic course of events can cause considerable difficulties on board. In the years from 1955 to 1959 De Carolis and Odaglia [8] recorded an average frequency of 1.04% infarctions in Italian seamen. Shishlova and Galich [24], writing about infarction in Russian seamen, report that approximately 50% of myocardial infarctions appeared when the patients were in good physical condition and did not show any symptoms of angina pectoris. Mazzoli [16] and Parodi [20] concerned themselves with varicosity and other peripheral vascular diseases in seamen, which in their opinion occur relatively often and can prejudice fitness for future duty at sea.

Mundal et al. [38] investigated latent ischaemic heart disease in sea captains. Of 110 apparently healthy Norwegian captains on ocean-going ships, a near maximal bicycle exercise test revealed a pathological exercise electrocardiogram for 10.0%, while the corresponding results for a comparable group of Oslo men and a group of Norwegian sea pilots were 4.6% and 11.8%, respectively. The significant difference in prevalence between the captains and Oslo men could not be explained by differences in serum lipids, blood pressure or a family history of coronary heart disease. The captains were taller and more physically fit than the Oslo men, but they were significantly heavier and had a more rapid age decline in physical performance capacity and a higher prevalence of heavy smokers. 10 of the 11 captains with a pathological exercise electrocardiogram were, or had been, heavy smokers (≧20 cigarettes/day). A high caloric intake in relation to caloric expenditure, heavy smoking and poorly defined factors such as stress, irregular workhours and varying climatic conditions are factors to be considered as explanations for these findings. The claim by captains that they have a higher risk than average for developing coronary heart disease was to some extent corroborated in the study.

General experiences show that masters, elderly mates and engineers seem to be more prone to cardiac disorders especially angina pectoris and infarction, but there are no reliable figures available. Lack of physical exercise and general hypodynamia is an outstanding fact in the life of ship captains and watchkeeping officers. These circumstances together with the at least temporary high mental load may be one of the reasons, or even the main reason, for the increased risk of this group.

3.8.5 Preventive Aspects

According to Toschev's investigations [25] the average loss of working hours in the Bulgarian merchant fleet through cardiovascular diseases amounted to 4%–5% of the total hours lost through illness. As nowadays the ships of most countries do not carry a doctor, the sudden occurrence of disorders which suggest a cardiac disease may cause major problems for the captain or the officer responsible for medical care on board. Due to the very poor medical training given to most of the officers, it is often very difficult for them to arrive at a diagnosis. In individual cases, distinguishing between angina pectoris and infarction may be possible by trial with a nitrate preparation in accordance with radiomedical advice. Technically it would be possible to make ECG recordings at sea to be transmitted by radio to a medical advice centre for evaluation. Kohfahl and Koch [13] report that ECG telemetry has been introduced into the German Search and Rescue Systems (Lifeboat Association). The ECG is made on board the SAR vessels and transmitted via radio to Cuxhaven Hospital for evaluation. A similar system is said to have been applied successfully on freighters of various other nations (Shani [23]; Avdeeva [5]).

Even though the tracings from individual ECG leads do not enable one to diagnose an infarction with certainty, such systems could certainly be useful on board and might avoid the necessity of diverting the ship to a port with all the associated consequences and costs.

The medical disposal which is given following a myocardial infarction varies from country to country. Many regard infarction as a permanent bar to seafaring; others leave the decision to the conscience and judgement of the examining doctor. The poor prognosis of a re-infarction on board with scant facilities is a prime consideration. The possibility of sudden unpredictable death together with the difficulty in such circumstances of quickly obtaining a suitable replacement crew member must also weigh heavily in the decision. In a survey of questions concerning fitness for duty at sea in the case of cardiac and circulatory system disease, Wittwer [32] maintains that having had an infarction renders one unfit for duty at sea. There are very few references available dealing particularly with rehabilitation rates after infarction in seamen. Aleinikova et al. [7] report a rehabilitation rate of 50% in all cardiovascular diseases. Vieweg and Lee [27] found a significantly higher reinfarction mortality in U.S. naval and Marine Corps personnel.

Most authors studying cardiovascular diseases in seamen agree on the following points:

- The excessive consumption of cheap tobacco on board may be a major risk factor.

- The number of seamen with cardiovascular diseases grows with increasing age and the associated long years of service on board (maximum in the age group between 40 and 50 years).
- Obese subjects comprise the majority of patients.

As on land, the increase in cardiovascular diseases at sea will be difficult to halt. A full clear explanation to patients suffering from hypertension or obesity and to cigarette smokers of the risks involved may be beneficial. For the doctor each examination for fitness for duty at sea should be an occasion to warn these high-risk patients about the dangers of cardiovascular diseases, particularly myocardial infarction, and the need to take urgent corrective action. The promotion of sporting activities on board and increased participation in spare-time physical training, could also contribute to halting the increasing incidence of cardiovascular diseases among seafarers.

The Framingham and other studies (Kallio et al. [35]; Kannel et al. [36]; Mann [37]) show that there are several clear risk factors such as hypertension, heavy smoking, hypercholesterolaemia and obesity. On the other hand there is the paradoxical result of a recent risk factor intervention trial which showed that special preventive care will not necessarily be followed by the desired significant reduction of the risk of CHD [17]. However, it seems clear in the trial results that stopping cigarette smoking will lower the risk of CHD and mortality.

References

1. Aarsberetninger 1971–1981. Danmarks Rederiforenings Laegekontor (ed). København 1972–1982.
2. Aleinikova, L.I., M.S. Denisuk and S.A. Sinitsin: Reabilitatsia plavsostava s serdechno-sosudistoy patologiey kak problema na vodnom transporte. (Rehabilitation of the crew with cardio-vascular pathology in seafaring). Bull. Inst. mar. trop. Med. Gdynia *25*, 2/3/4, 226–228 (1974).
3. Apanasenko, G.L.: O tipe samoregulyatsii krovoobrashcheniya i ego izmeneniyakh u moryakov pod vliyaniem plavaniya. (Self-regulation types of blood circulation and their changes among seafarers caused by sea-voyages). Gig. Tr. prof. Zabol. *17*, 7, 38–40 (1973).
4. Apanasenko, G.L. and E.I. Gura: Vliyania razlichnykh uslovii plavaniya na funktsionalnoe sostoyanie apparata krovoobrashcheniya. (Influence of different seafaring conditions on functional state of blood circulation apparatus). Voen.-med. Zh. 2, 71–74 (1973).
5. Avdeeva, T.: Kardiogramma cheres okean (ECG over the ocean). Morskoy Flot 6, 38–40 (1978).
6. Barnatskii, V.N., A.G. Kuznetsov and V.A. Kotenko: Profilaktika gipertensivnykh sostoyanii u plavsostava v okeane. (Prophylaxis of hypertension in crews on sea). Kosm. Biol. aviakosm. Med. *11*, 4, 85–87 (1977).
7. Barnatskii, V.N., V.A. Kotenko and B.I. Goryaev: Profilaktika arterialnykh gipertonii u moryakov. (Prophylaxis of arterial hypertension in sailors). Vrach. Delo 2, 50–53 (1981).
8. De Carolis, F. and G. Odaglia: Rilievi clinico-statistici sull'infarto miocardico nella gente di mare. (Clinical-statistical study on myocardial infarction in seamen). In: Atti del primo congresso internazionale sull' assistenza di malattia e la tutela infortunistica della gente del mare nei paesi della c.e.e. Genova, Napoli, Trieste: Casse marittime per gli infortuni sul lavoro e le malattie 1960. Vol. 2, pp 420–434.
9. Di Nardo, U.: Compartamento dell'apparato cardio-circolatorio di naviganti in clima tropicale. Osservazioni cliniche ed elettrocardiografiche. (Behaviour of the cardio-circulation system of seamen in tropical climates. Clinical and electrocardiographical observations). Atti della "Sezione studi" del C.I.R.M. 51–61 (1960).
10. Filikowski, J.: Effect of obesity on the morbidity of seamen. Bull. Inst. mar. trop. Med. Gdynia *30*, 1, 5–8 (1979).
11. Guida, G.: The pathology of the seaman (Report on the activity of the C.I.R.M. "Studies Section": 1959–1967). Atti della "Sezione Studi" del C.I.R.M. 19–23 (1967).
12. Jungmann, H.: Untersuchungen zur Tropenakklimatisation an Schiffsbesatzungen. Z. Tropenmed. Parasit. *13*, 2, 137–158 (1962).
13. Kohfahl, M. and P. Koch: ECG-telemetry in sea emergency cases. In: Abstracts. Telemetry of the cardiovascular system. International Symposium. September 5–7, 1979. Erlangen 1979.
14. Kraemer-Hansen, H.: Diagnosenverteilung bei Seeleuten. Auswertung der Erkrankungsbögen der Abteilung für Schiffahrtsmedizin am Bernhard-Nocht-Institut für Schiffs- und Tropenkrankheiten in Hamburg aus den Jahren

von 1966 bis 1975. Dissertation, University of Hamburg, 1977.
15. Manual of the International statistical classification of diseases, injuries, and causes of death. Vol. 1 and 2. Based on the recommendations of the Ninth Revision Conference, 1975, and adopted by the 29th WHO Assembly. Geneva: WHO 1977 and 1978.
16. Mazzoli, N.: Le flebopatie degli arti inferiori fra la gente del mare. (Phlebopathic diseases of the legs of seamen). In: Atti del primo congresso internazionale sull' assistenza di malattia e la tutela infortunistica della gente del mare nei paesi della c.e.e. Genova, Napoli, Trieste: Casse marittime per gli infortuni sul lavoro e le malattie 1960. Vol. 2, pp 514–521.
17. Multiple risk factor intervention trial. Risk factor changes and mortality results. J. Amer. med. Ass. *248,* 12, 1465–1477 (1982).
18. Muzyka, V. I. and T. I. Levina: Cardio-vascular system of maritime seamen during changes connected with quick changes of climate. In: VII International Symposium on Marine Medicine, 23–30 Sept. 1976, Odessa. Moscow 1976. p 396.
19. Otterland, A.: The mortality among seafarers. Atti della "Sezione Studi" del C. I. R. M. 39–52 (1963).
20. Parodi, V. M.: Le vasculopatie periferiche nella gente di mare. (Diseases of the peripheral blood-vessels of seamen). Lav. e Med. *13,* 4, 1–11 (1959).
21. Pons, R.: La pathologie du marin et sa prévention. Rev. int. Serv. Santé Armées *49,* 7/8, 579–586 (1974).
22. Rizzo, N. and A. Tumbiolo: Analisi dei valori pressori di un gruppo di marittimi. (Analysis of blood pressure among a group of seamen). Atti della "Sezione studi" del C. I. R. M. 89–94 (1967).
23. Shani, E.: Personal communication 1980.
24. Shishlova, L. A. and Z. M. Galich: Course and results of myocardial infarction in seamen. In: VII International Symposium on Marine Medicine, 23–30 Sept. 1976, Odessa. Moscow 1976. p 407.
25. Toschev, G.: Dynamik der Herz-Gefäßkrankheiten unter den Bedingungen einer Dispensairbetreuung der Schiffstransportarbeiter. In: Fourth international symposium on marine medicine, Varna, October 15–17, 1970. Sofia 1972. pp 214–219.
26. Vasilev, N. F.: Pokazateli funktsionalnogo sostoyaniya serdechno-sosudistoy sistemy i koagulogrammy u moryakov. (Indexes of functional state of the cardiovascular system and the coagulogram in sailors). Vrach. Delo 7, 26–29 (1980).
27. Vieweg, W. V. R. and D. A. Lee: Coronary artery disease: Its impact on naval and marine corps personnel. Milit. Med. *139,* 187–191 (1971).
28. Vinnikova, V. N. and L. M. Matsevich: Concerning the question of hypertension and ulcer morbidity of seamen. Bull. Inst. mar. trop. Med. Gdynia *25,* 2/3/4, 221–224 (1974).
29. Vuksanović, P. and H. Goethe: Diseases and accidents among seamen. – An international comparison of distribution of diagnoses. Bull. Inst. mar. trop. Med. Gdynia *33,* 1/2, 13–33 (1982).
30. Waskiewicz, J. and T. Banaszkiewicz: The evaluation of the state of the circulatory system in the officer personnel of the Polish ocean lines. I. A general characterization of the investigated population. II. Changes in ECG rest recording and in phonocardiographic recording. Bull. Inst. mar. trop. Med. Gdynia *32,* 3/4, 153–158, 159–167 (1981).
31. Watson, N.: Personal communication 1983.
32. Wittwer, N.: Beurteilung der Seetauglichkeit bei Herz- und Kreislaufkrankheiten unter besonderer Berücksichtigung der Hypertonie. Verk.-Med. *14,* 6, 189–202 (1967).
33. Wittwer, N.: Ergebnisse elektrokardiographischer Untersuchungen sowie Cholesterolwertbestimmungen bei Seeleuten automatisierter Schiffe. Verk.-Med. *22,* 10, 355–358 (1975).
34. Wolf, J.: Veränderungen des Blutdrucks bei Beschäftigten in der Hochseeschiffahrt. In: Fragen der Schiffahrtsmedizin. Vorträge aus dem Intern. Symp. vom 28.–31.3. 1963 in Heiligendamm. Sonderheft des Medizinischen Dienstes des Verkehrswesens II. pp 175–181.

Addendum

35. Kallio, V., H. Hämäläinen, J. Hakkila et al.: Reduction in sudden death by a multifactorial intervention program after acute myocardial infarction. Lancet p 1091 (1979).
36. Kannel, W. B. et al.: Sudden coronary deaths. The Framingham study. Ann. N. J. Acad. Sci. *382,* 3–21 (1982).
37. Mann, G. V.: Diet heart question. New Engl. J. Med. *297,* 644–650 (1977).
38. Mundal R., J. Erikssen and K. Rodahl: Latent ischemic heart disease in sea captains. Scand. J. Work Environ. Hlth *8,* 178–184 (1982).

3.9 Urologic Diseases

P. O. Oliver

In this chapter commonly occurring urologic diseases which may affect either passengers or ship's crew are covered. It should, however, be understood that certain of the methods of treatment advised could be carried out only on a passenger liner or other ship carrying a doctor. The extent of the treatment given in a merchant ship would depend entirely on the training and competence of the ship's officer responsible for health care and the content of the medical chest aboard the ship. Some of the more complicated surgical procedures discussed could, of course, be carried out only by a specialist in urology ashore.

The kidneys are concerned not only with the excretion of the end-products of metabolism and of foreign products and their metabolites but also with the maintenance of the tissue fluids at a constant composition. In doing so they assist in maintaining the pH and volume of the urine within physiological limits. The clinical features of renal disease arise from disturbances of renal function or as a result of pathological changes in the renal tract. There is often no close relationship between the disease process and the disturbance of renal function (Robson [10]). Diagnosis frequently results from abnormalities in the urine or blood and for this reason careful examination of the urine is essential in order to determine abnormal urinary constituents or bacteriological involvement. Likewise, chemical analysis of the blood with estimates of glomerular function are useful procedures in estimating renal dysfunction.

Valuable information can however be obtained by simple observation, measurement of urinary flow, and clinical testing of the urine. Oliguria, with a urinary output of less than 400 ml per day, is an indication of renal failure whereas polyuria, with a urinary flow of 3–4 litres per day, may be suggestive of diabetes mellitus, chronic renal disease or diabetes insipidus. Nocturia may indicate bacterial cystitis. The colour and appearance of urine may prove significant. Red urine usually indicates the presence of red blood cells whereas a dark brown urine leads to a suspicion of obstructive jaundice. Milky urine may suggest chyluria; bright green or blue, the presence of methylene blue from proprietary kidney pills.

Radiological investigation, including excretion urography, renal pyelography and angiography, plays a part in the diagnosis of renal disease. Additional information can be obtained by direct inspection of the urinary tract by cystoscopy or urethroscopy coupled with ureteric catheterisation. The more recent developments of radio-isotope and computerised scanning are useful adjuncts in diagnosis. In certain cases renal biopsy is of value. The importance of correct diagnosis in seafarers suffering from renal disease cannot be overemphasised and no seaman should be allowed to be at sea until all underlying renal disease has been eliminated. A recent study of the causes of medical attendance aboard British merchant vessels demonstrated the high incidence of diseases of the genito-urinary system in seafarers (Oliver [6]).

3.9.1 Urinary Tract Stone

The high incidence of urinary stone in the seafaring community has long been recognised as a major source of disability. It is estimated that around five new cases per annum occur in every 10000 of the population in the United Kingdom, with a preponderance of males over females of 2:1. Of particular significance to seafarers is the fact that over half of all cases will suffer a recurrence within 10 years, and although the majority of stones are passed spontaneously, some 30% will necessitate surgical removal. A variety of conditions are frequently associated with stone formation, all of which may, to some degree, contribute to its causation. Persistent crystalluria due to oversaturation of urine with aggregation of acids and salts often associated with climate or occupation, particularly in conditions involving excessive sweating and reduced urinary output, places seamen at high risk. Other factors such as urinary infection and stagnation, biochemical changes and metabolic or genetic abnormalities are significant.

There are only a very few nautical medical publications dealing with kidney disease in general and urinary stone in particular. Ejsmont [4] stated that 8.1% of 446 Polish seamen treated in hospital for diseases of the urinary system suffered from urinary stone. Arduini and Rizzo [1] found urinary stone in 4.35% of hospitalised Italian seamen, while Renke and Bublewska [8] reported on another group of seamen admitted to hospital, 5.9% of whom suffered from urinary stone.

In a study on the occurrence of urolithiasis in the Royal Navy, Blacklock [2] found that especially the engine staff and the officers were prone to this condition. The incidence rate was almost twice as high as that among other occupational groups on board.

Arduini and Rizzo [1] reported a much higher frequency rate in ordinary seamen than in officers; also the sickness rate of the engineers was much higher than the sickness rates of the firemen and mechanics.

Pellegrinelli [7] stated that, of all insured Italian seamen in the period from 1957–1958, 0.836% suffered from kidney disease. Of all nephropathies the most frequent was kidney stone, which made up 60.8%.

Nearly all of the authors discussed the reason for the frequent occurrence of urolithiasis. Macro- as well as microclimatic loads, especially during tropical voyages, are considered a main cause.

They report that kidney stone was predominantly diagnosed in seamen who are repeatedly on longer tropical voyages.

The majority of patients presenting with stone disorders have calculi consisting of calcium oxalate or calcium phosphate, the greatest number being idiopathic in origin and resulting from increased urinary calcium oxalate associated with changes in pH and urinary volume. The diagnosis of urinary calculi is rarely in doubt as the dull ache located in the lumbar region, often accompanied by severe renal colic, is unmistakable. As the calculus passes down the ureter, pain may be excrutiating and radiate down into the scrotum. Such symptoms are usually associated with haematuria and, occasionally, obstruction to the urinary flow.

Patients suspected of having a renal calculus require radiological examination of the urinary tract, preferably by intravenous pyelogram, and urinary analysis to determine biochemical constituents and associated infection. The immediate treatment of severe kidney pains or colic involves bed rest, warmth to the site of the pain and administration of pain-relieving drugs such as pethidine 100 mg or morphine hydrochloride 15–30 mg by injection, repeated at intervals of 2–3 h if necessary. Fluid intake should be increased to at least 4 litres daily and more under tropical climate conditions. Antispasmodic drugs, like atropine sulphate 0.9 or 1 mg intramuscularly, may be of value. Surgical intervention is necessary if the stone has not moved for several months or there is evidence of hydronephrosis. Large stones remaining in the kidney always require removal if permanent kidney damage is to be prevented. It is unusual for stones larger than 1 cm in diameter not to require surgical removal.

All cases of renal or ureteric calculus should undergo full investigation and treatment before the patient is considered fit for seagoing duties. An isolated attack of renal colic with the successful spontaneous passage of a calculus after a period of observation, provided urine and kidney functions are normal and there is no clinical or radiological evidence of remaining calculi, should not be an obstacle to further sea service. A history of recurrent calculus formation renders such an individual permanently unfit for seagoing service.

3.9.2 Urinary Retention

This can present as a serious and not uncommon emergency at sea in the elderly male, as a result of prostatic hypertrophy. Acute retention may also be caused by other forms of bladder neck obstruction, urethral stricture or accidental injury. Rarely, severe prostatitis causes obstruction. In such an event urgent catheterisation may prove essential. Clinical examination usually reveals a tender, distended bladder, and should there be no previous history, morphine hydrochloride 15 mg by injection should be administered coupled with a hot bath. Failure of these conservative measures necessitates catheterisation using the smallest catheter that will relieve the obstruction.

Normally a 14–16 F 5-ml Foley catheter, using an aseptic technique coupled with continuous drainage, will suffice. Most difficulties in male catheterisation can be alleviated by adequate lubrication and urethral anaesthetic using 1% lignocaine containing chlorhexidine (lidothesin gel). Such a procedure reduces the spasm around the membranous urethra, which is the commonest cause of difficulty. Should urethral catheterisation prove unsuccessful then suprapubic drainage should be carried out. The catheter is introduced 3 cm above the symphysis pubis, precisely in the mid-line, local anaesthetic being infiltrated into the skin and subcutaneous tissue down to the bladder wall. A 1-cm incision is made over the intended site and the catheter introduced. A suprapubic balloon catheter is desirable but, if not available, a large-bore intravenous cannula can prove effective. Long-term catheterisation should not usually be necessary although cases may occur on passenger vessels on long sea voyages. The smallest catheter that will be effective should again be used so as to avoid irritation of the bladder and urethra produced by too large a catheter and inflated balloon with resulting by-passing of urine. Most of the new silicone catheters will safely stay in place for several months if necessary. Regular bladder washouts should be unnecessary provided an adequate fluid intake in excess of 3 litres daily is maintained by mouth. Antibiotics have little influence in preventing infection and are better reserved for the treatment of infection should it occur. In certain circumstances non-sterile intermittent self-catheterisation may be recommended in patients suffering from loss of bladder tone with chronic retention and high residual urine volume.

A history of urinary obstruction from whatever cause requires full renal investigation before an individual can be considered fit for a seagoing career. Failure to effect permanent relief is a ground for rejection. Passengers with a history of prostatic obstruction should take extreme care before embarking on a sea voyage unless they are confident that adequate medical facilities are available on board.

3.9.3 Urinary Tract Infection

Urinary infection is a common clinical problem and one which frequently occurs in structurally normal urinary tracts. Although symptoms may indicate involvement of the lower urinary tract such as bladder or urethra, it is usually considered that the kidneys and upper urinary tract are inevitably involved.

Acute pyelonephritis is characterised by infection in the renal parenchyma and pelvis of the kidneys and is associated with severe constitutional symptoms, such as fever and rigors. Symptoms of urinary infection with renal pain, frequency of micturition and haematuria are apparent. The condition should not be confused with acute appendicitis, and urinalysis should normally establish the true diagnosis. Treatment should be directed to eradication of the urinary infection by the early commencement of appropriate antibiotic therapy, for example, ampicillin, co-trimoxazole or nitrofurantoin. Chronic or recurrent urinary tract infection is an indication for long-term chemotherapy in the form of ampicillin 250 mg twice a day or nitrofurantoin 50 mg twice a day. Co-trimoxazole 480 mg daily is a useful alternative.

Investigation of urinary tract infection in adults should always require the quantitative bacterial culture of a mid-stream urine specimen together with a determination of red and white blood cell concentrations. Catheterisation should be avoided. Men of all ages with a urinary tract infection should be fully investigated to exclude an underlying obstruction to the renal tracts, such as prostatic hypertrophy. Seafarers with a history of uncorrected recurrent renal infection should not be permitted to remain at sea.

With the increasing number of women being employed at sea, the incidence of cystitis has steadily risen. The high incidence of lower urinary tract infection in women during the reproductive years is now recognised although significant bacteruria is often lacking. Symptoms consist of increased frequency of micturition associated with dysuria. Treatment of recurrent cystitis in women can prove immensely difficult and maintenance antibiotic therapy may be necessary for several months to prevent recurrence. A regular daily dose of cephalexin 250 mg or nitrofurantoin 50 mg may prove effective. Particular attention should be paid to personal hygiene and avoidance of triggering factors such as vaginal deodorants.

3.9.4 Haematuria

The appearance of blood in the urine to any significant degree is usually apparent to the naked eye, although certain other causes of a red urine, such as intermittent porphyria and drug-induced changes, should be excluded. Careful urine microscopy is essential to establish the correct diagnosis, particular care being taken to exclude false-positives. Normal urine contains less than five red blood cells per mm^3. Multistix blood tests are reliable in carrying out routine screening procedures, although they do not prove that the blood is glomerular in origin. The distribution of the haematuria may be significant as an initial blood-stained urine is suggestive of a lower urinary tract source whereas a uniformly blood-stained urine is characteristic of an upper renal source. Kidney involvement is confirmed by the presence of red blood cell casts in the urine. The classical description of painless intermittent haematuria as an indication of neoplasm and painful haematuria as due to infection may be misleading.

Red cells may be found in the urine in a variety of clinical conditions involving the urinary tract which can be diagnosed by the presence of characteristic symptoms and signs in addition to haematuria. Inflammation of the kidney and urinary tract, acute glomerulonephritis, tumour and renal calculi will each present a classical picture. Haematuria as the sole presenting symptom may be indicative of renal tumour or tuberculosis, bladder papilloma or malignancy, prostatic benign enlargement or carcinoma. In those individuals who have been resident in the tropics, schistosomiasis should not be overlooked. No individual with a history of haematuria should be permitted to return to seagoing duties or to embark as a passenger on a long sea voyage without thorough renal tract investigation to determine the underlying pathology and without the common causes of haematuria, being excluded. Particular care should be taken to recognise patients on anti-coagulant therapy or suffering from thrombocytopenia; such patients present a serious hazard at sea should a sudden and catastrophic haemorrhage occur without appropriate medication being available.

3.9.5 Proteinuria

The presence of protein in the urine, confirmed by the use of the dipstick test (Albustix) or salicyl sulphonic acid, is always evidence of disease of the renal parenchyma and is unusual in disease of the lower renal tract. Small amounts of protein may occur in severe urinary infection or associated with macroscopic haematuria. It is not uncommon in carrying out routine medical examinations of apparently healthy young adults to detect varying amounts of albumin in the urine. Extreme lordosis in young persons will cause proteinuria. Such postural or orthostatic proteinuria is usually regarded as benign but may be suggestive of early glomerulonephritis. Further investigation is necessary and the patient should be required to empty the bladder before retiring and then to collect the early morning sample of urine on awakening, and a further specimen later in the day. The diagnosis is confirmed if the early morning specimen is free of protein and the daytime specimen positive. A follow-up test 1 year later is advisable to detect those patients who may later develop glomerular disease.

Some protein is normally found in the urine in severe chronic kidney disease, as a complication of heart failure and in the course of a febrile illness. In the nephrotic syndrome large amounts of protein may be excreted – the daily output is normally in excess of 5 g and may exceed 10–15 g. The majority of cases are due to glomerulonephritis, though some are drug induced or associated with carcinomata.

Persistent proteinuria, even in a young person, should never be regarded as a benign condition until full renal investigation, including kidney biopsy if necessary, has proved negative. Chronic renal disease is a disabling condition and is a contra-indication to seafaring. All cases of proteinuria detected at pre-engagement medical examination should, therefore, be thoroughly investigated before an assessment of fitness for seagoing duties is made.

3.9.6 Prostatic Disease

Benign prostate hypertrophy is a common disabling condition at sea as a result of the increasing age of the seagoing community, both crew and passengers. The enlarged prostate causes progressive obstruction to the urinary outflow from the bladder by compressing and constricting the urethra, causing urinary obstruction, retention and hydronephrosis. In the early stages the patient presents with a sudden desire to micturate but has difficulty in doing so, with eventual tenderness and distention of the bladder from a slow build-up of residual urine. Nocturia may be a troublesome symptom. The anatomical size of the prostate, determined by rectal examination, is often unrelated to the severity of symptoms. Although benign hypertrophy is considered to be due to hormonal imbalance, hormonal therapy has proved disappointing, and prostatectomy remains the treatment of choice. The decision to undertake an open operation or transurethral resection, TUR, depends largely on the surgeon's skill and particular experience. The mortality and morbidity from TUR is halved compared with open operation and the duration of hospital stay thereafter significantly reduced. Grossly enlarged prostates are best treated by open surgery. However, transurethral resection should still be regarded as major surgery and complications, such as frequency of micturition, may persist for some months. A small proportion of patients (less than 5%) suffer from impotence postoperatively. The treatment of cancer of the prostate remains controversial and many urologists now consider that when a patient is free of symptoms or the symptoms can be relieved by resection, no further treatment is indicated. Oestrogen therapy should be held back until metastases or complications develop. Orchidectomy is increasingly recommended and has met with success, radiotherapy being reserved for those patients with painful bone metastases.

Acute inflammation of the prostate is relatively uncommon, although when it occurs it is extremely troublesome, with accompanying pyrexia, dysuria and perineal pain radiating down to the testes and inner thigh. Untreated it may lead to septicaemia or prostatic abscess. Parenteral antibiotics are effective, such as co-trimoxazole (Septrin) 960 mg every 12 h or gentamycin 2.5 mg/kg daily in divided doses every 8 h.

Chronic prostatitis is a symptom complex which is not well understood and which may be associated with a psychoneurotic personality. With a high incidence of sexually transmitted disease, chronic prostatitis is common amongst seafarers. Symptoms are recurrent discomfort in the prostate area associated with urgency, dysuria and pain on ejaculation. Treatment should commence with a prolonged course of antibiotics of at least 36 months, such as co-trimoxazole and, if this fails, tetracycline derivatives such as doxycycline (Vibramycin) or minocycline (Minocin) are of value. Repeated prostatic massage may prove beneficial.

3.9.7 Urethral Stricture

Post-gonorrhoeal stricture has become much less common since the introduction of the antibiotic treatment of gonorrhoea. Most strictures develop during the first year after a gonorrhoeal infection, but they may not give rise to difficulty in micturition for 10–15 years. In the majority of cases dilatation of the urethra once every 5–6 months is a satisfactory form of treatment, although unsuitable for seafarers. With the introduction of the fibroscopic endoscope, urethroscopy has become a relatively easy and valued procedure, although the earlier claims for stricture success with the urethrotome were over-optimistic as recurrence commonly occurred. To assess cure a follow-up over a 3-year period is essential before seafaring is resumed.

3.9.8 Kidney and Bladder Tumours

The classical picture of renal tumour – haematuria and dragging pain in the loin with a palpable mass – is unmistakable and confirms that the disease is in an advanced stage. Particular care should be taken to recognise early findings such as raised ESR, anaemia, weight loss and hypertension, so that an early diagnosis can be established with beneficial results. Renal scanning is now an invaluable procedure. Nephrectomy, in the absence of metastases, is the treatment of choice. Removal of a kidney for reasons other than malignancy need not be a bar to seafaring and selected individuals, following a successful nephrectomy, may be considered fit to continue at sea, although unsuited for service in the tropics or engine room.

Bladder tumours are histologically similar to those found in the renal pelvis and ureter and are usually transitional cell carcinomata. Some are benign, such as a bladder papillomata, and are successfully treated by diathermy, although the risk of recurrence after apparently adequate treatment is ever-present. It is generally unwise for patients with a history of bladder tumour, however successfully treated, to serve at sea.

3.9.9 Renal Tuberculosis

Tuberculosis of the kidney tends to occur in young people and is invariably secondary to tuberculosis elsewhere, resulting from blood-borne infection. Regrettably, the incidence of genito-urinary tuberculosis has not fallen in line with that of pulmonary tuberculosis. Unlike the latter, where radiography has proved such a valuable diagnostic procedure, genito-urinary tuberculosis is difficult to diagnose. The disease usually manifests itself with haematuria and dysuria in addition to which the general symptoms of tuberculosis, i.e. malaise, pyrexia and weight loss, may be apparent. Urine is often sterile on examination or may show evidence of secondary infection typical of a bacterial cystitis. Tuberculous cystitis is always secondary to a tuberculous focus in the kidneys which is usually recognisable on radiological examination following an intravenous pyelogram. Urine culture, either from the bladder or both ureters, demonstrating acid/alcohol fast bacilli should confirm the diagnosis and enable early treatment to commence, even before final culture is conclusive. Standard oral treatment of tuberculosis in the form of rifampicin, isoniazid and pyrazinamide is effective and should be continued for at least 6 months. Nephrectomy or epididymisectomy is indicated only in the cases where the tuberculous lesion is well advanced and tissue destruction extensive. Surgery may be of value in relieving the complications of urethral stricture and fibrotic bladder following chemotherapy. Very careful appraisal and follow-up studies for at least 2 years should be undertaken before considering an individual fit to return to seafaring duties. The risk of relapse is always present and the difficulties of diagnosis formidable in a seagoing situation.

3.9.10 Disorders of the Testes

3.9.10.1 Undescended Testes

It is estimated that 0.7% of testes remain undescended into the scrotum after the 1st year. The seminiferous tubules develop between the 5th and 9th year and it is therefore advisable to recommend orchidopexy before the age of 6 years if fertility is to be preserved.

Despite the awareness of the need for early corrective surgery, cases of undescended testes are still encountered in the course of routine pre-engagement medical examinations in young adults. Such individuals should undergo orchidectomy in view of the high risk of malignancy. The annual incidence of testicular tumour is more than 2 per 100000 males and this is increased 35 times if the testicle remains undescended. In addition to the removal of the undescended testis, surgery should aim to give the genitalia a normal appearance by insertion of a plastic testicular prosthesis. Unilateral orchidectomy does not affect fertility or testosterone function. No person should be permitted to embark on a seagoing career with an undescended testis not corrected by surgery.

3.9.10.2 Torsion of the Testis

Sudden severe pain originating in the testicle, scrotum or groin in a young man in his teens or early twenties is typical of this condition. Care must be taken not to confuse this sudden emergency with that of an acute epididymo-orchitis, which is uncommon in this age group. Torsion of the testis is attributed to congenitally abnormal attachments permitting a twisting of the mesentery of the testis within the tunica vaginalis. Unless there is conclusive evidence of a urinary tract infection, surgical exploration is essential. Failure to relieve the torsion within 4 h of onset of symptoms may result in serious and irreparable testicular damage. Under seagoing conditions it is better to risk an unnecessary operation of this nature, where the surgical risks are minimal and recovery, following antibiotic therapy, likely.

3.9.11 Medical Standards for Seafarers

All entrants and former merchant seafarers seeking to re-enter the merchant navy should have healthy kidneys, ureters, bladder and urethra [5]. Urine should be free from abnormal constituents. All applicants having proteinuria, glycosuria or another urinary abnormality should be referred for investigation. The loss of one kidney, prostatic disease or enlargement, urinary obstruction from any cause, or a history of recurrent stone or urinary incontinence should cause rejection. Boys who have suffered nocturnal enuresis should have been dry for at least 2 years before acceptance.

Any chronic nephropathy involving the danger of renal insufficiency is sufficient to certify unfitness for duty on board. Also, passengers starting a cruise on a passenger liner should not suffer from a renal insufficiency. Although some of the cruise liners have dialysers on board and Beermann [3] has reported positively on relevant experience on board, it should urgently be recommended that these people be prevented from seafaring unless appropriate precautions are taken.

References

1. Arduini, M. and N. Rizzo: Etiologia e profilassi della calcolosi renale nei naviganti. Atti della "Sezione Studi" C. I. R. M. 47–59 (1962).
2. Blacklock, N.J.: The pattern of urolithiasis in the Royal Navy. J. roy. nav. med. Serv. *51*, 2/3, 99–111 (1965).
3. Beermann, G.: Medizinische Erfahrungen während einer Kreuzfahrt mit Dialysepatienten. Dtsch. Ärztebl. *78*, 4, 132 (1981).
4. Ejsmont, W.: Higiena pracy na statkach a stan zdrowia marynarzy w polskiej marynarce handlowej. [Occupational hygiene on ships and the health status of seamen in the Polish merchant marine]. Warsaw: Państwowy zaklad wydawnictw lekarskich 1966.
5. Medical and Visual Standards. General Council of British Shipping (Ed.). London 1976.
6. Oliver, P.O.: A study of the causes of medical attendance aboard British Merchant Ships. Publ. Hlth (Lond.) 95, 74–81 (1981).
7. Pellegrinelli, G.: Rilievi clinico-statistici sulle nefropatie nei marittimi. Lav. e Med. *16*, 31–35 (1962).
8. Renke, W. and A. Bublewska: The level of glycine in urine of persons affected with urolithiasis (considering persons working on the sea). Bull. Inst. mar. Med. Gdansk *21*, 1/2, 139–145 (1970).
9. Renke, W., Z. Kasztelan and A. Winnicka: Further research on glycine content in urine in cases of oxalic urolithiasis (considering urolithiasis in seamen). Bull. Inst. mar. Med. Gdansk *24*, 1/2, 73–78 (1973).
10. Robson, J.S.: Diseases of the kidney and urinary system. In: Davidson's principles and practice of medicine, 12th edn. Ed.: J. Macleod. Edinburgh: Churchill Livingstone 1978. pp 421–457.

3.10 Mental Disease

R. Dolmierski

The seaman has to adapt to continually changing conditions in which the work and rest periods scarcely differ (Dolmierski [12]). The monotony of life is often hard to bear and the continual noise and vibration and the possible hazards of the cargo, among other factors, are undoubtedly frequent causes of disturbance, particularly in the form of neuroses (Dolmierski and de Walden [7]).

In the long term a combination of nervous tension, worry and homesickness may cause a reaction, the harmful effect of which is sometimes greater than that of a single mental shock. These factors may be connected with work, family worries or environmental conditions and have unpleasant effects ranging from nervous tension to psychoneurotic behaviour (Bilikiewicz [1]). Over-fatigue, lack of sleep, the unsettled way of life and other factors also lead to psychoneurotic reactions.

Atmospheric and climatic influences are important contributory causes of neuroses which are often underrated by doctors. Sexual trauma and the lack of continuity in the sex life are also very important aspects in the evaluation of the seaman's mental health. In the same way, one has to consider internal factors which do not arise from change of environment, but are rather an expression of the attitude of the given person towards his surroundings. Difficulty in making social adjustments may also play a part in the development of neurosis (Dolmierski and Nitka [6]).

In dealing with seafarers, it is considerably more difficult to assess mental health than it is to diagnose organic disease. The physician will find that often he is consulted by patients of a different race, culture and language. As part of the disorder the patient may not wish to talk about his symptoms and, consequently, crew mates will be unaware of his suffering and unable to contribute to the history of the disease. The majority of cases will not be examples of florid, mental disorders but they will fall into the category of borderline disturbances which are inevitably difficult to assess.

In evaluating the mental state of the patient, the usual history taking and observation of the patient will also present difficulties. His behaviour, personal hygiene, means of self-expression and relationship to the rest of the crew will vary from ship to ship according to race and culture. It may be time consuming and require great thoroughness to evaluate and put in proper perspective observations such as level of mood, restlessness or anxiety.

The system of periodic routine medical examination will have excluded seafarers suffering from chronic mental disorder. Typical cases usually present as acute functional disorders. For the most part they are connected with somatic conditions such as infection, trauma or poisoning or with alcohol misuse. They are sometimes due to growing conflicts during long voyages but one has to remember that the conflicts often stem from mental disorders which have begun to develop earlier.

3.10.1 Neuroses

Neuroses are the most frequently diagnosed mental illnesses among the crew of seagoing ships.

Neurotic symptoms usually develop slowly. At the beginning, the patients usually complain of getting tired quickly, are sensitive and easily irritated, and have difficulty in concentrating. Small problems are blown up to enormous proportions. Habitual introspection with associated hypochondria is characteristic of the state of mind. The vegetative symptoms gradually grow; there is headache and vertigo, a feeling of weakness, changes of skin perception such as hyperaesthesia and numbness, reduction of appetite and insomnia (Kepiński [15]). One observes a high sensitivity to noise, anxiety state, frequent diarrhoea due to nervousness and increased perspiration. Complaints of impotence are also characteristic. Sufferers are highly aware of their condition and demand treatment. Usually – with or without consulting the doctor – they take too much medication (Galuszko [13]). In every consultation one must proceed carefully, to avoid suggesting new symptoms to the patient and confirming him in his opinion that he is seriously or even incurably ill. Persons suffering from neurosis frequently feel the need to be ill. It must be emphasised that one should never neglect neurotic complaints, as they are often precursors of serious somatic disease of the central nervous system. Therefore, when the patient presents typical symptoms of neurosis, he must never be neglected, but always painstakingly examined (Dolmierski and Nitka [8, 9]). The most frequent neuroses found among seamen are those of sexual, anxious, depressive and hypochondriac origin.

3.10.1.1 Sexual Neuroses

Under this heading are included only disorders of psychogenic origin which disturb, hinder or prevent normal sexual intercourse. All cases of organic disease or deformity of the genital organs are excluded. Seafarers frequently suffer from sexual neurosis resultant from deprivation during long voyages followed by contact with casual partners when in port. There is much ignorance about what should constitute a normal healthy sex life and this is compounded by a great deal of misinformation in magazines and other media. Many of these temporary disorders resolve spontaneously when a relationship is established with a satisfactory partner. Cases which do not resolve should be referred to a physician specialising in the subject. Self-treatment can lead to the patient taking stimulants which are ineffective and not only make the condition worse but also perpetuate it.

3.10.1.2 Anxiety Neuroses

These neuroses are characterised by anxiety, disturbances in concentration, insomnia, nightmares, increased heart rate, palpitations, increased muscle tension and diarrhoea. The neurosis is manifested by feelings of acute anxiety regarding imminent misfortune leading the patient to panic.

3.10.1.3 Depressive Neurosis

Depressive neurosis appears as a result of a chronic pathological condition of the central nervous system or after an extended period of misfortune (Dolmierski and de Walden [10]). Sometimes it is not very different from cyclophrenic depression, but it has a more benign course and psychotherapy leads to a considerable improvement.

3.10.1.4 Hypochondriac Neurosis

Hypochondriac neurosis is characterised by an excessive preoccupation with and exaggeration of one's own ailments, in particular organs or over the whole body. The patient feels ill and devotes his whole attention to his symptoms. He complains of problems so varied that they cannot be classified in any one group of disturbances. This neurosis has many features in common with neurasthenia and hysteria.

3.10.1.5 Treatment of Neuroses

One basic method of curing neuroses is psychotherapy. In more serious cases pharmacological treatment is indispensable, but the drugs must be chosen by the physician. With tranquillisers, the period of use must not be too long (Bilikiewicz [1]).

3.10.2 Functional Psychotic Syndromes

A characteristic symptom of the functional psychotic syndromes is the appearance of disturbances of consciousness. Acute functional syndromes are mostly caused by serious somatic diseases affecting the central nervous system, psychosomatic diseases or deterioration in chronic disease processes.

The most frequent causes are infectious diseases like typhoid fever, epidemic typhus, acute rheumatic arthritis, pneumonia, influenza, malaria and some other tropical diseases; disturbances of the circulatory system; alcoholism; abuse of drugs; drug poisoning and other ailments, particularly disturbances of the thyroid gland, kidney and liver diseases and functional disturbances appearing after sunstroke. Acute mental disorders often result from organic diseases of the brain complicated by acute psychotic syndromes. Of special importance here are: meningitis and encephalitis, epilepsy, brain tumours and head injury. Reactive factors also play a considerable causal part in the appearance of acute mental disorders.

3.10.2.1 Delirium

Delirium is the most frequent of all mental disorders on board ship. The course of delirium consists of three phases. The first prodromal phase is very difficult to diagnose. The patient feels ill, restless and anxious, has headache and vertigo, and is oversensitive to noise; his moods change from gaiety to tears, and he talks excessively. The restlessness gradually increases, the anxiety becomes intensified and the patient wakes up because of realistically terrifying dreams, which continue to frighten him in the waking state. This phase lasts some hours or days, changing gradually to the second phase.

The second phase is characterised by visual hallucinations. The patient gradually loses his orientation in time, place and environment and shows great anxiety and unrest, trying to escape from hallucinations he is experiencing. The content of the hallucinations is mostly coordinated. The patient sees animals, for instance mice and rats, and receives reproaches, abuses and threats, often related to his job, home etc. The content of the hallucination may be suggested by the people around and by the environment. The degree of disturbances in consciousness varies; sometimes the disturbances are difficult to observe, but more often contact with the patient is absolutely broken. The duration of this phase varies greatly, but is normally within the range of 1–6 weeks.

The character of the third phase depends on the cause of the delirium. In some cases great psychomotor agitation turns into a coma ending in death. However, this outcome is very rare; more frequently mental disorders lessen in intensity (often connected with a drop in body temperature), the level of consciousness improves and the hallucinations weaken. The patient falls into a very long final sleep, from which he awakes wearied. Gradually he begins to recognise his surroundings and regain his orientation and emotional equilibrium.

Delirium on board ship is mostly caused by chronic alcoholism. Although it is sometimes triggered off by sudden abstinence, one should not give the patient any alcohol. One dangerous cause-dependent symptom is psychomotor agitation, which should be treated with chlorpromazine hydrochloride in a dose of 300 mg/day, preferably intramuscularly. The patient should not be left alone, even for a short time, because in his psychotic state he may jump overboard. He must be admitted to hospital for treatment in the nearest port.

3.10.2.2 Obnubilation

The most frequent causes of obnubilation are organic lesions of the brain and epilepsy, which quite often appear as complications in somatic diseases. A characteristic trait of obnubilation is the sudden and unexpected onset, in the case of epilepsy directly after the epileptic fit. There is psychomotor agitation and confusion about time, place and identity. Sometimes, however, the behaviour of the patient is quite normal, the only symptoms being imprecise orientation, slowing down of mental activity and reduction of the intellectual powers. The obnubilation may last anything from 10–20 min to many weeks. Most frequently it ends just as suddenly as it began, sometimes after a deep sleep. The psychotic experiences will be forgotten completely.

As in delirium, the medical treatment is causal. After an epileptic fit epilepsy should be treated first. The patient has to be put ashore in the nearest port and, depending on the cause, hospitalised or sent home.

3.10.2.3 Reactive Psychoses

We speak of a reactive state in the case of disorders caused by mental trauma, meaning that the disorders appear as a reaction to environmental stimuli. It is not always a case of a single serious trauma. Among seamen many traumas of low intensity are most frequently found, the individual's reaction depending on the resistance of his central nervous system. For these traumas to act pathogenically, the body must be susceptible to them. Thus the reactive factor never acts alone. Individual differences mean that not every person reacts in the same way to a mental trauma.

To reactive psychoses belong: reactive depressions, expressed by disturbances in concentration, retardation in brain function (bradyphrenia), fixed ideas (monoideism), inability to arrive at a decision and suicidal intentions.

The basic form of medical treatment is psychotherapy. In more serious cases a pharmacological therapy is necessary, consisting of administration of tranquillisers. In contrast to cyclophrenic depression, in reactive depression thymoleptics should not be prescribed.

3.10.3 Mental Disorders with an Organic Background

In this context only posttraumatic mental disorders are dealt with in which there has been a temporary or permanent lesion of the brain and the causal link between brain lesion and mental disorder is evident.

3.10.3.1 Cerebral Trauma

Cerebral trauma is the consequence of head injury but may also be an indirect consequence of trauma elsewhere, e.g. that resulting from a jump with the legs kept straight. It may or may not involve lesions of soft tissues and bones. The most frequent forms of cerebral lesions are concussion, oedema and contusion (Dolmierski and Nitka [5]). Cerebral concussion is diagnosed when the patient has headache, vertigo, nausea and vomiting after a short, sudden loss of consciousness. Brain oedema, however, is characterised by a gradual increase in severity of intracranial pressure, the symptoms of which are headache, nausea, vomiting, disturbances of consciousness, pulse oscillation from quick to slow (less than 60/min) and respiratory disturbances. Cerebral traumas may involve loss of consciousness – not necessarily at the time, but possibly shortly before or after the trauma.

3.10.3.2 Cerebral Concussion

Immediately after cerebral concussion and severe trauma there are disturbances of consciousness. Cerebral functions are briefly interrupted; the patient has difficulty in concentrating, easily becomes weary, shows affective instability and complains of headache and vertigo. After the symptoms have worn off, vomiting occurs and the cerebral functions regain their equilibrium. Amnesia is characteristic and is sometimes retrograde.

The unconscious patient must be placed on his side so that the saliva can more easily drain from his mouth. One should observe the pupils, looking particularly for differences in diameter. The patient must be rested and in the case of psychomotor agitation given sedatives, ideally 25 mg chlorpromazine hydrochloride intramuscularly and 100–200 mg phenobarbitone sodium. In the case of bradycardia 80–100 mg frusemide should be given.

3.10.4 Intoxication and Addiction

3.10.4.1 Alcoholism and Alcoholic Psychoses

The use of alcohol is a generally accepted habit. We speak of alcohol misuse when consumption, in terms of frequency, circumstances or quantity, oversteps the customary dietetic and social standards in the given culture. Excessive consumption of alcohol not only affects the subject's health, but during working time, particularly at sea, endangers his own safety and that of the whole crew. A great number of accidents at sea are due entirely to excessive use of alcohol (Dolmierski et al. [3]). Drinking at sea is in all merchant navies a very old and harmful tradition. Alcoholism as a disease is classified by the WHO into the following categories: a) episodic excessive drinking, characterised by irregular, relatively short bouts of drinking; b) habitual excessive drinking, in which the bouts are more frequent; and c) alcohol dependence understood as addictive and chronic alcoholism. The feature differentiating simple excessive drinking from addiction is the ability to control consumption and not fall victim to physical dependence.

3.10.4.2 Chronic Alcoholism

Chronic alcoholism is characterised by changes in the central nervous system, the circulatory system and the parenchymatous organs. The psyche undergoes change; symptoms of the psycho-organic syndrome appear; intellectual capacity decreases, interests become narrower. Eventually interests and concerns disappear completely, the finer feelings are blunted and psychodegradation sets in (Bilikiewicz [1]). The archetypal drinking humour is nothing more than organic euphoria. The feeling of contentment comes from the company in which the alcoholic is drinking: alone at home he becomes bitter, irritable and brutal and neglects himself.

Alcoholics have no feelings of responsibility. They minimise their problem and promise improvement, but the promises are always vain. The alcoholic neglects not only himself, but also, and primarily, his family, becoming insensible to their feelings. Medical treatment consists of measures to reverse the dependence on alcohol and requires specialist consultation (Dolmierski and Nitka [11]). Stimulants and sedatives (including tranquillisers and other neuroleptics) are given.

3.10.4.3 Acute Alcohol Intoxication

Intoxication is a direct toxic effect of alcohol on the body. It is first expressed by an increase in physical and mental activity, i.e. by generalised intensification of feeling, talkativeness and movement, but these manifestations give way to muscle weakness and lowered psychomotor drive. Gait becomes unsteady and speech indistinct, perception and concentration suffer, the subject has a lower opinion of his own performance and irritability and aggressiveness increase. Conflicts arise with the people around, sometimes leading to unlawful behaviour. The tolerance to alcohol is considerably lower in people who misuse it, and similarly low in organic diseases of the central nervous system.

3.10.4.4 Pathological Inebriation

Pathological inebriation usually occurs in chronic alcoholics, but sometimes in people who do not misuse alcohol or in those with a very low degree of tolerance. The occurrence of these disturbances often results from fatigue, excessive heat (as in a tropical climate) or general diseases. The behaviour of the patient may seem normal, but he becomes irritated and impetuous. Drinking only a small quantity of alcohol often leads to acute disturbances of consciousness of a quite severe type with psychoses involving hallucinations and fantasies. The subject may have a fit of rage, attacking everybody and destroying everything around him. His perception is limited and he is confused. This agitation lasts only a short time, some few hours, before he falls asleep to wake up oblivious of what has happened.

3.10.4.5 Acute Alcoholic Hallucinations

Acute alcoholic hallucinations, which occur more rarely than pathological inebriation, are almost always auditory and mostly of an accusing, persecuting and commanding character. They are usually voices of enemies, sometimes of friends, and are accompanied by anxiety and unrest. The patient becomes aggressive and fights with "enemies". This condition lasts from several weeks to several months.

The patient must be kept secure and under continuous supervision. Treatment is with neuroleptics, e.g. chlorpromazine hydrochloride at a total dosage of about 300 mg during 24 h by intramuscular injections. The patient must be put ashore in the nearest port for treatment by a specialist.

3.10.4.6 Alcoholic Paranoia

Alcoholic paranoia is quite common among seamen and is characterised by the systematic appearance of delusions which cause jealousy, mostly regarding infidelity by the spouse. The patient constantly controls and checks the suspected person's behaviour, making himself very disagreeable. The evidence of infidelity can be anything – a glance, a smile, a word. Confessions of imaginary transgressions are often forced by beating and other mistreatment of the partner. Other functions remain absolutely unaffected, and the patient is able to work normally.

The treatment is exclusively specialist and prophylactic; his comrades should not talk with the patient about his delusions.

3.10.4.7 Narcomania and Drug Dependence

Narcotics may be used illegally by young people frequently out of curiosity or the desire to show off. Even physicians are sometimes reckless in prescribing narcotic drugs, to relieve pain and thereby causing addiction. The transition to addiction is rapid: first appear character disorders, abulia, lack of dutifulness and feelings (particularly the finer feelings) and a narrowing of interest (eventually limited to obtaining narcotics). The ability to work gradually decreases. Narcomania often leads to suicide. Among the most common addictions are those to morphine and cocaine, which have a clinical course differing from that in other narcotic addictions.

Specialist help is needed in gradual lowering of the narcotic dose and in giving sedatives. We note that drug dependence is much more frequent than narcomania. Under drug dependence is to be understood continuous or periodic use of a drug in order to obtain a general feeling of well-being or to avoid an undesirable state of mind. In the course of increasing dependence on a given drug, tolerance develops, leading to ever larger doses. The mechanisms of the formation of dependence are similar to those in narcomania. Therefore one should not irresponsibly give drugs which may lead to dependence.

3.10.5 Psychoses

3.10.5.1 Schizophrenia

Under the heading of schizophrenia is a group of assorted disease syndromes characterised by specific intellectual, emotional and behavioural disorders and damage to the personality structure. Among the most significant of the various symptoms (Weitbrecht [17]) are personality disorders and disappearance of the finer feelings and of the ability to alter one's mood. Emotional life is completely ruined. The patient has no sense of being mentally ill, and is indifferent to everything happening around him. The behaviour of the patient is abnormal and egocentric: even a short conversation shows eccentricity, lack of detachment and maladjustment to the situation. The psychomotor drive is usually lowered (Kretschmer [16]). The patient does not apply himself to his work but performs it without concern carelessly and superficially.

A man who prior to becoming ill was ambitious and full of energy is completely changed; listless, lacking drive and interests. Superimposed on this chronic process are acute mental disorders. Depending on the dominant clinical symptoms, three types of schizophrenia may be distinguished: hebephrenic, characterised mainly by disorders in the emotional sphere; paranoid, with auditory hallucinations and delusions; and catatonic, characterised by disorders of the psychomotor drive (Hopkinson [14]).

In the case of acute disorders the patient should be kept secure and isolated, and should be treated within 24 h; he should be put ashore at the nearest port for specialist treatment. At this time he should be given divided doses of chlorpromazine hydrochloride (maximum 300 mg) by intramuscular injections.

3.10.5.2 Cyclophrenia

Cyclophrenic disorders are manic-depressive psychoses. The two stages can occur together or separately.

Depression Syndrome. The depression syndrome is quite common and in spite of routine medical examinations may also occur at sea (Dolmierski and de Walden [10]). Among the most important symptoms are despondency, inhibition of mental functions and lowered psychomotor drive. A characteristic symptom is anxiety, often similar to that occurring with cardiac infarction. However, the single most dangerous symptom of depression is the inclination to suicide, which is often committed or attempted.

Foremost one must bear in mind the possibility of suicide; the patient should be isolated and kept under continuous supervision. He should be given one to three 25-mg tablets of thioridazine hydrochloride three or four times per day, until he is hospitalised. He must without fail be put ashore at the nearest port for specialist treatment.

Manic Syndrome. This syndrome is characterised by exaggerated general feelings, accelerated thinking and intensified psychomotor drive. The patient feels happy, content and very optimistic. There is a lack of reserve in his behaviour; he behaves insultingly to other people, is quarrelsome and gets into conflicts. His mental processes are rapid and chaotic, his inhibitions disappear, he abuses alcohol, becomes sexually very aroused and in general behaves in a shameless way. In a severe case he sometimes attacks people around him.

Sedate and hospitalise the patient in the nearest port for specialist treatment.

3.10.6 Personality Disorders

A personality is a complex of characteristics, tendencies and habits which determine the subject's reactions and way of thinking

(Bilikiewicz [1]). The formation of personality, normal or abnormal, depends on various biological, genetic factors and on external environmental influences. The border between normal and pathological is here indistinct. One accepts, not taking into consideration the aetiology of disturbances, that all character deficiencies are included under psychopathy.

At present we believe most cases of pathological alterations of the character to result from organic lesions of the central nervous system. The most typical symptoms of pathological alterations of the character are irritability, sudden rages, the tendency to impulsive actions and affective discharge in the form of fits of fury due to narrowing of the area of consciousness/awareness (Cramer [2]). Other peculiarities are similar to those in psychopathy, i.e. lying, stealing, laziness, lack of discipline and inability to live together with other people, all to the detriment of good relationships. Furthermore, the patient can show lack of reserve, cruelty, a tendency to addiction (particularly to misuse of alcohol and drug dependence), sexual extravagances and unethical or criminal behaviour. The atmosphere on board ship, particularly during very long voyages, is disturbed by individuals with a pathologically altered character, whom we used to evaluate from the point of view of morality instead of treating them as ill owing to lesions of the central nervous system. Such individuals should be subjected to specialist examination, and if symptoms and signs of an organic lesion of the nervous system are found they must not continue to work in an occupation as arduous as that of seamen.

3.10.7 Treatment of Mentally Ill Crew Members on Board Ship

The attitude of society to a mentally ill person is an indicator of the cultural level. It is obvious that a mentally ill person cannot work at sea, as this profession requires the appropriate mental characteristics, including great resilience. Anyone developing a mental disorder should be placed in the ship's hospital (if there is no hospital, in a separate cabin) under continuous supervision.

Mental disorder is here taken to include not only cases of acute psychosis with great psychomotor agitation, but also, for example, depressive states, which very often lead to suicide attempts, sometimes successful. Medication consists of neuroleptics (available on board ship in special medicine chests), mostly chlorpromazine hydrochloride at 150–300 mg/24 h in three doses of 50–100 mg injected deep into muscle. One should remember that high doses of neuroleptics lead to orthostatic disturbances, manifested as a sudden decrease in arterial pressure, and if this occurs the patient's head must be lowered. It may be necessary to give him drugs which improve circulation, and if they have no calming effect, one can give one injection of phenobarbitone sodium 200 mg intramuscularly. Should the agitation persist, the patient is to be tied carefully to the bed, the bonds securing the lower and upper extremities and the chest. When the patient calms down he can be released. Even when the violent phase has passed, one should not keep the patient on the ship, but put him ashore in the nearest port for hospitalisation or transfer him to another ship with a doctor on board. Conversation with the patient should be of a calming nature; his delusions should not be discussed for fear of aggravating the situation. Psychiatric treatment on board is difficult, and therefore only emergency measures are possible. Detailed instructions can be obtained by radiomedical advice, and specialist treatment in the nearest port.

References

1. Bilikiewicz, T.: Psychiatria kliniczna [Clinical psychiatry]. 5th ed. Warsaw: Panstwowy Zaklad Wydawnictw Lekarskich 1973.

2. Cramer, A.: Strukturen des vorsprachlichen Eindrucks- und Ausdrucksverhaltens in der Leidensgebärde. Nervenarzt 42, 607–609 (1971).
3. Dolmierski, R., K. J. de Walden-Galuszko and J. Nitka: Alkoholism a zdolność do pracy w Polskiej Marynarce Handlowej. [Alcoholism vrs. work ability in Polish merchant marine]. Ann. Acad. med. Stetinensis, Suppl. *10,* 95–100 (1973).
4. Dolmierski, R., K. J. de Walden-Galuszko and J. Nitka: Analysis of cases of mental disturbances in the light of present regulations and rulings of the medical appeal board in years 1971–1972. Bull. Inst. mar. Med. Gdansk *24,* 243–51 (1973).
5. Dolmierski, R. and J. Nitka: A preliminary appraisal of the state of the central nervous system in the seamen of the Polish merchant marine. Bull. Inst. mar. trop. Med. Gdynia *26,* 1, 17–24 (1975).
6. Dolmierski, R. and J. Nitka: Estimation of the occurence of neurotic disorders in sea economy workers exposed to the action of electromagnetic waves. Bull. Inst. mar. trop. Med. Gdynia *27,* 1, 57–61 (1976).
7. Dolmierski, R. and K. J. de Walden: Environmental factors causing neurosis in seamen. Bull. Inst. mar. Med. Gdansk *23,* 1/2, 7–11 (1972).
8. Dolmierski, R. and J. Nitka: Häufigkeit der Neurosen unter den Besatzungen der polnischen Handelsmarine. Verk.-Med. *25,* 5, 219–222 (1978).
9. Dolmierski, R. and J. Nitka: Neurosen und Leistungsfähigkeit auf See bei der polnischen Handelsmarine. Verk. Med. *25,* 5, 223–228 (1978).
10. Dolmierski, R. and K. J. de Walden: Ocena kliniczna przyczyn samobójstw u marynarzy. [Clinical evaluation of the cause of suicides among seamen]. Psychiat. pol. 3, 255–258 (1972).
11. Dolmierski, R. and J. Nitka: Stosowanie Esperalu w leczeniu alkoholizmu u marynarzy. [Usage of Esperal in alcoholism therapy of seamen]. In: Zagadnienia zdrowotne w gospodarce morskiej. Warsaw: Państwowy Zaklad Wydawnictw Lekarskich 1980. pp. 117–119.
12. Dolmierski, R.: Zaburzenia nerwicowe marynarzy. [Neurotic disorders in seamen]. Ann. Acad. med. Stetinensis, Suppl. 10, 79–84 (1973).
13. Galuszko, P.: Niektóre problemy powstawania nerwic u marynarzy floty handlowej. [Some problems concerning the sources of neuroses among seamen of merchant marine]. In: Pamietnik 28. Naukowego Zjazdu Psychiatrów Polskich, Lublin 1963. Warsaw: Państwowy Zaklad Wydawnictw Lekarskich 1965, pp. 69–75.
14. Hopkinson, G.: Delusions of infestation. Acta psychiat. scand. 46, 111–119 (1970).
15. Kepiński, A.: Psychopatologia nerwic. [Psychopathology of neuroses] Warsaw: Państwowy Zaklad Wydawnictw Lekarskich 1972.
16. Kretschmer, W.: Reifung als Grund von Krise und Psychose, Untersuchung zum psychiatrischen Entwicklungsgedanken. Stuttgart: Thieme 1972.
17. Weitbrecht, H.-J.: Psychiatrie im Grundriß. 3rd ed. Berlin, Heidelberg, New York: Springer 1973.

3.11 Other Diseases (Neurological, Ophthalmic, ENT and Other Conditions)

W. H. G. Goethe

3.11.1 Neurological Diseases

In nearly all studies of the incidence of illnesses affecting seafarers, neurological disease is shown by comparison to be uncommon. As indicated already in Chap. 3.1, group VI (diseases) of the ICD [17] includes diseases of the eyes and ears with those of the nervous system. Figures can be misleading unless this is understood. Kraemer-Hansen [16] found that diseases of the central and peripheral nervous systems were diagnosed only occasionally in foreign seafarers treated at a West German out-patient clinic, the rate being 2.06% (excluding eye and ear diseases). Dolmierski et al. [6] reported similar findings in Polish and foreign seafarers treated at Gdynia. Matthiensen [18] found only 0.4% when he examined medical log books of ships without a doctor, so presumably ships' officers can diagnose neurological disease only very rarely. Somov et al. [23] analysed the sickness data of 640 seafarers from the far east of the USSR. Vascular disorders of the brain were found predominantly in older officers. Chondrosis intervertebralis occurred more frequently in ordinary seamen (deck) and catering personnel. Neurosis was more common among young seafarers. The authors concluded that factors such as age, length of service at sea, rapid changes of climatic zones, ability to adapt and length of voyage were important in the development of certain diseases of the nervous systems.

Dolmierski and Nitka [7], in their study of the central nervous system based on EEG screening, indicate that a large number of abnormalities could not be interpreted with certainty although they indicated an underlying brain dysfunction. The study does not contain any specific details of the pathology.

Our own experience of sick seafarers in an out-patient clinic in Hamburg shows that true neuritis, neuralgia and central nervous system disorders are in fact, diagnosed only very rarely when strict criteria are applied. On the other hand, lumbago, sciatica, myalgia and similar conditions in the so-called "rheumatic group" occur more frequently. It is often difficult to make a positive diagnosis in these conditions where symptoms outweigh signs and the pathology is uncertain. However, they should not be classified as neuralgic disorders, as is the case in many studies.

3.11.2 Ophthalmic Diseases

According to the ICD, disorders of the eyes belong to group VI (diseases of the nervous system and sense organs) whereas accidental injuries to the eye region are to be found in group XVII [17].

Epidemiological publications on the frequency of diagnoses in seamen contain scarcely any details on ophthalmic diseases and accidents. In the study by Kraemer-Hansen [16] ophthalmic diseases and accidents have a frequency rate of 4.75%. Matthiensen [18] reports a rate of 3.1% and Dolmierski et al. [6] show an average annual rate of approximately 1.5%. Similar figures from various Italian sources are given by Molfino [20]. He also points out that ophthalmic and ENT diseases are mostly included in the group of "neurological diseases and diseases of the sense organs". Consequently, ophthalmic and ENT diseases often do not appear in the comparative statistics as separate figures. Offer-Ohlsen [22] found that diseases of the eyes account for about 3% of all diagnoses in Norwegian seafarers. In detail, conjunctivitis predominated at 55%, while "eye aches" at 20% and refraction disorders at 17% were the other major complaints.

Several authors dealt with the importance of eye injuries caused by accidents and their secondary effects. Bietti and Vanni [4] gave practical advice on urgent first aid for injuries of the eyes. They distinguish between four kinds of basic injury:

1. Injuries caused by foreign bodies at the conjunctiva and the cornea and injuries caused by penetration;
2. Contusions of the eye-ball;
3. Thermal burns;
4. Acid burns caused by contact with chemicals.

The authors discuss the rather restricted diagnostic and therapeutic possibilities aboard. Zorn [25] investigated the problem of eye injuries and the subsequent medical treatment on board. He believes that eye injuries happen more frequently on board than is acknowledged. Considering that occasional slight injuries are not recorded at all and that in many countries accidents are only notifiable if there is an unfitness for duty lasting more than 3 days, it can be assumed that eye injuries make a total of approximately 8%–10% of the occupational accidents of seafarers. Zorn investigated the possible treatment of eye injuries and diseases in relation to the content of the ship's medicine chest available on board vessels of different nations.

Elze [9] points to the need for immediate medical treatment of acute eye diseases and injuries on board and the required medical facilities. The ship's crew or at least the ship's officer in charge of medical care should have had the necessary training in the immediate medical first aid measures to prevent permanent damage in case of acid burns of the eye. Furthermore, he gives instructions on how to treat perforating injuries and contusions of the eye-ball, glaucoma, arc eye etc.

Hager [14] emphasizes that the medical training of ships' officers should include the treatment of eye diseases and injuries. He is of the opinion that an adequately equipped ship's medicine chest and even the facilities of radiomedical advice are useless if the ship's officer in charge does not possess the required basic skills which include: description of the state of the eyes after examination, opening of the eyelids with eyelid retractor, rinsing of the conjunctival sac, administration of eye-drops and ointment, description of the state of the cornea upon lateral reflection, removal of foreign bodies from the cornea with medical instruments, assessment of intraocular pressure by palpation of the eye-ball and assessment of visual fields or visual acuity. Also de Bary [2] reports on the hazards involved with eye injuries and the subsequent medical treatment. He deems it absolutely necessary that iron particles should be completely removed from the eye as they may otherwise cause rust rings on the cornea which are scarcely reparable later on and may lead to permanent impairment of vision as a secondary effect.

Friemann et al. [10] and Friemann and Overhoff [11] describe a specific kind of eye disease in relation to the fishing industry. It is a quickly developing keratitis which predominantly occurs with the handling of herring oil during the loading process. The irritation is caused by saprogenic ptomaine, particularly dimethylamine and trimethylamine. This type of corneal damage was also mentioned by Kersten and Mansch [15].

Statistical data show (see above) that diseases and accidents of the eyes are not frequently diagnosed in seamen in out-patient clinics ashore. It is evident from the total number of diagnoses involving seamen from many countries that presbyopia and the need for reading glasses rank first, followed by conjunctivitis of differing origin. Frequently seamen, particularly from Asia, present with a developing or an already advanced pterygium. This condition is also frequently found during the course of a general medical examination.

Ch'en and Huei-ying [5] report on the occurrence of pterygium in Chinese fishermen. These patients complain often of conjunctival irritation and want the pterygium to be removed.

Injuries of the eyes rank only third in the frequency distribution curve. They are mostly caused by foreign bodies at the conjunctiva and the cornea. Perforating injuries and, surprisingly, glaucoma very seldom occur.

3.11.3 Ear, Nose and Throat Diseases

In the ICD, ENT diseases are to be found either under "diseases of the respiratory system" (VIII) or "diseases of the nervous system and the sense organs" (VI). So, ENT diseases do not appear as an individual group of diseases.

Ear diseases were found by Kraemer-Hansen [16] to have a frequency rate of 2.87%. Dolmierski et al. [6] state an average rate of 1.3%. The study of medical log books by Matthiensen [18] showed a fairly high frequency rate of 7.8%.

Only one specific publication on the importance of ENT diseases in seafaring can be found. De Bary [3] published a review of "ear troubles at sea". His experiences have predominantly been with ear diseases on board DC tankers. Nevertheless, his findings may be representative for seafaring in general. Otitis externa was the most frequent diagnosis, followed by wax obstruction. The much more dangerous otitis media fortunately occurred infrequently. He gave instructions for diagnosis and therapy at sea.

A specific kind of ear disease which particularly affects the engine room staff is labyrinthine deafness caused by noise. Various authors from many countries have studied this problem. Goethe et al. [12] report on the reduction of hearing capacity owing to noise exposure, especially among the engine room crew. Most surprisingly, this condition was also found in deck personnel without any specific explanation having been found as to how they could have been exposed to high levels. Grewe and Rodegra [13] studied the results of more than 6800 audiometric screenings and found bilateral hearing loss due to noise in 136 cases. In 24 cases the loss was severe enough to be classified as a prescribed occupational disease.

Nowak [21] reports on a considerable number of cases where hearing loss due to noise on board was diagnosed, especially in older persons. Menyakin and Poperetskaya [19] examined 553 fishermen and seamen and found that 43.7% had suffered noise damage in varying degrees from slight to severe.

According to personal experience in a seamen's out-patient ward, the most frequent ear diseases were wax obstruction and otitis externa. Acute otitis media was not frequent. Occasionally chronic otitis media with perforation of the tympanum and persistent discharge was seen.

Seamen frequently complain of nose disorders. Seafarers from Asia, tropical and subtropical countries are especially prone to nasal congestion which is often caused by polyposis or deviation of the septum. Surgical treatment may be indicated but in many cases this is put off because of the lack of time and other difficulties. Nose bleeding is very rarely seen in the seamen's out-patient ward itself. According to the patients' complaints, post festum nose bleeding seems to occur on board more frequently. Diseases of the throat are mostly diagnosed as pharyngitis and laryngitis accompanying head colds. They may also occur together with bronchitis. There are only a very few cases of septic tonsillitis and/or quinsy; patients with these disorders nearly always have a high fever and, therefore, require intensive treatment.

There are only a few publications dealing with nose and throat diseases of seamen. Durante [8] mentions in his study on the "physiopathology of the respiratory system among fishermen" the occurrence of throat diseases and tonsillitis. He analysed the sickness data of 635 seamen suffering from diseases of the respiratory system and found infections of the pharynx in 67 and tonsillitis in 76. Diseases of the nose are not specifically mentioned. Balestrieri and D'Alessandro [1] observed a more frequent occurrence of tonsillar disease in seamen.

Epidemics of upper respiratory infections and infectious pharyngitis sometimes occur. Ulewicz and Dolmierski [24] described their observations of such an epidemic on board a passenger ship. In total, 282 persons fell ill – 84 crew members and 198 passengers. Treatment was effected with procaine penicillin and tetracycline. The presumptive diagnosis of streptococcal infection was proved ashore by means of serological tests.

3.11.4 Other Pathological Conditions or Disorders

In most of the international statistics on the frequency of diagnoses (see Chap. 3.1) the group of "symptoms and ill-defined conditions" (group XVI of the ICD) is about halfway down in the list. In many instances, this group of diseases does not appear at all and, obviously, the authors in those studies tried to classify them in other groups.

Symptoms of uncertain origin are often defined in the seamen's out-patient wards as general weakness, fatigue, exhaustion, pains and paraesthesia in the limbs or trunk and similar vague complaints. In rare instances, these disorders may be caused by malnutrition, but presumably they are mostly due to the boredom and frustrations of shipboard life, the mental stress and the social isolation from other people ashore. Sometimes shipping doctors describe these conditions as "tankeritis". Apparently, this term derives from the fact that tankers are at sea for long periods with only very short calls at remote ports. Very often the crew members have no chance to go ashore and to establish social contacts. The seafarer is then virtually locked in his small environment which may be likened to a cage even if it is (sometimes desirably) gold-plated. Feelings of frustration which may lead to ill-defined disturbances are the consequence. Nowadays this applies not only to tankers but to the shipping industry in general.

References

1. Balestrieri, N. and A. D'Alessandro: Osservazioni sulle tonsillopatie dei marittimi. Atti del Centro di Studi e Ricerche per l'Assistenza sanitaria e sociale dei Marittimi C.I.R.M. Rome 1961, pp. 87–92.
2. Bary, J. L. J. de: Diagnosis and treatment of injuries and diseases of the eye at sea. [Circular letter]. Fawley 1960.
3. Bary, J. L. J. de: Ear troubles at sea. [Circular letter]. Fawley 1960.
4. Bietti, G. B. and V. Vanni: Nozioni pratiche sui soccorsi di urgenza nelle lesioni traumatiche dell'apparato oculare. Atti del Centro di studi e ricerche per l'Assistenza sanitaria e sociale dei Marittimi C.I.R.M. Rome 1961, pp. 19–28.
5. Ch'en, Li and Y. Huei-ying: Eine statistische und histopathologische Untersuchung des Pterygiums bei Fischern und Bauern. Med. Sowjetunion Volksdem. *6*, 9, 1851 (1959).
6. Dolmierski, R., J. Filikowski and A. Kotlowski: Activities of WHO Pilot Health Centre for Seafarers in Gdynia. Bull. Inst. mar. trop. Med. Gdynia *31*, 3/4, 149–156 (1980).
7. Dolmierski, R. and J. Nitka: A preliminary appraisal of the state of the central nervous system in the seamen of the Polish merchant marine. Bull. Inst. mar. trop. Med. Gdynia *26*, 1, 17–24 (1975).
8. Durante, E.: Contributo allo studio della fisiopatologia dell'apparato respiratorio nei marittimi. Atti della "Sezione Studi" del C.I.R.M., Rome 1968, pp. 211–220.
9. Elze, K. L.: Akute Augenerkrankungen und deren Behandlung auf See. In: Jahrestagung der Deutschen Gesellschaft für Verkehrsmedizin, Hamburg, 11–13 April 1975, pp. 61–63.

10. Friemann, W., W. Overhoff and J. R. Walter: Augenerkrankungen in der Industriefischerei. Arch. Gewerbepath. Gewerbehyg. *17,* 1-56 (1959).
11. Friemann, W. and W. Overhoff: Keratitis als Berufserkrankung in der Ölheringsfischerei. Klin. Mbl. Augenheilk. *128,* 4, 425-438 (1956).
12. Goethe, H., E.-G. Schmidt, E. Zorn et al.: Lärmbelastung auf See- und Binnenschiffen, Untersuchungen zur effektiven Lärmbelastung der Besatzungen. Ed.: Bundesanstalt für Arbeitsschutz und Unfallforschung, Dortmund. Bremerhaven: Wirtschaftsverlag NW 1979. (Forschungsbericht 201)
13. Grewe, H.-E. and H. Rodegra: Untersuchungen über die Lärmschwerhörigkeit des Maschinenpersonals. Hansa *112,* 21 (1975).
14. Hager, G.: Die Grundausbildung von Schiffsoffizieren zur Behandlung von Augenerkrankungen und die dazu notwendige Standardausrüstung auf Seeschiffen. In: Fragen der Schiffahrtsmedizin. Vorträge aus dem Intern. Symp., Heiligendamm, 28-31 March 1963. Medizinischer Dienst des Verkehrswesens II. pp. 159-164 (1963).
15. Kersten, E. and L. Mansch: Zur Möglichkeit berufsbedingter Hornhautschädigungen in der Futterfischindustrie. Z. ärztl. Fortbild. *55,* 20, 1191-1194 (1961).
16. Kraemer-Hansen, H.: Diagnosenverteilung bei Seeleuten. Auswertung der Erkrankungsbögen der Abteilung für Schiffahrtsmedizin am Bernhard-Nocht-Institut für Schiffs- und Tropenkrankheiten in Hamburg aus den Jahren von 1966 bis 1975. Dissertation, University of Hamburg 1977.
17. Manual of the International Statistical Classification of Diseases, Injuries, and Causes of Death. Vols. 1 and 2. Based on the recommendations of the Ninth Revision Conference, 1975, and adopted by the 29th WHO Assembly. Geneva: WHO 1977 and 1978.
18. Matthiensen, R. P.: Diagnosenverteilung bei Erkrankungen in der Schiffahrt. Auswertung von Schiffskrankentagebüchern und ein Vergleich mit dem statistischen Material der SBG sowie der Ortskrankenkassen. Dissertation, University of Hamburg 1969.
19. Menyakin, R. P. and V. I. Poperetskaya: Profesionalnye ismeneniya organa slukha i ravnovesiya u moryakov i rybakov. [Occupational changes of hearing and vestibular system in seamen and fishermen]. In: Vestn. Oto-rino-laring. 1, 39-42 (1980).
20. Molfino, A.: Aspetti di patologia oculare nella gente del mare. In: Atti del primo congresso int. sull'assistenza di malattia e la tutela infortunistica della gente del mare nei paesi della c. e. e., Genoa 3-5 Oct. 1960, Vol. 2, pp. 537-549.
21. Nowak, R.: Die Lärmschwerhörigkeit des Schiffsmaschinenpersonals. Z. ges. Hyg. *17,* 7, 488-492 (1971).
22. Offer-Ohlsen, D.: The Norwegian seafarer – the picture of health? Analysis of health – and medical reports from the merchant navy. Lecture. Symposium "Safety of life at sea". Oslo, 20-21 Oct. 1980. Research program associated with The Royal Norwegian Council for Scientific and Industrial Research. System for Sikkert Skip. Manuscript.
23. Somov, O. G., M. N. Baishtruk, D. I. Bobrikova et al.: Questions of neurological morbidity among crew members. In: VII International Symposium on Marine Medicine, Odessa, 23-30 Sept. 1976. Moscow 1976, p. 420.
24. Ulewicz, K. and R. Dolmierski: Pharyngitis epidemic on a passenger ship. Bull. Inst. mar. trop. Med. Gdynia *27,* 1, 105-108 (1976).
25. Zorn, E.: Probleme der Diagnose und Behandlung von Augenverletzungen und -erkrankungen auf See. Klin. Mbl. Augenheilk. *165,* 2, 369-376 (1974).

3.12 Dental Problems in Seafaring

H. Bäter

Diseases of the teeth, mouth and jaw can affect the general state of health considerably and it often happens that, on account of this, a ship has to make an emergency call at a port or a fishery protection vessel has to be asked to assist. Very often it needs only a short inspection of the cavity of the mouth in order to achieve an early diagnosis and to apply effective treatment. Therefore the alarming increase of dental diseases, and with it the problems on board arising from such diseases, is surprising.

In fact, the regular medical fitness examinations as they have been carried out since 1946 in many seafaring countries are of great value in fighting dental diseases. However, in 1973 the Joint Committee of the World Health Organization (WHO/ILO) made it quite clear that the "problem of the continuously increasing number of dental diseases with seafarers cannot be solved by them" [7].

3.12.1 Morbidity

Papers by Evjen [4], Otterland [12] and Matusov [11] were based on the first statistics which the WHO published in 1975 showing the most frequent diseases of seafarers. According to these statistics, dental diseases took fourth place in frequency after coronary diseases, accidents and venereal diseases.

These statistical data induced further countries to carry out dental examinations in seamen. In 1975 Sandbekk [15] examined Norwegian seamen, who make up 2% of the Norwegian work-force and are thus the biggest seafaring group worldwide in relation to the national population. He found dental caries in 96% of the seamen examined.

Trunov et al. [16] reported that diseases of the mouth were among the most frequent on the general list of seamen's complaints. The longer the voyage lasts, the higher is the frequency of the complaints as an effect of prolonged exposure to the adverse conditions on board and failure to adapt to them. Diseases of the mouth and their complications constitute 30%–35% of all cases where seamen ask for medical assistance in foreign ports. Among diseases of the mouth, dental caries is by far the most frequent. The second place is occupied by such complications of dental caries as pulpitis and pericementitis. Amphodontosis resp. periodontitis – lesion of the periodontal tissue – is often found and requires great care on the part of the doctors. Stomatitis, gingivitis and other lesions of the mucous membrane of the mouth are not infrequent.

Although intensified international and national efforts have been made to solve the problem of diseases of the mouth, recent publications by Goethe et al. [5], Zorn [18], Kaerger [8], Klafstad [9] and Bormann [2] show an improvement in only very few countries. In fact, a deteriorating situation can be observed in most countries. At present in some of the statistics on distribution of diagnoses, diseases of the teeth, mouth and jaw already take second place behind accidents on board ships. The number of cases on board ships is significantly higher than among a comparable group of the population ashore. The causes of these diseases are complex and partly concern the specific life on board with its extremely long and irregular working hours, its abuse of sugar, alcohol and tobacco and quick turnarounds in port. All of this causes physical and psychological stress.

Especially for seamen on fishery factory vessels, tankers, container ships or other cargo ships in line shipping, life on board can lead to total social neglect due to monotony and isolation over a long period. The fact that a seaman often cannot leave the ship for months is also a reason for total neglect of the care of the teeth.

Schmidt [14] gives an extensive report on the experience with dental treatment on board fish factory ships. These ships of the GDR have a ship's dentist on board who is responsible for the stomatological care of the entire fishery fleet in his area.

Of 2740 seamen who were examined between 1974 and 1976, Bäter [1] found two-thirds to have moderate or bad oral hygiene, one-third to have evident odontolithiasis and 50% to be in need of dental care. In addition to this, one-third were suffering from parodontopathias.

Even worse findings were made by Wianz [17], who examined 422 fishery men: 64% were suffering from odontolithiasis and 53% from parodontosis.

In a clinical-statistical study on parodontopathias, Sacco and Galassi [13] found that 92.5% of 1500 examined seamen had a parodontic alteration or a mucosal lesion; 65% showed gingivitis purulenta or haemorrhagica, 21.7% an atrophic-hypertrophic parodontosis with pyorrhea alveolaris, 11% gingivitis-stomatitis with alterations and 2.3% an epithelial defect.

3.12.2 Oral and Dental Care

It is therefore obvious that a high proportion of dental disease is due to lack of oral hygiene.

WHO has demanded repeatedly an extensive education in dental diseases and oral hygiene for seamen in order to convince them of the necessity of regular dental care and treatment.

As stated above, a further cause of increasing dental disease is the constantly reduced times in port which nowadays are calculated in hours, leaving the seamen little opportunity for thorough dental treatment. Because of this, and because very few dentists ashore are prepared to treat seamen without advance notice, the only measure they are offered when suffering from severe tooth-ache is extraction of the tooth. This is also one of the reasons why many seamen postpone a necessary dental examination as long as possible. The result can be a severe and sometimes dangerous abscess during a voyage.

WHO claim that seamen ashore should have precedence over other patients in urgent cases. The recommendations of Marchenko [10] go much further. He not only proposes dental treatment for seamen before the beginning of each voyage but also suggests that they should be visited and treated by mobile dental stations during their voyage. These mobile stations should be installed on board bigger passenger ships or a dentist should visit smaller ships carrying portable instruments with him, staying on board ship until all crew members have been treated. Afterwards the dentist could board another ship. Dental control and treatment in this way would be very effective; however, up to now this practice has been implemented mainly in countries of the Eastern bloc. From first publications it can be concluded that the German Democratic Republic in particular is working on a further development of this system. Bormann [2] reports on 11726 cases of dental treatment at sea which were carried out in 1969. By this method, the number of carious dentitions could be reduced from 81% to 50%. Some shipping companies of Western countries have developed and carried out similar programmes.

Research in various countries has shown that changes in the social security system have no significant effect on the standard of dental health of their seamen. (Seamen in some of the countries of the Eastern Bloc are an exception.) Bäter [1], for instance, found only 50% of all gaps between teeth of West German seamen to be closed prosthetically whereas foreign seamen, who generally have to pay far more money for this kind of treatment, had hardly less dental prostheses. Apart from a certain indifference toward gaps between teeth, one of the reasons for this obvious lack of prosthetic treatment may be lack of time, which does not allow a seaman to undergo a difficult and long procedure of prosthetic treatment. In most countries, appointments months ahead are necessary for this kind of treatment. The treatment itself is so extensive and time consuming that in order to complete it a seafarer would have to stay ashore.

It seems that in most countries seamen, being a social minority, are neglected. Often the seamen feel that no provision is made for their dental problems, with the result that more and more emergency treatment on board proves necessary.

3.12.3 Dental Care on Board

In general one of the deck officers is in charge of the medical treatment on board. He is entrusted with this task by the captain of the ship before the beginning of a voyage.

A deck officer has to undergo medical training during his nautical studies ashore. There are few countries, however, which in addition to theoretical medical training, demand a course of practical work in a hospital, but no country demands practical examination in basic dental medicine.

The officer in charge of medical treatment usually obtains his dental knowledge from the medical guide which should be part of the medical chest according to national regulations on medical equipment on board. On many ships the "International Medical Guide for Ships" [6] is available. On ships of certain flags, however, no medical guide is provided and no dental medicines or equipment are available. In severe cases the officer will ask for additional radio-medical advice. The medical chest of ships of the German Federal Republic contains, among other things, eugenol (oil of clove), provisional fillings and antiseptic mouth washes as well as dental forceps, excavators, mirrors and probes. The ships of some other countries carry similar dental facilities, but others do not have adequate provisions.

The aim of emergency treatment can only be to relieve the toothache and to prevent a deterioration in the patient's condition until he is able to undergo appropriate dental treatment ashore.

Most of the time the dental therapy is restricted to the application of strong analgesics and to provisional closure of the carious defects. Even a provisional closure, however, requires skill and some diagnostic knowledge. In the case of an early pulpitis, the officer in charge will succeed in relieving pain with the help of eugenol, as this medicine will protect the pulp from thermic and chemical influences and has an alleviating effect.

In the case of a pulpitis necroticans, however, he will increase the patient's pain to an unbearable state by this method as the gas pressure of the putrescent tooth can then no longer escape.

The officer in charge of medical treatment would undoubtedly be under great stress if required to extract a tooth. During 10 years of being a radio officer at sea I never heard of an extraction of a tooth by a ship's officer. This precautionary measure seems to me sensible and advisable now, knowing the dangers of unskilled anaesthesia, a broken root left in place or even a mandibular fracture after extraction. For these reasons the medical guide of the German Democratic Republic (DDR) "Health Safety on Board" strictly prohibits extraction of teeth by officers (Ebert [3]). Therefore dental treatment on most ships is restricted to relieving the patient's pain and to tranquillising the tooth for some days. In most cases, trepanations by excavator, antibiotics and cold compresses can slow the process until the next port is reached. In an extreme case, ships could call at a port as an emergency within hours or days in order to land the patient. This, however, causes technical difficulties and is expensive so that a captain would agree to this decision only as a last emergency measure.

3.12.4 Dental Problems in Fishery

Seamen on modern fishery factory vessels, on the other hand, are entirely dependent upon themselves, often having to stay within the fishing area for up to 6 months. During such a long voyage a captain may try to extract a tooth himself when conservative treatment has failed.

Under favourable circumstances there will be a fishery protection vessel near the fishing area carrying a fishery protection doctor for emergency cases on board. Most of these doctors are surgeons and owing to their special training they are able to carry out a simple conservative treatment or even an extraction. From their journals it can be seen that fishery protection doctors complain frequently about increasing numbers of calls for help from fishermen suffering from dental diseases. Quite often a call for help is not sent out until the patient develops a serious condition because of incorrect aid or lack of treatment over a long period. During some of the voyages of the German fishery protection vessels, more than 50% of the emergency treatments were for diseases of the teeth of fishermen.

3.12.5 Final Remarks

Summarising the above, it has to be stated that, despite intensified national and international efforts, diseases of the teeth, mouth and jaw in seafaring have increased considerably in number as well as severity. They take second place after accidents on board and show – in contrast to the latter – an increasing tendency.

There is no denying that seamen tend to be indifferent and neglectful where the care of their teeth is concerned. However, recent findings also show that dental treatment of seamen is not satisfactory owing to unfavourable factors in seafaring, such as very short times in port and reduction of personnel on board, leaving little or no time for conservative or prosthetic treatment.

References

1. Bäter, H. H.: Untersuchungen des Gebißzustandes bei deutschen und ausländischen Seeleuten und daraus abzuleitende Empfehlungen. Dissertation, University of Hamburg 1979.
2. Bormann, H.: Entwicklung, Aufgaben und Bedeutung der stomatologischen Betreuung. In: Medizinischer Dienst des Verkehrswesens der DDR, Rostock 1969.
3. Ebert, H.: Gesundheitsschutz an Bord. Leitfaden für Kapitäne und Schiffsoffiziere. Berlin: VEB Verlag Volk u. Gesundheit 1980.
4. Evjen, A.: Unpublished report to WHO Regional Office for Europe. Copenhagen 1959.
5. Goethe, H., P. Vuksanović and A. Backhaus: Die medizinische Betreuung der Deutschen Hochseefischer in den Jahren 1948 bis 1975. In: Fischereischutzboote und Fischereiforschungsschiffe der Bundesrepublik Deutschland. Ed.: Bundesministerium für Ernährung, Landwirtschaft und Forsten, Bonn, Hamburg. Hamburg: Paul Moehlke 1975.
6. International medical guide for ships. Geneva: WHO 1967.
7. Joint ILO/WHO Committee on the health of seafarers. Geneva: WHO 1973.
8. Kaerger, E.: Zahnärztliche Behandlung von Seeleuten. Hansa *114*, 15/16, 1477–1478 (1977).
9. Klafstad, J.: Personal communication 1981.
10. Marchenko, A.: Forms of organising dental health services to mariners. In: VII Int. Symposium on Marine Medicine, Odessa, 23–30 Sept. 1976. Moscow 1976. p. 381.
11. Matusov, A.: Provision of medical services for sailors in the merchant navy. Leningrad 1971.
12. Otterland, A.: A sociological study of the mortality in merchant seafarers. Stockholm: Scandinavian University Books 1960.
13. Sacco, S. and C. Galassi: Studio clinico-statistico delle malattie parodontali nei lavoratori del mare. In: Atti del primo congresso int. sull'assistenza di malattia e la tutela infortunistica del-

la gente del mare nei paesi della c.e.e. Genoa, 3–5 Oct. 1960. Genoa: Casse Marittime per gli infortuni sul lavoro e le malattie 1960. Vol. 2, pp. 636–639.

14. Schmidt, L.: Ein Schiffsstomatologe im Nordmeer - Erfahrungsbericht. Z. ärztl. Fortbild. *75*, 483–489 (1981).
15. Sandbekk, O. W.: Tannhelse og bruk av tannlegetjenester blant sjöfolk i utenriksfart. Norske Tannlägeforen. Tid. *87*, 275–281 (1977).
16. Trunov, J. I., N. V. Pavlov, L. M. Shafran et al.: Analysis of stomatological morbidity among seamen and its prophylaxis. Bull. Inst. mar. trop. Med. Gdynia *25*, 2-3-4, 236–240 (1974).
17. Wianz, E.: Die zahnärztliche Versorgung von Seeleuten der deutschen Hochseefischerei. Dtsch. zahnärztl. Z. *37*, 4, 391–396 (1982).
18. Zorn, E. W.: Betrachtung über die Schiffahrtsmedizin und ihre Entwicklung in Deutschland. Der Seewart *37*, 3, 93–98 (1976).

3.13 The Sick Seafarer Ashore

W. R. Anderson and W. H. G. Goethe

The ship's master must make all decisions on the need for medical care for his crew when at sea. In the event of illness or injury it is extremely important for him to decide as soon as possible whether the patient can be cared for aboard or should be removed from the ship. When in doubt, his first priority is to obtain radiomedical advice from a reliable source. If advised to evacuate the patient he may request air/sea rescue if the ship is within an acceptable distance of that facility. If not, it may be necessary to divert his ship to the nearest port. A major port is always preferable because many of the smaller ports are without adequate medical facilities and suitable means of subsequent repatriation.

The treatment of seafarers in foreign ports presents significant social/medical problems. The WHO drew attention to these problems at a Conference on Health and Welfare of Seafarers in Marseille in 1959. Evjen [4] made a full detailed report of the discussion. During the 37th session of the WHO in 1965 these problems were discussed again [6]. The WHO report estimated a total population of about 750000 seafarers to which could be added 250000 fishermen. Thus one million people working at sea were at risk, of illness and injury and they might require medical treatment aboard, at home or in foreign countries.

The Joint ILO/WHO Committee on the Health of Seafarers has also dealt with this matter repeatedly. In the report of the session in September 1973 [11] the Committee pointed out the importance of establishing medical centres in ports for the treatment of sick seamen of all nationalities. It particularly referred to the activities of the Pilot Health Centres for Seafarers in Gdynia (Poland) and Auckland (New Zealand). According to Dolmierski et al. [2] and Dolmierski [3], a total of 10484 consultations were given to foreign seamen and fishermen of more than 16 nationalities. Of these, 8309 were for general medical and surgical conditions, while 2175 were specifically for diseases of the mouth, including dental conditions.

Goethe and Vuksanović [5] also emphasized that seafarers on articles represent a population at risk in regard to medical care. They pointed out that nowadays few doctors work on merchant ships. Medical care at sea is given by laymen who may or may not be competent to deal with any emergency. In general, seafarers are treated by doctors only when in port. Ram [10], in his survey of Maritime Health Problems, noted a great tendency for ships' officers to avoid personal responsibility in medical matters and to rely on advice from port doctors as much as possible.

During the European Nautical Medical Meetings in 1978 in Germany [8] and 1979 in Great Britain [9] the participants dealt comprehensively with the subject of medical care and hospitalization of seamen in foreign ports and the problems of medical care overseas.

It is surprising that there are so few publications on this problem, which affects all maritime countries. Most authors, such as Haralanov and Angelov [7], deal only with national aspects.

A special problem which has nearly been

solved by the signatory states is the treatment of venereal diseases. The so-called Brussels Agreement [1], signed by a great number of seafaring nations in 1924, states that the nations who signed the agreement ought to establish free treatment centres for seamen suffering from a venereal disease. In 1972 the WHO published a World Directory of Venereal Diseases Centres at ports in which the addresses of the centres and the doctors as well as the opening hours are listed [12].

3.13.1 The Seamen's Doctor

In his home country a sick seaman normally consults his family doctor or the doctor of his shipping company. This doctor will treat the seaman himself or admit him to hospital. According to the customary practice no problems normally arise. The situation becomes quite different as soon as the seaman falls ill on board and the ship, as is usual nowadays, has no ship's doctor and treatment has to be given by the captain or another officer on board. This treatment normally comprises only urgent first aid measures. The patient will be sent to a doctor in the next port. In ports where there is no special medical centre for foreign and home seamen irrespective of nationality, the representative of the owner looking after the ship will choose a doctor known to him, either sending the seaman to him or asking the doctor to come on board. In most countries seamen cause problems for a general medical practice because they present very specific difficulties. The main problem is the language barrier. As the international language in navigation nowadays is English, it is necessary for a doctor who wants to treat seamen successfully to speak medical English fluently and as far as possible to know other major languages.

Besides this there are some other difficulties concerning the treatment of seamen. The specific conditions on board like working conditions, watch systems and environmental load such as noise, vibration, macro- and microclimate, gas, dust and vapours demand a wide knowledge if the doctor is to deal satisfactorily with the sometimes very atypical complaints of the patients and to decide whether the seaman can continue his duty on board or not.

Often ships nowadays remain only a short time in the port so that usually there is very little time left for special investigations and treatment. The seamen's doctor must be able to perform laboratory examinations, ECG, X-raying etc. with no delay and to make a diagnosis quickly. Normally all these measures have to be taken in one or two days, sometimes in a few hours.

Owing to the lack of time, a long and extended investigation is impossible. Usually the decision whether the seaman can stay on board or must sign off is expected by the captain or by the ship's agent as soon as possible. This decision is of great importance for the patient as well as of great economic importance, because the costs of repatriation and the replacement of the ill seaman can be very high.

When seafarers are sent to a doctor by an agency, very few take with them any information about their medical history, previous treatment or reports of medical investigations carried out at other ports. Indeed, it is often very difficult to obtain an adequate history of the present complaint unless the seafarer can speak some English or an interpreter is available. With the reduced number of crew members, it is usually not easy for the captain so send an officer to act as interpreter. The doctor is therefore seriously handicapped in making a diagnosis and deciding upon treatment. He will often have to repeat investigations which have been done at another port. This results in a considerable loss of time and extra unnecessary costs.

The sick seafarer's problems may vary from one country to the other. When the seamen's doctor does not speak English and there is no interpreter available, language barriers reduce medical history to basics. In some ports interpreters may be available. Church groups and seamen's service organizations as well as consulates may be asked for help regarding interpretation and general assistance to sick seafarers.

A very simple thing like medical reporting may create considerable problems. Generally a typewritten report in English is issued after treatment. There are many complaints by masters and owners that the seamen's doctors do not always issue a typewritten report in understandable language. The report normally contains the diagnosis, laboratory findings, X-ray findings and instructions for further treatment. This information is necessary for the seamen's doctor in the next port or in home country in order to continue the proper treatment. X-ray films and other original documents should be given to the patient as well, as he rarely returns to the doctor who performed the initial examination.

Unfortunately, the company or the master very often do not issue the forms which should be filled in by the doctor, so that the doctor must use his own form. Some forms in use by certain companies, on the other hand, are such sophisticated questionnaires that the seamen's doctor will not fill it in or use it. Up to now it has proved to be impossible to agree internationally on one special form for this purpose. The Joint ILO/WHO Committee on the health of seafarers recommended in 1981 a special form consisting of 3 pages "Medical Report Form for Seafarers" and urged the "... adoption of a standard medical form for use by doctors examining and treating seafarers which would be an important step in improving medical care for seafarers, and the Joint Committee recommends that the Medical Report Form for Seafarers should be used to facilitate the exchange of information regarding the sick or injured seafarer between the ship's master and the doctor/hospital on shore [13]."

Up to now this medical report form has not been generally introduced.

The modern merchant service has changed. The ships are larger, the crews are smaller, there is usually one man for one job. Containerized cargo and new methods of bulk loading and discharging have changed port turnaround time from days to hours. The doctor no longer has adequate time to make in depth studies of a seaman's medical problem while the ship is in port. The first decision is: Can he be treated on board or must he sign off for treatment ashore. Once the sick seaman has been removed from the ship there are three alternatives: the seaman may be repatriated to his home immediately for further care, he may be admitted to a hospital or he may be placed in a hotel or seamen's home for subsequent out-patient medical care.

3.13.2 Personal Experiences of Practice at a Port Clinic in the U.S.A.

Early recognition of potential medical problems is essential. Too frequently a seaman requests medical care while in port and is told that there is insufficient time or that he can see a doctor in the next port. Most doctors familiar with seamen's habits realize that many visits to the doctor are a means to get off the ship for a few hours. However, many of these seamen may have a potentially serious medical problem that cannot be adequately treated on board. It behoves all doctors to anticipate this progression or degeneration in the case of a patient who is a seaman. An example: An engineer visited a doctor in a European port because of fatigue. Medication was prescribed. His report was completed and sent to the ship. The patient arrived in an American port. The fatigue persisted. He presented his report from the prior visit; the diagnosis was leukaemia. The haemoglobin was 9.5 g. Three weeks later the haemoglobin was 8.2 g. It is obvious that he should not have embarked on a prolonged voyage. This man could have been repatriated from the European port to his home in less than 1 h by air rather than a 12-h tiring flight from America. There was a total lack of communication between the doctor, the patient and the owner's representative.

Unlike the population ashore, seafarers do not have the advantage of being able to consult their own doctor readily when worried about their health. As a result minor symptoms which persist are often exaggerated when there is an opportunity to attend a doctor in a port in a foreign country. A shipping doctor is aware of this tendency but in addition he must watch carefully for the occasional real malingering patient.

A malingerer may have such a well-documented illness that a doctor cannot, in good faith, send the seaman back to the ship. An example: A European ship arrived in an American port for bunkering. The master requested medical care for a seaman who was coughing blood. The ship arrived at 03.00 and was sailing at 07.00. Chest X-rays were taken and showed evidence of tuberculosis, activity undetermined. An erythrocyte sedimentation rate was 20 mm/h. A sputum smear was non-diagnostic. The patient was admitted to hospital for further evaluation. The ship's destination was Hong Kong. The day after admission the patient admitted that he had had adequate treatment in his homeland and that he faked haemoptysis to get off the ship. He was aware of his abnormal chest X-ray and was very confident that he would be removed from the ship for medical reasons.

Quite frequently a master will collaborate with a seaman to request medical pay-off so that the man would be repatriated at the expense of insurance underwriters rather than company expense. A common ploy for this type of patient is a urinary tract stone history with severe pain and haematuria. On one occasion a Greek seaman actually shaved his fingertip to produce sufficient blood to cause the haematuria. His ruse was uncovered when dried blood was found under his finger-nail. He also readily admitted that he was not ill. Malingerers will continue to tax the brains of the medical profession. When malingering is suspected the doctor should notify the owner through the agent that this seaman should have a thorough evaluation on return home and be reprimanded and possibly pay his repatriation expense at his home port. It is useless to return these men to their ship only to try their charade again.

The seaman's doctor must determine if a seaman is not fit for full duty on board because of illness or disabling injury. A recommendation to remove or sign off the disabled seaman is given to the master through his agent or his consulate. Normally the master will follow this advice. But the master may elect not to sign off his crew member and the doctor has no recourse except to give any advice and medication that may be of value for use on board. Such refusals are not common but do occur and frequently have disastrous results, including permanent disability and death which would not have occurred had the seaman been left ashore.

Many masters will not accept a seaman with recommendations for light duty or no duty for a few days, e.g. the Australian Seamen's Union Agreement states that a seaman who is temporarily unfit or limited in any way must be repatriated. There are similar union agreements within the major maritime powers. But such agreements do not exist in all countries, especially not among those ships manned by third world nations' crews. Captains of those ships usually prefer to keep the man on board even if he is temporarily unfit or fit only for light duty.

Frequently an injured seaman arrives having been treated in another port and obviously needs daily care which cannot be given on board but he does not necessarily need hospitalization. The master may request treatment so that the seaman may rejoin the vessel within a reasonable time. These seamen may be treated as out-patients while living in a hotel or a seamen's home. Many fractures become permanent disabilities if adequate physiotherapy is unavailable. Corneal abrasions and ulcers heal with adequate daily care but cause blindness without such care. These are examples of maladies that may be treated on an out-patient basis.

The seaman who becomes ill or injured in the service of a ship while in foreign waters presents the doctor ashore with many associated problems in addition to the medical infirmity. The seaman must clear immigration. Should he not be admissible for non-medical reasons, the immigration service will issue a detention order. The detained seaman then must be treated while he is technically under guard. In some countries the detainee cannot be treated as an out-patient in a hotel or seamen's home.

The quarantine or public health service must screen the patient with particular attention to any medical conditions that are excludable. In the United States the quarantine service determines if an excludable condition exists. Should their decision be positive, the service then issues a class A medical detention order and presents this to the immigration department, which in turn detains the seaman for medical treatment. The order to detain crewmen under the immigration and naturalization act of the USA is specific:

> Any alien crewman afflicted with feeble-mindedness, insanity, epilepsy, tuberculosis in any form, leprosy, or any dangerous, contagious disease, or an alien crewman suspected of being so afflicted shall, upon arrival at the first port of call in the United States, be paroled to the medical institution designated by the district director in whose district the port is located, in the custody (other than during the period of time he is in such medical institution) of the agent of the vessel or aircraft on which such alien arrived in the United States and at the expense of the transportation line for a period initially not to exceed thirty days, for treatment and observation.

Other countries are less strict in this respect.

3.13.3 Hospital Treatment

The seriously ill and injured should be hospitalized for total care. The doctor should try to anticipate the length of hospitalization. The agent should be advised to contact the owners to pre-arrange repatriation. Too frequently a patient will be ready for repatriation and must wait an additional week because no travel arrangements have been completed.

The seaman's doctor should assess the long-term prognosis of the patient. Some owners will, on request, fly a mother, wife or other relative to the patient. This gesture may be the turning point in recovery. Should there be no hope for recovery, the doctor should attempt to have the patient repatriated while still alive so that he may die at home. Extensive dramatic surgery should not be attempted when death is inevitable. The death of a loved one away from home always creates doubt in the family thoughts.

The need for hospitalization could be markedly reduced by instituting a more comprehensive screening programme prior to sailing. Early recognition of medical problems before sailing or at a port nearer home is essential in maintaining good health among seamen and also would create a substantial financial reward for the owner.

The seaman is discharged from the hospital after obtaining maximum benefits. He may be transferred to a hotel or seamen's home for follow-up care or be repatriated to the home port or be returned to his ship. In any case, a medical report should accompany the patient and should include diagnostic impressions, X-ray and laboratory findings, required medications and recommendations for follow-up care. Should he return to his ship and need medication, a sufficient supply should be given to complete the voyage. In review the ten most common causes for hospitalization are:

Acute trauma, fracture, laceration etc.
Cardiac disease, coronary artery disease etc.
Peptic ulcer disease with bleeding or perforation
Hypertension, uncontrolled
Acute infections, respiratory etc.
Urinary tract stones
Diabetes
Alcoholism with pancreatitis, delirium tremens and psychosis
Hepatitis
Psychosis

3.13.4 Repatriation by Air

International air travel between major cities of the world has made a great contribution to the repatriation of sick seamen. A seaman can be repatriated half way around the world in 24 h by jet travel. The doctor must decide which patients can be repatriated immediately for further care. Safety and comfort are of paramount importance. The doctor should be aware of the regulations of the airlines regarding transportation of patients. Most airlines have a medical director who decides if and when a particular patient can be transported. Most airlines request a medical report from the attending physician. These remarks refer to those patients who obviously are ill or injured, such as stretcher patients or those needing assistance in walking.

The shipping industry is experiencing an economic crisis. Many ploys are used to save money. Third world seamen are rapidly replacing crews on ships under flags of convenience. Masters frequently attempt to bypass medical care in order to repatriate seamen who are in need of medical care. Incidents have occurred where a psychotic seaman has disrupted the flight plan of an international airline. The man was subdued by airport security and hospitalized for psychiatric care. All nations have a similar set of immigration and quarantine regulations that may vary but basically serve the same purpose.

The doctor must determine the need for an escort for the patient en route. The escort should be advised of any visas necessary for the trip. Escorts should be chosen with respect to their medical qualifications and informed of the patient's condition and any problems anticipated en route. Prior authorization should be received from the owners before embarking on expensive elective procedures such as open heart surgery with coronary bypass. A seamen's doctor should consider the availability of medical care in the seaman's homeland before repatriation. Aftercare of many medical problems is essential. Hypertension and diabetes must have continued control. It is frustrating to hear tales of despair from seamen who have not been offered ongoing medical care in their homeland.

3.13.5 General Recommendations

As the seaman belongs to a population at risk relating to health, special attention should be given to his medical care in port.

The following points of view should be considered:

1. A foreign seaman does not fit into a general medical practice or into a general out-patients' ward which is adjusted only to the native population of the country.
2. The seaman should be treated by a seamen's doctor who is familiar with the characteristics of seafaring and with the problems on board. This may be a private practice, a community practice or a special out-patient clinic for seamen.
3. For a seamen's doctor it is necessary to have good nautical medical knowledge and some multilingual ability as well as to show understanding for the ethnological background of his patient.
4. There should be easy, quick access to diagnostic facilities such as laboratory tests, ECG and radiology.
5. Shipping companies and their agents should be informed that an interpreter must accompany the patient whenever

there is a language barrier. A list of interpreters in the locality who can be called upon at short notice is also useful.

6. All case notes including personal details, medical history, previous treatment and investigation results should be sent to the doctor by the ship's captain. These should be returned to the captain after the consultation either by the patient or through the agent. Use of the WHO medical report form is strongly advised for this purpose.
7. The seamen's doctor should give the sick seafarer his report and his prescription for further treatment on board typed in English. Without these measures further successful treatment of the patient on board is not possible. Medicine must be supplied or prescribed in sufficient quantities.
8. This information should be passed on by the ship's captain to the doctor in the next port if further treatment is necessary.

References

1. WHO Study Group: The agreement of Brussels, 1924, respecting facilities to be given to merchant seamen for the treatment of venereal diseases. Geneva: WHO 1958.
2. Dolmierski, R., J. Filikowski, A. Kotlowski: Activities of WHO Pilot Health Centre for seafarers in Gdynia. Bull. Inst. mar. trop. Med. Gdynia *33*, 3/4, 149–156 (1980).
3. Dolmierski, R.: Progress report for 1980 on the activities of WHO Pilot Health Centre for seafarers in Gdynia (Poland) 1981.
4. Evjen, A.: Medical facilities ashore. Conference on health and welfare of seafarers, Marseille, 16–21 February 1959. Geneva: WHO 1959.
5. Goethe, H., P. Vuksanović: Sicknesses, injuries and health care on board – medical education of shipboard personnel. In: International workshop on human relationship on board, Bremen, 21–22 January 1982. Ed.: H. Böhm. Bremen, pp 119–130.
6. Health of seafarers: a study of the nature and extend of the health problems of seafarers and the health service available to them. Geneva: WHO 1965.
7. Haralanov, V., B. Angelov: Medical service in the Bulgarian water transport system. In: III International symposium on marine medicine, Leningrad 1968. Moscow, pp 160–164.
8. Medical care and hospitalisation of seamen in foreign ports. In: Proceedings of the European nautical medical meeting, Hamburg, 24–28 May 1978, Ed.: H. Goethe.
9. Proceedings of the second European nautical medical officers meeting, West Sussex, 10–14 Sept. 1979.
10. Ram, J.: Maritime health services at sea. SAPANUT J Israel Shipping Res Inst 6, 2, 4–8 (1976).
11. ILO/WHO Joint Committee: Report on health of seafarers. 5th session. Geneva: ILO/WHO 1973.
12. World directory of venereal-disease treatment centres at ports. Geneva: WHO 1972.

Addendum

13. Joint ILO/WHO committee on the health of seafarers. Sixth report. Geneva: ILO/WHO 1981.

4 Preventive Medicine Aboard

4.1 Health Education of the Seafarer

Y. Stenko

4.1.1 Safety and Health Training

Attention should in particular be paid to all aspects of personal safety and survival at sea in emergencies. These subjects are dealt with well in two publications of the U.K. Department of Trade [5, 6]. Seafaring has always been a dangerous occupation which can have an adverse effect on health either through disease or injury. Therefore, every seafarer should know the dangers inherent in his work. He must also know and strictly observe the specific requirements and safety rules necessary to prevent avoidable accidents. All crew should be taught how to rescue and transport casualties from bilges, narrow passages and through confined spaces. It is also necessary that they should be trained in the technique of mouth-to-nose and mouth-to-mouth artificial respiration.

On fishing ships the work is particularly dangerous and the crew should be properly trained in the special techniques of trawling, sorting and processing of fish. In addition to working procedures, fishermen must know the varieties of dangerous fish (sharks, electric fish etc.) and be aware that some fish can inflict poisonous stings.

Methods of health education are diverse and depend on the place and establishment where it is organized. A basic knowledge of health protection and major hygienic norms should be provided by doctors and specialists in maritime colleges and special marine training institutions. For senior officers and ship command personnel, special training courses and practical classes should be organized (Morozov [4]). At the same time, it is necessary to pay attention to the organization of control of personal and vessel hygiene observance by all the members of the crew and the passengers, and also to ensure a knowledge of international conventions and rules of environmental protection, both at sea and in ports. To this end, manuals such as the Ship Captain's Medical Guide, various visual aids (teaching models, posters), colour slides (Stenko [7]) and publications by WHO, ILO and the Alliance of the Red Cross and Red Crescent Societies are utilized. In a number of countries, this activity involves the participation of specialized medical naval institutions such as the Transport Medical Institute in the People's Republic of Bulgaria, the Institute of Marine and Tropical Medicine in Hamburg (FRG), the Institute of Marine and Tropical Medicine in Gdansk (PPR), the Water Transport Hygiene Research Institute of the USSR Ministry of Health, the Department of this Institute in Odessa and marine hospitals and clinics in ports of many countries of the world. Numerous public organizations are involved in health education activity. In several countries there exists a special network of establishments – houses or rooms of health education where the training of medical personnel for health education work is provided by the state and general health education measures are organized for the population, including sailors (lectures, exhibitions, radio broadcasts, films etc.).

4.1.2 Organisation and Means

Health education work on vessels is provided first of all by medical workers (where there are ships' doctors) or by the senior command staff. For this purpose, vessels can be equipped with printed propaganda matter e.g. popular science literature (Lamoureux [3]), booklets, leaflets, memoranda and slogans; visual aids e.g. posters, slides, films and photo albums; and finally, oral propaganda e.g. radio lectures and programmes on video equipment.

While organizing health education on vessels, attention should be paid to health protection during the work on board. Besides general hygiene norms, which are obligatory for the crew and the passengers, a sailor must be aware of safety rules to protect his health at work.

Many of the injuries at work are caused by slips, trips and falls, sometimes from a considerable height. Injuries can also be caused by falling objects or broken hawsers. Hence, general health education should be organized during routine activity such as cargo handling work and ship work during the voyage. During routine work a sailor should be made aware of the effect of tropical and polar climates and, thus, of suitable clothes, headgear, footwear and work schedules (Dolmierski et al. [1]).

Workers in noisy ship compartments (engine compartment, auxiliary machinery compartment etc.) should use hearing protectors such as ear plugs or ear muffs. A warning notice must be placed at the entrance to such places.

Specific work conditions and safety measures to be observed during storms should be explained to the sailors. Such work is extremely difficult, particularly during a high wind and rolling and pitching, which is made even more dangerous by low air temperature.

During cargo handling work, the danger of working near open holds, tank necks etc. should be explained. The safety regulations for cargo loading or discharge must be strictly observed.

On tankers and gas carriers the crew should know the norms of personal hygiene and the measures to prevent the toxic effects of gasoline, benzene, ammonia etc.

During work on deck the crew should know the characteristics and breaking strains of ropes and hawsers. Care should be taken during lifting and lowering ship's boats. Sailors, more often than others, have to rescue people from the sea. Thus (and also for self-protection during accidents and in emergency situations), sailors must swim well and know the rules of life-saving together with resuscitation techniques. This knowledge should be periodically reviewed and practised.

Specific work during a voyage can include various types of activity characteristic of the ship concerned. Fishing, whaling, research, hydrography and other ships all have work peculiar to them.

The most modern safety measures can be wasted if those concerned have not been trained in their use [5; 6]. Thus, knowledge of evacuation from ships and behaviour in lifeboats on the open sea and on uninhabited shores are integral elements of health education on vessels. Particular attention should be paid to the psychological training of the crew and the passengers. A shipwreck victim faces the following dangers: freezing, drowning, thirst, hunger, exhaustion, sea sickness, dehydration, injuries etc. Therefore, every sailor and passenger should be aware beforehand of all the necessary measures to be taken in an emergency.

A knowledge of modern marine medicine allows us to provide detailed characteristics of shipboard factors capable of changing human physiological functions and in several cases affecting sailor's health. Conditionally, these factors can be subdivided into the following groups:

1. Factors connected with ship work, causing fatigue;

2. Factors connected with rest and relaxation during leisure time, including sleep;
3. Factors connected with physical elements of the habitat environment, e.g. the round-the-clock effect of vibration, noise, rolling and pitching, high frequency and ultra-high frequency radiation, etc.;
4. Factors connected with chemical elements of the shipboard environment, e.g. emission of chemical compounds of polymers contained in varnishes, paints and glues used in the decoration of cabins and compartments, and also the process of transport of chemicals;
5. Socio-psychological factors connected with the isolated habitat of sailors;
6. Stress factors: fires, survival of a shipwrecked victim.

Therefore, health education should involve appropriate literature, vivid posters and leaflets concerning the above-mentioned factors which influence the sailor during his stay on board the ship.

Harmful habits of smoking and alcohol consumption (see Chap. 4.4) should be particularly highlighted in health education work. Anti-smoking health education campaigns in different countries are organized with the help of various techniques: posters, leaflets, radio and TV programmes and state legislation such as warning notices on cigarette packets and their limited sale. Tobacco smoking is the most common dangerous habit representing a mass chronic routine intoxication. This problem was emphasized in the decisions of the 63rd session of WHO Executive Council [2]: "This is one of the most serious problems of modern health care and a major problem of premature death which can be avoided." It has been established that the risk of developing cancer is ten times greater among smokers than non-smokers. Lip and larynx cancer are observed four times more often in smokers, while pancreatic cancer occurs twice as often. Death resulting from duodenal ulcer is three to four times more frequent in smokers, than in non-smokers, while fatal myocardial infarctions are seen four times as often. Out of 100 adult TB patients, 95 are smokers.

4.1.3 Smoking and Alcohol

An anti-smoking campaign pursues two purposes: 1) prevention of the development of the habit itself, 2) the giving up of smoking by sailors who are already addicted. Effective health education should be given to deal with smoking. Illustrated posters and pamphlets should be displayed prominently on board: medical treatment alone cannot succeed. There should be a strong desire on the part of the smoker to give up the habit. The sailor's wish, the doctor's will and medical treatment taken together can yield the desired effect. Anti-smoking campaigns are organized by such UN organizations as WHO, UNESCO and UNICEF and also by many governmental and nongovernmental organizations.

Alcohol addiction represents one of the serious health risk factors for sailors. Elaboration of a system of anti-alcohol education work is a task for health education. Four groups of non-specific factors favouring alcohol addiction in sailors are:

A. *Disruption of the personal environment by absence from home and frequent changes of ship*
a) Family problems
b) Alcohol addiction among the family members
c) Harmful psychological background in the family
d) Inadequate level of education of parents and unsatisfactory family upbringing

B. *Somato-neurological factors*
a) Congenital mental diseases
b) Severe somatic diseases and infections of the nervous system in early childhood
c) Organic cerebral defects
d) Mental deficiency and infantilism

C. *Pre-existing individual and psychological peculiarities*
a) Neurosis
b) Unstable, emotionally labile type
c) Parabehavioural personality development

D. *Moral and ethical personal immaturity*
a) Negative attitude towards training and a low level of education
b) Absence of socially meaningful motivations
c) Limited scope and instability of interests, lack of hobbies and spiritual interests
d) Uncertainty in matters of professional orientation, short-term contracts
e) Behaviour affected by poor motivation, escape from responsibility
f) Loss of "life perspective"

An anti-alcohol campain among sailors can be organized with two main objectives:
1. Prevention of alcohol addiction
2. Control of established alcohol addiction

Each of the above objectives is characterized by its own content of health education.
1. The content of medical anti-alcohol education aimed at prevention of alcohol addiction is defined by the modern notion of alcohol as a substance possessing narcotic properties.
2. Description of signs of alcohol addiction is included in one of the major sections of the anti-alcohol campaign aimed at alcohol addiction control. Timely identification and more adequate treatment of alcohol addicts depends on a knowledge of these signs among sailors. Educational texts should describe the alcohol syndromes, such as the hangover, the obsessive inclination to drink more, the loss of a sense of proportion, the diminished tolerance for alcohol and the character changes when drunk. Health education should reserve an important place for a thorough description of the effect of alcohol on the nerve cell. The primary aim of health education is to stimulate an interest in these problems and by greater self-awareness to encourage seafarers to moderate drinking habits and if necessary to seek medical advice.

4.1.4 Monotony and Other Psychological Factors

The monotonous life aboard together with boredom from the same companions and insufficient information about the family and relatives in many cases may result in depression and anxiety among sailors. The described factors leading to mental overstrain in sailors can be subdivided into the following groups:
1. Long-term separation from the home country;
2. Rigid psychological dependence on the type of ship and character of the voyage;
3. A feeling that the work to be done never finishes;
4. Considerable volume of monotonous working processes;
5. Constant alertness in case of emergency;
6. Increased feelings of anxiety and concern by the crew for their general health and sexual life.

This is a very incomplete list of factors capable of inducing neurotic reactions in sailors. (See also Chap. 3.10). The preventive approach to health education envisages a method of mental self-discipline on vessels and relaxation techniques in particular. This method represents an effective means of prevention of nervous, cardiovascular and other diseases. Records and tape-recordings with exercises are used on vessels for individual training or practice. Both group and individual training can be organized.

In view of the predominantly male composition of the crew, sexual hygiene and related questions should be dealt with. The problem of sexual relations has philosophical, social, physiological and biological aspects. A comprehensive approach to the problem demands the separation of health education into two areas of concern: life on board, where abstinence represents a normal condition for sailors, and life on shore, where a sailor should possess knowledge of personal hygiene and the methods of VD prevention.

References

1. Dolmierski, R., J. Filikowski, I. Golebiowska et al.: Morski poradnik medyczny. [Medical guide for seafaring]. Warsaw: Państwowy Zaklad Wydawnictw Lekarskich 1981.
2. Executive Board 63rd Session. WHO Chronicle *33,* 7, 337 (1979).
3. Lamoureux, V. B.: Guide to ship sanitation. Geneva: WHO 1967.
4. Morozov, A. A.: Study of hygienic knowledge and practice of personnel engaged in fishing and fish processing at sea as a means of evaluating the standard and effectiveness of health education in the fishing fleet. In: VII International symposium on marine medicine, Odessa 23–30 Sept. 1976. Moscow 1976. p. 265.
5. Personal Safety on Ships. Prepared by the Department of Trade and the Central Office of Information. London: Colibri Press 1979. Dd 803473 1 Pro 12510.
6. Personal Survival at sea. Prepared by the Department of Trade and the Central Office for Her Majesty's Stationery Office by Collier/Searle Ltd. Dd 596696 Pro 11369.
7. Stenko, Yu. M.: Meditsinskaya pomoshch v more. [Medical aid at sea]. Min. of Fishprod. USSR. Moscow 1975.

4.2 The Seafarer's Personal Hygiene

Y. Stenko

4.2.1 Life Situation on Board

The concept of personal hygiene involves not only the care of a seafarer's body but also the care of his cabin. Each individual should have a sound knowledge of the hygienic measures necessary to maintain a healthy condition of the skin, mouth, nose, head, hands and nails as well as the anal and genital regions. Cabin hygiene implies clean berth and linen, pure air and adequate lighting. In addition it is necessary to know about the special requirements of hygiene in tropical areas and in very cold climates.

The mode of life (sailor and passenger) on board is characterized by its own peculiar "habitat" conditions, which differ from those ashore (Ebert [2]; Naeve [4]; Stenko [6]). They include the constant influence of changing time zones (abnormal daily biorhythms), the changing seasons (entering the southern hemisphere and vice versa – abnormal annual biorhythms), the continuous effect of ship noise and vibration, the ship's motion, limited living space (vessel size: from 50 to 200–300 m long and from 5 to 100 m wide, with differing numbers of decks, from 2 to 20), relative hypodynamics (depending on the vessel size and sailor's occupation, from 1500 to 12000 steps a day) and the chemical effect of the environment (release of gaseous substances from polymers, dyes and linoleums).

Every sailor should have a separate berth. An ideal condition is an individual cabin or a cabin shared by two sailors. All berth linen should be changed every 10 days or every 7 days in tropical conditions. If possible, linen changes should be organized even more frequently. Other bedclothes and mattresses should be aired as often as twice a months. To maintain body hygiene, vessels are equipped with baths, showers and washrooms. Washrooms with hot and cold water are preferable; moreover the potable water storage should provide no less than 100 litres/day/person. On small vessels the potable water norm is reduced to 40 litres/day/person.

The work in merchant ships may sometimes be dirty and sweaty. Therefore it is important that regular showers should be taken to remove excessive sweat, dust, oils and oiled products. The skin pores are thereby enabled to fulfil their secretory and thermoregulatory function. This is most important for the skin/air interchange, which is equivalent to from 12% to 18% of the total gas exchange through the human lungs. In some countries cold water baths and showers with massage are recommended to promote a hardening of the physical condition.

One more skin protective function should be mentioned. Exposure of the human organism to direct sunlight is not always harmless owing to the high dose of ultraviolet irradiation, which causes sunburn. Sunlight-irradiated cuticle cells gradually accumulate pigmented granules hindering ultraviolet ray penetration inside the body. Moderate tan is obviously useful but excessive sun irradiation is undesirable for those individuals who tolerate the heat only poorly.

To maintain adequate vessel sanitation, laundries and dryers are installed. There should be a store of washing materials which are available to every sailor and they should be sufficient to maintain proper sanitation in the galley, washrooms, cabins, lavatories and urinals and in the communal rooms of the ship.

All seafarers should have a check-up by a dental surgeon every 6 months. Meantime, mouth and teeth hygiene should be observed. It is better to brush teeth after sleeping and in the evening before sleep. It is recommended that the mouth should be rinsed after meals and false teeth should always be kept clean.

Of all skin microbes, 95% are observed under the nails. One gram of finger-nail dirt contains up to 380 million microbes, including pathogenic ones. Helminthic ova are often identified there. Thus, it is necessary to keep the hands and nails clean by washing in soap and hot water and using a nail brush. Hand and toe nails should be regularly cut. Hands should be thoroughly washed with soap before meals. The hands and bodies of the workers in food stores, mess rooms and the galley should be particularly clean. The working clothes of such workers should also be clean at all times and changed as necessary when soiled.

Fingers can be contaminated after visiting lavatories and using toilet paper. Hence, hand washing with soap is necessary after urination and defaecation.

One fly can harbour up to 6 million microbes of 44 pathogenic species. Microbes survive up to 2–3 days on the body and feet of a fly. Some microbes (up to 28 million) are observed in the fly intestinal tract. Flies defaecate up to 50 times a day. In the fly intestinal tract, dysenteric pathogens can survive up to 3 days while those of typhoid fever can survive up to 7 days. Thus elimination of flies in cabins, and particularly in food installations, results in a radical decrease in infectious intestinal diseases.

After some intestinal diseases, particularly those which were not severe or remained unidentified, a sailor can become a pathogen carrier. In such cases the sailor, particularly if he is engaged in food preparation and distribution or has contact with potable water reservoirs, can be a source of danger to the crew and the passengers. Therefore, any sailor who has had intestinal disease (typhoid fever, dysentery and so on) should be kept from food preparation and its distribution and from potable water until a medical authority provides him with a certificate proving that he is not an infectious carrier.

It must be ensured that food workers have no skin eruptions, cuts and pustules, because they can be a source of infection to the members of the crew. Therefore, personal hygiene of the body, hands, nails and the head hair by food handlers and other catering staff must be strictly observed. Such workers should also observe normal cleanliness when not on duty. Food galley wastes should be removed every day. After a shift, those who have worked in the engine room or on deck should have a bath or take a shower.

Cabin sanitation should be maintained at a high standard. Cabins should be swept or washed every day. Litter should be collected in special bins or litter collection places. Minimal norms of dry household litter per person per day constitute 0.002 m^3 and solid food waste can be 0.003 m^3.

Cabin lighting should be adequate. It should be remembered that dirty windows and port holes decrease illumination intensity by up to 50%–70%. Artificial illumination with incandescent lamps should be sufficient for reading and be no less than 250 lux.

4.2.2 The Impact of Climate

Under tropical conditions of high external temperature and air humidity but where a system of air conditioning is operating, the temperature-humidity gradient will affect the organism when a person leaves or enters a cooled cabin. The primary reaction of the organism at the moment of entering an area with a lower air temperature represents a reflex reaction to cooling, manifested by skin vessel contraction and skin cooling as a result of cold blood stimulation of both skin exteroceptors and interoceptors of deep tissues, organs, veins and arteries. Depending on the intensity of external temperature stimulation, verious thermoregulatory mechanisms come into action, characterized by skin depot-to-depot blood redistribution, an increase of arterial blood pressure, reflex slowing of the pulse rate and increased heat production. The greater the strain is on the thermoregulating system, the more vividly the primary organism reaction is manifested. This is confirmed by the fact that during air temperature drops of 20 °C (a change of temperature conditions from 40° to 20 °C) the primary reaction is so great that it involves muscle fibres ("gooseflesh") in addition to skin vessels. So-called cold shock can develop.

When sailors are on deck under conditions of high air temperatures the thermoregulation processes adapt to maximal heat exchange. Enhanced heat exchange continues during the first 5–15 min after a person enters an area with a lower air temperature, owing to thermoregulatory inertia, already "adjusted" to maximal heat exchange. This enhanced heat exchange during the first 5–15 min can be explained by the fact that the whole body is covered with perspiration when the sailor leaves a high temperature environment.

Considerably raised water conduction, exceeding air heat conduction by a factor of three and its thermal capacity by a factor of four, results in better evaporation from the skin in those who enter a cooled installation where the decrease of solar temperature by 5°–30 °C results not only in a more intense body heat exchange but also in supercooling.

Rapid change of heat exchange modes is of great significance. Thus, during work on deck a sailor's body receives heat from the warmed deck and bulkheads, and also as a result of intensive solar radiation, and releases heat mainly through evaporation of sweat. When entering a compartment with a cooler temperature, in addition to the continuing loss of heat through the sweat evaporation, there is a loss due to radiation and convectional cooling, the former being more intensive.

Microclimatic conditions in ship compartments (Table 1) are characterized by a combination of four parameters: temperature, relative air humidity, air speed and mean radiative temperature of the bulkheads.

The body is characterized by broad adaptive potential. An unfavourable effect of cold climate can be eliminated by a proper organization of leisure time and heating (Stenko [5]).

To prevent the cooling down of the body and the feeling of freezing during breaks it is necessary to raise the room temperature to a value between 15 °C and 20 °C and to decrease the air speed to 0.5 m/s.

4.2.3 Clothing

Sailors' clothes must be waterproof, adequately protecting the body from cold and

Table 1. Estimated microclimate values in vessel compartments

Compartments	Navigation area	Air temperature (°C)	Relative humidity (%)	Air speed (m/s)
	Summer period			
Cabins, public, medical and service compartments	Northern	20–22	70–40	0.15–0.2
	Moderate	22–23	60–40	0.20–0.3
	Southern	23–24	60–40	Up to 0.5
	Tropics	25	60–40	Up to 0.5

wind; footwear should have felt insoles. There must be facilities for drying the clothes, footwear and gloves and they should be capable of ensuring dry clothes and footwear in 5–6 h time, i.e. 1 h before the next shift (Dolmierski et al. [1]).

4.2.4 Sleep and Rest

A major part of the cabin rest period should be devoted to sleeping. There is nothing worse than inadequate sleep. If sleep is frequently inadequate, the nervous system impairment develops in the form of irritability, undue tiredness and the appearance of various diseases. Thus, it is not by chance that modern marine medicine attaches great significance to normal sleep in the maintenance of health. There must be attention to such things as linen, cabin illumination, relative quiet etc.

During sleep and rest in a cabin in rough weather, the level of energy loss increases by 10%–30% (over 4 points) compared with normal sea conditions. This is due to the necessity of stabilizing the body in space with the help of a greater number of muscles than are normally used. In such cases the head should always be above the level of the legs. Naturally, this position is hard to maintain during considerable pitching or rolling. Thus, cabin couches are fixed perpendicular to the berth to allow for the various sleeping positions which are necessary.

4.2.5 Smoking

Smoking in cabins is not recommended. As is known, 20% of all noxious substances released from a cigarette are consumed by the smoker, while 30% are destroyed or remain in the butt and 50% pass into the air. Anti-smoking health education work is generally needed.

4.2.6 Physical Exercise

Body hygiene, a proper mode of life, rational diet, physical exercise – these are the elements of personal hygiene.

The smaller is the waist line, the longer is life. Gaining weight means ageing. The limited space on a ship and the absence of the physical diversions ashore result in a poor state of physical fitness. Hence the need for physical exercises and sports on vessels. It is established that over 80% of sailors enjoy sports and take part in various physical exercises, preferably games – table tennis, volley ball, basketball, mini-soccer, hygienic gymnastics or weight lifting.

Recently, sports rooms or cabins, equipped with velo-ergometers, trainers and other facilities, have been installed on many vessels. Specific marine exercises should also be developed, climbing the sea-ladder, ropes etc. During time in port it is useful to organize sports competitions with other ships' crews.

4.2.7 The Interior of the Cabin

Sailors keep their personal clothes and footwear in their cabins; the clothes should be regularly cleaned and pressed. One has to remember that, on ships, these clothes and uniforms are constantly swinging and rubbing owing to the ship rolling and pitching, and they get damp due to raised air humidity. Thus, regular drying and proper up-keep of clothing are necessary.

A cabin interior decorated with plants and flowers creates additional comfort, a good psychological mood and makes up for the monotony of life at sea. Sometimes a sailor is separated from his home, family and relatives for a long time. When he leaves land his physiological functions become adapted to the monotonous ship's life and a specific marine mode of life develops (Stenko [6]). During a long voyage the number of external stimuli decreases, while some such stimuli become habitual.

The amount of sex and other blood hormones stabilizes at a certain constant level. As a result of sexual fantasies, film shows etc., this level can be elevated, resulting in natural ejaculation during sleep. This is a normal function of a healthy body. Decoration of the cabin walls with erotic pin-ups should be discouraged because they are a disturbing influence in the absence of normal outlets for sexual energy, especially at night. Daily exercise and a shower at bedtime encourage a relaxed mood. During tropical voyages and shore leave sailors should wear caps and sun glasses. In view of the fact that a heating microclimate is created at a distance of 30–50 cm from the open deck surface which is due to the raised surface temperature of the deck and secondary air heating plus direct solar radiation, the wearing of long woollen socks is necessary. They will protect the feet and shins from overheating. Wearing heavy clothing in tropical conditions inhibits thermoregulation; sensible clothes (shorts, shirt with short sleeves and open collar without a tie) prevent the sailor from overheating. But strong sun radiation should be taken into account.

Any small personal article, such as a handkerchief, smoking pipe or mouthpiece, sandals and shaving articles, can, when used by more than one person, become a source of infection. Thus, they should be individual.

In view of close daily mutual contacts of the crew members during their work, in cabins and public places, strict observance of the personal hygiene norms by every sailor will lead to a satisfactory health status. By strengthening his body, man can cope with many hardships. The sea favours people with strong bodies and high morale.

References

1. Dolmierski, R., J. Filikowski, I. Golebiowska et al.: Morski poradnik medyczny. [Medical guide for seafaring]. Warsaw: Państwowy Zaklad Wydawnictw Lekarskich 1981.
2. Ebert, H.: Health protection on the GDR sea-going ships without medical personnel. Bull. Inst. mar. trop. Med. Gdynia *28,* 3/4, 125–128 (1977).
3. International medical guide for ships. Geneva: WHO 1967.
4. Naeve, W.: Schiff ohne Schiffsarzt. Erkrankungen und Verletzungen der Besatzung eines Frachtschiffes im Liniendienst Europa-Südamerika. Münch. med. Wschr. *113,* 24, 909–913 (1971).
5. Stenko, Yu. M.: Meditsinskoe posobie dlja kapitanov. [Medical guide for captains]. 2nd ed. Moscow: Advert. Bureau of Min. Merch. Mar. Moscow 1970.
6. Stenko, Yu. M.: Psikho-gigiena morjaka. [Psycho-Hygiene of seamen]. Leningrad: Meditsina 1981.

4.3 Food Hygiene Aboard Ship

Dilwyn T. Jones

4.3.1 Introduction

Food hygiene principles on ships are, in the main, the same as on land. However, the application of those principles is more difficult at sea and outbreaks of food poisoning are likely to be more dramatic because of the isolation of the ship and the consequent serious effect if even a small number of the crew are rendered unfit to work. The ship's community is a semi-closed one and there is restricted opportunity to replenish stores: Hence the importance of good storage facilities. Space is always short on board, with the result that food preparation, cooking and storage areas are liable to be too small for the reasonable practice of good food hygiene unless a very positive attitude has been shown at the ship design stage. The extremes of temperature experienced in a ship trading worldwide must be allowed for in ventilation and refrigeration capacity, while the movement of the ship requires specific design features and the constant vibration in a ship under way renders some otherwise favoured materials unusable.

Nevertheless, it must be accepted that a ship's canteen or dining room is merely a floating restaurant and must achieve standards as good as in any catering establishment ashore. This can be achieved only by skill, knowledge and energy of the highest order. Personal and continued scrutiny of food hygiene methods by the responsible ship's officer, together with strong support from management ashore, are essential. It is a serious error to limit hygiene inspections to the times when the ship is in port – only random inspections at sea will reveal the true state of affairs.

Responsibility for the maintenance of good ship's catering is sometimes placed in the hands of a Catering Committee but food hygiene should always be the responsibility of only one officer, otherwise there may be differences of opinion, leading to confusion among the staff. Such sole responsibility must be matched by giving the authority to act immediately when correction of bad practice is necessary.

Throughout this chapter, the term "food" is used to indicate both food and drink.

4.3.2 Epidemiology

Ulewicz et al. [14] considered that a ship creates a sui generis epidemic environment, more favourable for the development of infectious diseases than ordinary conditions of human life and work ashore. This tends to be supported by their survey work, which showed that ships' crews had the same carrier rate for *Salmonella, Shigella* and some enteropathogenic serotypes of *E. coli* as shore staff but had a higher incidence of overt disease. This indicated to the authors that conditions on board ship were more favourable to the development of gastrointestinal disease outbreaks.

Routine monitoring of the microbiological state in food areas on ships is limited by the small amount of laboratory equipment usually kept on board. However, swabbing of work surfaces and equipment can be carried out in port and some of the results of such surveys have been disturbing. It was shown in one instance (Poultney [12]) that passengers would have been better advised to eat off the toilet seats than off the cafeteria tables.

The lack of microbiological expertise and equipment on board makes it very difficult to mount a thorough investigation of gastrointestinal outbreaks between ports. Any determination of the causative organism and its method of spread will frequently depend upon clinical examination and a detailed consideration of the symptoms and signs and of their timing in relation to the consumption of suspect foods. A careful study of the foods served at each meal and a listing of the foods eaten by each crew member or passenger, whether suffering from the condition or not, may, with luck, demonstrate which food is responsible. On most occasions, however, there is no such good fortune and food preference charts will go no further than an indication that certain foods must be viewed with suspicion. It may even be possible to allocate different degrees of suspicion to the foods but, without certainty, it can be difficult to persuade those responsible that changes should be made. On a ship with no surgeon, the investigation may have to be delayed until the ship arrives at the next large port and then the success of the enquiry will depend on the accuracy of the memories of those on board. In many of these cases it is impossible even to assemble a list of suspect foods, except in the most general terms. Where ships' officers responsible for food hygiene have had sufficient training or have had a protocol prepared for them, they may carry out a preliminary investigation at the time of the attack and this could prove very useful.

In all cases, any outbreak of possibly food-borne illness should invariably be followed, as soon after the onset as possible, by a most stringent check of all food hygiene practices on board, together with a detailed examination of the gastrointestinal history of every food handler (N. B. the broad definition of this word is set out later in this chapter). There must be no half-measures or scruples about this and it is always advisable to ensure the support of the ship's master by consulting him beforehand, by telling him precisely what is intended and by keeping him informed at every stage. In this way, even an abortive investigation can be used for the cementing of good relations and the establishment of an educational programme on board, resulting in great benefit to all.

The organisms found in shipboard outbreaks of food-borne disease are the same as on shore, *Salmonella, Shigella, Staph. aureus* and *Vibrio parahaemolyticus* having all been incriminated at times. Attention has also been drawn to the importance of certain serotypes of enterotoxigenic *E. coli* – both heat-stable and heat-labile toxin being involved, together or separately (Hobbs et al. [4]); Wachsmuth et al. [15] and Lumish et al. [8] – and the method of spread on ships has been studied (Solodovnikov et al. [13]). It is apparent that good food hygiene is a primary defence against the problem (Hobbs et al. [4] and Hobbs et al. [6]). The occurrence on ships of viral gastroenteritis, such as that caused by the Norwalk agent, cannot be ruled out. The difficulty of isolating viruses makes shipboard investigation rarely practicable but evidence is slowly accumulating to suggest that viruses may be a cause of food-borne gastroenteritis (Appleton et al. [1]). Viruses do not replicate in food (Appleton et al. [1]), so it seems reasonable to consider that where temperature and humidity are associated with an increase in cases, a viral cause is unlikely.

Factors, other than food hygiene standards, which may be important in determining whether a person suffers a gastrointestinal infection on a ship include (a) climatic conditions (b) foods eaten and (c) resistance to infection of the person concerned. The latter factor may be influenced by (a) the previous exposure of the person to such infections (people from more "sanitised" countries are at greater risk), (b) dietetic irresponsibility, (c) overexposure to the sun, (d) lack of sleep and general non-adaptation to shipboard life and (e) upsetting movement of the ship (Parker [11]; Merson et al. [10]; Werner et al. [17] and Gangarosa et al. [2]). On cruise ships, there is a relationship between the incidence of food-borne diseases and the length of the cruise, its geographical location and the ambient temperature. It is also worth noting that survey work (Merson et al. [9]; Werner et al. [17]) has shown that the real number of cases in any outbreak (and, one suspects, on any cruise) is likely to be four or five times the number logged by the surgeon but this has been disputed (Parker [11]).

Eating ashore is very often blamed for illness on ships. In fact, the ports visited by cruise ships are such that they might be said to be carrying their passengers into risk of infection (Langley [7]). Too much should not be made of this. It is too facile an answer to a complex problem. Certainly, if shipboard standards of food hygiene are low or if outbreaks recur in the same ship on cruises to different waters or if primary illness occurs in people who have not been ashore or before the first port of call is reached, grave suspicion must fall on the ship. It is not uncommon to find, on investigation of a major outbreak, that there has been a number of minor outbreaks on the same ship during the previous few months, but these have been ignored by the ship's officers or regarded as a "normal" happening. This attitude should be strongly attacked and all ships' masters should be instructed by their companies to report even the smallest outbreak at the earliest moment.

Recent work has supported the traditional suspicion of some shipboard conditions and practices. That ancient companion of seafarers, the cockroach, has been shown (Merson et al. [9] and Wegner et al. [16]) to be sometimes contaminated with food poisoning organisms, including several serotypes of *Salmonella*. The liking of the cockroach for warm dark corners in the galley is well known, so it must represent a potential food poisoning threat but its actual involvement has yet to be shown. Hobbs et al. [5] demonstrated that galley cloths and cutting boards had high bacterial counts and recommended that they be thoroughly cleansed at the end of each day (the cutting boards being additionally subjected to hard wire brushing), then soaked overnight in a solution of sodium hypochlorite containing 130 ppm of available chlorine. Morning rinsing in water of potable quality renders them safe and pleasant to use. On the other hand, Goethe and Herrmann [3] took scratch samples from fixtures in a large number of seagoing ships and examined them bacteriologically. Only a third of the samples were free from *E. coli* but it was found that the *E. coli* count of the wooden surfaces was only half that of the plastic surfaces.

Gastrointestinal disease on ships is usually mild in character but is occasionally severe. In young children, old people and those already debilitated by other conditions, it is always potentially serious and may be life threatening.

The necessity of maintaining high food hygiene standards on ships, given the difficulties already discussed, underlines the need for shipboard food handlers to be highly trained. They should have to undergo a complete trade training, designed for work on ships, before going to sea, and attendance at refresher courses, at reasonably short intervals, should be an established practice.

If a ship's master is in doubt as to the safety of the food hygiene practices on his ship, he should apply to a Port Health Authority or similar organisation. Their staff are expert in this field and will investigate and advise willingly.

4.3.3 Food Handling and Food Handlers

The general principles of food handling – obtain the food from a good source, cook it thoroughly, handling it as little as possible, and eat it immediately or hold it below 6 °C or above 60 °C – are as applicable at sea as they are on shore but, once again, they are more difficult to apply at sea. The inevitable limitations on space make the provisions of sufficient refrigerated storage very difficult, while the variation in ambient temperature often makes generous refrigerated space absolutely essential. The same type of problem occurs with the separation of different types of foods. Shortage of space leads to a temptation to handle all foods in the same containers or on the same work surfaces but this must be firmly resisted. Of great importance here is the separation of raw and cooked foods and particularly of raw and cooked meats – no contact, direct or indirect, between these foods should ever be permitted. Expenditure on specially labelled containers and refrigerated spaces combined, perhaps, with a system of colour coding (Poultney [12]) is amply justified.

The general rules on the temperatures at which foods should be held can be summarised as follows:

All frozen foods	Below −18 °C
Milk, cream and all foods containing them	6 °C
Raw meat, poultry and fish (for short periods)	Below 6 °C
Manufactured or pasteurised meat or meat products	Below 6 °C
Fruit and vegetables	6° – 10 °C

These temperatures do not guarantee indefinite keeping qualities and producers' or manufacturers' instructions should always be carefully followed.

For buffets on deck, it is a temptation to prepare the food early and hold it on deck at ambient temperatures. This can be highly dangerous and the "below 6 °C or above 60 °C" rule must be rigidly applied, food being allowed to remain between these temperatures only for the short time it takes to prepare it. This principle applies just as strongly to food prepared early for seamen working awkward shifts. In all mass catering, the use of large joints of meat and huge specimens of poultry has economic advantages. There are health problems, however, in that the middle of the joint may not reach a sufficiently high temperature to kill off any pathogenic organisms. Therefore, it is better to cut the meat into smaller pieces for cooking but, if this is not possible, the cooking time must be adjusted. The temperature at the middle of any joint must reach at least 74 °C during cooking and anything, such as masses of moist stuffing, which makes this more difficult should be actively discouraged. This temperature (74 °C) is a useful figure to remember, as reheated leftovers must always be raised to at least that before being served.

It cannot be repeated too often that, with the exception of canned or otherwise preserved food and of fruit and vegetables, food must not be left at temperatures between 6 °C and 60 °C for any longer than is absolutely necessary. The ambient temperature in a galley will fall within this risk range – therefore it is dangerous to leave food in the galley for any length of time. This is especially important when food is thawing or cooling. Thawing must be carried out in a refrigerator and cooling after cooking must be as rapid as possible, the food being transferred to a refrigerator at the earliest practicable moment.

Unwashed salads and fruit from any source are often contaminated with coliform bacteria, amoebae and other parasites and, therefore, potentially with pathogenic organisms. They should, if to be eaten raw, always be washed in a solution of sodium hypochlorite providing 80 ppm of available chlorine which, after 30 s of immersion, will reduce the coliform count to negligible figures (Hobbs et al. [5]).

A food handler has been defined as a person who carries out any process in the sale of food or in the preparation, transport, storage, packaging, wrapping exposure for sale, service or delivery of food or who cleans any article or equipment with which food comes into contact and in the context of shipping applies to everybody in the catering department, especially to the cooks, the other kitchen personnel and the stewards. This rather legalistic definition serves to emphasise the point that anyone who touches, directly or indirectly, another person's food or drink is a food handler who must, during his work, keep himself and his clothing as clean as is practicable in the circumstances. This may not appear to be a particularly stringent requirement but, as in all food hygiene, the practical (as opposed to the totally theoretical) approach is to be preferred. Only in that way can the essential cooperation be obtained from those who actually do the work. For instance, insistence on snow-white cleanliness when a food handler is heaving large joints of frozen raw meat about is a nonsense – but it is absolutely correct to insist that he change into clean clothing and wash thoroughly before he goes back to work in the galley, handling food (raw or cooked) which is being prepared for consumption. Bodily cleanliness is just as important as clean clothing and all food handlers should be expected to maintain clean hands, face and head. Ambient temperatures on board tend to be high, especially in the tropics, and a casual approach to dress (or undress) is often the result. The food handler working in such temperatures must be even more careful to maintain personal cleanliness and to cover those parts of his body which may come into contact with food. Contamination of food with drops of sweat may also be a problem.

Good personal hygiene is greatly encouraged by an easy availability of washing facilities. Baths and/or showers must be plentiful and easy of access. Of particular importance to food handlers are the handwashing facilities – these must be so easily available that no food handler is ever tempted to wash his hands in a sink intended for the washing of food, utensils or equipment. Each food preparation area should be equipped with an adequate number of wash-hand basins, each fitted out with hot and cold water (delivered by mixer tap), soap, nailbrush and disposable towels or hand-drying machine. Constant care should be taken to ensure that these are used before starting work, after every handling of raw food, after any dirty job and, invariably, before handling any cooked or otherwise ready-to-eat food. In addition to these facilities in the food preparation areas, there must be handwashing basins easily available near each toilet. Of all food hygiene precautions, thorough washing of the hands after using the toilet is by far the most important. Health education plays a great part here and all food handlers should be taught the reasons why toilet/hand hygiene is so important. However, all that will go for nothing if the washbasins are not immediately available on leaving the toilet or if the basin is not fully fitted out. Response can be greatly improved by the use of posters giving the "Now wash your hands" message in those languages normally spoken by the food handlers.

It may be that if these precautions are faithfully observed, the chances of a food handler transmitting any food poisoning will be greatly reduced. However, it is a commonsense precaution to prevent the employment of a food handler who is suffering from, or carrying, any potentially food-borne disease. Medical screening, designed with the job in mind, is essential before signing on. In addition, there must be an invariable rule on board that any food handler who falls ill must report sick immediately, be taken off food handling work and not be allowed back to it until all possibility of his suffering from a potentially food-borne infection has been excluded by a qualified person. Especial care must be taken with gastrointestinal illness, and the mildest diarrhoea or nausea in a food handler should initiate the above procedure. Discharges from the nose, ear or mouth and skin conditions such as boils or other staphylococcal infections are other reasons for exclusion from work. Cuts on hands are a matter for judgement. If they are clean and covered with a clean, waterproof dressing, they may be allowed. Smoking, spitting or nailbiting in a food preparation area must be absolutely forbidden.

In deciding what degree of risk is present, it is reasonable to consider (a) the nature of the food (i.e. raw vegetables would not present any risk), (b) the way in which the food is packed, (c) any process to which the food will be subjected before it is eaten and (d) any possibility of contamination being passed secondarily to other foods.

4.3.4 Delivery of Food to the Ship

Careful selection and monitoring of food sources is of great importance but all that effort will be wasted if the method of transport from the source to the ship allows the food to deteriorate or be contaminated.

As with all food rooms and containers, delivery vehicles and barges must be clean and constructed in such a way that they may be kept clean. There must be no accumulation of dirt or refuse in the vehicle. If open food is carried, the vehicle should be covered and have an impervious floor or duckboards. Any ice used in packing the food must be made from water of potable quality and be uncontaminated. Any equipment in the vehicle which comes into contact with food also should be clean, but the degree of insistence here should have some regard to the form of packing or wrapping of the food.

The crew of the vehicle and any men who help to carry the food from the vehicle should be regarded as food handlers and be expected to have the same standards as any such person on the ship, bearing in mind what has already been discussed on the practical, rather than the theoretical, approach. If the food is so wrapped as to prevent contact between it and the body of the carrier, there is no risk, provided that the wrapping of the food is regarded as contaminated and not allowed into contact with open food during unwrapping or storage. If, however, the food is not well wrapped, the carriers should wear clean, washable protective clothing, designed to protect the food from any contact with their bodies.

4.3.5 Galley Design

The design of any cooking or food preparation area and the equipment used therein is always an important factor in the maintenance of good food hygiene. Where, as in ship's galleys, the available space is severely limited and there are other specific problems to be overcome, such as have been previously discussed, design becomes a crucial factor. From the earliest planning stages of any new tonnage, or of any major refit, one member of the design team should be experienced in food hygiene at sea. In some countries, e.g. West Germany, this principle is embodied in legislation but, legally required or not, it should always be followed. Apart from the benefits to health, such an arrangement is a real economy, as the later correction of built-in bad design is always highly expensive.

All surfaces – deck, deckhead and bulkheads – of all food areas must be easily cleanable. They must be hard, smooth, impervious and light in colour so that cleanliness can be easily monitored. Absorbent surfaces, such as cloth or other fibrous material or plaster, should not be permitted unless they can be hard sealed.

Equipment and work surfaces should be made of stainless steel with good welded joints. Other materials may be affected by the vibration of the ship, allowing cracks to open and food debris to collect.

A galley tends to be a warm place at the best of times but in the tropics it can become a furnace unless very efficient ventilation is provided. Even then, the ambient temperature is likely to be high and the principle of safe temperature ranges must be well understood by the staff.

The lighting of all food rooms must be such that there are no dark corners where dirt and debris can collect unnoticed and the work surfaces should have an illumination of at least 200 lux.

Condensation may be a considerable problem. The standard of ventilation is a crucial factor here but, even where ventilation is excellent, some condensation may occur and the design of the equipment and of overhead trunking and pipework must ensure that drips do not occur where food may be contaminated.

Efficient cleaning is of first importance and the galley design must make this as easy as possible. Thorough cleaning beneath equipment can be facilitated or made impossible by its design. Tubular construction with no under-worktop cupboards is sometimes recommended but may be too space consuming. The space beneath equipment should be either at least 15 cm high to allow easy access or completely eliminated by bedding and bolting down the equipment to the deck so that dirt, food debris, insects and rodents cannot obtain entry. Work surfaces should be regularly swabbed down with sodium hypochlorite solution. Wood chopping blocks should be examined regularly. They wear badly in use and the surface becomes so cut about that it is impossible to clean. Planing will establish a new surface and remove the health risk. The deck should be regularly washed down to remove grease and food debris. It has been the habit to use sea water for this, through special outlets, carefully labelled, located at not more than 45 cm above the deck. In polluted waters, however, even these can be dangerous in use, because of the possibility of the water splashing on to work surfaces or into containers (Merson et al. [10]). It is better, therefore, except in the unlikely event of absolute certainty that the water overside is unpolluted, to use only potable water for washing down. Drainage of all this water must be efficient – gulleys must be free running and easily cleaned out and washed through. They should be covered with easily removable, heavy plates of perforated metal.

The design of equipment for washing and sterilising utensils and crockery should be based on simple logic rather than good looks. Whatever scheme is used, there must be a capacity for removing food debris, with or without detergent, for rinsing and for bactericidal treatment. This can be efficiently carried out in three stages – first, removal of gross food debris by hand, second, washing in a detergent solution at not less than 60 °C and third, a bactericidal rinse. The latter can be by immersion for at least 30 s in water at not less than 82 °C or for at least 1 min in a lukewarm solution of sodium hypochlorite providing, at all times, more than 50 ppm available chlorine. It cannot be overemphasised that temperatures and concentrations of bactericidal agents are crucial factors and must be meticulously monitored. If a dishwasher is available, the first stage, i.e. removal of gross food debris, must still be carried out by hand before the dishes are placed in the machine. The washing phase should be maintained at more than 60 °C for at least 1 min and the rinse at more than 82 °C. After any of these methods, the utensils or crockery should be allowed to air-dry without wiping. If they must be wiped, the cleanliness of the cloths must be carefully monitored.

Some mention must be made of two potential design problems which are often ignored. First, on a ship it is quite impossible to avoid pipes and ducts being fixed on deckheads and bulkheads, even in the food preparation areas. It is, therefore, imperative, especially with sewage and other waste pipes, that the possiblity of leakage is avoided by a refusal to accept inspection or drainage points within the food areas and an insistence that any inevitable joints are regularly inspected. Second, it is impossible to maintain high standards of food hygiene if untrained staff are able to pass casually through the food areas. Therefore, good design will ensure that these areas cannot be used as a short cut from one part of the ship to another.

Waste and refuse collection and removal must be carefully planned, with the emphasis on removal. Refuse collection in the food areas can be in metal bins or in bags hung off the deck but removal, and immediate replacement with clean containers, must be carried out regularly and frequently. If metal bins are used, an area outside the food handling areas must be set aside where they can be cleaned and steam-sterilised. Refuse storage must also be located well away from any form of food handling. The area should be specially and clearly marked and the containers therein must be tight lidded and be rodent and insect proof.

All food storage, serving and preparation areas must also be protected, so far as is possible, against rodents and insects, crawling or flying. However, the best protection is sometimes unavailing and a constant surveillance should be maintained. In a modern ship, insects are likely to be the greater problem and a regular spraying programme, using residual and space insecticides, should be undertaken but the greatest care should be exercised to ensure that there is no contamination of food or surfaces likely to come into contact with food.

4.3.6 Ice-Making and Milk-Making Machines

Ice is a substance which is vastly misunderstood on some ships – because it is cold, it is thought to be totally harmless. Nothing could be farther from the truth. It is a truism that, in any shipboard outbreak of gastrointestinal disease, all ice sources, machines and storage methods should be subjected to the most careful scrutiny. Commercially bought ice should be particularly suspect and the sources checked thoroughly before purchase and during the period of supply. If ice is made on board, the water supplied to the machine must be of a potable quality and the machine must be maintained and serviced strictly according to the manufacturer's instructions. Removal of ice from the machine by hand should be roundly condemned. The use of a scoop should be encouraged by its ready availability and the use of posters. The shape and size of the scoop should be such as to permit the removal of a reasonable amount of ice in one operation and the material of which it is made should be impervious, smooth and easily cleaned – and it should be so cleaned, frequently and carefully. When not in use, the scoop should be kept in a container of sodium hypochlorite solution, on, or very near, the ice-making machine.

Machines for reconstituting milk have been the source of a number of outbreaks of disease. Although fresh milk, bought ashore and refrigerated aboard, must be carefully handled and the sources regularly monitored, it is preferred by most seafarers. This fact, and the availability of ultra heat-treated milk, which keeps for long periods, have greatly reduced the number of reconstituters in use. There are instances, however, when reconstituted milk is used, either out of preference or necessity. Dried whole milk is the usual "raw" material used and this must be stored in a dry, cool place, protected from rodents and insects. It must also be protected from taints and odours, which it picks up very quickly. The dried milk must be carefully loaded into the constituter to ensure that it all falls into the mixing vat, otherwise a mass of caked milk powder will form which, if the ambient temperature is high enough, will act as an excellent medium for the replication of organisms (Hobbs et al. [5]).

After use of any food or drink machine, it is of the utmost importance that it should be thoroughly cleaned and sterilised. Where a machine is in constant use, regular cleaning and sterilising, at least once every 24 h, should be instituted. Manufacturers of these machines usually issue excellent instructions for their maintenance and cleansing and these should be meticulously followed.

4.3.7 Refrigerated Stores

The temperatures at which various foods should be kept have already been discussed. The temperature maintained by ordinary refrigeration is commonly 4° – 6 °C while deep freeze units maintain a temperature no higher than – 18 °C. The maintenance of these temperatures is the reason for the not inconsiderable cost of installing the units and a refusal, on financial grounds, to fit adequate monitoring equipment to ensure that the temperatures are maintained, day and night, makes no sense. In fact, such refusal leaves matters worse than they would be if there were no refrigerated stores at all. In the latter case, staff can be educated to select foods and use cooking methods which do not rely upon low temperature storage; but if a refrigerated store is available in which the temperature can exceed the safe limit without anyone being aware of it, the staff may be dangerously misled. The permanent presence of an accurate maximum/minimum thermometer inside (or outside, showing the temperature inside) each refrigerated store is the minimum acceptable. Continuous temperature recording systems are even better. The sealing strips of refrigerator and deep freezer doors should be examined regularly. They are liable to perish, so decreasing efficiency and increasing cost.

In common with all other food areas, the deck, deckhead and bulkheads of these stores must be impervious, light in colour and easy to clean. There must be no smells within a store as food taint is a surprisingly pervasive and distasteful phenomenon. Such smells should be sought immediately on entering the store as, in some people, the sense of smell is rapidly diminished by inhalation of cold air.

The method of storage must permit good ventilation of the foods and efficient rotation. The need to keep raw and cooked foods apart is as important here as anywhere else. The shelving should be easily cleaned and made of materials which will not deteriorate at low temperatures. All foodstuffs in a deep freeze, if not already packed in sealed containers, should be kept in sealed individual plastic wrapping. Foods kept in refrigerators should be similarly wrapped or kept in covered containers although the requirements need not be as stringent.

Thawing of deep-frozen food should always be carried out in ordinary refrigerated spaces, never at ambient temperatures. This method of thawing may take longer, but it removes the possibility of a high ambient temperature causing rapid multiplication of organisms already in the food. Adequate thawing time must always be allowed for large joints and poultry.

Ship's refrigerated stores must not only be efficient, they must be big enough for all the demands that will be made upon them. Even in a small merchant ship, an amount of space is required which may seem overambitious to people with other plans. It is not normally difficult to make out a convincing case for adequate long-term refrigerated stores. Short-term daily-use refrigerated stores are more difficult. Uninformed opinion may not see the need for the refrigeration of food prepared in advance and not to be eaten for some hours but it is here that outbreaks of food poisoning often originate.

4.3.8 Unrefrigerated Stores

These stores are sometimes regarded as spaces where anything or everything can be stowed away without any regard for food hygiene, safety or even commonsense. This can be very dangerous. There should be different stores for different purposes.

Unrefrigerated stores for food are better labelled as cool stores. It is unnecessary for the temperature to be kept below 10 °C but it should not be allowed to rise much above 15 °C. Good ventilation will have a part to play here but, in hot climates, an element of artificial cooling may be necessary. These lower temperatures will be of particular value in preventing insect infestation in stored cereals, especially in the tropics. These stores should be dry and fitted with good quality shelving, made of impervious material and easily removable for cleaning. The problem of condensation must be carefully considered, as pollution of the food may well follow any carelessness. Pollution from routine cleaning of the deck can be avoided by ensuring that no food is stored less than 45 cm above it. All containers in the store should be rodent and insect proof and have tight-fitting lids. Efficient rotation of the foods is as necessary here as it is in the refrigerated spaces. Watch should be kept for any blown or pinholed cans and for evidence of damage by rodents.

The second type of unrefrigerated store is used for galley and dining room equipment, utensils, crockery and cutlery. The only requirements are a dry, well-ventilated atmosphere, cleanliness and protection against rodents and insects, which consider these spaces to be attractive harbourage and breeding sites. Detergents and other non-toxic cleaning materials are best given storage space of their own but, if they must be stored here, they must be in carefully labelled, tightly closed containers.

Lastly, specific and plainly labelled storage areas are needed for pesticides and other poisonous substances which may, from time to time, be needed in and about the food areas. Under no circumstances should such substances be stored with foods or with any articles which may come into direct or indirect contact with foods. The security of storage of these things should be the responsibility of one sufficiently senior member of staff whose efficiency and records should be regularly monitored.

References

1. Appleton, H., S.R. Palmer and R.J. Gilbert: Foodborne gastroenteritis of unknown aetiology: a virus infection? Brit. med. J. *282,* 1801 (1981).
2. Gangarosa, E.J., M.A. Kendrick, M.S. Loewenstein et al.: Global travel and travellers' health. Aviat. Space environ. Med. *51,* 3 (1980).
3. Goethe, H. and R. Herrmann: Ergebnisse hygienischer Untersuchungen in Kombüsen, Pantries und Vorratsräumen an Bord von Seeschiffen. Zbl. Bakt. I. Abt. Orig. B *171,* 177–183 (1980).
4. Hobbs, B.C., B. Rowe, M. Kendall et al.: Escherichia coli 027 in adult diarrhoea. J. Hyg. (Lond.) *77,* 393 (1976).
5. Hobbs, B.C., J.M. Ritchie and E.D. Ritchie: Food hygiene on board ship. J. Hyg. (Lond.) *60,* 259–278 (1962).
6. Hobbs, B.C., M.J. Colbourne and P.E. Mayner: Food hygiene and travel at sea. Postgrad. Med. J. *51,* 817–824 (1975).
7. Langley, A.R.: Shipboard hygiene – an owner's viewpoint. Paper. Conference of the Association of Sea and Airport Health Authorities, (U.K.), June, 1980.
8. Lumish, R.M., R.W. Ryder, D.C. Anderson et al.: Heat-labile enterotoxigenic escherichia coli induced diarrhea aboard a Miami-based cruise ship. Amer. J. Epidem. *111,* 4, 432–436 (1980).
9. Merson, M.M., J.M. Hughes, D.N. Lawrence et al.: Food – and waterborne disease outbreaks on passenger cruise vessels and aircraft. J. Milk Food Technol. *39,* 4 (1976).
10. Merson, M.H., J.M. Hughes, B.T. Wood et al.: Gastrointestinal illness on passenger cruise ships. J. Amer. med. Ass. *231,* 7, 723–727 (1975).
11. Parker, W.S.: Food poisoning at sea. Brit. med. J. *2,* 22 (1954).
12. Poultney, M.: Inspection of ships – a new approach. Paper. Conference of the Association of Sea and Airport Health Authorities, June, 1980.
13. Solodovnikov, Y.P., M.V. Turchinskaya, A.N. Ioyrish et al.: Izuchenie pishchevogo i bytovogo putey rasprostraneniya dizenterii na rechnykh sudakh. [A study of food and domestic routes of dysentery spread on river ships: a trial]. Zh. Mikrobiol. (Mosk.) *51,* 90–93 (1974).
14. Ulewicz, K., A. Kunert and P. Michniewski: Investigations on the carriage of salmonella and shigella bacilli among ship crews. Bull. Inst. mar. med. Gdansk *17,* 3, 291–296 (1966).
15. Wachsmuth, K., J. Wells, P. Shipley et al.: Heat-labile enterotoxin production in isolates from a shipboard outbreak of human diarrheal illness. Infect. and Immun. *24,* 3, 793–797 (1979).
16. Wegner, Z., W. Kruminis-Lozowska, J. Lalko et

al.: Study of the presence of Salmonella and other pathogenic bacteria in cockroaches on ocean-going ships. I. Basic investigations on isolation of bacterial strains from Blattella germanica (L.). Bull. Inst. mar. trop. Med. Gdynia *30,* 1, 59–67 (1979).

17. Werner, S. B., M. P. Hudgins, F. R. Morrison et al.: Gastroenteritis on a cruise ship - a recurring problem - Publ. Hlth Rep. *91,* 5, 433–436 (1976).

Additional References

Code of practice on the hygiene of food and fresh water supplies in passenger ships. London: General Council of British Shipping. 1981.

The food hygiene (docks, carriers, etc.) regulations, 1960. The food hygiene (markets, stalls & delivery vehicles) regulations, 1966.
The food hygiene (general) regulations, 1970.
The food hygiene (ships) regulations, 1979.
London: Her Majesty's Stationery Office.

Handbook on sanitation of vessel construction. Standards of sanitation and ratproofing for the construction of vessels. Ed.: U.S. Department of Health, Education, and Welfare. Washington: U.S. Government Printing Office 1967. (Public Health Service Publication No. 393).

Handbook on sanitation of vessels in operation. Sanitation features and facilities on vessels in operation. Ed.: U.S. Department of Health, Education, and Welfare. Washington: U.S. Government Printing Office 1963, (Public Health Service Publication No. 68)

Hobbs, B.C. and R.J. Gilbert: Food poisoning and food hygiene. 4th ed. London: Edward Arnold 1978.

Supplemental instruction guide for vessel sanitation. Inspection report. Ed.: U.S. Department of Health, Education, and Welfare. Center for Disease Control. Bureau of Epidemiology. Quarantine Division. Atlanta, 1976.

Lamoureux, V.B.: Guide to ship sanitation. Geneva: WHO 1967.

4.4. Alcohol, Drugs and Smoking in Seafaring

A. Backhaus, E. Zorn

4.4.1 Alcohol

It is, of course, a well-known fact that songs, shanties and novels concerning the lives of seamen contain many references to alcohol (Hitz [21]; Nolan [34]; Schadewaldt [37]; Wenzel [46]; Wodarg [50]). Alcohol has long been connected with life at sea, and the reason for this view is historical. Intemperance among seafarers in past centuries had many causes: the adverse social conditions of seafaring, the extremely bad living conditions on the ships of the day, the cold temperatures to be endured, the scarcity of good potable water and the lack of non-alcoholic beverages as well as, in some cases, the character of the crew members selected. In the reports of the British Admiralty in the seventeenth and eighteenth centuries complaints are voiced about the increasing intemperance on ships (Schadewaldt [37]), and in 1856 Fonssagrives, a French specialist in nautical medicine, wrote that alcoholism is the leprosy of seamen [13]. It was generally accepted that there were far more alcoholics among seamen than on land – the Bremerhaven physician Otto H. With also made this claim in 1858 [49]. Among elderly seamen delirium tremens was many times more frequent than among the population on land, e.g. in Germany in 1830 the figures were 18.1% and 2.8% respectively (Schadewaldt [37]). There are reports of alcoholic excesses in the German Imperial Navy during the last century, as well as in the navies of other nations. Ever since delirium tremens was first described, numerous examples have been reported, showing that it occurs in a higher percentage in the navy than among civilians (Marjot [29]).

It is extremely difficult to assess objectively alcohol consumption and alcoholism among seafarers today, as there are scarcely any representative data on the subject, and the few fragmentary data that we do possess are of only limited informative value.

Although there have even been some reassuring attitudes in medical publications about alcohol for seamen, the fact remains that every statistic proves that alcohol is not beneficial, but a danger to both professional seamen and those who sail for pleasure.

Many publications contain alarming figures about alcohol consumption on seagoing vessels (Cocking [10]; Wodarg [50]). According to an Australian statistic, up to 50% of the persons who accidentally drown have consumed alcohol and would be unable to drive a car. This article, entitled "Drinking and Drowning" [12], points out that not only people on the beach and crews of private boats but also many seamen have drowned after alcohol consumption – up to 2,3‰ blood alcohol level. Other authors have reported similar findings (Kubisch [28]; Naeve [32]). Norwegian statistics record that out of 100 patients at clinics specialising in treating alcohol addicts, 16 were sailors, though the percentage of sailors in the population was less than 5% (Brun-Gulbrandsen and Irgens-Jensen [6]; Kjølstadt [25]). Reports and thorough investigations in the navy, e.g. in the USA and West Germany, have shown that alcohol was the reason for most difficulties and offences concerning discipline and social life (Gunderson and Schuckit [16, 17]; Kanstorf [24]; Measey [30]; Schuckit and Gunderson [39, 40, 42]; Tetzlaff [43]).

The consumption of alcohol and the prevalence of alcoholism itself vary greatly between nationalities. Apart from national customs and economic factors, ideological and religious factors also have a certain limited influence. Habits regarding alcohol consumption that are present on land continue to be adhered to on board. Germans, and north Europeans generally, predominantly consume beer, whereas south Europeans tend to consume wine, and North Americans and Scandinavians, high-proof alcohol. Since Islam totally forbids the consumption of alcohol, alcoholism is very rare on ships with a Muslim crew. Alcohol consumption is also restricted on ships from the USSR and the People's Republic of China. Among Norwegian, Swedish and Finnish crews, alcohol consumption is probably far greater than on land, and alcoholism is a current problem (Brun-Gulbrandsen and Irgens-Jensen [6]; Kjølstad [25]). In the light of all the evidence, one can certainly make the assumption that the very different national characteristics have a considerable influence on alcohol consumption among seafarers.

Nevertheless, one cannot assess alcohol consumption simply on the basis of the nationality of the crew members, for the influence of the shipping company and the example set by the captain also play an essential role in determining the nature of life on board and thus also the extent of alcohol consumption. There are 'dry' as well as 'wet' ships, and whether a ship is dry or wet depends essentially on the orders of the company and the captain's example. Thus no seaman dependent on alcohol will be found on ships which belong to companies that forbid the sale of high-proof alcohol or even all alcoholic drinks and whose captains keep a tight control on alcohol consumption. The opposite is the case on the ships of those companies that adopt a very liberal or opportunistic attitude towards alcohol consumption and whose captains themselves are fond of alcohol. As a result, the differences between ships are considerable, and fragmentary data cannot be regarded as having general validity.

On board, just as in the world of work ashore, beer holds a special position. Seamen very often regard it as thirst quenching and refreshing, but not as an alcoholic drink.

During studies on work-load on board seagoing vessels (the 'Flensburg Study', 1972–1974), 180 probands were closely questioned on, among other things, their consumption of alcohol. Twelve percent were teetotallers; the remaining 88% drank between two and ten bottles of beer a day (average, ca. five bottles). A third also consumed concentrated alcoholic beverages on a regular basis – about one bottle a week.

In 1975 Zorn [51], in another study, found on German ships an average consumption of three to four bottles of beer per man and day and one to two bottles of spirit per week. The individual beer consumption differed between zero and ten bottles of beer per day. About 10 years earlier Backhaus [1] had reported an average beer consumption of five to six bottles per man and day.

According to the experience of the German Seeberufsgenossenschaft, alcoholism has the highest incidence rate among the seamen who are officially declared unfit for duty at sea. In 1981 a total of 117 seamen were declared unfit, 53 thereof for alcoholism or other addictions [44].

During the proceedings of the Maritime Court of Enquiry in Hamburg between 1965 and 1974, five cases of running aground or collision and 41 accidents with a fatal outcome were registered as essentially resulting from the influence of alcohol. In at least eight cases of fire on board, excessive intake of alcohol had played a decisive role. One can, however, assume with certainty that a not negligible number of unexplained accidents – especially those involving the disappearance of crew members from the ship – were caused by alcohol. There are undoubtedly many accidents caused by alcohol that are not attributed to it afterwards (Zorn [51]).

In an evaluation of 176 acutely fatal accidents on board or near to the ship in Hamburg harbour, blood concentrations of alcohol were between 1.5‰ and 3.0‰ in 80% of the victims (Naeve [32]). Approximately two-thirds of the accidents occurred during leisure time.

Reports of excessive alcohol consumption are often kept secret by the arcane nature of the seafaring community. Of 900 Polish seamen, 201 (22.3%) were registered as periodically drinking to excess, which also led to conflicts. There is a need for prophylactic measures against excessive alcohol consumption among 20%–30% of seamen, and approximately 3% are in need of treatment (Dolmierski [11]).

There is no doubt that overindulgence in alcohol poses a serious risk to the crew, the ship and the environment. It is, however, difficult to assess the extent of this risk, and comparisons with land and air traffic are scarcely possible. That a crew member is drunk need not necessarily and directly have an effect on the ship's safety, since the person concerned can usually be relieved by another crew member (this should be done if at all possible). The risk to safety as a result of alcohol consumption will increase quite considerably owing to the reductions in personnel and the introduction of bridge designs for one-man control as well as to the higher speeds of ships and the increased traffic in shipping lanes. From both a medical and a legal point of view it seems necessary to introduce as soon as possible, for both sea and inland shipping, a limit regarding the permissible concentration of alcohol in the blood. This would remove the legal confusion in the area, facilitate police measures and take the burden of proof (which poses a considerable problem) away from the investigating authorities and the court. It has been recommended that the level be set at 1.3‰ (Janssen [23]; Naeve [32]). Supervision to ensure that the permissible level is adhered to could, in conjunction with long-term explanation of the effects of alcohol, have a positive influence on the drinking habits of seafarers and thus make alcoholic intoxication among them a rare occurrence.

It is not possible to rule out a certain intake of persons of unsuitable character into the occupation of seafaring, although such instances are certainly less frequent than in previous centuries. Nevertheless, since examinations to establish the suitability of candidates scarcely take into account the psychological sphere, it is virtually impossible to exclude those with character defects, neuroses, low intelligence and other faults in personality structure. In such men, exogenous factors such as the monotony of life on board, the lack of worthwhile leisure activities and the build-up of tension among the all-male crew can result in alcoholism. Alcohol consumption will also be promoted by a variety of other factors, e.g. the low cost of alcoholic drinks on board, a possible lack of good non-alcoholic drinks, difficulties in making contacts when going ashore – which are supposed to be eased by alcohol – and, finally, the hackneyed belief that to be a real seamen one must drink a large quantity of alcohol.

There are persons, who need the relaxing effect of alcohol to start a conversation. That is not a problem for sailors only, but it may be so for them more frequently than for others. If this is true, people who need alcohol for this purpose should train themselves to use alcohol reasonably in creating friendship. Northern European culture and civilisation does not help much in this training, as opposed to other countries, such as Spain, Italy and Greece, where the reasonable use of alcohol is the normal situation. They drink not only wine, but also some stronger forms of alcohol, not for the toxic effect, but for the taste and for the spirit of hospitality and community (Backhaus [2]; Bonfiglio and Cicala [3]; Carev and Šokec [7, 8]; Cicala [9]; Kolb et al. [26]).

Loneliness is clearly not a problem restricted to ships, but it is common on ships and depresses seamen more than people on land. Naturally, ships with extremely bad accommodation and a large crew can give a feeling of isolation to those on board. The same effect can also be caused, however, where there is good accommodation and a small crew. The ship is a place of isolation. This can be felt in the continual company of the same crew: company not selected by the individual. It can also be felt in one's own accommodation, in small groups at work or in one's leisure time. At sea, the crew is cut off from all social contacts with people on land.

Today the facilities on board ships and in the network of organisations looking after seafarers are the best possible (Glass [15]; Haasz et al. [19]; Hiles [20]). If everybody cooperates, the addict cannot avoid treatment (Bourg et al. [4]). Forcing an addict to undergo treatment will not lead to success. Only when the circumstances permit no escape will the addict surrender himself to being saved. Among his many contacts are crew members, friends, staff of the company personnel office, trade union officials, the security authorities (e.g. harbour police and coast guard), the company doctor and the authority's doctor. Everyone should feel responsible. The best course is to speak to the addict personally, although this is not easy. Subsequently the authorities must be informed, not as a condemnation but as a suspicion.

A person thought to have an organic disease or even a venereal infection is sent home and not allowed to work until he is cured. There is no condemnation and no moral verdict. A similar attitude should be adopted and no other steps are necessary in alcoholism. Such a scheme has been developed and practised with good results in the USA (Brownell [5]; Molloy et al. [31]). It implies a fundamental change in our attitude to alcohol abuse.

Since we cannot hope for the cooperation of the alcohol addict in the early stage – the lack of cooperation (Gardner [14]; Schuckit and Gunderson [41]) is a symptom of his sickness – everyone from friends to authorities is responsible for the potentially fatal development of the illness, which at the beginning is still curable. Strict rules are needed which should be based on law. For example:

- The captain should report all difficulties probably caused by alcohol
- In all accident cases, an alcohol test should be given without exception
- A company should not be allowed to send someone who is under the influence of alcohol to a ship or to a doctor for routine examination
- Liver function tests should be obligatory. In the case of pathological findings, further investigations should be made to establish whether the person is an alcohol addict (Hitz [21])
- Every person who is an alcoholic or is suspected of being one should be treated as a sick person: he should not lose his job or pay, and free treatment should be given

A very simple test of alcoholism is to ask the seafarer to drink no alcohol for at least one week or even longer. No alcoholic can do without alcohol. It might be possible to promote a general interest in an alcohol-free week to prove that the participants are not alcoholics, but it would require the cooperation of the seafarers' organisations and the shipping company.

Alcoholism among adolescent seamen represents a special problem. Young seafarers who join a ship prior to their 18th birthday, coming directly from a protective family background, enter an environment where customs and attitudes directly demand the abuse of alcohol (Kjølstad [25]) and are especially at risk. The Institute of Research into Alcoholism in Oslo, which to a large extent is concerned with the danger to seamen of alcohol, has established that most alcoholics in seafaring already consumed alcoholic drinks when 14–16 years old and by the time they were 18 years old had experienced their first intoxication. It has been shown with certainty that the risk of addiction to alcohol is considerably greater when the abuse of alcohol began prior to the 18th year of life. Consequently the prevention of alcohol abuse among young seamen is of great significance.

A general attack on alcoholism in seafaring depends on observation of the following conditions:

- Suitable selection of applicants; discharge of crew members dependent on alcohol
- Provision of worthwhile leisure activities
- A wide-ranging supply of non-alcoholic drinks on board; no sale of alcoholic drinks at a reduced price
- Detailed explanation of the consequences of alcohol abuse and education that will produce a critical attitude towards the use of alcohol
- A move away from the belief that high alcohol consumption is part of being a seaman

Most shipping countries are aware that there is a problem with alcohol on board their ships. It is likely that only limited progress will be made anywhere until the attempted solutions are given the authority of international agreement.

With the exception of a few countries (Scandinavian states and the USA), it does not seem proven that alcohol consumption among seafarers today is, on average, much greater than among other population groups. It is apparent that alcoholism plays a relatively small role in causing accidents to ships, but has a more important effect in personal accidents on board and in cases of suicide. On modern ships and as a result of reductions in personnel, inebriation during the navigation of a ship carries a greater risk than in the past, and consequently alcoholism must be fought energetically.

4.4.2 Drugs

In the past the seaman had excellent opportunities to come into contact with drugs, especially during journeys to the Middle and Far East. Nevertheless, despite familiarisation with and possibly sporadic use of opium, hashish etc., there is no evidence of chronic abuse. After the Second World War the situation, also in relation to drug addiction the world over, changed drastically – drug abuse and dependence became a problem to be taken seriously, especially among adolescents. Sometimes seafarers are involved in the illegal importation and peddling of drugs and thus are partly responsible for the spread of drug abuse. In the process a few individuals probably become addicts themselves.

There is nevertheless, little evidence of drug abuse aboard ships of various countries (Haasz et al [18]; Nail and Gunderson [33]; Plag and Goffman [35]; Sarg jr. [36]; Schmidt [38]; Wietfeld [47, 48]). It appears that the custom of drinking alcohol has prevailed and seafarers have not to any extent been influenced by the fashions of drug abuse affecting mainly young people ashore in some countries. Cases of addiction to "hard" drugs are infrequent, but "soft" drugs such as cannabis have occasionally caused concern on passenger ships and the ships of some countries where the drug is easily available. Drug abuse and drug smuggling are generally firmly dealt with in most countries but there are some where the penalties are extraordinarily severe. This presents difficulties for any master who has confiscated illegal drugs found on board. He might wish to retain the drug for evidence at a subsequent disciplinary hearing on return to the home country, however, when calling at a foreign port en route he might run into trouble with port officials. The best course of action might be to jettison the drug while at sea.

4.4.3 Smoking

Although the monotony of the watch on board, the inability to use leisure time to good purpose and the cheap price of tobacco may be conducive to heavy smoking, the smoking habits of seafarers scarcely have any characteristics specific to certain ships. For this reason there are very few publications which deal with smoking and seafaring (Hoeffler [22]; Krause [27]). The cigarette advertisements like to show seamen smoking, but according to our own experiences, of roughly 30000 crew members from all nations at the port of Hamburg, 10% are non-smokers between the ages of 16 and 60, but 5% between 18 and 30.

In 1965, Vellar [45] compared in a comprehensive study the smoking habits of Norwegian seamen and men ashore. As a result of this survey, covering 8548 seamen and 9114 men ashore, it has been established that smokers are more frequent among seamen, the consumption of tobacco for each individual smoker is higher and a good many more of the smokers use cigarettes only. The young people who go to sea thus enter a milieu where smoking is very common and quickly pick up the habit.

The smoking habits – frequency of smokers and the amount of tobacco consumed – reach a maximum at the age of 30, both among seamen and men ashore. There has been no change in this pattern since the 1920s. Among men ashore, however, pipe smoking has increasingly been replaced by cigarette smoking, so that like seamen 96% of smokers ashore under 20, smoke cigarettes only.

With older men there is, in both categories, an increase in the number of men who stop smoking. One half of those who stop can give no certain reason for doing so; of the rest, those who have stopped for medical reasons constitute a large group, whereas economic reasons and anti-smoking propaganda carry very little weight. It can be concluded that in general the decision to give up smoking is an act of free will rather than medical necessity.

There are no special statistics for seamen, smokers and non-smokers showing the percentage of lung cancer or heart disease.

The habit of smoking is different in countries where people are normally indoors and countries where people are normally in the fresh air. Though modern accommodation on ships keeps the seafarers in rooms for relatively long periods, there may still be smoking areas in places open to the wind. It may be interesting to investigate this further. Smoking is an aspect of the personality of men. Smoking habits will rarely be changed by medical or hygienic arguments.

References

1. Backhaus, A.: Sozialhygienische Erhebungen zur Problematik der Freizeit der Seeleute. Dissertation, University of Hamburg 1968.
2. Backhaus, A.: Alcohol – joy and danger to mankind. 4th Triennial Conference, International Christian Maritime Ass. Berlin, 12–18 July 1981.
3. Bonfiglio, G. and S. Cicala: L'alcolismo nei marittimi italiani. Atti della "Sezione Studi" del C. I. R. M., pp 53–65 (1963).
4. Bourg, M., D. Vanhoove, A. Barreau et al.: La femme du marin alcoolique. Essai de compréhension ethnosociopsychiatrique d'alcoolisme dans le milieu marin breton. Societe medico-psychologique. Seance du 26 octobre 1981. pp 1014–1023.
5. Brownell, St. M.: The Navy alcoholism prevention program – worldwide. Alcoholism *2,* 4, 362–365 (1978).
6. Brun-Gulbrandsen, S. and O. Irgens-Jensen: Abuse of alcohol among seamen. Brit. J. Addict. 62, 19–27 (1967).
7. Carev, V. and P. Šokec: Alkoholizam i brod. [Alcoholism and ship]. In: Pomorska medicina. (Naučne rasprave). Beograd: Izdanje Mornaričkog glasnika 1975. pp 363–371. (Pomorska biblioteka. Sveska 26.)
8. Carev, V. and P. Šokec: Neki etiološki faktori alkoholizma na brodu. [Some etiological factors of alcoholism aboard ships]. In: Pomorska medicina II. (Naučne rasprave). Beograd: Izdanje Mornaričkog glasnika 1979. pp 315–320. (Pomorska biblioteka. Sveska 30.)

9. Cicala, S.: L'alcoolismo nei marittimi. Atti della "Sezione Studi" del C.I.R.M. pp 111–121 (1962).
10. Cocking, R.: Nearly one crew member in five aboard ship has a problem with alcohol, and the situation is getting worse all the time. Freighting World, 8 October 1975.
11. Dolmierski, R.: Alkoholismus unter Seeleuten der polnischen Handelsmarine. Verk.-Med. *30*, 1/2, 18–23 (1983).
12. Drinking and drowning. Brit. Med. J. 1, 70–71 (1979).
13. Fonssagrives, J.-B.: Traité d'hygiène navale. Paris: Baillière 1877.
14. Gardner, A.W.: Identifying and helping seafarers who are problem drinkers. Fawley 1982. Manuscript.
15. Glass, G.S.: The alcohol rehabilitation unit, National Naval Medical Center, Bethesda. Milit. Med. *139*, 486–488 (1974).
16. Gunderson, E.K.E. and M.A. Schuckit: Hospitalization rates for alcoholism in the navy and marine corps. Dis. nerv. Syst. *36*, 681–684 (1975).
17. Gunderson, E.K.E. and M. Schuckit: Alcoholism in the navy and marine corps: hospitalization rates by age and pay grade. Manuscript [1975].
18. Haasz, A., I. Haasz, S. Ćuk et al.: Pomorci i droge. [Seafarers and drugs]. In: Pomorska medicina II. (Naučne rasprave). Beograd: Izdanje Mornaričkog glasnika 1979. pp 321–325. (Pomorska biblioteka. Sveska 30.)
19. Haasz, I., S. Ćuk and A. Haasz: Alkoholizam u pomoraca. [Alcoholism among seafarers]. In: Pomorska medicina. (Naučne rasprave). Beograd: Izdanje Mornaričkog glasnika 1975. pp 357–362. (Pomorska biblioteka. Sveska 26.)
20. Hiles, F.M.J.: The prevention and treatment of alcoholism in the Royal Navy. I. A policy. J. roy. nav. med. Serv. *66*, 3, 180–185 (1980).
21. Hitz, D.: Drunken sailors and others. Drinking problems in specific occupations. Quart. J. Stud. Alcohol *34*, 496–505 (1973).
22. Hoeffler, D.F.: Smoking and health in the Navy. U.S. Navy Med. *71*, 2, 15–19 (1980).
23. Janssen, W.: Alkohol auf dem Wasser – Erfahrungen der letzten Jahre und Begründung der Notwendigkeit einer zukünftigen Grenzwertgestaltung für den Sicherheitsbereich an Bord von Schiffen. In: Unfall- und Sicherheitsforschung Straßenverkehr. Kongreßbericht Jahrestagung 1981 der Dtsch. Ges. f. Verkehrsmed. gemeinsam m. d. Dtsch. Verkehrswacht. Hamburg, 7.–9.5. 1981. Bundesanstalt f. Straßenwesen, Bereich Unfallforschung, Köln, i. Auftrage d. Bundesministers f. Verkehr (ed). Braunschweig: Waisenhaus-Buchdruckerei 1981. pp 44–45.
24. Kanstorf, G.: Ursachen und Auswirkungen mißbräuchlichen Alkoholgenusses in der Marine. Analyse und Folgerungen. Studienarbeit, Stabsoffizier- und Auswahllehrgang der Marine 3/73.
25. Kjølstad, Th.: Alkoholisme hos Sjømenn. T. norske Laegeforen. *84*, 18, 1243–1248 (1964).
26. Kolb, D., E.K.E. Gunderson and S. Bucky: Prognostic indicators for Black and White alcoholics in the U.S. Navy. J. Stud. Alcohol *37*, 1094 (1976).
27. Krause, L.: Trink- und Rauchgewohnheiten bei Hamburger Arbeitnehmern verschiedener Berufsgruppen. Arbeitsmed., Sozialmed., Präventivmed. *7*, 139 (1975).
28. Kubisch, G.: Blutalkohol und Ertrinken. Blutalkohol 2 (1963).
29. Marjot, D.H.: Delirium tremens in the Royal Navy and British Army in the 19th century. J. Stud. Alcohol *38*, 9, 1613–1623 (1977).
30. Measey, L.G.: Alcohol and the royal naval offender. J. roy. nav. med. Serv. *58*, 1, 52–55 (1972).
31. Molloy, D., J. Barron, R. Farkas et al.: A union alcoholism program working with many employers. Labor-Mgmt. Alcsm. J. (N.Y.) *9*, 234–245 (1980).
32. Naeve, W.: Bedeutung des Alkohols bei tödlichen Unfällen an Bord und im Hafen. Blutalkohol *13*, 27–38 (1976).
33. Nail, R.L. and E.K.E. Gunderson: Drug histories of navy amnesty cases. Milit. Med. *140*, 172–178 (1975).
34. Nolan, B.: Seamen, drink and social structure. Marit. Pol. Mgmt. *4*, 77–88 (1976).
35. Plag, J.A. and J.M. Goffman: Characteristics of naval recruits with histories of drug abuse. Milit. Med. *138*, 354–359 (1973).
36. Sarg jr., M.J.: Heroin use in the navy. New Engl. J. Med. *286*, 2, 111–112 (1972).
37. Schadewaldt, H.: Alkohol an Bord. Schiff und Zeit 2, 55–65 (1975).
38. Schmidt, L.: Gifte mit Wirkungen auf die Psyche in der Vergangenheit und Gegenwart. Med. heute *15*, 12, 365–367 (1966).
39. Schuckit, M.A. and E.K.E. Gunderson: Alcoholism among navy and marine corps officers. Navy Medical Neuropsychiatric Research Unit. San Diego, Cal. [abt. 1972].
40. Schuckit, M.A. and E.K.E. Gunderson: Alcoholism in navy and marine corps women: a first look. Milit. Med. *140*, 268–271 (1975).
41. Schuckit, M.A. and E.K.E. Gunderson: Early identification of alcoholism in navy psychiatric outpatients. Navy Medical Neuropsychiatric Research Unit. San Diego, Cal. [abt. 1972].
42. Schuckit, M.A. and E.K.E. Gunderson: Deaths among young alcoholics in the U.S. Naval Service. Quart. J. Stud. Alcohol *35*, 856–862 (1974).
43. Tetzlaff, M.: Disziplin und Alkohol. Dienstvergehen unter Alkoholeinfluß, dargestellt an

Beispielen aus dem Bereich der Marine. Truppenpraxis 10, 785–788 (1977).
44. Unfallverhütung, Schiffssicherheit, Gesundheitsdienst. Bericht 1981. See-Berufsgenossenschaft (ed) Hamburg 1982.
45. Vellar, O. D.: Røkevaner blant norske sjømenn og menn i land. (Smoking habits among Norwegian seamen and men ashore). Landsforeningen mot Kreft (ed) Oslo 1965.
46. Wenzel, K.-H.: Des Seemanns bester Freund ist der Rum. Hamburger Gerichtsmediziner legen Studie über "Trunkenheit am Ruder" vor. Ärztl. Prax. *26,* 100, 4349–4350 (1974).
47. Wietfeld, H.: Seemann und Betäubungsmittel. Kommandobrücke 184–185 (1964).
48. Wietfeld, H.: Tabletten können die Schiffsführung gefährden. Kommandobrücke 220 (1965).
49. With, O. H.: Gesundheitspflege auf Seeschiffen für Gebildete aller Stände, namentlich für Schiffsoffiziere und Auswanderer. Bremerhaven: v. Vangerow 1858.
50. Wodarg, W.: Psychische Krankheiten der Seeleute. Untersuchung über Selbsttötung. Alkoholismus und andere wichtige psychiatrische Erkrankungen anhand von 236 von der See-Berufsgenossenschaft gesammelten Seeamtsverhandlungen aus den Jahren 1960 bis 1973. Dissertation, University of Hamburg 1977.
51. Zorn, E.: Alkoholkonsum an Bord. Beobachtungen aus der Praxis. In: Verkehrsmedizinische Probleme in der See- und Binnenschiffahrt. Jahrestagung der Deutschen Gesellschaft für Verkehrsmedizin Hamburg, 11.–13. April 1975. pp 7–16.

4.5 Infectious Diseases – Vaccination and Passive Immunization

J. Huisman

4.5.1 Infectious Diseases

Study of the annual reports of two large European ports, London and Rotterdam, shows that most of the infectious diseases among seamen diminished greatly after World War II [1; 8]. However, not all infectious diseases have shown such a favourable decline; this is especially true of sexually transmitted diseases, which, after a steep fall in the period after the war, continue to pose a serious problem. A number of explanations can be suggested for the remarkable downward trend of many infectious diseases. For instance, the total number of men employed at sea decreased steadily during this period and the length of stay of ships in ports was, in general, shortened. This, together with the location of newly built ports (mostly with better environmental hygienic conditions) far from population concentrations in cities, diminished exposure to the sometimes poor local endemic situations. In addition, better medical supervision of seamen, better general sanitary conditions on board, catering systems providing high-quality food in a satisfactory hygienic condition and a steadily improving quality of drinking water ashore in the ports as well as on board are factors that undoubtedly played a role in this decline in the incidence of (notified) infectious diseases on board seagoing vessels.

Of the diseases transmitted to seamen by food or drinking water, *typhoid fever* is by far the most serious. Cases of enteric fever (and paratyphoid fever A and B) are regularly seen among seamen of different nations. Typhoid vaccination does not prevent infection after a large infective dose such as is often the cause of food-borne infections, and vaccination against paratyphoid A and B is of unproved value. Of much more practical importance are *food poisoning incidents* such as *salmonellosis,* especially on cruise ships [17], but even typhoid fever and shigellosis can sometimes occur on modern passenger ships (Davies et al. [4] and Merson et al. [12]).

The incidence of *gastro-intestinal illness* on passenger cruise ships amounts to 1% or less on 92% of cruises and 5% or greater on 2% of cruises (Merson et al. [11]). Most of the food poisoning incidents on cruise liners and freighters are caused by poor kitchen hygiene practice and deficiencies in water systems. On the basis of environmental surveys and accepted current standards of the U.S. Public Health Service and the World Health Organization, a detailed set of recommendations for food and water sanitation includes: a) improving availability and use of hand-washing facilities by food-service personnel, b) improving refrigeration facilities and practices, c) holding all perishable cold food at 7 °C (45 °C) at all times, d) upgrading facilities and practices for washing and sterilising dishes, glasses and utensils and e) instituting continuous chlorination or other acceptable water treatment methods and routine coliform testing of all potable water [17]. Some countries advocate periodic stool examinations of food service personnel for enteric pathogens (e.g. the German Federal Republic). Other countries (e.g. United Kingdom and The Netherlands) consider this (costly) practice of limited value. Cases of *chronic amoebiasis* and its complications (e.g. amoebic hepatitis and amoebic liver abscess) and *giardiasis* – mostly not acquired on board – are observed in seamen from countries with high endemicity.

Viral hepatitis is regularly diagnosed in seamen. Modern laboratory methods can differentiate between *hepatitis A, hepatitis B* and – by exclusion – *non-A non-B hepatitis*. Hepatitis B is often seen after tattooing and is significantly more often observed in seamen seeking advice in venereal disease clinics. Special measures for seamen who are chronic carriers of hepatitis B virus are not warranted. Interhuman transmission on board is, under normal conditions, highly exceptional. Prevention of hepatitis A in contacts of a still contagious case of the disease is possible with normal immunoglobulin. Hepatitis A can easily be acquired by direct (faecal) contact, food or water.

Tuberculosis is still a major problem in many countries in the world; *eo ipso* is this true for seamen of these countries. Many countries require a periodic chest X-ray examination of seamen to exclude cases of infectious pulmonary tuberculosis. Ships' crews live in relatively close personal contact and this is especially true on naval vessels where there often exists relative overcrowding. A number of minor outbreaks of tuberculosis have occurred on board naval vessels where personnel have been exposed to an unsuspected active case of pulmonary tuberculosis on board (Knight [9]). A constant medical vigilance for cases of pulmonary tuberculosis, not only among crews of naval vessels but also among merchant seamen, is important. Persistent coughing or a change in an already existing cough pattern should give rise to the suspicion of tuberculosis and is an indication for an X-ray examination of the chest. If a case of smear-positive pulmonary tuberculosis in a seaman is found, the other crew members should be X-rayed and this procedure should be repeated after 6 weeks to 3 months. Smear-positive patients should be treated ashore; cases of active non-infectious pulmonary tuberculosis may be treated while ambulatory on board if the national medical standards permit. However, many countries would not allow such a patient to be employed aboard ship.

Of all the acute infectious diseases, malignant tertian (falciparum) *malaria* is unquestionably the most important cause of death in merchant seamen and travellers. The case fatality among non-immune adults may exceed 10%. Falciparum malaria may present a very varied clinical picture which, in some cases, closely resembles enteric fever but diarrhoea is rare. Complications in severe falciparum malaria may develop with great rapidity and with no previous warning. Parasites are localized in enormous numbers in internal organs and any part of the body may be affected, and thus malaria can simulate nearly every acute condition (cerebral, spinal, abdominal, cardiac, respiratory etc.). Falciparum malaria should be excluded in all acute clinical conditions in seamen who have visited malarious areas of the world (blood films). Individuals who are partly immune, or who have been taking chemosuppressive drugs irregularly, may show an atypical clinical picture and a wide variation in incubation period. The other human malarias – vivax (benign tertian), malariae and ovale – are, generally, not life threatening except in patients with concurrent disease (Bruce-Chwatt [2]). The most important practical aspect for the prevention of malaria in seamen is an adequate regime of chemoprophylaxis, preferably taken under strict supervision. Proguanil is a very valuable preventive drug at the adult dose of one tablet of 100 mg daily; it is especially advised for the Middle East and Asia. Chloroquine can usually suppress malaria in a dose of 300 mg base per week. In some ports of the world where malaria is epidemic (e.g. the west coast of Africa) a daily dose of 100 mg may be taken by non-immune seamen. Chloroquine is, notwithstanding the rising resistance against it, the drug of choice for Africa, the South-west Pacific and Central and South America. In areas where chloroquine-resistant falciparum malaria occurs (for instance in many countries of the Far East and East Africa, as well as in Papua, tropical South America and Panama), a fixed combination of 500 mg sulfadoxine and 25 mg pyrimethamine (Fansidar) should be used, administered once a week. Alternatively half of these amounts may be given weekly for a maximum period of 6 months [3].

Prophylactic drugs should be taken from a few days before arrival in malarious zones and be continued at least 4 weeks after leaving these areas. The fact that ships anchor at the roads is not always a guarantee that malaria transmission will not occur; the flight range of female Anopheles mosquitos averages 2 or 3 km from their breeding place (Bruce-Chwatt [2]). Dramatic outbreaks of falciparum malaria on board among seamen not taking suppressive drugs have been described (Schultz et al. [16]).

4.5.2 Vaccination and Passive Immunization

4.5.2.1 Vaccination Against Smallpox

Notwithstanding the fact that the Thirty-third World Health Assembly in May 1980 officially declared that the global eradication of smallpox had been achieved [15], a number of doctors continue to (re-)vaccinate travellers and seafarers against this now non-existent disease. On the basis of available information – as from May 1982 – only Chad and Democratic Kampuchea may be requiring smallpox vaccination from travellers [18]. Unfortunately there are still instances where the action taken at ports and airports in some countries is not consistent with the requirements of the national health administration as notified to WHO [5]. In practice all countries now accept a doctor's certificate indicating that vaccination against smallpox was not performed because of medical reasons ("risk of complications"). These certificates should be authenticated by the health authorities as in the case of WHO vaccination certificates. Vaccination against smallpox should now be considered as an unnecessary prophylactic medical treatment and therefore be abolished. This is especially true for primary vaccinations because of the relatively high risk of serious complications (e.g. postvaccinal encephalitis).

4.5.2.2 Vaccination Against Yellow Fever

The areas in which yellow fever is endemic are in Central and (parts of northern) South America and in Africa between 15° N and 10° S (including the Sudan, Ethiopia and countries of West Central and East Africa). There is no evidence that yellow fever ever has been present in Asia or on the northern coast of Africa [3]. Vaccination against yellow fever is required of any person leaving from, or arriving at, a port or airport situated in these endemic areas. The yellow fever vaccine used must be approved by the World Health Organization and the vaccinating centre must have been designated by the health administration for the territory in which it is situated. The World Health Organization must be assured that the vaccines used for this purpose continue to be of suitable quality [7].

Yellow fever vaccine consists of an attenuated virus (17D), cultivated in chick embryos in eggs from avian leucosis-free flocks and is effective. The 17D vaccine used today is a freeze-dried preparation, which is reconstituted in sterile water immediately before use. The dose is 0.5 ml subcutaneously. Antibodies appear 7–10 days after vaccination and persist for many years. Revaccination is officially required at the end of 10 years. Yellow fever vaccine should not be given to children under 1 year of age since it may give rise to encephalitis in the very young. Sensitivity to eggs and egg products is also a contra-indication. This fact must officially be stated in the International Certificate of Vaccination. If the contra-indications are observed, reactions are extremely rare (occasionally a mild local reaction or a slight malaise occurs on about the 7th day after immunization). The International Certificate is valid from 10 days after primary vaccination but immediately in the case of revaccination. Certificates are required for travel to or through the endemic areas and for Asia and the Far East if the traveller enters from an endemic area.

4.5.2.3 Vaccination Against Cholera

It is now generally agreed that the requirement of a cholera vaccination certificate will not prevent the introduction of the disease into any country [5]. Since immunization against cholera is of very limited value, a change was made in 1973 in the International Health Regulations: it was agreed that cholera vaccination was no longer officially required for most countries, no matter where the traveller came from. This is the reason why many countries (including some located in endemic areas) no longer require a valid certificate of vaccination against cholera. On the other hand some countries do still require valid vaccination certificates from seamen.

The whole-cell cholera vaccine consists of heat killed, phenol- or acetone-preserved, serotypes of *Vibrio cholerae* of the classic Ogawa and Inaba strains. The vaccine should contain 4×10^9 organisms of each serotype per millilitre [13; 14].

The usual dose is 1 ml subcutaneously or 0.2 ml intradermally, followed by a second dose 1–4 weeks later. Most countries accept a vaccination certificate as "valid" from 6 days after the first injection of vaccine. Many countries require only one injection of cholera vaccine but some require two. It is wise to check with the latest WHO Weekly Epidemiological Bulletin. There are only a few contra-indications to cholera vaccination; bad general health is one and some authors also consider serious local or general reaction after previous (subcutaneous) vaccination as an indication to give the vaccine only intradermally. After vaccination one does indeed observe, occasionally, local tenderness and redness at the injection site. Fever, headache, general malaise and even diarrhoea may occur. The vaccination offers some protection over a 6 month period and reinforcing infections will be necessary every 6 months in countries where a valid certificate is required.

4.5.2.4 Typhoid Vaccination

Because ships may enter ports in countries where the general standard of sanitation is unsatisfactory, many shipping companies provide routine vaccination against typhoid fever. Vaccination is recommended for seamen travelling to areas outside Northern Europe and North America. The vaccine consists of killed, whole cells of *Salmonella typhi*, preserved with phenol or acetone. It usually contains 1×10^9 killed organisms. Two doses of 0.5 or 1 ml (depending on the type of vaccine used) are given with a 4-week interval. A single dose will give some protection. Some authors prefer two injections of 0.2 ml intradermally with a 4-week interval (Woodruff and Bell [20]). Reinforcing injections are desirable after 3 years. Vaccination protects 70%–90% of individuals against waterborne infections (i. e. small infecting inocula). Local and general reactions may occur after typhoid vaccination, especially when it is given in combination with paratyphoid A and B vaccine and cholera vaccine. Rare complications of the neurological cardiovascular and renal systems have been observed. Contra-indications are poor general health, acute infections and chronic illness. If vaccination is nevertheless judged necessary in these patients, monovalent typhoid vaccine, intradermally injected, may be considered, but a risk may arise as well. In some countries only the monovalent vaccine is used and recommended because there is evidence that the paratyphoid A component is not very effective in

TAB vaccine and the B fraction is usually of too low antigenicity to offer worthwhile protection against paratyphoid B infection.

The importance of local immunity in the gut in typhoid fever has stimulated research for a live, attenuated, oral vaccine. A promising attenuated strain is the gal mutant, Ty 21a, isolated and characterized by Germanier and Furer [6]. After neutralizing the gastric acidity with sodium bicarbonate a capsule containing 10^9 viable attenuated live cells is taken orally. This is repeated on days 3 and 5. Except for slight gastro-intestinal symptoms, no adverse reactions are seen. Vaccine organisms have been found in stool cultures from only half of the vaccinees, usually for 1 day. Controlled studies have established the efficacy of this type of vaccine (Wahdan et al. [19]). Oral immunization for typhoid fever is probably the most promising and optimal form of vaccination; the vaccine does not give adverse reactions, produces local intestinal immunity and is protective even in the face of high inocula (Levine and Hornick [10]).

4.5.2.5 Vaccination Against Poliomyelitis

Routine immunization against polio is advised for all non-immune seamen travelling to areas outside Europe and North America. Many seamen have been immunized against polio in infancy or at school age, predominantly with live oral poliovirus vaccine (OPV). One booster dose with OPV or IPV (inactivated polio vaccine) is advised at the start of a career at sea. Adults not previously vaccinated are preferably vaccinated with inactivated poliovirus vaccine (IPV). OPV may also be used but carries a slight risk of vaccine-associated paralytic poliomyelitis. IPV is given in three doses; two with a 1-month interval between them and a third dose 6 months later. IPV can be given as plain polio vaccine or in combination with diphtheria and tetanus immunization. As plain vaccine it is administered subcutaneously and as combination vaccine (DTP), intramuscularly.

Immunity after IPV is long lasting; booster injections may be given after 5–10 years. There are no specific contra-indications to IPV and postvaccinal reactions are extremely rare. OPV should not be given to unhealthy adults nor to anyone with acute or intercurrent illness, especially diarrhoea or other intestinal dysfunction.

4.5.2.6 Other Vaccinations

In many countries, BCG vaccination is given in infancy or at school-leaving age. It is not necessary to revaccinate against tuberculosis at the start of a maritime career. Seamen from those countries in which BCG vaccination is not performed on a routine basis do not need to be immunized against tuberculosis, but should be examined if they have been exposed to a known, smear-positive case of pulmonary tuberculosis and should have a yearly chest X-ray. Immunization against *diphtheria* and *tetanus* – also provided in many countries in infancy and at school age – does not need to be given routinely to seamen (at the most in combination with IPV). *Influenza* vaccine may be given to high-risk personnel (e.g. those suffering from chronic pulmonary conditions) or for economic reasons (uninterrupted work routine on board seagoing vessels). From 1982 onwards, an inactivated vaccine against *hepatitis B* will be available in many countries. This very expensive vaccine should at this moment, not be given routinely to merchant seamen because the risk of acquiring this disease is relatively low. Pre-exposure vaccination against *rabies* should be considered only under very special circumstances (e.g. for those in charge of the care of exotic animals being transported over sea).

4.5.2.7 Passive Immunization with Normal Immunoglobulin

Routine administration of normal immunoglobulin for the prevention of a clinical attack of hepatitis A is unrealistic; it should only be given to close contacts of an actual case of hepatitis A on board. Normal immunoglobulin should be given as early as possible after exposure, but it is still effective if given as late as 14 days after exposure. The dose is 0.02 ml/kg body weight, intramuscularly.

4.5.2.8 Passive Immunization with Specific Immunoglobulins

The indications for the use of specific immunoglobulins on board are very limited indeed. In exceptional circumstances its use (ashore) can be considered (human antirabies immunoglobulin together with rabies vaccination after exposure to a rabid animal, human antihepatitis B immunoglobulin after exposure to HBV-positive blood, human antitetanus immunoglobulin after wounds or burns in those who have not been actively immunized). From this summing up it is clear that, in general, the indications for the use of specific immunoglobulins are the same for seamen as for people living ashore.

References

1. Annual reports of the medical officer of health for the Port and City of London. London: Corp. of London Port Health Authority 1950–1980.
2. Bruce-Chwatt, L. J.: Essential malariology. London: Heinemann Medical Books 1980.
3. Control of communicable diseases in man. Ed.: A. S. Benenson. Official report of the Amer. Publ. Health Ass. Washington 1980. p. 31.
4. Davies, J. W., K. C. Cox, W. R. Simon et al.: Typhoid at sea: an epidemic aboard an ocean liner. Canad. med. Ass. J. *1061,* 877–883 (1972).
5. Functioning of the international health regulations for the period 1 January to 31 December 1979. Wkly. epidem. Rec. *55,* 49, 377–384 (1980).
6. Germanier, R. and E. Furer: Isolation and characterization of Gal E mutant Ty 21a of salmonella typhi; a candidate strain for a live, oral typhoid vaccine. J. infect. Dis. *131,* 553–558 (1975).
7. International Health Regulation 1969. 2nd ann. edn. Geneva: WHO 1974.
8. Jaarverslag 1945–1980. Ed.: Gemeentelijke Geneeskundige en Gezondheidsdienst. Rotterdam: Gemeentedrukkerij 1946–1981.
9. Knight, V.: Tuberculosis afloat. J. Amer. med. Ass. *203,* 154–155 (1968).
10. Levine, M. M. and R. B. Hornick: Immunology of enteric pathogens. In: Comprehensive Immunology. Vol. 8, part 1. Eds.: R. A. Good and S. B. Day. New York: Plenum Med. Books 1981. p. 249
11. Merson, M. H., J. M. Hughes, B. T. Wood et al.: Gastrointestinal illness on passenger cruise ships. J. Amer. med. Ass. *231,* 7, 723–727 (1975).
12. Merson, M. H., J. H. Tenney, J. D. Meyers et al.: Shigellosis at sea: an outbreak aboard a passenger cruise ship. Amer. J. Epidem. *101,* 2, 165–175 (1975).
13. Requirements for cholera vaccine. (Requirements for biological substances No. 4). Revised 1968. In: WHO expert committee on biological standardization. Twenty-first report. Annex 1. Geneva: WHO 1969. pp. 27–44. (WHO Technical Report Series No. 413).
14. Requirements for cholera vaccine. (Requirements for biological substances No. 4). In: WHO expert committee on biological standardization. Twenty-fifth report. Annex 2. Geneva: WHO 1973. pp. 18–21. (Technical Report Series No. 530).
15. Resolution WHA 33.3 In: WHO Handbook of resolutions and decisions. Geneva: WHO 1980.
16. Schultz, M. G., S. N. Cohen, W. Greifinger et al.: An outbreak of malaria on shipboard. Amer. J. trop. Med. Hyg. *16,* 5, 576–579 (1967).
17. Survey of the incidence of gastro-intestinal illness in cruise ship passengers. Morb. Mort. Wkly Rep. *23,* 65–66 (1974).
18. Travel information manual. A joint publication of fourteen IATA Airlines. Amsterdam, May 1982. p. 12.
19. Wahdan, M. H., C. Serié, Y. Cerisier et al.: A controlled field trial of live salmonella typhi Ty 21a oral vaccine against typhoid: three-year results. J. infect. Dis. *145,* 292–295 (1982).
20. Woodruff, A. W. and S. Bell: A synopsis of infectious and tropical diseases. 2nd edn. Bristol: Wright 1978. p. 18.

4.6 DDD – Disinfection, Disinfestation and Deratting

A. Backhaus

In the long run, prevention of disease is more effective than the best therapy. But preventive measures must be carried out at a time when there is no apparent danger to health. Disinfection, disinfestation and deratting (DDD) are unpopular measures, but by deratting, the plague has been restricted to small areas of the globe; in addition, yellow fever and malaria have been eradicated in those areas where the transmitting insects have been killed, and disinfection has been an invaluable weapon against cholera and salmonellosis.

These measures will be more effective if the crew understand why their private life is being disturbed, if the company realises why deratting – with its high expense – is ordered, and if the shipping agent is aware of the danger and subsequent expenses should insects do damage to the holds and cargo. DDD will accomplish very little if there is passive resistance on the part of the people concerned. Information and practical hints are essential to good results. People should be informed not only of the necessity for and effect of the measures intended, but also of the dangers associated with the chemicals used. There is no disinfectant which kills only bacteria and micro-organisms and is harmless to man. There are no statistics available on the number of people who have been killed by the processes of DDD, but there have been numerous fatal accidents and many cases of poisoning all over the world.

4.6.1 Disinfection

Disinfection was performed by man long before the word was used and before the invisible world of micro-organisms had been explored (Munro [28]). Salt, sugar, vinegar and oil have been used to store food since the beginning of civilisation. For instance, 50% sugar or 10% salt inhibits the growth of *Clostridium botulinum;* 5% vinegar almost totally disinfects salad, vegetables and fruits; oil on the surface of a liquid prevents the penetration of oxygen. In ancient times wine was covered with oil to keep it fresh, and the effect lasted for hundreds of years, as shown by old bottles which have been found in the sea. However, such an effect is possible only with aerobic micro-organisms.

Nowadays, chlorine (e.g. as hypochlorites), quaternary ammonium compounds, silver, ozone and UV radiation are in general use, but hot water and steam have not lost their importance ([26]; Longrée [27]; Snitko [34]). Disinfection is achieved by the denaturation of protein or of enzymes, by damage to the cytoplasmic membrane or by inactivation of DNA polymerase. But a disinfectant does not discriminate between micro-organisms and food or cargo; it can be absorbed by food residues and the surface of a container must therefore be cleaned before it is disinfected. The time of exposure to the agent is one of the vital parameters for disinfection and sterilisation (Baumgart et al. [10]; Bode [11]; Eggensperger [18]; Hahn [21]). Methods of disinfection in general are not altered for use on ships, but the construction of a vessel and the associated possibilities of infestation on board must be considered (Backhaus and Müller [4]; Pöhn [32]).

4.6.1.1 Specific Targets of Disinfection

Tuberculosis

Tuberculosis is not as frequent a disease as it once was, but, using the port of Hamburg as an example, there are approximately 100 cases on more than 10000 ships per year [23; 43]. Disinfection may be a problem if a sailor has been signed off for some weeks before information of his disease reaches the ship, and the cabin is already occupied by another. Although to date there has been no reported infection due to occupation of a particular cabin, disinfection is and should be done for bacteriological and psychological reasons. It would seem reasonable to fix a date, perhaps of 3 months after the day on which the diseased person has signed off, after which disinfection is not necessary. However, this decision must be made according to law and with the agreement of local authorities. In general, chlorine-releasing compounds are used for disinfection of tuberculosis-infected areas.

Hepatitis

Cases of hepatitis amount to approximately 40 a year per 10000 ships in the port of Hamburg. Disinfection is necessary in every case, and should be done first during the voyage, then completed by specialists in the next port. Here, again, chlorine-releasing compounds should be used [43].

Salmonellosis

The frequency of salmonellosis on ships is about the same as that of hepatitis. The affected person rarely feels ill; more than 80% of them are carriers only, and in 18% of cases the bacteria are detected only when some cases of diarrhoea have occurred during the last voyage and an examination of faeces is done for all crew members. The carrier is generally still on board. Disinfection of the sanitary facilities must be done first and the person excreting salmonellae must wash his hands regularly with disinfectant, until he is cured. Disinfection must be completed in the next port of call, and, according to the rules of most nations, be approved by the local authorities (Günther [20]; [43]).

Fungi

Fungi are ubiquitous, particularly on ships, so the first step in prevention is to construct showers, bathrooms, swimming pools and saunas in forms which provide no place for fungi to thrive, and using materials which can be disinfected. However, investigations on many ships have demonstrated that even on stone and plastic various fungi can be found. Regular disinfection after effective cleaning is the only way to reduce their number. Several chemicals are recommended. The disinfection procedure should cover several hours, in every case according to the manufacturer's instructions for use. It should be noted as well that the possibilities of disinfecting an area are limited by the danger of causing allergic reactions.

4.6.1.2 The Ship

Cargo holds may be contaminated by micro-organisms brought aboard with the cargo. Cargo which is packed and sealed is hygienic and presents no problems, but the cover of the cargo may be partly destroyed, insects may creep from the cargo to the holds, or moisture may drip, for example, from pallets of animal skins onto the floor (Asaj et al. [2]; Tomažić et al. [40]; Tomažić [41]). The disinfection of holds is requested by many agents before they send their cargo to a ship. It may be necessary to cleanse the ship not only of the visible remnants of old cargo but also of residual odours. If the new cargo consists of very different goods, a disinfectant must be used that will not spoil them.

A special problem arose with the introduction of containerisation. The containers must be cleaned and in many cases disinfected. This is generally done ashore. If it has to be done on the ship, the cleaning must be effective, for dust and other residue of the previous cargo will not only enter the interior of the container but also be found in the ventilation ducts between the walls of the container if a wall is damaged.

The galley of the ship has typical problems with the source of the food supply (Terbeck [39]). If all food is supplied from the home port, the difficulty of storage grows with the length of the voyage. If fresh food is bought in foreign ports, it might carry the danger of contaminating the galley. Investigations in galleys and store rooms have demonstrated by bacteriological examination that the number of micro-organisms per cm^2 was significantly higher after obtaining stores in foreign ports. Disinfection once a week with quaternary ammonium compounds effectively reduced the number of bacteria. Regular disinfection of galleys after cleaning is often done in port. The possibility of contamination is more probable at sea than in port, but to date disinfection at sea is an exception, not the rule. Diarrhoea among crew members or passengers is considered inevitable; it is nevertheless very necessary to disinfect the galley, pantry and provision store room. Diarrhoea depends to some extent on the number of bacteria to which one is exposed, and disinfection can reduce the number drastically, even if it is far from sterilisation (Graham-Rack and Binsted [19]).

The provision store may be contaminated by a variety of micro-organisms, brought on board with the provisions. The construction of the storage room should avoid places which are difficult to clean. Disinfection cannot be effective without cleaning. The micro-organisms hide in dust and dirty places and are sheltered by dirt from the disinfectant. Sanitary installations (shower, lavatory, swimming pool, sauna) may be contaminated by many micro-organisms, but the prevalent contamination is caused by fungi. Mycosis (athlete's foot) is the frequent result. Construction of such facilities has to avoid places where fungi can grow, but even the best floor and wall surfaces will not prevent growth of certain forms. Investigations on ships, often done by the Port Health Authority of Hamburg, proved frequent contamination. The situation in vessels is a special one, for tropical or subtropical climates are advantageous for the multiplication of fungi, which are brought on board the ship by crew members and passengers. Disinfection with fungicidal chemicals should be done regularly, ideally at least once a week; it is even more efficient to add fungicidal chemicals to the cleaning water every day. As fungi are generally not visible, the person responsible for the sanitary facilities may not believe that the clean tiled floor is contaminated. The possibility, even on board ship, of demonstrating with culture plates must be used. By such a demonstration the personnel will be made aware of the danger and can be motivated to disinfect regularly.

The swimming pool and the sauna are generally contaminated by many bacteria, including *Escherichia coli* in high number. The water is not changed continuously and the empty pool is rarely disinfected. One must be aware of the danger, in spite of the fact that so far no proved infections have been reported.

Ice cubes are sometimes contaminated, even though they have been made of potable water. The method of storage is the usual source of contamination by pathogenic micro-organisms; ice machines are seldom, if ever, cleaned and very rarely disinfected. The scoop for taking the cubes out of the machine is seldom stored in a hygienic way. In many places the ice cubes are simply removed with the hand; consequently the remaining ice cubes are contaminated and when used infect the water or other beverage and the ice tools (Backhaus [8]). Therefore, disinfection of ice machines and ice scoops is necessary. The danger can be reduced if Ag^- is added to the water from which the ice is made.

Fruits and vegetables, especially salad, that are bought abroad may also be contaminated by micro-organisms, worms and other parasites. Disinfection of uncooked foods, such as salads, is difficult, and the smell of disinfectant chemicals is unpleasant. Vinegar has proved to be an effective disinfectant for those fresh vegetables and fruits that are consumed without being heated. Soaking in 5% vinegar for 5 min kills most of the pathogenic bacteria such as *E. coli* and *Salmonella*. Vinegar does not spoil the taste and has been in use for the preparation of salad for thousands of years (Backhaus and Wolter [5]).

4.6.1.3 Conclusion

Crews are – if at all – only slightly trained in disinfection, and are not aware of the danger of contamination by micro-organisms. They should use disinfectants, and must be thoroughly taught that disinfection without cleaning beforehand is impossible and that no disinfectant kills micro-organisms instantaneously: the necessary time is indicated on the package of every disinfectant, and this information must be read and followed. Every effort should be made to demonstrate contamination with bacteria and fungi (Pöhn [32]). Dried bacteriological culture media have been developed, which are activated upon use. Such a demonstration can encourage interest in disinfection (Backhaus [3]).

4.6.2 Disinfestation

Most insects on board ships are pests which can transmit diseases such as malaria and yellow fever, spoil food and cargo, and even destroy the ship itself. They do damage to wood and may damage the insulation of electric installations, plastic material and textiles.

Insects crawl or fly aboard ship or are brought by the wind. They are brought with cargo, or in the clothing and hair of passengers and crew. They lay their eggs in cargo, food and on people (Bull [13]). They multiply very quickly: a pair of cockroaches brought on board at the beginning of a voyage can develop into an army by the time the port of destination is reached. The fight never ends, and negligence can be fatal to the crew and lead to destruction of the cargo. Even insects that do not transmit disease can make life miserable for human beings, if only by depriving them of sleep.

In the *Guide to Ship Sanitation,* Lamoureux [23 a] gives information on insect (vermin) control.

4.6.2.1 Transmission of Disease

Far more insects transmit disease than was previously thought. Even those that do not inject bacteria or poison through the skin by biting (as with malaria, yellow fever or the plague) can carry germs, and if they are killed and crushed against the human body the germs can enter the body through small cuts or wounds, as happens with typhus. The more known about the way of life and habits of these pests, the more can effective methods be developed to fight them.

Yellow Fever

The eradication of *Aedes aegypti* is the first and most effective step in the prevention of yellow fever. The mosquito was formerly found on many ships and was often responsible for the death of an entire crew. There are currently no reports on infestation; nevertheless, in some ports the health authorities investigate for infestation not only by rats but also by *Aedes aegypti*. The mosquitoes prefer to stay in the area of the deck, but may be found in the outer rooms as well, and this is where disinfestation must first be done. If the ship is destined for a country or port which is known to be infested, pesticides with a long-lasting effect should be used beforehand as a preventive measure.

Arbor Virus

Yellow fever is one of the best-known arbor viruses, but more and more are detected, the Argentinian haemorrhagic fever being one of the most dangerous. Many of these viruses are transmitted by ticks, in particular Congo virus. Fleas may also be dangerous, and disinfestation must be done for hygienic reasons.

Malaria

The *Anopheles* mosquito, which transmits malaria, has been found in private quarters, in holds and in sheltered places on the decks of ships. It may be carried by the wind from the shore to a ship passing far from the coast. Disinfestation is the best preventive measure, not only when in port but also when only passing by an infested country, as the open sea can be dangerous as well as river areas. The possibility of insects crossing long distances even in hostile surroundings should never be underestimated.

Typhus and Other Diseases Transmitted by Lice

Head lice, body lice and crab lice may all transmit disease. The germs are found in the body of the louse and are prevalent in their faeces; they are rubbed into itching skin when a person scratches. Disinfestation is done with pesticides, and must include clothing, bed linens and blankets. Shaving the head of the infected person may also be necessary.

Salmonellosis and Amoebic Dysentery

Infestation by cockroaches and flies has been proven as a cause of salmonellosis and amoebic dysentery, but every omnivorous creeping insect can transmit the germs of these diseases. Flies can be exterminated in the same way as mosquitoes and other pests; industry produces new pesticides every year. Galleys and provision store rooms, pantries and mess halls should be treated regularly with pesticides that have a long-lasting effect, but one must be aware when using them of their toxicity to man.

Anthrax

The skins and crushed bones of animals may be contaminated with anthrax. The insects which transmit the germ to man are generally overlooked. In one case, crushed bones were shipped from Asia to several ports in northern Europe. They were loaded on pallets, in blocks of 1 m^3 or larger. The bones had been contaminated with anthrax germs and the cargo was infested with the eggs of small Asian flies. The temperature in the hold was approximately 30 °C. After 6 weeks at sea the ship arrived at the first port. Millions of flies, their legs and wings contaminated with anthrax, left the hold and found their way under the clothing of crew members and dock workers. They were killed and squashed when the men scratched their itching skin. The swarm of insects was not only unpleasant but also dangerous (Huisman [22 a]).

Murine Typhus

Murine typhus is seldom seen on board ships today; no outbreak of plague has occurred in European ports for many years. However, rats infested with insects can be dangerous; a case which occurred in Rotterdam will serve as an example: Rats on board a ship had been infected with *Rickettsia mooseri*. The rats were attacked by dock workers, and during the episode fleas were transferred from the rats to the men, who subsequently fell ill with murine typhus. Therefore, every rat or mouse found should be killed and disinfested of its fleas or other insects, after which it can be sent for further investigation (Huisman [22 a]).

Cockroaches

Cockroaches are ubiquitous and multiply rapidly. They damage food, clothes and even books, and they transmit disease. They are omnivorous and deposit their adherent egg cases (oothecae) anywhere. The eggs are disseminated all over the world in ships, planes, automobiles and on people. The oothecae are more resistant than the adults to pesticides, making cockroaches masters at survival (Pleśtina [31]; Ulewicz et al. [42]). A ship is an ideal place for cockroaches. Food is freely available; there is a cargo residue in the holds; and there is sewage and waste in many corners. Small hiding places are open to them, such as tubes, chinks and slits. They can move freely about a ship using the ducts for ventilation and electrical connections. There is a great deal of moisture, and the temperature in the hiding places is ideal for breeding. Pesticides do not penetrate into the long connecting ducts, so that if adults are killed the newly hatched take their place. It is possible to fight cockroaches, but a short campaign has no positive effect (Bakić [9]; Černjul [14]; Dimitrov and Penev [17]). Long-term fumigation is successful using cyanide (3–5 days). It is necessary to take periodic samples and sometimes to add more of the fumigant to keep the concentration effective. Other pesticides that can be used are pyrethrum (natural or chemically synthesised and with a long-lasting effect), carbamates and chlorinated insecticides. These must have a flushing effect, or a chemical with such an effect must be added.

Spray, liquid or dust will never reach the farthest places; the cockroaches must be forced to come out. Pyrethrum was the first natural insecticide that had a flushing effect, but many others have since been synthesised. After being flushed out, the adults are killed when they come into contact with the effective concentration of pesticide. But cockroaches soon learn to avoid places which have been treated, and every spot must therefore be covered systematically; the smallest pathway should not be free of the chemical.

The application of pesticides must be renewed every 2–4 weeks for many months to ensure success, because the oothecae are not harmed by the initial treatment. The young emerge several weeks to a year later, and if there is a long-lasting effect, and if the pesticide has not been removed in cleaning, the newly developed insects will be killed on their search for food. Cooperation between the DDD specialist and the ship's staff is essential to the success of a campaign against cockroaches (Penev [30]).

4.6.2.2 The Hold

Pests can spoil cargo in many ways. Flies lay their eggs in fruit, which is then spoiled by the maggots, and worms may eat the entire fruit. Grain may be infested with beetles; there are one or two at first, but when the holds are opened at the port of destination nearly every kernel has been ruined by insects and maggots.

4.6.2.3 In-transit Fumigation

It would seem reasonable to have cargo disinfested ashore, before it is loaded onto a ship. But since agents and companies do not always do this, in-transit fumigation, especially of grain, is becoming more and more common, and this is done in the holds of the ship (Leesch et al. [25]); Redlinger et al. [33]). The only fumigant in use today is phostoxine. To date more than 5000 cargoes have been fumigated in transit; there were several fatal accidents at the beginning, but the technique is now said to be foolproof, and no mishaps have been reported recently.

Nevertheless, there are some countries and private companies which have strictly forbidden in-transit fumigation. In port the crew should leave the vessel while it is being disinfected. Only trained personnel remain on board and they take all necessary preventive steps. On the open sea, however, no one can leave the ship. The captain must have full knowledge of the facts about phostoxine (PH_3) at his disposal.

On the positive side, PH_3 is applied in a safe way; the gas forms only slowly after the fumigant has been sprayed. It can be smelled even at very low concentrations, below the danger level, and there is enough time for workers to evacuate an area. Technical instruments are available for ambient air monitoring. Fumigant residue is harmless if it is collected at the port of destination by trained personnel. PH_3 is very successful in combatting beetles and other pests if applied over a sufficiently long period of time, which is normally guaranteed by the length of the voyage.

On the negative side, although PH_3 has a penetrating odour, there have been cases where it was ignored. There is no simple way to distinguish between a harmless concentration and one that is toxic. Poisoning by a fatal dose is not realised immediately; symptoms appear after 12–48 h, but no medical help is available in most cases, and even then it would be too late and have no effect. Women and children are known to be more susceptible than men to PH_3 poisoning. The company, the captain and the countries involved must decide, on the basis of these facts, whether to take the risk of fumigating in transit.

There are other fumigants but the situation does not differ. Methylbromide is effective but it has no odour. The time between poisoning and the first symptoms is the same as, or even longer than, that for PH_3. Cyanide is effective but nearly impossible to use in the hold in transit. Its effect on insects is not as strong, and higher concentrations would be required. The fact remains that realistic knowledge of the danger involved may reduce the risk of fatal accidents.

4.6.2.4 Fumigation of Holds in Port

Fumigation is done in many thousands of ships a year to kill pests such as the copra beetle, with methylbromide and phostoxine as the main agents. The lethal effect depends on time, temperature, concentration and penetration of the fumigant.

There are countries that demand fumigation, even if there is no proof of infestation. To fumigate while the crew is on board is dangerous. Fatal accidents have occurred on all five continents. A man sleeping on board may not notice the penetration of the fumigant into his accommodation (Backhaus [7]; Brodniewicz [12]). Technical systems must be used to detect the fumigant in time, but they may be used without sufficient precaution or they may fail because of a technical defect. The cargo itself may be dangerous, however, after fumigation and ventilation. Cargo such as expellers that are in bags may be fumigated and ventilated without difficulties. But the same cargo in bulk retains the toxic fumigant far longer. The samples of air in holds and in sleeping quarters may seem to be free of toxic substances, but with a change in temperature or atmospheric pressure, toxic substances can penetrate from the holds to the accommodation (Backhaus [6]; [23]). The concentration of the fumigant must be checked continually. Methylbromide will adhere to the cargo if there is albumin and oil in the product, e.g. in expellers. Only when the cargo is unloaded and brought to a storehouse ashore or to another ship, is the ventilation ideal.

Very often there is no poisoning, but fumigation personnel and the crew can get careless. Fatal accidents have proven that we should be aware of the high risk, both at the time of and after fumigation of cargo. The literature quoted is only a small example of reports of poisoning.

4.6.2.5 Containers

The cargo in a container may be infested in the same way as cargo in the holds of a ship; containers do not prevent infestation by pests. As the container is thought to be water- and gasproof, it is taken to be the best place to fumigate. Containers can be collected in special places for the process, and ventilation seems to be no problem. This may be true for the new types of containers, but older ones are not gasproof and, with only one door, are poorly or not at all ventilated.

One container, fumigated with toxic gas on shore, then taken to the ship after being inadequately ventilated, may be harmless, but if 25% or more of the cargo on a container vessel contains residual fumigant the crew members may experience toxic effects. To avoid this, containers must be labelled with the name of the fumigant, the time of fumigation, and the type and amount of ventilation. The officer in charge and the captain must be informed of the number of fumigated containers and must receive specific data on the fumigant used, the symptoms of toxicity and appropriate first-aid measures.

Fumigated containers must be added to the list of dangerous cargo. They are disinfested with pesticides which are applied to the walls, the openings and the ventilation system. After disinfestation has been done repeatedly as a preventive measure, the container surface becomes not only fatal to insects, but also toxic to men. All those who have to work with containers must be thoroughly informed.

4.6.2.6 Conclusion

It is necessary to be aware of the danger both of insects and of pesticides and fumigants. Through knowledge, vigilance and patience it is possible to fight pests successfully, and at the same time prevent toxic effects on human beings from fumigants and pesticides (Pleśtina [31]; Vuković and Svetličić [44]).

4.6.3 Deratting

International health regulations [22 b] order the continuous fight against rodents in ports, on board ships and planes and in heavily populated areas. As long as men cross the sea by ship, rodents will try to go with them. Rats are curious; they adapt to every climate and to nearly all methods devised for killing them. Rats transmit plague, murine typhus, brucellosis and Weil's disease, via insects they carry and in their urine and faeces. It is hoped that plague has been eradicated, but other diseases are always being discovered – haemorrhagic fever will not be the last – and as rats can transmit many different diseases, they must be fought on board and in port. In some countries international and national regulations contain the word "rodents", in others the word "rats". There are mice on board ships as well. They can also transmit diseases and are more resistant to coumarin, but their number is smaller. It is reasonable to include mice in the programme of eradication. Knowledge of the species is important to effective killing. *Rattus rattus* and *Rattus norvegicus* behave differently. A method of poisoning which is effective with one can be useless with the other. The well-adapted strategy is as important as the poison itself. A specialist is needed to investigate and to find the effective method of killing a particular species, but some general rules and experiences can be reported here (Snitko [34]).

4.6.3.1 Prevention of Rats

Ratproof construction of ships has done more towards eradicating rats than traps and poison. Detailed information on the ratproofing of ships is given in the *Handbook on Sanitation of Vessel Construction* [21 a], in a special manual [32 a] and by Lamoureux [23 a]. The smaller the area of the ship in which rats can live and which they cannot leave, the more difficult it is for them, and the better the chances are of hunting them. If rats can reach every part of the ship, they can escape all danger: they will find sufficient food and water and have time and space to multiply. But ratproof construction has, so to speak, a psychological effect on rats. They do not like to be in places where they cannot find ways out. They have their own security system. They like small tunnels and many hiding places and avoid large open areas. They may not choose a ship without possibilities to hide and to escape. The communication system of rats is one of the best in the world. Messages about dangerous food or a dangerous place are sent from group to group. It is impossible to construct a ship without any hiding places for rats. They do not like the smell of gasoline, and they leave a ship in the dockyard if there is too much noise. But they adapt themselves, even to refrigeration holds, by growing a thick coat, and have been found in the modern system of transportation, in the container. However, it is always possible to collect garbage, to clean the deck and the holds and to take away any source of food from the kitchen or from the cargo. To keep a place clean is the fundamental rule of hygiene in general, but it is fundamental, too, to the prevention of rat infestation. Nearly every sailor and every captain knows in which ports rats thrive today. Unfortunately, it is nearly impossible to prevent the rats from coming on board (Bull [13]). They may gain entry by crawling up the mooring ropes and may enter via gangways.

The best means of controlling rats is to kill them as early as possible. A few may be caught in traps or killed by poison before they have a chance to multiply if immediate action is taken. If they have a chance to multiply in the ship's holds and accommodation quarters it is much more difficult to kill them.

4.6.3.2 Searching for Rats

Rodents leave tracks and faeces. Without a doubt they mark their path by urine as well, which is of importance regarding the contamination of food by germs; but urine is visible only with the help of a special lamp which is not generally in use.

Faeces are the clearest evidence of the presence of rodents, and provide more information than do tracks left by feet or tails. An examination of the faeces can help to determine the species. With experience one can say with great accuracy whether the animal is a rat or a mouse, young or old, and when the faeces were excreted. From the distribution of the faeces one can tell the approximate number of rodents and which species one is dealing with. Rodents also leave tracks in dust or in poison which has been distributed on the ship. Traces of coloured poison may be left on walls by the rat's tail. If there is even the suspicion of rat infestation, steps to derat should be taken immediately, even though the process of eradication may be expensive.

4.6.3.3 Control of Rats

Detailed information on rodent control is given by Lamoureux [23 a] and in a special chapter of the *Handbook on Sanitation of Vessels in Operation* [21 b].

If there are few rodents, traps are helpful, but different types are required for different species. Traps will reduce the number of rats but will not eradicate them (Lebedev et al. [24]); a rat dying of poison serves as a warning of danger to other rats, which will avoid the place and the poison. Their communication system is mysterious, but highly efficient. Consequently, any poison used must kill within a short time, as does sodium fluoroacetate (1080) (Cornwell [15]; [16]; [35]; [36]; [38]), or it must kill all the rats at once, as do gases such as cyanide. A third possibility is a poison which kills a long time after it is consumed, preventing the rats from establishing a connection between the food and death. Coumarin, which prolongs the coagulation time, is an example of this type. Any poison used must be safe to the people on board the ship; safety should be the foremost concern. Every poison that is administered to eradicate rats is dangerous to man; the quantity of coumarin or one of its derivatives which is lethal to rats is not lethal to human beings. Nevertheless, even coumarin must be put in a place where no other small animals or children can consume it. The compound 1080 is fatal in small quantities to rats, though the lethal dose for man is perhaps 10 times the lethal dose for rats. However, if the intention is to kill 50–100 rats, 1080 must be prepared in a quantity which can kill more than one man. The use of 1080 is permitted in only a few countries under strict rules and effective supervision ([1]; Swann [37]). Cyanide can be administered only by trained personnel.

Registration and control of used and unused packages is necessary. Cyanide, in the concentration necessary to kill rats, is fatal to man as well. Access to the ship must be constantly controlled. Every person and every pet animal must leave the ship. During ventilation, the gas leaving the ship must be examined to ensure that it is not dangerous to the surroundings. Gas concentration after ventilation must be checked more than once. Cyanide can escape from blankets due to an increase in temperature when a person is sleeping. Consequently the concentration of the gas must be checked when the temperature in the sleeping quarters is higher than 20 °C.

Coumarin requires 8–14 days to take effect. If a ship leaves port after only a short stay – today the normal occurrence – the effect of the poison will not have been ascertained.

Sodium fluoroacetate requires less time to be effective – 12–24 h if there is no way for the rats to avoid the poison. It is generally applied as a tasteless and odourless liquid. Cyanide can take effect within minutes or after several hours, but the time required for ventilation is much longer. The total amount of time needed for the use of cyanide is 24 h; in every case crew members must stay ashore for one night.

Corpses of rodents poisoned with cyanide or coumarin have not been proven to be dangerous, but a dog may be killed by eating a rat that has consumed 1080.

4.6.3.4 Conclusion

Ratproof construction of ships, general cleanliness and eradication of rats as early as possible are the best and most economical measures for preventing rat infestation. The method of killing depends on their number, their hiding places, their habits and the disease they carry. Although plague itself has been conquered, rats still transmit disease, and the damage they do to food and equipment must not be neglected.

References

1. Anweisungen für die Schiffsleitung falls Rattenbekämpfung an Bord eines Schiffes stattfindet mittels der chemischen Verbindung 1080. Rotterdam: Reinigungs- und Desinfektionsamt
2. Asaj, A., M. Vučemilo, D. Linić et al.: Suvremene mogućnosti dezinfekcije broda. [Contemporary possibilities for ship disinfection]. In: Pomorska medicina II. (Naučne rasprave) Belgrad: Izdanje Mornaričkog glasnika 1979. pp. 453–457. (Pomorska biblioteka. Sveska 30).
3. Backhaus, A.: Bakteriologische Kontrolle mit Eintauchnährböden und Trocken-Kultur-Medien. Hamburg 1978.
4. Backhaus, A. and H. E. Müller: Bakteriologische Längsschnittuntersuchungen auf Kauffahrteischiffen auf großer Fahrt. Hamburg 1978.
5. Backhaus, A. and R. Wolter: Desinfektion von Salat, Obst und Gemüse mit Essig. Hamburg 1978.
6. Backhaus, A.: 5. Fallbericht einer tödlichen akuten Methylbromidvergiftung. In: D. Weller: Methylbromid. IV. Medizinische Toxikologie (Fallbeispiele). Frankfurt: DEGESCH 1982. pp. 249–251.
7. Backhaus, A.: 7. Fallbericht einer tödlichen akuten Methylbromidvergiftung. In: D. Weller: Methylbromid. IV. Medizinische Toxikologie (Fallbeispiele). Frankfurt: DEGESCH 1982. pp. 255–256.
8. Backhaus, A.: Hygiene der Eiswürfel. Hamburg 1978.
9. Bakić, J.: Suzbijanje Blattella germanica L. na brodovima RM i objektima posebne namjene. [Extermination of the Blattella germanica (L.) on naval craft and places equipped and used for storing and preparing food]. In: Pomorska medicina II. (Naučne rasprave) Belgrad: Izdanje Mornaričkog glasnika 1979. pp. 711–731. (Pomorska biblioteka. Sveska 30).
10. Baumgart, J., M. Schmiedel and Th. Reinke: Mikrobielle Stoffwechselprodukte als Indikator der Haltbarkeit von Feinkosterzeugnissen. Alimenta 51–55 (1977).
11. Bode, R.: Darstellung der Desinfektionsmittelprüfung in Deutschland. Hyg. Med. 8/9/11 (1981).
12. Brodniewicz, A.: Poisoning of seamen with methyl bromide due to fumigation of a Polish cargo ship in Haiphong (Vietnam). Arh. Hig. Rada *18*, 19 (1967).
13. Bull, J. O.: Rodent and insect control in stored food crops. A contractor's view-point. Prog. Food Nutr. Sci. *4*, 3–4, 91–95 (1980).
14. Černjul, Z.: Pojava i značenje žohara na plovnim i stacionarnim objektima i njihovo suzbijanje. [The appearance and significance of cockroaches on board of floating and station-

ary objects and their repelling]. In: Pomorska medicina (Naučne rasprave). Belgrad: Izdanje Mornaričkog glasnika 1975. (Pomorska biblioteka. Sveska 26).

15. Cornwell, P. B.: Pest control in buildings. A guide to the meaning of terms. London: Hutchinson 1973.
16. Deratting procedures. In: Foreign quarantine manual of operations. Washington 26 August 1960.
17. Dimitrov, M. Iv. and Iv. Penev: Otnosno nyakoi savremenni metodi sredstva za borba s khlebarkite v korabite. [Modern methods and means in cockroach control on board ships]. Transp. med. Westi *22,* 1, 6–8 (1977).
18. Eggensperger, H.: Desinfektionswirkstoffe und ihre Wirkungsmechanismen. Dtsch. Apoth.-Ztg *113,* 21, 785–791 (1973).
19. Graham-Rack, B. and R. Binsted: Hygiene in food. Manufacturing and handling. London: Food Trade Press 1964.
20. Günther, M.: Salmonellose und ihre Bekämpfung durch personal- und betriebshygienische Maßnahmen. Dtsch. Z. Lebensmitteltechnol. *26,* 8/9 (1975).
21. Hahn, W.: Desinfektionsmittel – Wirkungsweise, Wirkungsspektrum und toxikologische Aspekte. Hyg. Med. 10 (1981).

21a. Handbook on sanitation of vessel construction. Standards of sanitation and ratproofing for the construction of vessels. Ed.: U.S. Department of Health, Education, and Welfare. Public Health Service. Washington: U.S. Government Printing Office 1965. (Public Health Service Publication No. 393).

21b. Handbook on sanitation of vessels in operation. Sanitation features and facilities on vessels in operation. Ed.: U.S. Department of Health, Education, and Welfare. Public Health Service. Washington: U.S. Government Printing Office 1963. (Public Health Service Publication No. 68).

22. Hickin, N. E.: Household insect pests. London: Hutchinson 1964.

22a. Huismann, J.: Personal communication 1978.

22b. International health regulations (1969). 3rd annotated edn. Geneva: WHO 1983. p 26–29.

23. Jahresberichte des hafen- und flughafenärztlichen Dienstes. Hamburg 1973/74, 1975, 1976/77, 1978/79.

23a. Lamoureux, V. B.: Guide to ship sanitation. Geneva: WHO 1967.

24. Lebedev, G. I., N. N. Rutkevich and V. A. Sednev: Deratizatsiya fentolatsinovoy pastoy na korablyakh i beregovykh obyektakh. [Deratisation by phenoated paste onboard and ashore]. Voen.-med. Zh. 7, 64–65 (1981).
25. Leesch, J. G., L. M. Redlinger, H. B. Gillenwater et al.: An in-transit shipboard fumigation of corn. J. econ. Entomol. *71,* 6, 928–935 (1978).
26. Liste der vom Bundesgesundheitsamt geprüften und anerkannten Desinfektionsmittel und Verfahren. 7th ed. Bundesgesundhbl. *21,* 16, 255–261 (1978).
27. Longrée, K.: Quantity food sanitation. New York: Wiley Interscience 1980.
28. Munro, J. W.: Pests of stored products. London: Hutchinson 1966.
29. Novaković, T. and J. Bakić: Mogućnost primene i efikasnost insekticidnih lakova u dezinsekciji brodova Ratne mornarice. [Possibilities of application and efficacy of insecticidal lacquers in disinfection of the navy ships]. Vojnosanit. Pregl. *37,* 5, 392–397 (1980).
30. Penev, Iv.: Prouchvaniya varkhu nyakoi metodi i sredstva za borba sas sinantropnite khlebarki. [Studies on certain methods and means in synantropic cockroaches campaign]. In: Nauchni trudove po transportna meditsina. Vol. 5. Ed.: Ministerstvo na transporta. Transporten meditsinski institut. Sofia: Meditsina i fiskultura 1979. pp. 34–46.
31. Pleština, R.: Toksikologija nekih antikolinesteraza što se upotrebljavaju u dezinsekciji. [Toxicology of some insecticides used in desinsection]. In: Pomorska medicina (Naučne rasprave) Belgrad: Izdanje Mornaričkog glasnika 1975. (Pomorska biblioteka. Sveska 26).
32. Pöhn, H.-Ph.: Exotische Krankheiten? Legionellose. Bundesgesundhbl. *22,* 25, 457–461 (1979).

32a. Rat proofing of ships. Ed.: U.S. Department of Health, Education, and Welfare. Public Health Service. New York: Stevens & Wood 1959.

33. Redlinger, L. M., J. M. Zettler, J. G. Leesch et al.: In-transit shipboard fumigation of wheat. J. econ. Entomol. *72,* 4, 642–647 (1979).
34. Snitko, V. M.: Gazovaya deratizatsiya i dezinsektsiya na morskom flote. [Deratisation and desinsection by gas in seafaring]. Voen.-med. Zh. 2, 51–53 (1979).
35. Sodium fluoroacetate. In: Operational memoranda on economic poisons. Savannah: Communicable Disease Center 1956.
36. Sodium fluoroacetate FCH_2COO Na AFL 1080. London: Associated Fumigators Limited
37. Swann, W. G.: Use of "1080" in the Port of London. Ed.: The Medical Officer of Health, Port and City of London. London 1970.
38. Technical sodium monofluoroacetate. In: Specifications for Pesticides. 2nd ed. Geneva: WHO 1961.
39. Terbeck, G.: Hygieneanforderungen im Küchenbereich zur Verhütung übertragbarer Krankheiten. Bundesgesundhbl. *20,* 25, 373–378 (1977).
40. Tomažić, D., I. Vodopija and M. Kožar: Dezinfekcija brodskog tereta. [Desinfection of ship's cargo]. In: Pomorska medicina (Naučne ras-

prave). Belgrad: Izdanje Mornaričkog glasnika 1975. (Pomorska biblioteka. Sveska 26).

41. Tomažić, D.: Dezinsekcija brodskog tereta u rasutom stanju. [Desinsection of ship's load in bulk]. In: Pomorska medicina (Naučne rasprave). Belgrad: Izdanje Mornaričkog glasnika 1975. (Pomorska biblioteka. Sveska 26).
42. Ulewicz, K., Z. Wegner and W. Kruminis-Lozowska: Study on the possibility of adopting a complex method in Blattella germanica (L.). Control on board ships. Zbl. Hyg., I. Abt. Orig. B *168*, 538–545 (1979).
43. Unfallverhütung, Schiffssicherheit, Gesundheitsdienst. Berichte. Hamburg: See-Berufsgenossenschaft 1972–1981.
44. Vuković, V. and B. Svetličić: Neki biološki i toksikoloski aspekti primjene suvremenih insekticida u pomorstvu. [A few biological and toxicological aspects of the application of insecticides with maritime affairs]. In: Pomorska medicina. (Naučne rasprave) Belgrad: Izdanje Mornaričkog glasnika 1975. (Pomorska biblioteka. Sveska 26).

4.7 International Health Regulations

Dilwyn T. Jones

Over the centuries, certain diseases have been responsible for pandemics which were sometimes so catastrophic that civilisation itself was threatened. Diseases such as influenza, malaria and typhoid have all caused international disasters in the past but it was the "quarantinable" diseases which so terrorised nations that governments were eventually forced to come together and agree measures to be taken against them. This was neither a quick nor an easy process – between 1851 and 1897 there were ten international sanitary conferences but signed and ratified conventions did not result until the last decade of the century. In the twentieth century, the first decade saw the establishment of the Pan American Sanitary Organization (and Bureau) and the Office International d'Hygiene Publique. The latter was responsible for worldwide international health matters until the World Health Organisation was set up in 1946.

The International Sanitary Regulations were adopted by the Fourth World Health Assembly in 1951. They set out to establish essential measures to be adopted by member countries in order to minimise international spread of disease but they also laid down maximum controls permitted to those countries, so that disturbance of international trade would also be minimised. The aim was to encourage countries to rely on their own internal health services rather than extreme measures at their frontiers and ports. Primarily, the Regulations set up a uniform system for controlling the spread of the quarantinable diseases, other infectious diseases and other health matters not being dealt with at all. These 1951 Regulations were amended over the years and consolidated as the International Health Regulations in 1969 [1] which were, in turn, amended with effect from 1 January 1974 and from 1 January 1982. It is this amended form which is dealt with in this chapter.

It is useful for doctors involved in nautical medicine to know how the system works, if only to know how much internationally disseminated information is the considered opinion of the experts at Geneva and how much is merely what the infected country wants the rest of the world to know.

Many countries have their own national regulations which, while they may be based on the International Regulations, are likely to differ in detail from them. Therefore, it is always wise, when approaching a port in an unfamiliar country, to spend a few moments talking on the radio to the Port Health Authority. In this way, much time and, possibly, embarrassment may be saved. This radio consultation should take place some hours before the estimated time of arrival at the port, so allowing plenty of time for any extra documentation or other procedures that may be required.

The Regulations are divided into parts and the remainder of this chapter is given over to some attempt to select and summarise each part. No attempt will be made to produce any legal interpretations and the chapter has no force in any law system. If more detailed or accurate information is needed, an approach should be made to the appropriate national health administration or to the World Health Organisation.

4.7.1 Part I – Definitions

Most of these are self-explanatory, but some might benefit from a little comment.

The definition of "arrival" dodges the real problem – it does not state which part of a port is the point of arrival. Some countries define it as the first crossing of the outer edge of the port area, others as the act of first mooring or anchoring within the port area and yet others as the act of passing some point arbitrarily designated as the quarantine point.

The definition of "container" is very specific and refers only to the 20-ft equivalent units, not to vehicles, conventional cargo packings, small parcels or boxes.

The "diseases subject to the Regulations" used to be referred to as "quarantinable diseases". It is of interest that the 1851 International Sanitary Code (drafted at an international conference but ratified by only three countries) dealt only with cholera, plague and yellow fever. Then, over the years, louse-borne typhus, relapsing fever and smallpox were added. Now, however, these three latter additions have been removed and the definition covers only the original three diseases.

"Free pratique" – that ancient phrase – is defined as permission for a ship to enter a port, disembark and commence operation. It is now so commonplace for a ship not to be approached for health purposes until it is well inside the port that this definition becomes something of a nonsense. A much better definition would be "permission for a ship to go alongside, disembark and commence operation".

The definition of "infected area" makes it clear that the limits of the area are defined by the government of the country concerned, not by any independent authority.

"Medical examination" of a ship is an important definition. It includes a visit to, and inspection of, the ship, scrutiny of vaccination certificates and/or passports and questioning of travellers but includes physical examination only if the circumstances of the individual case justify it.

4.7.2 Part II – Notification and Epidemiological Information

This deals with the means by which information is fed in to WHO by individual countries and them disseminated by WHO to all member states. It says that a state must inform WHO within 24 h of the first suspected case and then confirm it (or otherwise) at the earliest possible moment. Details of the case or cases, source and type of disease, the area infected and prophylactic measures taken must be notified by the state to WHO immediately they are available and updated thereafter, frequently and in detail. It is the responsibility of the state to decide when an area becomes free from infection, but the criteria for such a decision are laid down. A state must inform WHO of the measures which it intends to take against shipping coming from an infected area and it must also inform shipping companies of its vaccination requirements.

For its part, WHO publishes a Weekly Epidemiological Record and transmits daily epidemiological bulletins by radio as part of its duty to disseminate the information received from individual countries.

4.7.3 Part III – Health Organisation

This part lays down that every state must set up an organisation to ensure that each port has a supply of drinking water and food, an effective system for the removal of sewage and other wastes and a health organisation to monitor these functions and to deal with medical matters, especially infectious diseases. Deratting (and rat-proofing) is specifically mentioned as a function of the health organisation, as is the issue of Deratting or Deratting Exemption Certificates. WHO issues a list of ports worldwide which have been approved for these deratting functions.

4.7.4 Part IV – Health Measures and Procedure

The measures set out are the maximum permitted and must be started immediately, carried out as rapidly as possible and applied to all to exactly the same degree. There must be as little disturbance as possible to the person concerned and his health must not be damaged – neither must his baggage or the ship and its cargo. After the procedures are completed, the traveller and the ship's master are entitled to a certificate setting out what has been done and why it was necessary. A ship which is not infected or suspected may not be refused free pratique. A person under surveillance may not be restricted in movement in any way but he may be required to report regularly, especially if he is about to change his address. He may be subject to medical investigation but not to rectal swabbing. He may even be allowed to continue his voyage, information on his case being sent ahead to his next port of call.

The health authority must do all it can to ensure that a ship leaving port does not carry any infected or suspected people or any vectors of the diseases subject to these Regulations. The authority may medically examine any person before departure and, if the area is infected, may require vaccination certificates to be held.

A ship which is merely passing through a country's waters may not have any health procedures applied to it. A healthy ship, passing through a country's canals or waterways on its way to another country, may not be subject to any procedures except medical examination (and the same applies to the arrival at a port of any healthy ship from which the passengers and crew do not disembark). Even if there is a person from an infected area on board, procedures are limited to the placing on board of a sanitary guard and the ship must be permitted to take on fuel, water and stores. However, if the ship is infected or suspected, its passage through a canal counts as arrival at a port and it will have the full procedures applied to it.

Wherever practicable, free pratique should be granted by radio, before arrival, to a ship which represents no risk to the public health. However, the port health authority may retain the right to carry out medical examination of a ship or person on arrival, any further health procedures depending on the findings of that examination. Destination addresses in writing may be required from travellers. Any infected person may be removed and isolated by the health authority and must be so removed if the ship's master requires it. Any suspect person may be placed under surveillance until the end of the appropriate incubation period.

Once these measures have been completed, they should not be repeated at any subsequent port unless there has been a further incidence of disease or the measures have otherwise been shown to be ineffective. No ship may, for health reasons, be prevented from calling at a port. If, however, the port lacks the facilities to deal with the health problem, the ship may be ordered to the nearest port that does have them. Any ship which will not submit to these measures may be required to leave port, being permitted only to take on fuel, water and stores. It must not then call at any other port in that state.

Cargo and goods may be dealt with under these Regulations only when coming from an infected area and when there is reason to think that the goods may be contaminated with disease. Other than live animals, goods in transit may not be dealt with at all if remaining on the ship. If goods have been disinfected, the port health authority must issue a certificate, giving details, to the interested parties, including the ship's master. Baggage belonging to a healthy traveller may be disinfected or disinsected only if he is carrying infectious materials or vectors of one of the diseases subject to the Regulations. Printed matter may not be subjected to any health measure and postal parcels may be dealt with only in certain circumstances which are laid down.

4.7.5 Part V – Special Provisions Relating to Each of the Diseases Subject to the Regulations

4.7.5.1 Plague

For the purposes of the Regulations, the incubation period is 6 days. Vaccination against this disease may not be required on entry into any country.

Every country must maintain a deratting service and carry out regular examinations of rodents found in any plague-infected (or suspected) area. All precautions must be taken to prevent rodents getting on to ships. Every ship must be kept free of rodents or regularly deratted and must be in possession of a valid Deratting or Deratting Exemption Certificate issued by an approved port health authority. If such a certificate is not carried, an approved port health authority may inspect the ship and derat as necessary.

Before departure from an area infected with plague, every suspect must be isolated for 6 days. On arrival, any ship may be regarded as infected if it has a human case of plague on board or one occurs more than 6 days after embarkation or if there is a plague-infected rodent on board. It may be regarded as suspected if a case of human plague occurs less than 6 days after embarkation but there has been none since or if there has been abnormal mortality among rodents on board and the cause is unknown.

The health authority may disinsect and place under surveillance any suspect person and disinsect the baggage of any infected or suspected person or any other article considered to be contaminated. If there is, or has been during the 6 days prior to arrival, a case of pulmonary plague on board, all passengers and crews may be isolated for 6 days from the date of last exposure. If there is rodent plague on board, the ship must be disinsected and deratted, the method being laid down. When all these procedures have been completed, the ship must be regarded as healthy and given free pratique.

4.7.5.2 Cholera

For the purposes of these Regulations, the incubation period is 5 days.

If, on arrival, a case of cholera is, or has occurred, on board, the health authority may place any suspects under surveillance or isolation for 5 days from the date of disembarkation. It may remove, and dispose of, any materials (except food cargo) which it considers to be contaminated and must disinfect water tanks and food-handling equipment. When all this has been completed, the ship must be given free pratique. Any food carried as cargo may be subjected to bacteriological examination only by a health authority in the country of final destination. No one may be required to submit to rectal swabbing but a person who has come from a cholera-infected area within the 5-day incubation period and has developed symptoms suggestive of cholera may be required to submit to stool examination.

4.7.5.3 Yellow Fever

For the purposes of these Regulations, the incubation period of yellow fever is 6 days. Vaccination against yellow fever may be required of any person leaving an infected area for another country. If the person has a certificate which is not yet valid, he may nevertheless be allowed to leave, but at his destination he may be isolated until his certificate becomes valid or until 6 days after the date of last exposure, whichever is the earlier. A person having a valid certificate may not be treated as a suspect, even if he comes from an infected area. In all cases, the vaccine used must have been approved by WHO and the vaccination must be carried out at an approved centre. Every member of the crew of a ship trading into any port in an infected area must hold a valid certificate of vaccination.

Every ship leaving a port where *Aedes aegypti* still exists, for an area where it has been eradicated, must be kept free of it in all its stages. On arrival, a ship may be regarded as infected if there is a case of yellow fever on board or one has occurred on the voyage. It may be regarded as suspect if it left an infected area less than 6 days before arrival or, if arriving less than 30 days after leaving such an area, a vector of yellow fever is found on board. Any other ship must be regarded as healthy.

On arrival of an infected or suspected ship in an area where yellow fever vectors are present, any passenger or crew member who disembarks without a valid certificate of vaccination may be isolated for 6 days from the date of last exposure. Furthermore, any such ship (or any healthy ship from an infected area) may be inspected and any yellow fever vectors destroyed, and the ship may be required to keep at least 400 m from land until this is done.

When all this is completed, the ship must be given free pratique.

4.7.6 Part VI – Health Documents

Before arrival at the first port of call in any country, a ship's master must ascertain the state of health of all on board and, where the country requires it, must fill in and give to the Port Health Authority a Maritime Declaration of Health, countersigned by the ship's surgeon, if there is one. He must also provide any other health information required by the Port Health Authority.

Deratting and Deratting Exemption Certificates, the Certificate of Vaccination against Yellow Fever and the Maritime Declaration of Health are reproduced in the appendices to these Regulations and this format must be used. They must be printed in English and French and completed in one of those languages. The International Certificate of Vaccination must be signed by a medical practitioner in his own hand or by another person authorised by the national health administration. Official stamps are no substitute. If vaccination is contra-indicated on medical grounds, the vaccinator must so certify, with reasons, written in English or French "which health authorities should take into account", whatever that means!

No health document other than those set out in these Regulations may be required in international traffic.

4.7.7 Part VII – Charges

No charge may be made by a health authority for any medical or supplementary examination required to ascertain the health of the person examined or for any vaccination (or its certification) of a person on arrival. Any other charges for measures under these Regulations must conform with a national tariff, notified to WHO, and must be moderate and not exceed the actual cost of the service provided. Furthermore, there must be the same charges for each person or shipping company.

4.7.8 Part VIII – Various Provisions

Every ship leaving a port in an area where transmission of malaria or other mosquito-borne disease is occurring (of where insecticide-resistant mosquito vectors or disease are present or where a vector species is present which has been eradicated in the destination area) must be kept free from all stages of the mosquito concerned. A footnote draws attention to the need for nautical medical officers to be trained in the diagnosis and treatment of malaria and for all crews of ships in malarial areas to be given "supervised suppressant treatment during a suitable period of time".

Any ship carrying migrants, nomads, seasonal workers or pilgrims (and the people concerned) may be subjected to additional health measures as laid down by the states concerned. The standard of hygiene on such ships must not be inferior to that laid down in Annex V of the Regulations.

4.7.9 Part IX – Final Provisions

The eight articles in this part deal only with administrative provisions regulating the relations between WHO and the member states.

References

1. International health regulations (1969). 3rd annotated ed. Geneva: WHO 1983.

5 Special Fields in Nautical Medicine

5.1 Health Standards – Fitness for Duty at Sea

E. N. Watson

The International Labour Organisation has shown its concern for the health of seafarers by adopting ILO Instruments at the special maritime sessions of its conferences. The first of these Instruments, the Medical Examination of Young Persons (Sea) Convention No. 16 [3] was adopted at the 3rd ordinary session in 1921. Further attention was given to the medical examination of all seafarers at the 28th maritime session in 1946 when the Medical Examination (Seafarers) Convention No. 73 [4], which laid down certain requirements for these examinations and the related medical certificates, was adopted. These two Instruments still represent the base from which all subsequent developments have evolved.

Unfortunately, Convention No. 73 had a mixed reception and only 29 countries had ratified it by 1982. There is hope, however, that the Merchant Shipping (Minimum Standards) Convention No. 147 of 1976 [5], which requires only substantial equivalence with No. 73, will bring about wider implementation. Provision for the inspection of certificates by port state officials may add to the impetus.

The joint ILO/WHO Committee, writing in 1961 [10], regretted that the ILO Conventions and recommendations on seafarers' health had either not been ratified by all nations or not been fully implemented. It was felt that full implementation of Convention No. 73 by all seafaring countries would have considerably raised the general health standard of seafarers and forestalled many complaints, justified or otherwise, regarding unfit men being passed fit for sea. That opinion may be correct but it requires some qualification.

The essence of Convention No. 73 is the requirement that every seafarer must possess a certificate attesting "that he is not suffering from any disease likely to be aggravated by or to render him unfit for service at sea or likely to endanger the health of other persons on board". That advice, while excellent as a general statement, leaves open the determination of the many diseases which would preclude work at sea. It has rested with the competent authority in each country to determine the crucial issue of specific health standards. In consequence, differing sets of medical criteria have been evolved in the maritime countries and that position remains unchanged.

The lack of international criteria had been recognised by the World Health Assembly in 1948, when the Joint ILO/WHO Committee on the Hygiene of Seafarers was set up [7]. At its first session in December, 1949 the Joint Committee selected for early study a number of subjects, including the standard of fitness for seafarers. This was considered at the conference organised by the Regional Office for Europe of the World Health Organisation in Marseilles (in 1959) [2]. The prophylactic value of the pre-employment medical examination of seamen was generally acknowledged. However, it was agreed that although it was simple to set standards to exclude chronic somatic diseases, there remained many lesser medical conditions where it was extremely difficult, or impossible, to make such precise recommendations. The need to resolve the difficulty was reiterated at further ILO Maritime Meetings in 1967 [12] and 1970 [8] but the matter has remained in abeyance.

The difficulties of achieving an international consensus on health matters was well illustrated by reaction to the ILO/IMCO/WHO International Medical Guide for Ships [6] and the accompanying list of approved essential drugs. Despite its representation of modern medical opinion over the wide range of subjects at that time, national differences in medical practices and treatment resulted in many countries producing their own guides. This position remains unchanged and WHO still admits that the preparation of a drug list [13] of uniform, general applicability and acceptability is not possible. Each country is left with the direct responsibility of evaluating and adopting drugs according to its own policy in the field of health. This fact has considerable bearing when setting national medical standards and it militates against achieving international agreement.

It might appear extraordinary that after so many years it has not been possible to produce, and to agree, a set of international medical standards. However, those who have been involved in the complicated issues of setting national standards would not share that view. Even where it is possible to get agreement between the doctors involved in the task, their decisions may conflict with general legislation governing the rights of employed persons. Full medical facilities are taken for granted ashore but very few doctors work in merchant ships, with certain exceptions such as the Polish merchant fleet (Tomaszunas, et al. [14]). Medical treatment has therefore become the responsibility of designated ships' officers whose ability to diagnose and treat is commensurate with their limited medical training and knowledge. This circumstance excludes many medical conditions which could be permitted at sea under the supervision of a doctor. In consequence, practices and treatments which are used ashore but are unsuitable in the context of seafaring, can cause conflict with medical colleagues who frequently have little understanding of the medical and administrative problems affecting seafarers.

At national level, in an attempt to overcome these difficulties, the responsibility for supervising the health of seafarers is usually shared by government, seafarers' organisations and shipowners. Their tripartite agreements are often issued in the form of statutory regulations governing the various aspects of the medical examination to be carried out. The potentially hazardous nature of seafaring is given much consideration in deciding the objectives, content and method of the medical examination, together with detailed advice on diseases considered to be incompatible with seafaring. In addition to the inherent dangers of navigating in any kind of climate, weather and sea conditions, a ship has much moving machinery in the engine-room, on deck and elsewhere. It is not only a place of work requiring attention throughout the day and night, but also a temporary home in which the crew must eat, sleep and find recreation. The crew itself is a closed community divided by traditional hierarchy into the three departments, deck, engine-room and catering, which are supervised by the shipmaster and his officers. These officers are responsible for carrying out statutory regulations to ensure the safety of a ship. It follows that a seafarer unable to fit in or unwilling to take responsibility or to accept a reasonable measure of discipline, could impair efficiency and affect safety. Within the confines of such an ordered society day-to-day relationships tend to be formal and that, combined with the limited facilities for recreation, the separation from family and friends and rapid turnround in port, can lead to tension. Much has been done to ameliorate living and working conditions but some difficulties can never be completely overcome. The propulsion engines and generators produce noise and vibration which, although suppressed, are constantly present in the background. The ship's movement, external weather conditions, forced ventilation system and acoustic properties of the materials used in ship construction may add significantly to this discomfort.

A fuller description of life and work aboard can be found elsewhere but the current trend is towards employing fewer seafarers in a crew carefully adjusted in size to obtain maximum efficiency. This is particularly relevant in newer ships with much modern equipment where the crew is required to be more highly trained and skilled than in former years. Any illness aboard ship may throw an extra burden on the other crew members, who are obliged to take over the extra duties wherever possible in addition to nursing and treating the sick person. It follows that there can be no category of "light work" at sea. All jobs must be properly performed and all crew capable of carrying out strenuous tasks in the event of an emergency. Nevertheless, the extent of duties and their physical requirements have a definite bearing on the application of medical standards and doctors dealing with seafarers should understand fully the nature of each job if sensible decisions are to be made.

Serious illness occurring unexpectedly and perhaps at the least opportune time in ship operation presents great difficulty for the shipmaster. He would always obtain medical advice by radio which might enable him to remain on course without prejudice to the patient. Alternatively, he would if necessary divert his ship to nearby help from another ship or to port in circumstances where a life might be endangered. It is in the true interest of all that such costly diversions and delay should be avoided wherever possible by excluding seafarers of suspect health.

A comparison of the various national sets of medical standards shows much general agreement on the medical conditions which are regarded as a bar to seafaring. It is pertinent to reflect on how these lists have been drawn up. A great deal has been written and published on the medical aspects of seafaring and the bibliography published by the Department of Nautical Medicine, Bernhard-Nocht-Institute, Hamburg gives nearly six thousand references. Yet, surprisingly little has been written on the method employed in arriving at the lists. It would seem that the doctors responsible for examining seafarers in each country have drawn on their experience of morbidity and mortality to produce similar conclusions.

It has always been extremely difficult to elicit medical statistics on diseases affecting seafarers which would satisfy strict epidemiological criteria. This has been acknowledged at WHO/ILO conferences but, nevertheless, it has been possible to identify categories of diseases which are more prevalent. From these categories diseases liable to cause unacceptable consequences can be culled for addition to the basic list of chronic somatic diseases and disorders seriously affecting bodily function or the special senses such as eyesight and hearing. In addition, analysis of radio requests for medical advice has assisted in identifying intercurrent illnesses whilst on articles aboard ship (Brayley [1] and Schepers [11]).

The system used in applying medical standards varies from country to country. It is common to find that a single set of standards has been laid down which is applied strictly when examining young entrants but due allowance for age and the nature of the duties to be performed is made when assessing serving seafarers in accordance with those standards. In effect, that system has purposely avoided setting definitive standards for serving seafarers; an individual and arbitrary assessment is made in each case. Wherever a number of doctors is entrusted with the examination of seafarers, there should be accepted rulings to be observed in order that their decisions may be seen to be uniform and fair. A medical standard by definition should be a measure to which all decisions may conform. All too often many of the national sets contain positive, concise rulings that are vitiated by qualifying clauses which render them difficult to interpret and apply. That can lead to conflicting opinions on "fitness" from shipping doctors involved in any particular case and the difficulty may be compounded by additional views from family doctors and hospital consultants.

The overall responsibility within any industry rests with its management. It is less than satisfactory to burden lay managers and union officials with problems which they are not competent to solve. Wherever decisions are in accordance with unambiguous medical standards agreed by both sides, friction is kept to a minimum.

It could be argued that medical practice is so complex and the individual response to illness so varied, that it is not possible to devise firm medical standards for use in dealing with serving seafarers. That perpetuates the concept that arbitrary assessment by individual doctors is superior to a consensus ruling. If that is accepted, no further efforts should be made. However, there is an alternative method which could be explored. This would define a set of strict criteria for those entering the industry, bearing in mind the limited use and application of seamanship skills when applying for work ashore. A breakdown in health early in a career may cause difficulty in obtaining suitable retraining and, in that context, it represents wasted years. A similar breakdown in mid-career at a time when domestic and financial responsibilities may be at their height, must be avoided wherever possible. This is a rational approach to protect the interests of applicants to the industry, but different considerations apply when dealing with the inevitable impairment in health which will affect the serving seafarers. It is therefore necessary to have a separate set of standards for them. This set should be based upon the entrant standards but should also define for the commonly occurring diseases, the point in the progression of the pathological process where continued seafaring becomes unacceptably hazardous. Many of these common diseases are amenable to treatment which, if timely and successful, will enable a quick return to sea duty. However, it is necessary for the examining doctor to have an agreed ruling to ensure the compliance of the patient. This is also necessary when dealing with the more serious diseases which may result in a permanent bar to seafaring.

It is impossible to include specific advice on every medical condition which might be encountered. In order that such cases are not left to arbitrary decision, it is necessary to include a general statement of principles to be observed which may be used when assessing the suitability of persons suffering from the rarer diseases. This should, amongst other considerations, take account of the side-effects and incompatibilities of any required medication and include the therapeutic consequences of losing a medicine or being unable to obtain it abroad. The willingness or ability of the patient to comply with the treatment is another important issue. It should also exclude those suffering from a medical condition where the possibility of serious exacerbation requiring expert treatment could occur during the voyage.

It may be possible in a national fleet or in a shipping company to impose a condition of restricted service. By this means a particular type of ship or shipping trade may be avoided and the length of voyage may be adjusted to fit in with medical requirements. An acceptable degree of flexibility is thus introduced but the system can succeed only if used with discretion. In some countries it has been customary to place in the coastal trades seafarers who are no longer medically suitable for prolonged deep sea voyages. However, coastal work is often more arduous than other shipping trades and it may place an added strain on a seafarer of impaired health. It is also undesirable that the coastal trades should accumulate a significantly greater proportion of seafarers who are medically sub-standard. The benefit of a restricted service system is mainly to accommodate seafarers suffering from a remediable condition which needs close supervision and treatment over a short period.

Irrespective of the system chosen, it is essential that a procedure for dealing with appeals against decisions of permanent unfitness for sea service and restriction of service should be introduced. The ILO Convention No. 73 stipulates that such appeals should be lodged with a medical referee or referees who shall be independent of any shipowner or of any organisation of shipowners or seafarers. That arrangement is undoubtedly fair to seafarers but, unless the referee has a full knowledge of working conditions at sea and experience of nautical medicine, decisions unacceptable to shipping doctors will be made.

5.1.1 Differences in Regulations Concerning Specific Disorders

It is not my intention, nor is it possible here, to make widespread comparisons of the different sets of national medical standards. But it is instructive to look closely at the advice given in these sets when dealing with some of the more commonly occurring diseases such as diabetes mellitus, hypertension, ischaemic heart disease, myocardial infarction and epilepsy.

5.1.1.1 Diabetes

Most nations bar diabetics from entry into the shipping industry. Few would quarrel with that decision yet just as few are able to agree on advice regarding serving seafarers who develop the disease during their career. The insulin-dependent Swede may continue at sea unless the insulin doses prove difficult to adjust. A Frenchman may continue on certain types of voyage, provided the condition is stabilised by diet or oral treatment. A German requiring insulin is barred, but milder cases may continue on oral treatment only, if strict diet is not required. A Dutchman should be barred but the history of his previous employment on board ships would be a major factor affecting the assessment. A Briton would continue only if the condition could be controlled by food restriction without strict diet, insulin or oral treatment. A Norwegian requiring insulin would not be permitted to sail on foreign-going vessesl but might be allowed to continue in the coastal trades or on ferries in the North Sea.

That represents a considerable range of opinion on case disposal and given that the disease and its progression are similar in each country, an explanation for the diversity should be sought. To evaluate these rulings it is necessary to weigh various factors which include the basic knowledge of the disease process and its treatment, epidemiological studies and the occupational aspects.

The pathology of diabetes mellitus and the usual clinical course are common knowledge. The severity of the metabolic disorder is in direct proportion to the degree of insulin deficiency. About a quarter of all diabetics have a deficiency severe enough to require insulin injections to maintain whatever control of blood glucose is possible when balanced against carbohydrate and other energy intake. The life expectancy of affected persons, even those who are without symptoms, is reduced by the accompanying progressive arterial degeneration. Most diabetics will die not from fluctuations of blood glucose but from the manifestations of arterial degeneration. To accept that does not underestimate the consequences of marked fluctuations which may cause either ketosis or hypoglycaemia. Acute infection and serious injury are frequent precipitating causes. Both must be regarded as serious emergencies which need skilled urgent attention if tragedies are to be avoided.

If such cases are permitted to remain at sea, due consideration should have been given to several occupational factors. There is the impracticality of catering for individual food preferences or all the requirements of a prescribed diet as opposed to general food restriction. This is especially so when linked to the watchkeeping system which covers periods of duty throughout the night, when full catering facilities are not available. In addition, those responsible for the ship's safety in adverse weather in busy shipping lanes may for long periods be unable to leave their post. In such circumstances, carefully measured food and fluid intake is a secondary consideration and this may lead to temporary hypoglycaemia which, even if not severe enough to precipitate collapse, may mar judgement. Ever present is the knowledge that it is not always possible to gauge with much precision the degree of arterial degeneration affecting the peripheral and central blood vessels, so an extra mortality from unpredictable myocardial infarction and allied conditions must be accepted.

Most countries have decided against the employment at sea of insulin-dependent serving seafarers. It is likely that the decision has been based upon a concept of what medical surveillance can be expected to achieve. In making allowance for the other complications of diabetes which affect also the eyes, kidneys and neuromuscular system, it may be felt that it is not possible or, indeed, desirable that surveillance should embrace the monitoring of a severe disease process through to the point where life is endangered or severe disability appears.

The remaining three-quarters of all diabetics are mainly of the maturity onset type, the majority of whom are, or have been, overweight. It is generally accepted that overnutrition is the most important aetiological factor in this group. Most of these cases can be treated solely by restricting food intake. The success of this treatment depends on the willingness of the patient to maintain the altered eating habit. Those who are able and willing to comply succeed in leading an apparently normal life in which it is reasonable to suppose that the pathological process has been slowed to a degree acceptable under strict medical supervision. Most countries are prepared to allow continued service in such cases where the seafarer will play his part fully in following the treatment regime. However, there is always a minority unable to reduce food intake. It is common practice to prescribe oral hypoglycaemic drugs for these patients. The rationale of such therapy for seafarers is open to question. There is no suggestion of cure and major studies over a substantial period such as that by Meinert et al. [9] have shown that the prognosis is not improved by this treatment. The oral hypoglycaemic drugs have incompatibilities, side-effects and contra-indications to use. On balance, this should be weighed against the ability of these drugs to moderate fluctuations of blood glucose for a patient unable to control his appetite and therefore with an accelerated disease process.

With this view of the three categories of diabetic patients, it is possible to formulate a standard which is reasoned and compatible with an agreed overall philosophy which has been accepted by any group of doctors entrusted with the task. And yet, as already cited, there is little agreement between countries on case disposal although the medical position is common knowledge. There are differences in national medical practices and attitudes to disease but that is not a convincing explanation. The answer probably lies within the conflict of interests of those involved in the industry: shipowners, insurers, government, unions and seafarers. The medical interest and well-being of the seafarer should always be the paramount consideration. But, paradoxically, medical advice to that end is not always acceptable to a seafarer. Some can envisage no other sort of life, nor can they adjust to the thought of illness and unemployment ashore. Within a system of arbitrary assessment it is unfortunately usual that those who protest most vigorously, and who can rally most support from unions, politicians and doctors ashore, manage to remain at sea long after they have become medically unsound.

The shipowners are responsible, usually under law, for providing and paying for any medical attention required by the crew. They accept with good grace the cost of medical emergencies which cannot be foreseen but they expect crews to be free from the risk of predictable illness. The ship owners usually join with the seafarers' organisations in ensuring that an acceptable system of medical surveillance is maintained. Nevertheless, no system is trouble-free, and it is in those circumstances when doctors fail to agree that issues other than the purely medical may intrude.

Diabetes mellitus was chosen as a good illustrative example of the many difficulties which have to be resolved if a workable solution is to be reached. The resolution of those difficulties is fundamentally concerned with the identification of a definite stage in the progression of disease beyond which it is not possible to support the risks of the treatment regime and possible complications of the disease itself.

5.1.1.2 Cardiovascular Disease

The cardiovascular degenerative diseases present some similar problems. Most countries will not permit seafaring if there is evidence of organic heart disease or serious disorder of conduction, rhythm or rate. The diagnosis is usually firmly based and the disposal in these cases is clear-cut. Unfortunately, that does not apply when dealing with essential hypertension without other demonstrable evidence of hypertensive heart disease.

In the United Kingdom, as well as some other countries, coronary heart disease is the major cause of death in middle and old age. The seafaring population shares that fate. Hypertension is a major precursor to both ischaemic heart disease and coronary occlusion. In the natural progression of hypertension both these complications occur at a rate which is somewhere between double and treble that to be expected in the unaffected. Wherever hypertensive patients are allowed to continue working at sea, an increased mortality and morbidity must be accepted.

Once again there is much disparity between the national standards. Some countries will go no further than suggesting that the cause, severity and complications should be considered. Others state that any excess over 100 mmHg diastolic pressure is unacceptable, while yet others set figures for both systolic and diastolic pressures. The difficulty is the general reluctance of doctors to state what should be regarded as a normal blood pressure.

However, the introduction of the specific antihypertensive drugs has forced some general agreement on the level of pressure at which treatment for uncomplicated essential hypertension should be commenced. As a general guide when treating those under 65 it is regarded as reasonable and prudent to prescribe when the diastolic pressure reaches 100 mmHg recorded at the fifth phase. There is less agreement on the level at which raised systolic pressure should be treated but some studies suggest 165 mmHg. In setting a standard it may then be held that above the level of 165/100 mmHg the risks of complications have increased to an unacceptable degree. If that is fixed as a maximum permitted untreated level, the position is clear. But the question of accepting those treated with antihypertensive drugs at higher levels remains to be answered.

The cardiovascular degenerative diseases are progressive ill-understood disorders which are not amenable to curative treatment. Hypertension is a single manifestation which can be controlled but it requires daily medication, often for prolonged periods and sometimes for life, with powerful drugs which have well-documented side-effects and incompatibilities. For patients with well-controlled pressure the rate of strokes and kidney damage will be reduced but it has yet to be convincingly shown that the myocardial infarction rate is significantly reduced or the progression of the underlying degenerative process slowed. There has been a plethora of published work on all aspects of the use of the antihypertensive drugs and it is not possible to cover that ground here. It must be considered in great detail with the utmost care before a decision is reached. However, in the context of standards, certain aspects are important. Once treatment has been started, it must not be stopped abruptly. A guaranteed supply of the drug and confidence in compliance from the patient would be obligatory. Many hypertensive patients are considerably overweight and some are unwilling to moderate their food and alcohol consumption or to deal with other risk factors which may be present. Whether treated or not treated, they represent a "poor risk" group. And so, many specific factors must be delineated. These include decisions on whether there should be satisfactory control of personal habits and reduction to desirable weight before treatment is started with nominated drugs (some are unsuitable) for which a maximum permissible dose would have to be stated. Perhaps the most difficult problem is the assessment of the underlying disease process by ordinary clinical methods without repeated very specialised procedures. Angina pectoris may be suppressed and the heart rate slowed in treated hypertension. The true level of blood pressure will be unknown. The electrocardiogram is not a wholly reliable indicator. Various studies such as the Framingham survey have indicated the limitations of the ECG in detecting disease (Wilson and Junger [15]). It may be felt that these complex matters can be resolved satisfactorily and a rational standard formulated which fulfils the requirements of Convention No. 73 [4]. However, it is doubtful that this objective could be achieved and, if that conclusion is accepted, treatment with antihypertensive drugs at sea should not be permitted. In reality it constitutes the medical supervision of a serious disease by less than reliable methods which may not detect impending dangerous complications.

Most national sets of standards regard organic disease of the heart and major blood vessels as a bar to further seafaring. That decision is complicated by recent advances in surgical procedures such as heart valve replacement, coronary artery by-pass surgery and the repair of aortic aneurysms. The replacement valves used, whether prosthetic or tissue, are prone to develop serious incompetence. A prosthetic valve, which is usually supported by anticoagulant therapy to reduce the risk of emboli, may fail suddenly within hours or several days. Tissue valve failure is usually more gradual over several days or weeks. Transient ischaemic attacks with accompanying focal neurological disorder can occur in patients receiving either type of valve. These occurrences are often unpredictable and of too serious consequence to be considered safe for seafaring. The improved quality of life following these life-saving operations is not sufficient reason to put aside the known possible sequelae. The same consideration applies to coronary artery by-pass surgery which, although bringing symptomatic relief of anginal pain, does not exclude the risk of sudden occlusion of the graft or affect the progression of the already considerable degree of arterial degeneration. There is, as yet, doubt that the general prognosis is significantly improved or the rate of sudden death reduced to an acceptable level. Whatever the final outcome of balancing the conflicting opinions from various studies, it is highly unlikely that the level will be acceptable. For the same reason the degree of arterial disease which is necessary to produce an aortic aneurysm would preclude a seafarer even after a successful repair. Peripheral vascular disease causing intermittent claudication is in the same category and it has been shown to be associated with increased risk of arterial disease affecting the heart and brain.

In most countries myocardial infarction precludes further seafaring. No condition exemplifies better the disparity between the disposal of seafarers and workers ashore. It is current practice that an landsman should be encouraged to return to work as soon as possible after the acute phase has passed. It is recognised that the prognosis is unpredictable no matter how favourable the clinical assessment may suggest. It is virtually impossible to arrange life insurance during the first year following the infarction and thereafter, obtainable only on penalty of very heavy extra premium. The percentage of sudden deaths and lesser complications reported varies but, even at the lowest figure most countries feel that the risk is too high for seafaring.

5.1.1.3 Peptic Ulcers

In dealing with peptic ulceration the natural history of the disease is the paramount consideration in setting a standard. This diathesis is uninfluenced by any type of treatment. Before the advent of H_2-receptor blocking drugs and the widespread use of endoscopy, it was customary to allow a return to seafaring after a period ashore following healing of the ulcer in an initial attack. With any recurrent ulceration, the seafarer could choose between staying ashore or seeking a surgical cure. There is no indication that treatment with cimetidine has altered the position. Although about three-quarters of all ulcers will heal within 6 weeks given adequate dosage of cimetidine, just about the same number will relapse within a year of stopping the treatment.

During remissions of the disease, daily treatment with a low dose of cimetidine will keep a patient free of symptoms. However, a significant number of cases will relapse during long-term treatment and the high relapse rate after stopping the treatment will be unaffected. This is an unresolved problem which may be acceptable in the management of patients on land but is not tolerable at sea. Intestinal haemorrhage or perforation while at sea are dreaded complications which carry a high mortality.

5.1.1.4 Epilepsy

In most standards epilepsy is a complete bar to service at sea. Among serving seafarers when cases occur, a few are caused by organic disease, some by alcoholism but most are classified as idiopathic in origin. In many of these cases, fits can be suppressed for most of the time by a single anti-epileptic drug provided that the patient will regulate his life and comply unswervingly with daily medication. In a fresh case, the dose and frequency of administration needs careful adjustment to balance suppression of fits against possible side-effects of the drug. This therapy will extend over an indefinite period until at least 2 years have passed without a fit. The drug may then be gradually withdrawn over a trial period. Administratively, it is not possible to accommodate absences of such length although, medically, some could be re-admitted on the completion of this prolonged treatment.

5.1.2 Conclusion

This chapter has presented a philosophy for medical supervision and, by selected examples, attempted to demonstrate a method of setting definitive medical standards for seafarers. It is polemic, dogmatic and unashamed if it succeeds in promoting new thought and discussion for a very important but neglected subject. Many of the sets of standards in force at present contain enough waivers and qualifying clauses to make them ambiguous and difficult to apply with any consistency. A stricter interpretation of Convention No. 73 [4] is needed to meet the requirements of modern ships employing fewer seafarers in more specialised jobs. But, to be successful and acceptable, it should be linked to proper financial provision for those who suffer a breakdown in health during their career, together with facilities for retraining in work ashore.

The framework of international conventions and recommendations has been available for many years. It rests with the occupational physicians engaged in nautical medicine to accept the challenge. The seafarers of all countries, their unions and employers have a right to expect international medical standards to ensure a uniform, consistent high level of health protection.

References

1. Brayley, N.F.: A review of three years experience of medical advice to seafarers by the casualty officer, Royal Navy Hospital, Plymouth, via Portishead Radio (W/T Medico Portishead). J. Roy. nav. med. Serv. *66,* 2, 93–106 (1980).
2. Conference on the health and welfare of seafarers. Marseille: WHO, Regional Office for Europe 1959.
3. Convention concerning medical examination of children and young persons employed at sea. Convention No.16. Geneva: ILO 1921. pp.67–69.
4. Convention concerning medical examination of seafarers. Convention No.73. Geneva: ILO 1946. pp.633–637.
5. Convention concerning merchant shipping (Miniumum standards). Convention No.147. Geneva: ILO 1976.
6. International Medical Guide for ships. Ed.: ILO, IMCO, WHO. Geneva: WHO 1967.
7. Joint ILO/WHO committee on the hygiene of seafarers. Report on the first session. Geneva: WHO 1950. (Technical Report Series No.20).
8. Maritime Conference 1970. Geneva: ILO 1970.
9. Meinert, C.L., G.L. Knatterud, T.E. Prout et al.: A study of the effects of hypoglycemic agents on vascular complications in patients with adult-onset diabetes. II Mortality results. Diabetes *19,* Suppl. 789–830 (1970).
10. Nature and extent of the health problems of seafarers. In: Joint ILO/WHO committee on the hygiene of seafarers. Third report. Geneva: WHO 1961, pp.3–5. (Technical Report Series No.244).
11. Schepers, B.-F.: Die funkärztliche Beratung von Seeschiffen am Stadtkrankenhaus Cuxhaven. Notfallmed. *7,* 1146–1158 (1981).
12. Seafarers' health and welfare. Geneva: ILO Joint Maritime Commission 1967. JMC/20/5.
13. Selection of essential drugs. Geneva: WHO 1977. (Technical Report Series No.615).
14. Tomaszunas, S., J. Filikowski, A. Jankowski: The organisation of health service for seafarers in Poland. Bull. Inst. mar. Med. Gdansk *24,* 3/4, 265–274 (1973).
15. Wilson, J.M.G. and G. Junger: Principles and practice of screening for diseases. Geneva: WHO. (Publ. Health Papers No.34).

5.2 Toxicology in Seafaring – Dangerous Goods

L. M. Shafran

Serving as the basis for the development of shipboard toxicology for the last two decades has been the increasing importance of chemical factors in relation to a) the characteristics of work and rest of seagoing personnel of modern ships of all types and descriptions, and b) environmental pollution. Shipboard toxicology is part of preventive toxicology, dealing with the interreaction between the organism and chemical factors under specific conditions of shipboard environment (Tiunov and Savateev [19]).

Notwithstanding the great variety of indices such as quality and quantity, sources and nature, as well as properties of shipboard chemical factors, these can be integrated from the point of view of hygiene into three main groups: a) dangerous chemical goods, b) polymeric and synthetic materials c) chemically harmful substances in everyday life and work (Fig. 1). As can be seen from the diagram, one of the leading trends in shipboard toxicology is the study of the properties of dangerous goods and their toxic affects on the body resulting in biological changes, as well as the working out of effective measures for ensuring the safety of personnel, ships and port structures and for protecting the environment during shipment, handling and storing of dangerous goods (Andronov and Shafran [2]; Zorn [25]; Kolkovski [10]).

Included as dangerous goods are substances and articles which, in carriage, may be the cause of explosions, fires or damage to vessels, structures, warehouses or buildings, as well as loss of life, injury, poisoning, burns, irradiation or diseases of men and animals. In a wider toxicological sense the deleterious effect of noxious substances is understood as not only their ability to cause acute and chronic poisoning but also a) their capacity for acting selectively on some organs and physiological systems, macromolecules and metabolic links, b) their capacity for affecting the ability of the organism to react and c) their blastomogenic, embryotoxic, teratogenic and mutagenic effects (Sanotskii and Ulanova [16], Kagan [9]). However, in marine cargo handling operations and hygiene, a still wider use has been found for the primary definition as it includes in practice the whole variety of adverse effects connected with the carriage of dangerous goods by sea. It also presents a reasonable basis for studying the effects of particular goods or the whole range of dangerous cargoes carried by sea and can therefore be used effectively in maritime hygiene.

In recent years an ecological trend in shipboard toxicology has developed, finding its reflection in the work on environmental protection in ships carrying dangerous goods (Navaz [15]; Ulewicz [22]; Voitenko and Shafran [23]). Up to the present time, however, except for the well-developed studies on the prevention of pollution of the sea by oil, little progress has been made in investigating the effects of dangerous goods transported by sea.

5.2.1 Definitions and Criteria of Hazard

The dominant hazardous properties of many cargoes are flammability, liability to

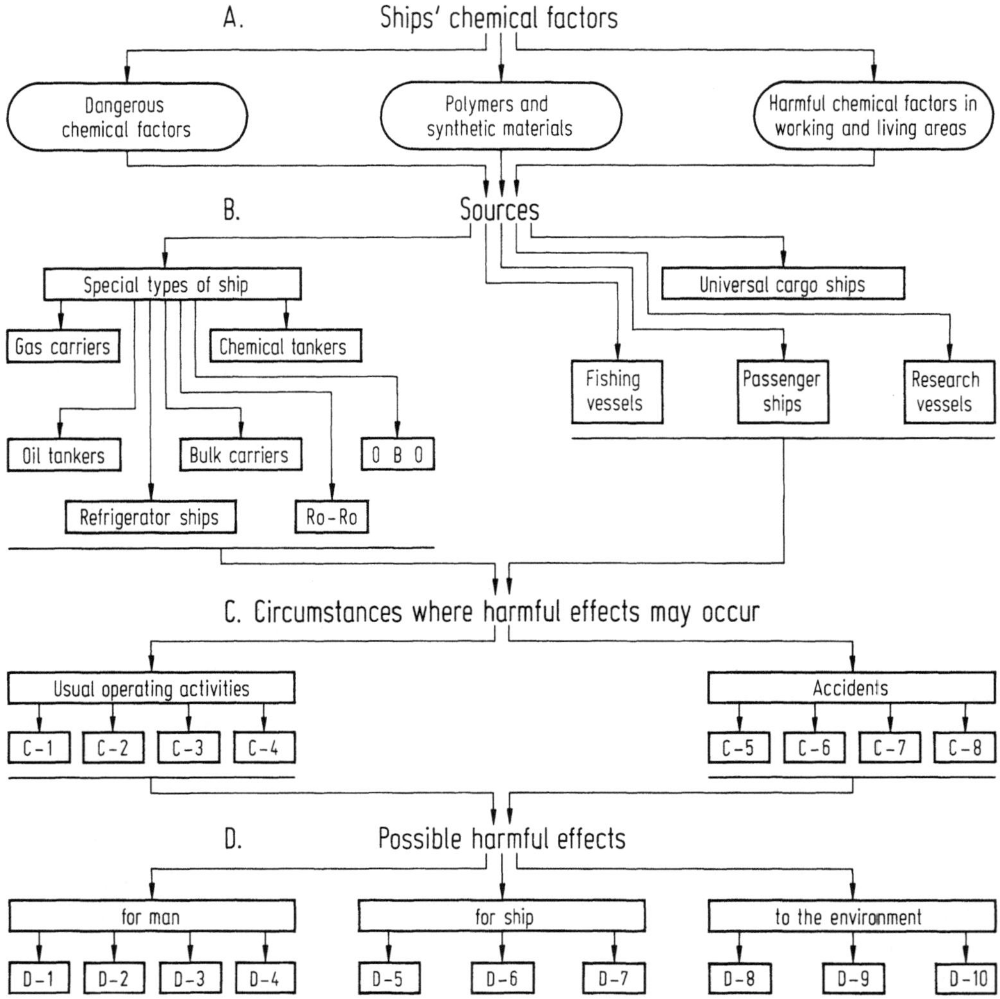

Fig. 1. General system (schematic) of ship's chemical factors showing sources, conditions and possible harmful effects. *C-1*, loading/unloading; *C-2*, sea voyage; *C-3*, tank washing; *C-4*, fumigation; *C-5*, corrosive effects; *C-6*, fire on board; *C-7*, explosion; *C-8*, water in holds; *D-1*, acute poisoning; *D-2*, chronic poisoning (diseases caused by poisoning); *D-3*, slowly developing toxic process; *D-4*, toxic effect causing a change in the normal ability of the organism to react (disadaptation); *D-5*, fire on booard; *D-6*, explosion; *D-7*, corrosive effect; *D-8*, atmosphere; *D-9*, sea; *D-10*, coast

explode and toxicity, and goods can easily be categorized according to these properties. Other goods disclose their hazardous properties only under specific conditions (for instance, goods which emit toxic gases and vapours when they come into contact with water or fire and goods which have been infected before shipment with pathogenic bacteria, spores, viruses etc.). In all these cases, the goods are to be regarded as dangerous, bearing in mind that their hazardous properties could appear in emergency situations.

Considering the fact that the exhibition of hazardous properties by various goods depends both on the goods themselves and on the specific conditions of transportation, which usually differ from those in industry, agriculture and everyday life, it is necessary to define such basic concepts as transport hazard and transport toxicity.

From the viewpoint of toxicology and

hygiene, transport hazard is the totality of properties of the cargo which define its ability to have adverse effects on the human body, the vessel and the environment under specific conditions of transport. The amount of cargo, the type of packing, the stowage location on board, the nature of adjacent cargoes and the direction and duration of the voyages, as well as many other factors of marine transport, have a considerable bearing on the transport hazard.

Transport toxicity is a more individual and specific concept involving the ability of the goods during their transport, storage and handling to have various kinds of toxic effect on the human organism and on the environmental flora and fauna. Naturally, the goods with toxic properties are given more specific attention by the marine sanitary service and the shipboard medical personnel.

The variety of hazardous properties of shipped goods was duly reflected in the integral classification of dangerous goods (Table 1) approved and accepted by the International Maritime Organization (IMO). This classification has been evolved in compliance with Regulation 2 of Chapter VII of the International Conference on Safety of Life at Sea (1960) and served as the basis for the International Maritime Dangerous Goods Code [8], which is the principal document specifying conditions regarding overseas transport of dangerous goods.

Table 1. International classification of dangerous goods

Class	Description
1.	Explosives
2.	Gases: compressed, liquefied or dissolved under pressure
3.	Inflammable liquids
4.1.	Inflammable solids
4.2.	Inflammable solids, or substances, liable to spontaneous combustion
4.3.	Inflammable solids, or substances, which in contact with water emit inflammable gases
5.1.	Oxidizing substances
5.2.	Organic peroxides
6.1.	Poisonous (toxic) substances
6.2.	Infectious substances
7.	Radioactive substances
8.	Corrosives
9.	Miscellaneous dangerous substances, that is any other substance which experience has shown, or may show, to be of a dangerous character

The IMO Dangerous Goods Code consists of a general description and alphabetical index of dangerous goods, and contains regulations for carriage of all classes of dangerous goods, as well as special regulations for carriage of dangerous goods in standard containers, tank containers, Ro-Ro ships, ferries and container ships. Each cargo label should contain: description and properties of the substance, type and kind of container and packing, maximum amount of substance in container, shipping specifications and danger signs.

Medical information on dangerous goods, including their toxic properties, methods of first aid, treatment and prevention of poisoning have been given in the Medical First Aid Guide for Use in Accidents Involving Dangerous Goods [14]) issued jointly by the IMO, the World Health Organization (WHO) and the International Labour Organization (ILO).

The acceptance of the IMO Dangerous Goods Code by the majority of maritime countries and the use of its basic statements in the elaboration of the respective national regulations played an important part in solving a number of problems in the ensuring of safety of navigation and safety of life at sea.

Such hazardous properties of goods as explosive risk, fire hazard and radioactivity are assessed according to specially elaborated criteria. With regard to the assessment of the toxic properties of substances, the UNO Committee of Experts [21] proposed criteria for the classification of dangerous goods depending on their physical state and the route of exposure (Table 2).

Consideration of the criteria indicated in Table 2 is of vital importance for the pre-

Table 2. Criteria for classification of dangerous goods depending on degree of toxicity, physical state and route of exposure

Route of exposure	Criterion (measure)	Danger group		
		I	II	III
Through mouth (perorally)	mg/kg	< 5	5–50	50–500[a] 50–2000[b]
Through skin (percutaneously)	mg/kg	<40	40–200	200–1000
By inhaling:				
Vapor and gases	mg/m³	<50	50–200	200–1000
Dust	mg/m³	< 0.5	0.5–2.0	2.0–10.0

[a] For solids
[b] For liquids

vention of accidents among seamen and dockside workers, especially in emergency incidents involving real danger of acute poisoning. At the same time, it must be taken into account that the median lethal doses (LD_{50}) and concentrations (LC_{50}) have been established in toxicological experiments on laboratory animals and may differ substantially from those with respect to human beings, depending on their specific and individual features, as well as on the specific shipping conditions. The latter are of paramount importance because, as emphasized by Chaigneau [4], the toxicological principle of classification of vapours and gases can be evaluated only relatively because their toxicity varies with the rise of temperature, reduction of oxygen content and presence of carbon monoxide and carbon dioxide and other gases in the surrounding air, i.e. environmental conditions typically existing in ships' spaces.

5.2.2 Shipping Conditions and Toxic Effects of Dangerous Goods

The ship is an industrial and communal entity, the distinctive features of which have a pronounced influence on the toxic effects of dangerous goods and other chemical factors on seamen. Pertaining to these features, as shown by Shafran et al. [18], are:

1. Unity of work and rest zones of the crew, owing to the limited size of the ship and superstructure – habitat of the seamen
2. Prolonged and continous adverse effects present at sea due to the weather along with the influence of physical, chemical and socio-psychological, occupational and everyday-life conditions on board
3. The dynamic nature of the complicated range of adverse environmental factors acting on seamen, among which the major component cannot always be discerned
4. Constant stress in the work of seamen which, in combination with the general lack of physical activity, makes them more prone to any toxic effects.
5. Conditions of continous relative social isolation when living within a small group of men, combined with general sensory deprivation. This may cause the seaman to overestimate possible dangers and to over-react in emergencies.

Apart from this, there are conditions which influence the potential toxic danger on board ship. These are the purpose and type of the ship, the duration of the voyage and the sailing area, and specific features appertaining to the working activities of various professional groups within the ship's complement.

It is important to bear in mind toxicological hazards during loading of goods, passage by sea with the cargo on board, discharging of goods, stripping, washing or gas-freeing of holds and tanks, and also passage by sea in ballast with degassed or undegassed tanks. The last stage is important with respect to tankers, gas carriers and bulk chemical carriers.

The handling of dangerous goods in ports involves the accumulation of large amounts of toxic substances within limited areas or spaces (cars, piers, holds) and their transfer by lifting cranes, vehicles and dockside workers, which creates a risk of damage to the containers and packing and thus a risk of poisoning a great number of seamen and workers in a short time. During these handling operations, the principal sources of gas emission and dust formation are the goods stowed on shore. When discharging the goods, a short intensive release of vapours and gases may take place upon opening the holds, owing to the accumulation of fumes during the voyage following contact of chemical substances with water, intensive oxidizing processes during the voyage, or damage to containers and packing etc. All these factors must be taken into consideration when elaborating measures to ensure safety in handling dangerous goods.

The passage by sea with cargo on board is the chief part of the overall transport process and the longest period when the seaman is likely to come into contact with the carried goods. During this period, noxious substances are emitted into the surrounding atmosphere exclusively from the ship's sources, and the estimated concentration of vapours and gases depends on the period of time the goods are stowed on board, as well as on the climatic and geographical conditions of navigation (especially on the metereological factors).

Any forthcoming change of cargo or repairs to the ship demand special preparation of the cargo spaces, which is known on dry cargo vessels and bulkers as cleaning of holds, and in tankers as stripping, washing and degassing of tanks. Although these stages are of relatively short duration, they include intensive labour-consuming operations with considerable expenditure of energy on the part of the members of the crew. These operations are also characterized by a sharp increase in the concentration of noxious fumes and dust in the air, not only in the cargo spaces but often in the crew accommodation areas as well, whereby the toxic substances are not only inhaled but also find their way into the organism through the skin.

From the above it can be seen that consideration of specific sailing conditions and peculiarities of each processing stage in the carriage of dangerous goods is a necessary requirement to ensure safety of seamen when noxious chemical factors are present on board.

5.2.3 Kinds of Toxic Effect of Dangerous Goods; Principal Clinical Syndromes

The variety of kinds and conditions of contact of seamen and dockside workers with dangerous goods brings about the multiple character of display of toxic effects, along with physical, chemical and biological properties specific to each substance. Both direct and indirect consequences of chemical injury can considerably hinder diagnosis and treatment of developed pathological states and disease conditions. Depending upon the active doses and concentrations, the individual features of the organism and the conditions of contact, dangerous goods and their components can cause the following kinds of toxic effects:

1. Accidents involving acute poisoning and critical conditions
2. Chronic poisoning and occupational diseases
3. Certain symptoms, syndromes, prepathological states, reduction of adaptive reserves and changes in reactivity.

In addition, under the action of shipboard toxic factors the quantitative indices and structure of diseased states of seamen may change. As the first group of the above-mentioned effects is most important in carriage of dangerous goods in all-cargo vessels, it will be necessary to consider its characteristics in some detail.

According to their type of toxic action, all dangerous goods can be conventionally subdivided into substances having a predominantly local or systemic (resorption) effect. In the first case, a reaction of skin and mucous membranes at the place of contact is evident, whereby burning, irritation or an inflammatory effect in noted. Evidence of the local effect will not exclude resorption symptoms which can develop as the poison is absorbed and circulates in the organism.

Sometimes, under the action of irritants or toxic agents, the nervous system may be damaged; this can cause serious lesions and even have a fatal outcome.

As a rule, under conditions of acute poisoning with toxic components of dangerous goods, a selective action of the toxic agent on the functional systems of the organism is noticed. However, detection of a specific action is hindered because most of the toxic agents have mediatory, indirect effects (Albert [1]). Besides in intoxication with some chemical substances, the characteristic features are the development of the pathological process in phases and the occurrence of a latent period, the manifestation and duration of which depend on the amount (dose, concentration) and properties of the toxic agent and on the rate of its biotransformation and elimination from the organism, as well as on the toxicity of the formed metabolites (Luzhnikov et al. [13], Tiunov [20]).

Most important in the development of the toxic effect and in the clinical picture of poisoning is the route of exposure. Under shipboard conditions, when carrying dangerous goods, poisoning occurs most often by inhalation and also through the skin, as was shown convincingly in the comprehensive study by Schepers [17]. However, descriptions are known of cases of mass poisoning by pesticides when eating food products contaminated during carriage by sea (Weeks [24]). Similar cases have been periodically described in the literature up to the present time.

In spite of the fact that practically all chemical substances have specific toxic effects, the collective intoxication symptoms following acute poisoning are usually confined to a number of basic clinical syndromes, among which the most significant diagnostically, under shipboard conditions, are the following: neurological syndrome, disturbance of respiration, circulatory disturbance, hepatic and renal insufficiency, and gastric disturbance. Their characteristics are described in detail in all handbooks on clinical toxicology (Luzhnikov et al. [13]; Golikov [7]; Ganzhara and Novikov [6]; Locket [11]; Ludewig and Lohs [12]; Braun and Dönhardt [3]), thus making it quite unnecessary to elucidate them in this section.

The diagnosis of acute poisoning when carrying dangerous goods by sea is greatly facilitated by data obtained on the contact of the crew members with known chemical substances stowed on board, by the absence among the crew of persons with aggravated diseases, the differential diagnosis of which could be made difficult, and by the crew personnel undergoing compulsory periodic medical examinations at which aggravated diseases can usually be revealed. Typical complaints among a number of crew members or dockside workers at the same time under conditions of contact with dangerous goods must always alert the ship's administration and the medical staff to possible poisoning from the components of the goods in hand. This is especially important under passage at sea, where there are minimum possibilities to render skilled (and specialized) medical aid. Therefore, early diagnosis of poisoning is the most important aspect of medical treatment.

5.2.4 Medical First Aid and Treatment of Poisoning

The general first aid measures for poisoning include:

1. Withdrawing the patient from contact with the toxic agent without any delay;
2. Reducing the content of toxic substance in the organism;
3. Provision of skilled medical aid;
4. Prevention of probable complications.

Apart from this, even while giving the initial treatment to the patient, it will be necessary to exclude the possibility of new cases of poisoning by warning the personnel and by temporary stoppage of work until the causes of the accident can be discovered.

All measures of treatment of acute poisoning may be divided into three main groups: ensuring rapid evacuation of toxicants from the organism, specific (antidotal) therapy and symptomatic treatment (Ganzhara and Novikov [6]).

Unabsorbed toxic agent may be evacuated from the gastrointestinal tract by gastric lavage, by the use of cleansing and syphon enemas and by purgatives, as well as by astringents, envelopers, absorbents and neutralizers. The techniques of the necessary procedures are set forth in the Medical First Aid Guide for Use in Accidents Involving Dangerous Goods [14]. Gastric lavage was regarded as being inappropriate for shipboard use by laymen.

The removal of toxicant from the organism is accelerated by forced diuresis, effected by an excessive water intake and the use of diuretics and uragogues.

Stimulation of respiration also makes for the evacuation of intoxicants from the organism through the respiratory tract. This is achieved either by pharmacological agents or by applying artificial respiration with the use of special apparatus or mouth-to mouth and mouth-to-nose respiratory methods. At the same time, use should be made of oxygen therapy and hyperbarbic oxygenation in a high-pressure chamber (on salvage and rescue service ships). Also, the respiratory centre is stimulated by giving the patient mixtures of oxygen and carbon dioxide to inhale.

When in hospital, to which the patient must be sent as soon as possible, these measures should be supplemented by applying haemodialysis, haemosorption and replacement of blood.

Of great importance in the complex treatment of poisoning is antidotal therapy, the agents and possibilities of which are steadily growing. Antidotes should be given to the patients right at the initial stages of the first aid treatment, and by means of them it is possible to prevent the development of intoxication or to minimize the pathological process. It is important that antidotes should be given only when the source of poisoning is definitely known.

All antidotes are divided into a number of main groups depending on their mechanism of action. Thus, activated charcoal and ion-exchange resins are the typical representatives of the physicochemical group. Pure chemical action is characteristic of dithiols, aminopolycarboxylic and aminopolyphosphoric acids. The group of functional antidotes includes agents which are counterpoisons by their pharmacological effect or antimetabolites (Conner et al. [5]). For instance, the primary oxidation of ethyl alcohol delays the formation in the organism of toxic products from methanol, which brings about the antidotal effect of ethanol in intoxications with methanol. Neostigmine and pyridostigmine, which are inhibitors of cholinesterase, serve as antidotes for poisoning with antidepressants, and when cholinesterase is depressed by organic phosphorus compounds, antidotes such as atropine and pralidoxime are its reactivators.

Symptomatic therapy is aimed at restoring the functions disturbed by the toxic agent and at the prevention of complications. This type of treatment is often predominant because there are, as yet, no antidotes for a number of toxic agents and in cases of poisoning with unknown chemical substances symptomatic therapy is the only kind of treatment available. Coping with the distrubances of respiration and oxygen deficit in the organism, arresting the disturbances of haemodynamics and cardiac action, controlling psychoneurotic disturbances and hepatic and renal insufficiency, restoring water - salt and acid - base balance, as well as maintaining homeostasis and using means for preventing infection - all these measures comprise the strategy and tactics of symptomatic treatment of poisoning, which measures are within the capacity of the shipboard medical staff.

5.2.5 Means for Prevention of Poisoning

Ensuring safe shipping, storage and handling in ports of chemical goods is a quite practicable task, provided the totality of preventive measures is planned and strictly followed. This will include organizational, technological and sanitary measures. The carriage of dangerous goods by sea should be organized as envisaged by the IMO Dangerous Goods Code. If the chemical substance to be carried is not included in the Code list, then the consignor should present written information on the degree and kind of risk, and, if necessary, provide individual means of protection, such as gas masks, instruments for detection of noxious vapours and gases in the air, etc.

Knowledge by the ship's administration and the members of the crew coming in contact with the goods of the hazardous properties of the goods being carried allows for timely provision of safety for the crew, the ship and the environment.

The technology of cargo handling operations, the stowage of cargo on board and its compatibility with other goods carried by the vessel, as well as sufficient mechanical ventilation of the cargo spaces during the voyage and in the course of handling the goods at ports must be in compliance with international and local hygiene regulations, so that the concentrations of noxious vapours, gases and dust within the working zones do not exceed the maximum permissible concentrations. The various national regulations may differ slightly from the international recommendations but as a rule they ensure the prevention of acute poisoning among seamen and dock workers.

In solving the problems of safety for men when carrying and handling dangerous goods, great importance should also be attached to sufficient lighting of the working places, provision of guards and warning notices.

Special attention should be drawn to the availability of individual appliances for the protection of respiratory organs and to the provision of adequate overalls, as well as to the necessary drugs and antidotes in the ship's first aid dispensary. The organization of storing and washing the overalls should be subject to permanent checks by the ship's administration and the medical staff.

A comprehensive approach to solving the problems of prevention of poisoning will guarantee success in the safe carriage of dangerous goods by sea.

References

1. Albert, E.: Isbiratelnaya toksichnost. [Selective toxicity]. Moscow: Mir 1971.
2. Andronov, L. P. and L. M. Shafran: Voprosy gigieny truda moryakov i reglementatsiya morskikh perevozok opasnykh gruzov. [Problems of seamen's hygiene of work and regulations for carriage of dangerous goods by sea]. In: Trudy III Mezhdunarodnogo simpoziuma po morskoy meditsine. Leningrad, 26–28 June 1968. Moscow 1969. pp. 44–47.
3. Braun, W. and A. Dönhardt: Vergiftungsregister. Haushalts- und Laborchemikalien, Arzneimittel. Symptomatologie und Therapie. 2nd ed. Stuttgart: Thieme 1975.
4. Chaigneau, M.: Classification des gaz délétères. Ann. Anesth. *21*, 6, 683–688 (1980).
5. Conner, Ch., N. J. Robertson, M. J. Kelly et al.: Rational use of emergency antidotes. Top. Emergency Med. *1*, 3, 27–42 (1979).
6. Ganzhara, P. S. and A. A. Novikov: Uchebnoe posobie po klinicheskoy toksikologii. [Manual on clinical toxicology]. Moscow: Meditsina 1979.

7. Golikov, P.S.: Neotlozhnaya pomoshch pri ostrykh otravleniyakh. Spravochnik po toksikologii. [First aid in cases of acute poisoning. Handbook on toxicology]. Moscow: Meditsina 1978.
8. International maritime dangerous goods code. Vols. 1–4 and supplements Ed.: IMCO, London. London 1972.
9. Kagan, Yu. S.: Obshchaya toksikologiya pestitsidov. [General toxicology of pesticides]. Kiev: Zdorovye 1981.
10. Kolkovski, P.: Khimicheskiyat factor v usloviyata na transporta. [Chemical factors in transport]. Transp. med. Vesti *20*, 1/2, 20–23 (1975).
11. Locket, S.: Clinical toxicology. The clinical diagnosis and treatment of poisoning. London: Henry Kimpton 1957.
12. Ludewig, R. and K. Lohs: Akute Vergiftungen. Ratgeber für toxikologische Notfälle. 6th ed. Stuttgart: Fischer 1981.
13. Luzhnikov, E.A., V.N. Dagaev and N.N. Firsov: Osnovy reanimatologii pri ostrykh otravleniyakh. [Fundamentals of reanimatology in cases of acute poisoning]. Moscow: Meditsina 1977.
14. Medical first aid guide for use in accidents involving dangerous goods. Eds.: IMO, WHO, ILO. London: IMO 1982.
15. Navaz, M.Z.: The carriage by sea of hazardous cargoes, requiring environmental control. Parts I and II. Holl. Shipbuilding *20*, 112–114 and 198–202 (1971).
16. Sanotskii, I.V. and I.P. Ulanova: Kriterii vrednosti v gigiene i toksikologii pri otsenke opasnosti khimicheskikh soedinenii. [Criteria of harmfulness in hygiene and toxicology when assessing hazardous properties of chemical compounds]. Moscow: Meditsina 1976.
17. Schepers, B.-F.: Gesundheitsgefährdung durch Chemikalien an Bord deutscher Seeschiffe unter besonderer Berücksichtigung gefährlicher Ladung. Dissertation, University of Hamburg 1978.
18. Shafran, L.M., L.P. Andronov, L.V. Basalaeva et al.: Razrabotka aktualnykh gigienicheskikh problem sudovoy toksikologii. [Elaboration of topical hygiene problems of shipboard toxicology]. In: X Ukrainskii syezd gigienistov. Tezisy dokladov. Vol. 2. Kiev 1981. pp. 118–119.
19. Tiunov, L.A. and N.N. Savateev: Nekotorye voprosy korabelnoy toksikologii. [Some problems of shipboard toxicology]. Voen.-med. Zh. *6*, 64–66 (1962).
20. Tiunov, L.A.: Osnovnye mekhanizmy metabolizma ksenobiotikov v organizme cheloveka i zhivotnykh. [Principal metabolic mechanisms of xenobiotics in men and animals]. In: VINITI. Itogi nauki i tekhniki. Toksikologiya. Vol. 12. Moscow 1981. pp. 5–64.
21. The transport of dangerous goods. Recommendations of the United Nations Economic and Social Council's Committee of Experts. New York: UN 1977. ST/SG/AC. 10/1/Rev. 1. pp. 372.
22. Ulewicz, K.: Sea-going vessel as biological ecosystem. In: VIII International symposium on Marine Medicine, Varna, 24–28 Oct. 1978. p. 241.
23. Voitenko, A.M. and L.M. Shafran: Voprosy sanitarnoy okhrany vozdukha v svyazi s perevozkoi na sudakh i pererabotkoi v portakh opasnykh khimicheskikh gruzov. [Problems of sanitary protection of air linked with shipping and handling in ports of dangerous chemical goods]. In: Gigiena naselennykh mest. Respublikanskiy mezhdunarodnyy sbornik. 20th ed. Kiev: Zdorovye 1981. pp. 72–75.
24. Weeks, D.E.: Endrine food-poisoning. A report on four outbreaks caused by two separate shipments of endrine-contaminated flour. Bull. Wld. Hlth Org. *37*, 499–512 (1967).
25. Zorn, E.: Gefährliche Güter. Toxikologische Problematik an Bord. Hansa *108*, 5, 435–437 (1971).

5.3 Health Problems on Tankships Carrying Oil, Gas or Bulk Chemicals

A. Ward Gardner

5.3.1 Introduction

There are three main types of tankships: those which carry crude oil and petroleum products, gas tankships and chemicals carriers. The very large crude carriers (VLCCs) are 200000–300000 dead weight tonnage. These ships usually have long voyages. Much smaller tankships deliver product from refineries to petroleum terminals. These ships tend to have short voyages, often in busy shipping lanes, and then load or unload product as quickly as possible at the port. In the subsequent parts of this chapter the petroleum and gas carriers will be discussed in one section and chemical carriers in another.

5.3.2 Hazards in Petroleum and Gas Carriers

The cargoes carried on these ships will often be flammable, toxic and liable to explode (Page and Gardner [31]). This implies a high potential for unfortunate incidents. So the standards of education of crew members, the safety precautions and the knowledge of hazards must also be high. Basic occupational health concepts imply that people must have knowledge of the hazards to which they are or may be exposed and that they should understand how the ship's operations can be conducted safely both for themselves and for others. An international safety guide for oil tankers and terminals [19] and a book by Page and Gardner [31] on petroleum tankship safety will be found useful in dealing with these hazards.

Quite a number of authors have dealt with the general work and life conditions and the specific hazards on board tankers (Amirov and Gasanova [1]; Duck [9]; Farrell and Eng [12]; Gasanova et al. [13]; Goethe [16]; Herrmann [17]; Matsevich [24]; Nikilov and Nefeudov [29]; Page [30]). They mentioned the special role of work hygiene on board tankers to avoid intoxications by inhalation. Matsevich [24] pointed out that the gas concentration of the air during the loading and unloading process of benzene was sometimes higher than the threshold limit value (TLV). Shishlovskaya et al. [38] reported on the hazards to crew members and to shoreside personnel occurring during the cleaning of tanks. On account of thorough measurements performed on board, Svedung [39] found out that during loading, if the wind conditions were unfavourable, inconveniently high concentrations of primarily hydrogen sulphide may occur on deck as well as in the engine room and living quarters. The air in cleaned and well-ventilated cargo tanks contained such a high concentration of harmful substances, primarily benzene, that according to the author, use of breathing protection – preferably fresh air masks – is warranted during all work in these tanks. If the tanks are not well cleaned of oil remnants and sediments it is not possible with moderate fan capacities (that is approximately one air change per hour) to obtain an acceptable air quality in the tanks.

There are only a very few publications concerning possible hazards to tankship crew members by dangerous cargo. The available statements are contradictory. Shafran et al. [37] reported that significant changes were discovered in the total number of leucocytes and the ratio of unusual forms in addition to changes in the contents of polynuclear aromatic compounds, glucogene and lipoids as well as in the activity of the acid and alkaline phosphates in the plasma. Kirjakov et al. [21] examined the crews of five tankers and identified leucocytopenia in 13% and thrombocytopenia in 7% of the examined seamen. They furthermore mentioned considerable rises of glucose-6-phosphate and cholesterol levels, a considerable fall of albumins, a rise of the β-globulin in the electrophoreses, an increase of ammonia and other changes. Tomaszunas et al. [41] found in 184 crew members on board tankers a reduced number of white blood cells, as well as an increased urine phenol level and a lower percentage rate of organic sulphates in urine.

These findings are not confirmed by other authors. Andreani and Strambi [2] also examined tankship crews and made the following subdivisons: crew members serving for more than 10 years, crew members serving less than 2 years duty on board. They could not trace significant differences in the numbers of white blood cells, red blood cells, cholesterol level and total protein level. In their comparative study of data of medical examinations in 201 tankship and 205 non-tankship crew members, Goethe et al. [15] could not attest hazards affecting the haematological and biochemical values. There were no pathological differences in number with respect to red blood cells and haemoglobin percentage. There was, however, a significantly slight increase of white blood cell numbers in tankship crew members compared with the findings in non-tankship crew members. The differential blood cell count showed decreased numbers of eosinophils and differences were found in alkaline phosphatase levels. These levels were lower than in non-tankship crew members, and the same applied in respect of acid phosphatase. It was a striking result of the subjective part of the examinations that tankship crew members seem to suffer more frequently from nausea, lack of appetite, uncomfortably sweetish taste and the feeling of being disturbed by bad odour than non-tankship crew members.

These varied findings by different authors show no consistent pattern or relation with known hazards. Under the specific environmental conditions and unfavourable work hygiene on board some tankships it appears that there may be in some people short-term alterations of the biochemical and haematological values. Collins et al. [7; 8] and Eddy et al. [10] studied the specific environmental load. The authors found out that besides the considerable thermal load in tropical waters, the continuously changing climatic conditions and the need for acclimatisation seem to be a repeated and strong stress factor. A study by Rodahl et al. [35] on work physiology dealt with the work-loads of crew members, especially of deck officers, during defined processes of work and/or activities, under unfavourable weather conditions and calls at ports. The stated very high load corresponds with that described by the authors for non-tankship personnel.

In spite of the fact that no specific diseases were found in tankship crew members, the distribution of diagnoses seems to differ slightly from that of the dry cargo ships. The few cases of poisoning, figuring as accidents, are excluded (see Chap. 3.1). Goethe [14] found that the rate of skin diseases (17.7%) was higher on tankships than on board other merchant vessels. Skin diseases were the most frequent of all registered diagnoses of tankship crew members. In his study on the health status of ocean-going oil tanker seamen, Nakamura [28] found very low blood pressure and low cholesterol levels with slight obesity. He did not, however, find signs of specific hazards.

Carter [3] examined the absences of tanker crews and found more frequent absences in ratings than in officers. Higher rates of absence were found in the engine room crew members than in the deck crew. The study unfortunately does not contain any comparative data.

Clark and Montgomery [4] reported on the special problems on board tankers operating in arctic zones. A most remarkable report on the medical aspects of the shipwreck of the tanker "Boehlen" as well as the details of the rescue and medical care of injured and hypothermic crew members was delivered by Le Chuiton et al. [22]. The injured seamen were admitted to the Naval Hospital Clermont-Tonnerre in Brest. The authors mentioned that the oiled surface on the water was thought to have slowed the process of hypothermia. Shafran et al. [37] found clearly marked disturbances of the compensatory mechanisms of the body caused by unfavourable working and living conditions on liquid gas carriers which may have pathological effects on the cardiovascular system. The authors did not state whether there was any correlation between the disturbances and the cargo. Paulsen [32] performed a general study on work-places and work hygiene aboard tankers, pointing particularly to safety problems. He did not mention special hazards.

A further discussion of the hazards can be found in the works listed in the references (Amirov and Gasanova [1]; Andreani and Strambi [2]).

The principal hazards of oil/petroleum tankships are:

Oxygen deficiency	flue gas nitrogen carbon dioxide
Toxic effects by inhalation	hydrocarbons hydrogen sulphide benzene organic lead compounds
Skin contact	light and middle distillates (gasoline, kerosene, light diesel oil); benzene and organic lead compounds may also enter the body via the skin but the likelihood of this route of absorption being of importance is very low compared with inhalation

5.3.2.1 Oxygen Deficiency

Flue gas or nitrogen may be used in 'tank inerting' so as to drive out oxygen from the ship's tanks. Carbon dioxide may be used for fire-fighting purposes to produce inert gas blanketing. Asphyxia will be the consequence to any person who enters such areas of oxygen deficiency who is not getting oxygen from a breathing apparatus or fresh air line.

Entry into Confined Space. Entry into any confined space, particularly if the atmosphere may be deficient in oxygen or if it has contained any toxic gas or vapour, is potentially hazardous. There should *always* be a strict system for checking that:

1. The atmosphere contains sufficient oxygen;
2. The concentration of toxic substances is below the Threshold Limit Values (TLV);
3. There is breathing apparatus, a lifeline and a harness ready for immediate use at the entrance to the compartment;
4. There is a crew member keeping watch *at all times* outside the space who can summon help if the need arises;
5. There is a written procedure with a check-list to ensure that these precautions are carried out. This check-list must be approved and signed by a senior officer *before* anyone is allowed to enter a confined space.

Ballast tanks are often thought to be safe to enter without going through the check-list above. This is not so. Oxygen can be depleted or absent in such tanks as it is used to make rust (iron oxide) in the presence of iron and water. Deaths have resulted from failure to appreciate this danger when crew members have not followed the precautions for confined space entry. Tanks in ballast are *not* safe to enter simply because they do not contain petroleum products or other cargo. Oxygen lack is a serious risk in *any* confined space where iron and water are present.

5.3.2.2 Toxic Effects of Hydrocarbons

Hydrocarbons can cause harm to people in two main ways:

1. By inhalation;
2. By skin contact.

In each case the problem can be further classified under two headings:

1. Short-term effects;
2. Long-term effects.

Inhalation of Hydrocarbons

Following inhalation, the toxicity of hydrocarbons as a class is not great, with the important exception of benzene (C_6H_6). With this one exception, volatility and risk are closely related; the more volatile the hydrocarbon, the greater the likelihood of inhalation leading to poisoning by 'gassing'. Remember too that a rise of temperature will lead to an increase in volatility.

Short-Term Effects by Inhalation. Inhalation of hydrocarbon vapours will, in the presence of adequate oxygen, produce a slow anaesthetisation of the person exposed. The rate of change in the person's condition will be roughly proportional to the amount of hydrocarbon inhaled, and will therefore depend upon both the concentration of the hydrocarbon inhaled and the time for which it is breathed.

Beginning with a stage of excitation, the effects give rise to 'drunken' behaviour, slurred speech, staggering, confusion and loss of consciousness. Further inhalation will lead in due course to arrest of breathing and heart beat and finally to death.

The hydrocarbon vapour can be breathed out again in fresh air. The effects are, therefore, reversible if caught in time and treated correctly.

Oil Mists or Sprays. Oil mists or sprays, if inhaled in high enough concentrations, may cause irritation of the lungs which may lead to pneumonitis. Even medicinal mineral oil will cause such a reaction. However, this is not unique to petroleum oils, since the excessive inhalation of many compounds may cause the development of chemical pneumonitis.

Long-Term Effects by Inhalation. There are, with the exception of benzene, no long-term effects which are directly due to inhalation of hydrocarbon vapours. However, permanent damage can easily result from lack of oxygen or from the complications of becoming unconscious, all of which may be associated with hydrocarbon vapour inhalation.

Benzene is in a risk class by itself in terms of the long-term hazard from inhalation of very low amounts of the vapour. It should also be noted that some commercial grades of toluene and xylenes frequently contain considerable amounts of benzene. Toluene and xylenes should therefore be viewed with the same concern as benzene, until, or unless, they are known to be benzene-free.

Many gasolines also contain benzene, sometimes up to 10%. In any case, the amounts should be known so that suitable precautions can be taken.

Skin Contact with Hydrocarbons

Hydrocarbons are best kept off the skin. The short-term effects may be to cause dermatitis or oil acne, and with certain hydrocarbons, the long-term effects may be to cause skin cancer if contact is prolonged. There is no substitute for personal cleanliness and tidy working in preventing oil contact, and thus preventing any possibility of short- or long-term effects.

Short-Term Effects on the Skin. The lighter hydrocarbons such as gasoline and kerosine can cause skin defatting which may lead to dermatitis. Heavier hydrocarbons, such as lubricating oils, can cause plugging of the pores and hair follicles which may go on to a condition known as 'oil acne'.

Long-Term Effects on the Skin. Heavier hydrocarbons, particularly those containing polynuclear (polycyclic) aromatic compounds, in contact with the skin for prolonged periods may give rise to skin cancers, particularly to scrotal cancer.

Precautions Against Skin Effects. The following preventative measures are recommended whenever any petroleum product is handled:

1. Avoid all unnecessary contact with the oil. Contact can be minimised by protective gloves and other protective clothing.
2. If contact with oil does occur, it should be removed from the skin as soon as possible. Towels should be clean when used and an adequate supply of them available. Harsh soaps should be avoided since they may cause dermatitis.
3. Solvents such as kerosine and gasoline should not be used to remove oil from the skin. Oil should be removed by washing with soap and water, or with a preparation designed for skin cleansing. *Never* use hydrocarbons as skin cleaners.
4. Crew members should be encouraged to take showers at the end of a day's work in order to remove all traces of oil from the skin.
5. If waste or rags are used to wipe oil from the skin or off machinery, sufficient quantities of them should be available so that the cleaning materials can be changed frequently and therefore kept relatively clean. Oily rags should *not* be kept in overall or trouser pockets.
6. Seafarers should be encouraged to wear clean work clothes, since oil-soaked outerwear or underclothes may hold the oil in contact with the skin longer than would otherwise occur. It may be advisable to provide one locker for work clothes and a separate one for other clothes in order to avoid contamination of the other clothes with oil.
7. Prompt medical advice should be sought for any skin disease at an early stage in its development. Once dermatitis appears in an individual, it may be possible to prevent it from becoming more severe by transferring the man to a 'clean' job until the dermatitis subsides.

Benzene (C_6H_6) (Benzol)

Benzene is a clear, colourless liquid, with a pleasant aromatic odour. Its TLV 'C' varies between countries but is usually in the 5–10 ppm range (10 ppm: 30 mg/m^3).

Inhalation Hazard. The effect of short-term inhalation of benzene vapour is anaesthetisation, similar to that caused by other hydrocarbons. Benzene vapour is also irritant in high concentrations. However, the important problem with benzene is that it is a serious and insidious destroyer of blood-forming organs, even when inhaled in low concentrations. Repeated exposure to low concentrations of benzene can lead to serious illness. *Benzene vapour must not be inhaled.* Where benzene vapours occur, breathing apparatus must be worn. Deck officers, pumpmen and others who may handle benzene frequently should be under medical supervision so suitable tests which indicate benzene exposure can be carried out.

When benzene is being handled, the accommodation spaces should be tested at regular intervals for benzene vapour, using a suitable detector. The concentration of vapour must be maintained below the TLV; note the 'C' notation after the TLV, indicating that the TLV is a ceiling value. Closed loading systems are advisable for benzene.

Skin Contact Hazard. Benzene can be absorbed through the intact skin but there is little danger of absorption by this route provided contact with the liquid is not prolonged. The main danger associated with benzene spills on clothing is that the vapours are released into the breathing zone and the inhalation hazard is increased.

Bitumen

The only likely hazard from bitumen is a burn. Bitumen burns are not usually serious, because bitumen is carried at a relatively low temperature. Unless the bitumen burn is on the face, the best treatment is to cool the burn at once by showering for 10 min in cold water. The resultant hard bitumen should be left on the skin, covered with dry gauze and left. When the bitumen drops off, healed skin will be found. On the face, after cooling as above, the bitumen should be removed by swabbing with medicinal liquid paraffin. Then treat as a heat burn in the usual way.

Cut back bitumens may contain creosote – a coal tar derivative with many polynuclear aromatic compounds in it. These polynuclear aromatics are liable to cause skin cancer following prolonged exposure. It therefore follows that as cut back bitumens are potentially carcinogenic they should always be kept off the skin.

Crude Oil

Crude oil is a mixture of hydrocarbons of all kinds. Its composition will vary with source. Crude oil may, and usually will, contain other substances, some of which are toxic, e.g., hydrogen sulphide. It is not easy to generalise about the toxicity of crude oils. However, the effects of inhalation of crude oil vapours will be approximately similar to the combined effect of the inhalation of gasoline vapour and of other toxic vapours which may be present. For example, when considering a sour crude, approximate details of its toxicity will be found under gasoline and hydrogen sulphide.

Gasoline (Petrol)

Gasoline is a mixture of hydrocarbons in the boiling range 30° – 200 °C (390° F). The composition varies widely. Its TLV is 100–200 ppm (0.05%). Make sure that the benzene content is below the TLV.

Many additives are used – usually in small amounts – but some, such as tetraethyl lead (TEL) and tetramethyl lead (TML) can, under some circumstances, be hazardous.

TML and TEL are added to gasoline to give it 'anti-knock' properties. TML and TEL are extremely toxic. The quantities in which they are added to gasoline are so small that they do not normally increase the toxicity of the gasoline. Nevertheless, the addition of these compounds does increase the hazard when tank cleaning. The reason for this is that these lead additives tend to accumulate in the sludge and scale in the tank. Dangerous concentrations may build up if the tank is continually carrying leaded gasoline. Deaths have occurred whilst cleaning shore tanks which are continually in leaded gasoline service, when known precautionary measures have been neglected.

Benzene may also be present in gasoline. The amount should be known and appropriate precautions taken.

Inhalation Hazard. Because gasoline is very volatile, high concentrations of vapour can readily occur in enclosed or confined spaces. such as cargo tanks or pumprooms. The short-term effects of gasoline inhalation are described under inhalation of hydrocarbons.

It is apparent from Table 1 that, contrary to some popular belief, a concentration of 2000 ppm (about 20% of the lower flammable limit) is *not* safe for even short exposures. The lower limit for immediate toxic effects is of the order of 900–1000 ppm. For safety, personnel must not enter cargo tanks or pumprooms unless the vapour concentration is below the TLV of 100–200 ppm (making sure that the benzene content is below the TLV).

Skin Contact Hazard. Gasoline on the skin can cause defatting and may thus lead to

Table 1. Human Response to Inhalation of Gasoline Vapours

Concentration (ppm)	Exposure time	Effects
160–270	8 h	Slight, but not generally objectionable, irritation of eyes and throat
500	1 h	No significant complaints
900	1 h	Slight eye, nose and throat irritation; some dizziness and unsteadines
2000	1 h	Symptoms of anaesthesia begin in 30 min
10000	10 min	Nose and throat irritation in 2 min, dizziness in 4 min and definite symptoms resembling alcoholic intoxication in 4–10 min
11000	5 min	Nose and throat irritation in 20 s; dizziness and drunkenness in 5 min

dermatitis. Skin contact should therefore be avoided. In addition, certain gasoline additives may cause skin allergy.

Kerosine (Paraffin)

Kerosine is a mixture of hydrocarbons in the boiling range 150° – 225 °C. The composition varies widely, but compounds of the paraffin, naphthene and olefin series generally predominate. Its TLV is 100–200 ppm (making sure that the benzene content is below the TLV). Kerosine has a low degree of toxic hazard when handled normally on tankers.

Inhalation Hazard. Because of low toxicity and volatility the inhalation hazard is negligible unless the cargo has been heated, in which case the increase in vapour pressure may give rise to toxic concentrations of vapour.

Inhalation of oily mists or sprays should be avoided. Mists or sprays may be encountered when oil is being loaded.

Skin Contact Hazard. The main problem with kerosine is dermatitis, and this is the hazard which will be of most importance to seamen. In addition to its defatting action on the skin, kerosine may also cause some irritation. Kerosines of naphthenic and aromatic origin have been shown to be more irritating than kerosines of paraffin origin, but all types may cause dermatitis. On prolonged contact the skin becomes red, dry and scaly, and ultimately begins to crack. When in this condition, the skin is susceptible to bacterial infection. Dermatitis problems are best prevented by avoiding unnecessary contact with kerosine. The skin should not be cleaned of oil, tar or paint by the use of kerosine.

Eye Hazard. In contact with the eyes, kerosine causes only slight transient irritation.

Lubricating Oils

The composition of lubricating oils varies widely. Before being sold to the customer, lubricants will also have varying amounts of additives of all kinds.

Lubricating oils and greases are a relatively harmless class of materials. No unusual hazard is involved in their carriage, provided that ordinary care is taken both to keep them off the skin and to avoid inhalation of their vapours (if heated) or of their mists. While all types of lubricating oil have not been systematically evaluated for their toxicity, experience has shown that there are no striking differences in their toxic effects on the body. In general, they have a low order of toxicity when taken internally.

Lubricating oils are often loaded through the tank lid and the free fall of liquid can produce mist or spray. These usually have no unpleasant effect on persons on deck, or on those peering down the tank lid. If the mists are found to be a problem, or when personnel have to be exposed to concentrated mists, breathing apparatus should be worn.

Additives used in lubricant formulations vary in their toxicity. This is generally of a low order. The presence of an additive in a lubricant does not usually necessitate any more special handling precautions than those required for kerosine.

Local Effects. The main potential problem associated with the handling of lubricating oils is dermatitis resulting from frequent and prolonged contact. This is characterised by acne (red or black spots at the pores), mainly on the back of the hands, forearms and thighs. The hair follicles and sweat pores become infected with the formation of small boils or pimples (oil folliculitis). For the occasional person who develops an individual sensitivity to lubricating oils, very severe skin reactions may develop, requiring special medical attention. In general, however, dermatitis need not be a problem if unnecessary contact with the oils is avoided and good personal hygiene is observed.

An additional aspect of skin contact is that of the danger of skin cancer. Cases of human skin cancer have resulted from contact with certain lubricating oils and waxes. In these instances, the skin contact was severe and prolonged over many years. The sensible approach, therefore, is to keep lubricating oil off the skin.

Experimental evidence indicates that washing with soap and water after application of a cancer-forming oil to the skin greatly reduces its tumour-inducing activity. There is thus a good experimental basis for recommending frequent washing whenever oils are handled.

Petroleum Products

The lighter petroleum liquids can cause defatting of the skin and can thus give rise to a dermatitis of occupational origin. Prevention is by keeping these substances off the skin. They should *never* be used to clean the skin on account of the risk of defatting.

Middle distillates such as kerosine and light diesel oil can, if left on the skin or particularly if soaked into clothing which is worn when in this condition, give rise to oily plugs in the skin follicles. These tiny black plugs in the pores are usually found over the fronts of the thighs and on the forearms and give rise to 'oil acne'.

5.3.2.3 Toxic Effects of Hydrogen Sulphide (H_2S) (Sulphuretted Hydrogen)

Hydrogen sulphide is a colourless gas with an odour of rotten eggs. Its TLV is 10 ppm (14 mg/m^3). Very low concentrations can be detected by smell (0.1 ppm). Smell should *not,* however, be used as a guide to the presence or absence of hydrogen sulphide because in high concentrations the gas paralyses the sense of smell. The effect of this will be that although hydrogen sulphide may be present in high concentrations, it cannot be detected by smell. The dangers of using smell as a guide will therefore be obvious.

Most crude oils contain some hydrogen sulphide - those which contain 10 ppm (or more) as a liquid are classed as sour crudes. There is a very real danger of poisoning by hydrogen sulphide when loading or discharging sour crudes. Precautions must be taken to ensure that vapours containing hydrogen sulphide are not breathed. Closed loading systems are recommended for ships carrying sour crudes. In the absence of these, breathing apparatus must be worn by those engaged in the loading operation. These precautions apply equally to ballasting after the discharge of sour crude oil from a tank.

The short-term effects of hydrogen sulphide are damage to the brain and the kidneys. Eye irritation may also be felt. In high concentrations a few breaths may be enough to produce unconsciousness, followed swiftly by death.

Table 2 shows how different concentrations of hydrogen sulphide gas will affect the human body.

Table 2. Human response to inhalation of hydrogen sulphide

Concentration (ppm)	Exposure time	Effects
50–100	1 h	Irritation of eyes, nose, throat and breathing passages. Longer exposures to concentrations of the order of 100 ppm, induce a gradual increase in severity of these symptoms, and death may occur within 4–48 h
200–300	1 h	Marked irritation of eyes, nose throat and breathing passages. Longer exposures to concentrations would probably not be tolerated
500–700	0.5–1 h	Loss of consciousness and possibly death
700–900	Few min. to 0.5 h	Unconsciousness and death will occur rapidly
1000–2000	Few min.	Immediately fatal

Long-Term Effects. Repeated exposures to low concentrations of hydrogen sulphide may cause some irritation and coughing. However, hydrogen sulphide does not accumulate in the body, and long-term poisoning is, therefore, not a problem.

Local Effects. The irritating effects of hydrogen sulphide are most pronounced in the eyes. Pain, sensitivity to light and other visual difficulties may also occur.

5.3.2.4 Toxic Effects of Carbon Dioxide (CO_2)

Carbon dioxide is a colourless gas which is heavier than air. It will be found on board, mainly in association with fire-fighting equipment. Its TLV is 5000 ppm (9000 mg/m^3).

The main hazard from carbon dioxide will arise when it has been used to extinguish a fire or to prevent a fire occurring in a pumproom or engine room. Carbon dioxide extinguishes fire by displacing the air – the oxygen content of the space is therefore reduced. If there is insufficient oxygen for a fire to burn, there is certainly insufficient oxygen for a man to live.

Crew members must not be allowed to enter compartments where carbon dioxide has been used as a smothering agent, until an adequate supply of oxygen has been assured. If entry is essential in the presence of high concentrations of carbon dioxide, then breathing apparatus must be worn.

The secondary hazard from carbon dioxide is frost-bite. As liquefied carbon dioxide leaves the applicator of a fire extinguisher or of a fixed installation, it expands and cools considerably owing to the latent heat of evaporation. The applicators become so cold that if touched by the human flesh they will 'burn'.

5.3.2.5 Toxic Effects of Organic Lead Compounds

Tetramethyl and tetraethyl lead (TML, TEL) are used as anti-knock compounds in gasoline to raise the octane number. These organic lead compounds can be found in tank scale and in tank sludge in higher concentrations than in the gasoline. So, entry to all tanks which have contained leaded gasoline *must* be controlled and, unless the threshold limit values are not exceeded, no entry must be permitted except to persons wearing breathing apparatus.

Any operation which disturbs scale or which moves sludge will increase the concentration of organic lead in air – so these operations greatly increase the dangers to people. It is therefore of the utmost importance for the safety of all crew members who may be involved that such operations are conducted under expert ship officer, medical and hygiene supervision. Urine lead levels can be used for biological monitoring of organic lead exposure.

5.3.2.6 Toxic Effects of Sodium Hydroxide (Caustic, Caustic Soda)

Sodium hydroxide may be found in tankers in the white crystalline form, or as a solution in water.

Sodium hydroxide is usually used as a cleaning agent on ships. However, a contaminated caustic solution, known as spent caustic, is sometimes shipped in cargo tanks and is jettisoned when at sea. Spent caustic contains many of the by-products and waste from a refinery that cannot be safely dumped into estuarial water through the refinery's effluent plant. Spent caustic may contain hydrogen sulphide, hydrocarbons and other sulphur compounds. It must therefore be treated as a high corrosive, toxic and flammable liquid.

Hazards. The short-term effect of caustic soda is to burn body tissue with which it is in contact. It is highly corrosive to the skin and the *eye,* in the crystalline form and when it is in a water solution. It is also an irritant if vapours are breathed which contain caustic soda.

Caustic can cause severe burns. It is one of the worst possible chemicals to get into the eye where it can cause much damage. Therefore, when handling caustic, even in weak solutions, *eye protection* must be worn. A tiny splash of concentrated caustic solution in the eye may cause, and has caused, loss of sight.

First Aid. If contamination occurs, immediate showering, with prior and special attention to the eyes, must be carried out to remove contamination. The eyelids should be held apart and the eyes washed out with water for at least 10 min, timed by the clock. This step must not be skimped or hurried. Unless all traces of the chemical are removed, burning will continue. Because of the severe pain, the victim may not willingly open his eye. The lids must therefore be held open while washing is carried out.

Similarly, showering of the skin must be carried out for at least 10 min, timed by the clock, using copious amounts of water. Contaminated clothing should be removed whilst under the shower. Burned areas of skin should then be treated as heat burns.

If caustic gets into the eye, medical aid must be sought at the earliest possible moment, because serious consequences may follow such an injury. *Prevention is easy. Cure may be impossible.*

5.3.2.7 Working on Petroleum Tankships

The larger tankships which carry crude oil round the world often have long voyages and only one day in loading and discharge ports. This means most crew members are excessively busy during loading and discharge and that during the long sea voyages they can settle to a routine which may become boring. Many of these seafarers follow creative hobbies in their spare time, but a few find the time difficult to fill and usually decide to leave this kind of job. For anyone who has personal or family problems, the lines of communication are long and home seems far away. The importance of regular radio-phone calls and mail in preventing breakdowns of all kinds hardly needs to be stressed. Coastal tankship seafarers face an entirely different set of problems: the difficulty here may be to get enough sleep and rest between the ports of loading and unloading, and to find time for leisure activities.

5.3.3 Chemical Carriers

A wide range of chemicals are transported by ships. An "International Maritime Dangerous Goods Code" and supplements [18] list the substances and the hazards. IMO have produced a medical first aid guide for use in accidents involving dangerous goods [26].

In 1971 IMCO published a "Code for the Construction and Equipment of Ships Carrying Dangerous Chemicals in Bulk".

Several amendments were published subsequently [5].

This code contains the technical details for the design and operation of chemical tankers from safety aspects. The National Academy of Science, USA published a report for the United States Coast Guard on the evaluation of the hazards of water transportation of bulk industrial chemicals, indicating in detail the toxicological hazards to crew members [11].

These documents give most of the information which will be required for the safe operation of chemical carriers.

The manifold health problems occurring during work on board chemical tankers have been described by several authors (for example Johnson [20], Trennt [42]). A series of studies performed by several Norwegian authors (Mowe et al. [27]; Riis Simonsen [34] and Wermundsen and Mowe [43]) show results of extensive chemical-technical, safety-technical, physiological and occupational medical examinations and a large variety of detailed individual information on the chemical hazards, the health problems of the crew and the hazards occurring during the process of loading and unloading as well as on the general load of the crew. The biochemical examinations in chemical tanker crews showed quite a number of abnormal transaminase results. A significant correlation with the length of service on board chemical tankers could not be determined. The frequency rate of pathological transaminase values was higher after 1 or 2 years' service on board than after 10 years' service. Of the examined seamen, 29% showed abnormal values. A large number of the seamen, however, consumed alcohol and this is known to affect transaminase results.

Following a thorough study of the transport of dangerous cargoes for several years within the German Federal merchant fleet Zorn et al. [44] and Schepers [36] came to the result that the biggest risk of intoxications or of chemical injuries of the skin exists on board tankships, predominantly chemical tankers. During the investigated period, 35 seafarers suffered from intoxications due to dangerous cargo (from 22 tankers), predominantly on board chemical tankers, and five out of seven fatal intoxications occurred on board tankers. Most chemical injuries of the skin also happened on board tankers – 43 out of 68 cases. Severe chemical burns were commonest on chemical tankers – 10 out of 12 cases. The increase of the rate of chemical intoxications was due to an increased rate of accidents on board chemical tankers.

The problems associated with the carriage of chemicals were discussed at the 2nd European Nautical Medical Officers' meeting (1979) in Great Britain. It was emphasised that the crews of chemical tankers are more exposed to the risk of hazards than are the crews of other vessels. The Joint ILO/WHO Committee on the Health of Seafarers was already in 1974 intensively concerned with the question of medical examinations of tankship crews carrying chemicals in bulk [25]. In a resolution the committee recommended that special medical examinations should be given to all crew members serving on board chemical tankers. These examinations should include clinical, laboratory and other tests as appropriate. Finally, it should be remembered that *all* chemicals which are carried should be identified for what they are – proprietary names will not do. The hazards *must* be clear to all crew members [40] who have to load, handle and discharge the dangerous goods so that appropriate and adequate safety precautions can be applied. Failure to take these elementary and essential steps can have serious consequences.

5.3.4 Occupational Hygiene Considerations

In tankships and chemical carriers particular attention must be paid to designing in safety and to designing out hazard. This principle applies, of course, to all ships, but is especially important when hazardous cargoes are carried. Coker and Gardner [6] have produced a set of occupational hygiene guidelines for ship construction.

References

1. Amirov, R.O. and A.M. Gasanova: Labour conditions in the oil-tankers and the floating means used in the oil-extracting industry in the sea. Bull. Inst. mar. trop. Med. Gdynia *25*, 2-3-4, 409–412 (1974).
2. Andreani, D. and E. Strambi: Osservazioni sulla crasi ematica di marittimi imbarcati su navicisterna (1). Atti del Centro Studi e ricerche per l'assistenza. Sanitaria e sociale dei marittimi 7–20 (1959).
3. Carter, J.T.: Absence attributed to sickness in oil tanker crews. Brit. J. industr. Med. *33*, 9–12 (1976).
4. Clark jr. W.R. and C.H. Montgomery: Arctic Tanker Medicine. Ind. Med. *39*, 3, 132–136 (1970).
5. Code for the construction and equipment of ships carrying dangerous chemicals in bulk. 1977 edition incorporating and amendments. London: IMCO 1977.
6. Coker, D.T. and A. Ward Gardner: Occupational health guidelines for ship construction. Shipping World and Shipbuilder *172*, 339–341 (1979).
7. Collins, K.J., T.P. Eddy, D.E. Lee et al.: Nutritional and environmental studies on an ocean-going oil tanker. 1. Thermal environment. Brit. J. industr. Med. *28*, 237–245 (1971).
8. Collins, K.J., T.P. Eddy, A. Hibbs et al.: Nutritional and environmental studies on an ocean-going oil tanker. 2. Heat acclimatization and nutrient balances. Brit. J. industr. Med. *28*, 246–258 (1971).
9. Duck, B.W.: Some medical aspects of tanker safety. School of Navigation, University of Southampton 1966.
10. Eddy, T.P., A.L. Stock and E.F. Wheeler: Nutritional and environmental studies on an ocean-going oil tanker. 3. Energy balances and physique. Brit. J. industr. Med. *28*, 330–341 (1971).
11. Evaluation of the hazards of bulk water transportation of industrial chemicals. A tentative guide. Revised edition. Committee on Hazardous Materials. Washington, D.C.: National Academy of Sciences 1970.
12. Farrell, T.R. and C. Eng: Chemical tankers – the quiet evolution. The Royal Institution of Naval Architects 147–165 (1974).
13. Gasanova, A.M., N.G. Trifel and P.J. Datiev: Work and leisure on oil tankers. In: III. International Symposium on Marine Medicine, Leningrad, 1968. Moscow 1969. pp. 34–36.
14. Goethe, H.: Arbeitshygiene auf Tankschiffen. In: Fragen der Schiffahrtsmedizin. Intern. Symp., Heiligendamm 28–31 March 1963. Medizinischer Dienst des Verkehrswesens II. pp. 89–92.
15. Goethe, H., R. Herrmann, R. Geister et al.: Die Frage der toxikologischen Beeinflussung der Besatzung von Tankschiffen. Eine vergleichende Pilotstudie über Tankschiff- und Nichttankschiffahrer. Arbeitsmedizin, Sozialmedizin, Präventivmedizin *11*, 2, 46–51 (1976).
16. Goethe, H.: Gesundheitliche Probleme bei Tankschiffbesatzungen. Bull. Inst. mar. Med. Gdańsk *17*, 3, 241–248 (1966).
17. Herrmann, H.: Arbeitsmedizinische Probleme bei der Seeschiffahrt insbesondere der Tankschiffahrt. Hansa *103*, 14, 1218–1220 (1966).
18. International maritime dangerous goods code. Vols. 1–4 and supplements. London: IMCO. 1972.
19. International safety guide for oil tankers and terminals. London: Witherley 1978.
20. Johnson, J.E.: Safe and efficient operation of chemical tankers. Lecture. Symposium "Safety of life at sea". Oslo 20–21 Oct. 1980. Research program associated with The Royal Norwegian Council for Scientific and Industrial Research. System for Sikkert Skip.
21. Kirjakov, K., P. Kolkovskij, P. Petrov et al.: Occupational petroleum intoxication among tanker fleet crews. Bull. Inst. mar. Med. Gdańsk *17*, 3, 249–254 (1966).
22. Le Chuiton, M., B. Dartigues, J. Blade et al.: Incidences médicales du naufrage du pétrolier "Boehlen". Méd. et Armées 5, 243–248 (1977).
23. Malizia, E. and M. Cecconi: Consigli terapeutici per i marittimi a bordo di navi trasportanti sostanze tossiche. L'Assistenza radio-medica 2, pp. 12 (1968).
24. Matsevich, L.M.: Uslovia truda na neftenalivnykh sudakh i mery ikh ozdorovlenia. [Work conditions on tankships and steps to their improvements.] In: XXIV moskovskaya nauchno-prakticheskaya konferentsia po problemam promyshlennoy gigieny 1969 g. Ed.: Sektsia gigieny truda morskogo nauchnogo gigienicheskogo obshchestva. Moscow 1969. pp. 115–116.
25. Medical examinations of crew members on tankers carrying chemicals in bulk. Report of the joint ILO/WHO committee on health of seafarers. Geneva: WHO Executive Board 1974. pp. 6–7.
26. Medical First aid guide for use in accidents involving dangerous goods. (MFAG). Chemical Supplement to the International Medical Guide for Ships (IMGS). London: IMO 1982.
27. Mowe, G., O.R. Simonsen and B. Wermundsen:

Sjøfolk i kjemikaliefart. Hovedprosjektet del I. Kjemiske miljø – og helseproblemer blant mannskap på skip som frakter flytende kjemikalier i bulk. HD 710/770701. Oslo: Yrkeshygienisk Institutt 1974. pp. 162.

28. Nakamura, F.: Health status of ocean-going oil tanker seamen. Bull. Tokyo med. dent. Univ. *20,* 3, 221–224 (1973).
29. Nikilov, S.H. and P.V. Nefeudov: About the health measures in tanker fleet. In: VII International symposium on marine medicine, Odessa 23–30 Sept. 1976. Moscow 1976. p. 249.
30. Page, R.C.: Bulk carriage of liquid chemicals by sea. Ann. occup. Hyg. 14, 205–211 (1971).
31. Page, R.C. and A.W. Gardner: Petroleum tankship safety. London: Maritime Press 1971.
32. Paulsen, J.: Gasskipet som arbeidsplass – praktisk erfaring med samarbeid mellom sjö og land. In: Foredrag ved 3S-konferansen om sikkerhet til sjös, Oslo, 21 November 1978. pp. 70–76. (System for Sikkert Skip. Rapport 78/4).
33. Proceedings of the second European nautical medical officers meeting held in the United Kingdom, West Sussex, 10–14 September 1979. London 1980.
34. Riis Simonsen, O.: Sjöfolk i kjemikaliefart. Hovedprosjektet del II. Tekniskhygieniske undersökelser om bord paa 19 skip som frakter flytende kjemikalier i bulk. HD 709/770701. Oslo: Yrkeshygienisk Institutt 1974.
35. Rodahl, K., A. Bolling and O. Tenfjord: Arbeidsfysiologiske undersökelser paa M/T Texaco Bergen. Oslo. (System for Sikkert Skip).
36. Schepers, B.-F.: Gesundheitsgefährdung durch Chemikalien an Bord deutscher Seeschiffe unter besonderer Berücksichtigung gefährlicher Ladung. Dissertation, University of Hamburg 1978.
37. Shafran, L.M., E.B. Yanushevskaya, V.I. Vigovskij et al.: Changes in the functional state of the cardio-vascular system and electrolytic metabolism in the body adaption process during voyages on liquid gas carrier vessels. Bull. Inst. mar. trop. Med. Gdynia *25,* 2-3-4, 415–419 (1974).
38. Shishlovskaya, K.Ya., B.Ya. Brodskaya, O.V. Verzilova et al.: Hygienic requirements for cleaning operations on tankers. Bull. Inst. mar. trop. Med. Gdynia *25,* 2-3-4, 300–302 (1974).
39. Svedung, I.: Air quality on board a tanker. In: Human factors in the design and operation of ships. Proceedings of the First International Conference on Human Factors in the Design and Operation of Ships. Gothenburg, February 1977. Stockholm: Garmat Service 1978. pp. 633–653.
40. Threshold limit values for chemical substances and physical agents in the workrooms environment. Cincinnati: ACCIH.
41. Tomaszunas, S., J. Uselis, A. Krynicki et al.: Working conditions on tankers and seamen health. Bull. Inst. mar. Med. Gdańsk *16,* 3/4, 209–218 (1965).
42. Trennt, W.: Uns Scheep. Probleme der Chemikalienfahrt. Das Tankschiff vom Rohöl zur Phosphorsäure. Lecture. Nautischer Verein Kiel. 28. 11. 1974. p. 5.
43. Wermundsen, B. and G. Mowe: Sjøfolk i kjemikaliefart. En yrkeshygienisk og medisinsk undersøkelse vedrørende transport av flytende kjemikalier i bulk på norske skip. Rapport fra forprosjektet 1973–1974. Oslo: Yrkeshygienisk Institutt 1975.
44. Zorn, E., B.-F. Schepers and H. Goethe: Gesundheitsgefährdung durch Chemikalien an Bord deutscher Seeschiffe unter besonderer Berücksichtigung gefährlicher Ladung. Zbl. Arbeitsmed. *30,* 1, 12–19 (1900).

5.4 The Fishing Fleet

R. R. Renfrew

Since man first ventured offshore to catch fish, ships have slowly evolved from those constructed from readily available materials, powered by paddles or sails and designed to suit local conditions, to the modern diesel-engined, highly sophisticated vessel with a world-wide, all-weather fishing capability.

Whereas, formerly, fish had to be landed almost as soon as they were caught and, later, either salted on board or iced down in the fish hold to prevent decomposition, ships are now sailing which catch and either can or freeze the fish and turn the offal into fish meal.

The introduction of the 200-mile limits, the quota system and the escalating costs of fuel have brought about further changes over the past few years. Large vessels are being slowly phased out and are being replaced by small, fuel-efficient ships fitted with electronic systems of navigation and fish finding. One has only to glance through the pages of a publication such as Fishing News International to realise the diversity of fishing vessels world-wide. These vary from those with the lone operator fishing with multiple hooked lines or crab or lobster pots to the giant factory freezer with a crew of over 90 men and women on board. Depending on the size of the vessel a fishing trip can last from as little as a few hours to as long as several months. These variable factors make it quite impossible to discuss the health problems of fishermen in other than general terms in a chapter of this size.

5.4.1 Medical Standards

During any fishing operation, men must carry out their tasks on an unstable platform, often cluttered with nets, wires, ropes and moving machinery such as winches, and with fish and fish slime on the decks. The working area of the average fishing vessel is on the foredeck and this is commonly open to the elements. Here, the net is brought in, the fish are spilled out into compartments on the deck and the net is returned to the sea. The fish are then sorted, gutted, washed and taken below decks to be packed in ice.

Of necessity, the fisherman wears thick warm clothing and waterproof protective suits or smocks, which become stiff in cold weather. This combination will slow him down and adversely affect his agility.

The fisherman must thus be capable of working in a hostile environment, in cold wet conditions and for long periods at a time.

It is important, therefore, that new entrants to the industry should be physically fit and have good eyesight. High medical standards must be recognised and strictly applied by the examining physician. Examinees with conditions which would normally cause rejection, for example herniae and hydroceles, should be re-examined following a successful operation.

Muscular development and co-ordination must be good and there should be no deformity which could impede movement.

Deck personnel should have at least 6/6, 6/9 unaided vision initially, whilst cooks, engineers and others must have a visual acuity, using aids if necessary, sufficient to allow them to carry out their duties efficiently. When visual aids are worn, spares should be carried on each trip to sea.

Further medical examinations should be undertaken at regular intervals and also after injury or serious or prolonged illness. This will not only ensure that good standards of fitness are maintained but that early detection of physical and mental illness takes place. Those conditions common in the industry – gastritis and peptic ulcer, bronchitis, hypertension and the sequelae of excessive consumption of alcohol – are easily detected by clinical examination.

Medical standards for merchant seamen are discussed in Chap. 5.1. As fishing is known to be more hazardous and arduous than service with the merchant fleets, there is no valid reason why these standards should not also be applied to fishermen.

5.4.2 Accidents

Fishing is known to be one of the most hazardous of occupations. The Standard Mortality Ratio (SMR) gives an estimate of the occupational risk after standardising for age. This was calculated for all fishing vessels in the U.K. for the years 1959 to 1963 and covered the age groups from 15 to 64 years. For fishermen, the SMR was found to be 1726, whilst for coal miners in the comparable period, the figure was 373 (Schilling et al. [5]). The SMR for fishermen represents a risk factor of 17 against the male working population within the same age groups. These findings are not solely confined to the United Kingdom. Joensen [3], reviewing the literature, claims that the mortality rate amongst British and Danish fishermen is considerably higher than amongst workers in any other trade whilst Goethe and Vuksanović [1] have shown that the accident rates amongst German fishermen were two and a half times higher than those in their merchant fleet in the period 1954 to 1972.

The Comission of the European Communities has recently published a study of the accidents to fishermen which were reported during the years from 1977 to 1980 [4]. This study was intended to involve eight countries, all of which have active modern fishing fleets. Unfortunately, two countries failed to supply returns and one did not supply returns after 1978. In all 6731 accidents were reported and analysed over the 4-year period. It must be accepted that all accidents were not reported as there are fluctuations in the numbers from year to year which could not be accounted for by better safety standards.

The published figures show that one-third of all the accidents are the results of falls and slips on board, whilst another third involve the fishing gear. A high proportion of the accidents take place during the fishing operation when the deck crews, which form the bulk of the men at risk, are at work, and on the working deck space of the ships where most of the activities connected with the fishing operation take place.

Hands and fingers suffer most frequent injury whilst contusions, sprains and fractures are the commonest results of trauma.

Most accidents occur when the injured person has been at work continuously for 2–4 h, which may indicate an element of fatigue, and the bulk of them occur during the daylight hours. This latter finding is of little significance as a high proportion of ships fish only during the hours of daylight.

The figures do not suggest that inexperience or increasing age result in higher accident rates, as would be expected.

Again contrary to expectations, the highest percentage of accidents occurs during wind forces of 0 to 3 (wind speeds of less than 1 knot to 7–10 knots) and in sea state of 0 to 3 (wave heights from flat calm to 1⅔ ft), that is, during very good weather conditions. In bad weather the ships cease fishing and ride out the gales and the men who were asked all stated that during bad weather they were more aware of the dangers and tended to take a lot more care.

Excessive fatigue considerably increases the possibility of accidents in any hazardous occupation and slips and falls are often the result of muscle fatigue. Whilst there is no doubt that fishermen remain on duty for longer periods than many shore workers, modern fishing vessels are designed to cut down the amount of physical effort which must be undertaken by the crews. Hydraulically operated power rollers and strategically placed winches take away much of the back-breaking work. The ropes, wires and nets are rolled on to drums when out of the water and so constitute less risk to the men. Notwithstanding these factors, fishing is still hard work. The period spent on deck depends on the time taken to haul, to carry out any net repairs and to shoot the gear once again, together with the time taken to gut, wash, sort and stow the fish. When the decks are cleared up, meals and rest periods can be taken before the next haul takes place. The number of daily hauls varies considerably with the type of vessel. Some ships fish through the whole 24 hours, when a system of duty watches is employed, whilst others, usually the smaller ships, fish during the hours of daylight and anchor for the night. Rest periods, therefore, tend to be short and broken, which results in increasing fatigue over the whole trip. The Report on Trawler Safety 1969 [6] recognised these factors and recommended that, whatever the type of fishing, crewmen should be allowed at least 6 h of unbroken rest daily, and that they should have shore leave between trips of at least 2½ days. In practice, at present, crews have more than 60 h shore time between trips. This allows for not only adequate rest but for the men to catch up with their social and family life. Rest periods for countries other than the U.K. are prescribed, some by law and others by agreement. In France there is a minimum of 8 h rest whilst on the fishing grounds, in Germany, 8 h and in Iceland, 12 h.

5.4.3 General Medical Problems

Schilling et al. [5], writing on the mortality of fishermen in Great Britain, gave the following standardised mortality ratios for fishermen for the period 1959 to 1963 for England and Wales:

Coronary heart disease	130
Hypertension	215
Cancer of the lung and bronchus	191
Cancer of the stomach	189
Accidents not at work including Suicide	169
Bronchitis	147

The authors also reported a tendency for the men to suffer from gastro-intestinal illness, notably gastritis and peptic ulcer, possibly attributable to a combination of overindulgence in alcohol and tobacco and to stress. The SMRs, where available, for Scotland showed appreciable variation attributable to the difference in fishing methods between the individual countries of the U.K. Since the publication of the figures in 1969, tremendous changes have taken place within the industry in the U.K. and these figures can no longer be an accurate reflection of the pattern of disease amongst fishermen. However, they do give a clear indication of the necessity of regular physical examination for all fishermen for early detection of disease.

To the above list should be added the problems associated with obesity. Skippers and engineers in trawlers are usually overweight. Their duties confine them to the bridge or engine room, their exercise is very limited and, often, they are unable to go below for proper meals and so they exist on tea and sandwiches of monstrous proportions. This regime inevitably gives rise to obesity and is, in turn, linked to hypertension. It is very noticeable that, where skippers are involved in the fishing operations, as in the smaller vessels, obesity is not a problem.

5.4.4 Diseases Specific to Fishermen

Probably the commonest conditions found amongst fishermen are various types of skin lesions, notably those caused by infections and allergies and some by infestations. Facilities for washing may be primitive in the smaller ships whilst in the larger vessels the use of such facilities is limited because of the need to conserve the available fresh water supplies. Although sea water is readily available, special sea water soaps are necessary for adequate cleansing of the skin. Ordinary domestic dishwashing detergents are effective with sea water and are commonly used by the fishermen for hand washing. In susceptible people this can carry a risk of establishing dermatitis.

The hands are always vulnerable to pricks from wire strands, fish bones and fish spines and when, as a result of these, infection from the fish slime is carried into the deeper tissues, septic lesions of varying degrees of severity ensue. This type of injury is so commonplace that it is usually ignored but adequate cleansing and a first aid dressing could prevent much morbidity.

Antibiotics are now carried on most ships and their use has drastically cut down the number of cases of palmar space infections which have to be dealt with.

5.4.4.1 Salt Water Boils

Grit and sand brought up in the nets, together with dried salt, lodges in the cuffs of the waterproof clothing worn by fishermen and causes chafing and minute abrasions of the skin of the wrists and the backs of the hands which become infected.

The condition appears first as multiple small irritating papules on the wrists and the dorsum of the hands. These soon become pustules and some enlarge further to form boils. The whole area becomes inflamed, indurated and painful.

Treatment. The area affected should be thoroughly washed with soap and water, dried and dressed with 10% ichthammol (ammonium sulpho-ichthyolate) in glycerine, twice daily. Alternatively after washing and drying, the lesions can be swabbed with spirit and then covered with a dry dressing. Antibiotics are usually unnecessary unless large boils develop.

Prevention consists of thorough washing of the wrists and hands at the end of each watch on deck. The cuffs of waterproof clothing should be scrubbed with fresh water inside and out at regular intervals, and when the cuffs become badly worn or cracked the garment should be repaired or discarded.

5.4.4.2 Dogger Bank Itch or Curly Weed Rash

This is a contact eczematous dermatitis found amongst the men who fish in the North Sea. The causal agent is a seaweed-like *Alcyonidium,* known to fishermen as 'curly weed', which grows in shallow waters. It is found in profusion in the Dogger Bank area, hence the derivation of the name, but it has spread to the waters off the West of Scotland and to some parts of Greenland and Norway. The disease occurs in men who have become sensitised whilst fishing in the North Sea but it has been seen in those women who are employed ashore to clean and repair certain types of nets used in that area. The process of sensitisation can take many years or it can occur after only a few trips but, once established, even if the man is kept ashore it requires only brief contact with fishing gear used in the area to precipitate an attack. Deep water fishermen are only rarely affected but if they are, history taking will reveal that they have fished at some time in the areas of the North Sea in which the 'weed' grows and that they have recently been fishing in the other areas mentioned above. The curly weed is prevalent during the months between March and November and it is during this time that the majority of new cases occur. The rash usually appears as a dermatitis affecting the dorsum of the hands, the wrists and the forearms. Once established, further contact causes the rash to spread to the face, especially to the forehead and around the eyes. Oedema of this area and conjunctival inflammation are features at this stage. Ultimately, the whole body may become involved.

The parts affected are itchy, reddened, oedematous and often excoriated. When the rash becomes eczematous, the weeping and drying of the area causes painful cracks to appear in the skin.

Treatment. The only effective treatment is to remove the patient from all further contact with the curly weed and it is usual to advise transfer to ships fishing in deep waters. In the early stages, the rash will clear up when the man comes ashore for a short period, but, in established cases, further treatment will be required.

Treatment on board is by the administration of an antihistaminic drug and the application of hydrocortisone ointment 1% to the affected part. The conjunctivitis will be relieved by the use of β-methasone sodium phosphate 0.1% eye drops with or without neomycin. In established cases a daily bath to which is added 20 ml of liquor picis carbonis is recommended, together with the application of an ointment made up as follows:

Liquor picis carbonis	2%
Ung. hydrocortisone 1%	25%
Ung. aquosum	to 100%

Further contact with curly weed must be avoided. Oral steroids are rarely necessary in the treatment of this condition.

5.4.4.3 Fish Erysipeloid

This skin disease normally occurs during the warmer months of the year. Although most frequently seen in the fish process workers ashore, it is not unknown at sea. The disease arises from infection introduced by minor pricks and abrasions caused by the bones and spines of fish. The causal organism is commonly *Erysipelothrix rhusiopathiae,* which is found in fish slime. The area around the minor wound becomes inflamed. The inflammation spreads rapidly and the lesions closely resemble erysipelas although the oedema is not so marked. Lymphangitis and lymphadenitis are often a feature.

Treatment. The treatment of choice is penicillin, either oral or by injection. If oral penicillin is used, it is best to give double the standard dose for the first 48 h. Patients allergic to penicillin should be given co-trimoxazole (each tablet contains trimethoprim 80 mg and sulphmethoxazone 400 mg).

Prevention. As with other skin complaints originating from fish slime, thorough skin cleansing is the best method of prevention.

5.4.4.4 Haddock Rash

This condition is fairly common in those areas where the preponderance of the catch consists of haddock. These fish seem to ingest grit when feeding and when gutting is carried out on large numbers of fish, this grit abrades unprotected skin and these abrasions become infected. The lesions are seen as inflamed weeping areas between the fingers and on the backs of the hands.

Treatment. The affected part should be well washed before the application of dressings and antibiotics should be given.

Prevention. The condition can be prevented by the use of protective gloves. Thick plastic gloves are better than cotton gloves but they must be in a sound condition to prevent the grit getting through to the skin.

5.4.4.5 Acute Tenosynovitis of the Wrist (Jumbo Wrist)

When the fisherman returns to sea after a long period ashore or where he is involved in prolonged gutting following large hauls of fish, the repetitive movements required by the gutting operation may cause tenosynovitis of the wrist.

In order to gut a fish efficiently, the fish is held at the tail section, ventral side upwards, by one hand, whilst with the other hand the knife is inserted into the abdomen and an incision is made right up to the head of the fish. This involves a movement of the wrist through an arc of about 75 degrees. A similar movement is made to cut out and remove the guts, liver and the dorsal vein. Constant repetition of this movement causes the inflammation of the tendon sheath.

There is localised pain, swelling and crepitus, usually in the dorsum of the hand and wrist. The grating can be felt by the examiner when he lays his hand on the affected part and asks the patient to flex and dorsiflex the wrist.

Treatment. The only effective treatment is immobilisation of the hand and wrist. This can be done conveniently at sea, using a padded splint, whilst ashore the treatment of choice is a scaphoid plaster cast. Immobilisation should be continued for 7–10 days. An elastic adhesive bandage applied from the hand to just below the elbow will relieve the symptoms and support the part but the patient must not be allowed to continue gutting, otherwise the condition will be aggravated and the period of immobilisation will be prolonged. The condition frequently recurs after further periods of heavy fishing and gutting.

5.4.4.6 Fishermen's Conjunctivitis

Whilst the nets are being dragged along the bottom of the sea, they collect not only fish but stones and boulders and various types of marine growths.

A particular type of marine benthos resembles a suet dumpling and has finger-like structures protruding from it. These growths are known by colloquial names such as tits or duffs by the fishermen.

As the net is brought on board, the weight of the contents ruptures these growths and a fluid containing microscopic silicaceous particles is released. If this fluid enters the eye it sets up an intense irritation. The conjunctivae become rapidly infected and soon subconjunctival oedema occurs. The sclera then appears to be covered by red blisters and there is marked photophobia and pain. Later the eyes close up.

Treatment. Immediate treatment is to wash the eyes with either warm plain water or with normal saline. Eyedrops containing β-methasone sodium phosphate 0.1% w/v and neomycin sulphate 0.5% w/v should be instilled three or four times daily until the condition subsides.

5.4.4.7 Poisonous Stings

Fishing in the warmer waters of the tropics and subtropics is not without additional hazards. Certain fish, jelly-fish, marine growths and sea snakes can produce painful and often major reactions in the fisherman coming into contact with or being bitten or stung by them.

Doctors in these areas are well experienced in dealing with casualties from these bites and stings and although these conditions are mentioned for the sake of completeness, no attempt will be made to advise specific treatment other than to say that in the event of collapse, normal resuscitative manoeuvres should be undertaken.

5.4.5 Medical Training

Unlike workers ashore, the fisherman at sea does not have ready access to medical aid and hospitals. Consequently, he must be prepared to deal with any accident or medical emergency until such aid can be obtained.

As a life-endangering situation, which requires immediate treatment, may arise in any part of a ship at any time, it is essential that all fishermen be given a basic first aid training, preferably as part of an induction course. This training should include the arrest of bleeding from various sites, artificial respiration and the treatment of the unconscious patient.

All fishing vessel officers should be given further medical training, based either on their own country's medical guide for seafarers or on the International Medical Guide for Ships, as part of the courses leading to the award of certificates of competency. The length of the courses and the depth of the training can be varied in accordance with the certificate of competency which is awarded. When fishing activity is restricted to coastal waters and prompt medical assistance is available, the degree of training need not be so great as when no restrictions are imposed.

The aim of the training is to give ships' officers such knowledge as is required in order to provide care for sick or injured crew members, either until they are fit or until they can be put under medical care ashore, to make proper use of the radiomedical advice facilities available for seafarers and to prevent the spread of disease on board.

When the course is taken at, or in association with, a hospital, those organising the course must monitor the content carefully as there is a danger that the staff will give instruction in practices suitable for a hospital situation but totally unsuitable for a small ship.

5.4.6 International Standards of Medical Care

In the interest of safety at sea, each major country of the world lays down standards of competence in seamanship and navigation which must be attained before a man is allowed to take command of a vessel sailing out of sight of land. These standards vary little from country to country and they apply to small fishing vessels just as much as to the large ocean-going ship. The crew of a fishing vessel is a small community which, from the minute it leaves its home port until it returns, is not only subject to the rigours imposed by the environment but by the very nature of the work undertaken by that crew, has a very high risk of trauma. Illness can strike any member of the crew at any time as in any community but medical assistance is available only through a radiomedical advice facility. The doctor's ability to come to a diagnosis then depends entirely on the observations of a layman. Unfortunately, there is no internationally agreed standard of medical training for ships' officers nor indeed of medical stores which must be carried on fishing vessels and on which a crewman's life may depend.

This was realised by the member states of the E. E. C. and some 9 years ago a Working Group of Maritime Medical experts was set up under the auspices of the Joint Committee on Social Problems in Sea Fishing to study means of harmonising the medical scales carried on fishing vessels, medical standards for new entrants to the industry, regular medical examinations for ships' crews to ensure that the men can carry out their duties without detriment to themselves or the safety of the ship and finally to produce an acceptable training syllabus to cover the treatment of both injury and illness.

During the discussions, it emerged that even within the member states of the E. E. C., medical standards varied considerably. Some countries require a thorough pre-employment medical examination and chest X-rays whilst others have no such requirement. Some countries produce a complex medical guide whilst others have a simple guide, virtually a first aid manual, and rely on the International Medical Guide for Ships (IMGS) [2] for further information. Some countries have long medical training for officers, some of it in a hospital setting to varying standards according to their professional ticket and taken as a block course. Others have hour-long lectures at weekly intervals throughout their professional training period. The contents of medical chests vary from one country to another and the drugs supplied in them vary in accordance with medical teaching in the country concerned.

The recommendations of this Committee include:

1. A new entrant to the industry must receive a strict medical examination to ensure that he is capable of doing the work required of him at sea. Regular physical examinations must be carried out at intervals not exceeding 2 years to ensure that he maintains a high standard of physical fitness.
2. All members of a ship's crew must be trained in simple life-saving procedures such as control of bleeding, dealing with an unconscious crew member and resuscitation techniques so that a casualty can be kept alive until more skilled assistance is obtained.
3. Ships' officers must receive medical training based on their national medical guide or on the IMGS so that they can deal with any accident which may happen on the ship, recognise the more common emergencies and if in doubt take a history and make simple observations sufficient to assist the doctor giving medical advice by radio to make a diagnosis.
4. Medical scales should be harmonised so that they contain drugs and dressings in sufficient quantities to deal not only with the emergency but also with those common ailments which are to be found in any community ashore.

If the recommendations of the Committee are accepted by the member states, a great step forward will have been made. The quality of life at sea will be improved as the men will be fit enough to face the hazards of fishing, injuries and illnesses should be dealt with quickly, much unnecessary suffering will be prevented and finally, through regular medical examinations, the illnesses to which fishermen seem to be particularly prone can be diagnosed and treated at an early stage and thus a useful working life may be prolonged.

References

1. Goethe, H. and P. Vuksanović: Distribution of diagnoses, diseases, unfitness for duty and accidents among seamen and fishermen. Bull. Inst. mar. trop. Med. Gdynia *26,* 2, 133–158 (1975).
2. International Medical Guide for Ships. Ed.: ILO, IMCO, WHO. Geneva: WHO 1967.
3. Joensen, H. D.: Arbejdsmiljøskader inden for fiskerierhvervet. Ugeskr. Laeg. *141,* 49, 3396–3400 (1979).
4. Research on the circumstance of industrial accidents in sea fishing. Ed.: Commission of the European Communities. Directorate-General, Employment, Social Affairs and Education. 1977 – v/33/82; 1978 – v/34/82; 1979 – v/35/82; 1980 – v/36/82.
5. Schilling, R. S. F., J. Walford and R. Wood: The mortality of fishermen in Great Britain. In: Trawler Safety. Final report of the committee of inquiry into trawler safety. Ed.: President of the Board of Trade. London: Her Majesty's Stationery Office 1969, p. 117–125.
6. Trawler safety. Final report of the committee of inquiry into trawler safety. Ed.: President of the Board of Trade. London: Her Majesty's Stationery Office 1969.

Additional Reference

Fishing news international – a monthly publication for the fishing industry. London: Heighway Publications.

5.5 The Female Seafarer

O. W. Tenfjord

5.5.1 Introduction

Sea transport is as old as mankind. Over the centuries the vessels have gradually become larger and the voyages longer. In olden times, life on board was hard, the living quarters were crowded and primitive and the travellers were exposed to wind and weather. The staple food and water supply soon became insufficient on long voyages and the work was physically hard. The accident, disease and death rates were high. Therefore, work at sea was naturally accepted as a male occupation and not suited to females.

However, great changes have taken place, particularly during the last century. The transition from sail to motor was a revolution, sailing time being cut down considerably and safety improved. The ships were built larger and more spacious. National legislation and international agreements gradually helped to improve working and living conditions. Common sleeping quarters were replaced by cabins with four, and later two, bunks. On many modern ships every member of the crew has his/her own cabin with shower-bath and toilet. These improvements helped to pave the way for women to seek employment at sea. They appeared first of all as cabin cleaners and attendants on passenger liners in the second half of last century, and later as members of the catering department. Cleaning, washing, making beds and cooking were typical female occupations, similar to their home work and duties, so they were readily accepted on board in these capacities. Mixed crews became customary on passenger liners and ferry boats.

At the beginning of the 1930s women appeared for the first time on cargo ships carrying a limited number of passengers, usually 12. They replaced the mess- and galleyboys for two reasons. In the first place, the difference in wages at that time was negligible and, secondly, they were better suited to this type of work. After the Second World War, women appeared as radio officers and in greater number in the catering department of the merchant marines of many Western countries. They had already served for years in other capacities, e.g. as nurses ([4], Fraser [5]).

Today, the main concern is the problem of accepting women as crew members on deck and in the engine room – the typically male departments on board. However, experience has proved that these difficulties can be overcome (Münster [14]). It depends largely upon their skill, knowledge and conscientiousness. They have to adapt themselves to the prevailing conditions and they cannot expect to be treated as "ladies". The campaign for equal rights and equal opportunities for both sexes has been, and will continue to be, of great help to them.

Since 1960 the German Democratic Republic has employed a limited number of women as process workers on fishing factory vessels (Stiewe [19]). Generally, very few data are available about the number of women working at sea. However, statistical data have been published in Norway every year since 1964, giving details about the number of women and men and their occu-

Table 1. Males and females serving on Norwegian ships (1st November of each year)

Year	Females	Males	Total	Females as % of total
1964	3972	60177	64149	6.2
1965	4017	58770	62787	6.4
1966	4362	58269	62631	7.0
1967	4362	57893	62255	7.0
1968	3921	53583	57504	6.9
1969	3338	45930	49268	6.8
1970	3379	42794	46173	7.3
1971	3255	41204	44459	7.3
1972	3340	40632	43972	7.6
1973	3094	38368	41462	7.5
1974	3012	36726	39738	7.6
1975	2791	33373	36164	7.7
1976	2626	32643	35269	7.4
1977	2750	32462	35212	7.8
1978	2432	29474	31908	7.6
1979	2432	28861	31293	7.3
1980	2777	31929	34706	8.0

pation on board Norwegian ships. A census is held every 1st November [1]. Table 1 gives particulars relating to the census of the years 1964–1980:

It is evident that there has been a steady increase in the proportion of women serving on Norwegian ships, from 6.2% in 1964 to 8% in 1980. About 30% of the personnel in the catering department have been women. The proportion of female radio officers has increased from 17.7% in 1964 to 30.2% in 1980. In 1980, six women worked as mates and 34 as subordinates (ratings) on deck and in the engine room. A similar trend is reported by Münster from West Germany (Münster [14]).

5.5.2 Females and the Ship's Community

Why do women seek employment at sea? For several reasons – some like to join their husbands who are seafarers, some want to travel and see the world, others have more practical reasons – they need money. Some make a few trips, others become professional seafarers. They will, on board, face a community and a culture which is somewhat strange to them. This has been developed and maintained throughout centuries by men and is characterized by its special language and a form which is rather rough and vulgar. The appearance of women in this community caused temptation, created tension and gave rise to jealousy, rivalry and severe interpersonal conflicts – and resulted in a great number of pregnancies which usually had to be paid for by the companies. As a concession to the shipowners, the Norwegian Government decided in 1959 to pay the cost of repatriation of female seafarers who were pregnant. The number who were repatriated in the period 1964–1980 is recorded in Table 2.

Table 2. Number of pregnant females repatriated from Norwegian ships in overseas service

Year	Number repatriated	Total females in overseas service	Repatriated as % of total
1964	199	5581	3.56
1965	259	6017	4.3
1966	240	6755	3.6
1967	216	6348	3.4
1968	210	6198	3.4
1969	173	5650	3.1
1970	131	5432	2.4
1971	138	5733	2.4
1972	106	5444	2.0
1973	96	5505	1.8
1974	86	5503	1.56
1975	47	4856	0.97
1976	37	4917	0.75
1977	39	5139	0.76
1978	30	4382	0.7
1979	21	4121	0.5
1980	21	4143	0.5

The highest absolute and relative figures occurred in 1965. That year, 259 were repatriated, representing 4.3% of the total female population in overseas service. Later on, there was a steady decrease and the figures reached the lowest level in 1980, with 21 and 0.5% respectively [1]. This substantial reduction is certainly a result of the common use of contraceptives.

There is no doubt that, whatever prob-

Table 3. Distribution, by major disease category, of females and males signed off sick from Norwegian ships in overseas service between 1954 and 1970

Diagnostic category	Total females	As % of total	Total males	As % of total
1. Tuberculosis	44	0.2	879	0.6
2. Venereal diseases	54	0.3	3506	2.4
3. Other infective diseases	106	0.5	1780	1.2
4. Malignant neoplasms	100	0.5	630	0.4
5. Respiratory system	2574	12.9	13248	9.0
6. Circulatory system	448	2.2	5973	4.0
7. Digestive system	1933	9.7	26748	18.0
8. Nervous system, mental diseases	2794	13.9	18850	12.7
9. Genito-urinary system	3053	15.2	5483	3.8
10. Complications of pregnancy and childbirth	2002	10.0		
11. Musculoskeletal system	2767	13.8	18071	12.2
12. Skin	1167	5.8	9272	6.3
13. Eye diseases	60	0.3	1200	0.8
14. Ear diseases	181	0.9	2299	1.5
15. Asthenia	59	0.3	219	0.1
16. Nutrition and metabolic	80	0.4	647	0.4
17. Blood, blood-forming organs	84	0.4	215	0.1
18. Accidents	1932	9.6	34565	23.3
19. Others, ill-defined conditions	580	2.9	4686	3.2
	20028	99.8	148261	100.0

lems the women may have created, they have been greatly beneficial to the ship's community and have contributed largely to normalizing the life on board and helping to make the atmosphere more sober and homelike [4].

Today, women are received on board without objections, even if they are not always accepted as equal partners. Women from the countries of the Third World will, however, be unable to work on ships registered in those countries. Their status in their own community makes it impossible.

5.5.3 Health Problems

5.5.3.1 Merchant Marine

Health problems are reflected in morbidity and mortality rates. Without access to these data it is difficult to make an evaluation of the risks and hazards for women working at sea and to take the necessary preventive steps.

There are hardly any reliable statistical data available concerning diseases among seamen (Vuksanović and Goethe [20]) and this is even more the case with female seafarers. One of the very few sets of data relates to Norwegian women [2]. During the 17-year period 1954–1970, 20028 women and 148261 men were signed off sick and repatriated from ships in overseas service. The main diagnostic categories are presented in Table 3.

The women who were repatriated constitute a heterogeneous group with regard to the seriousness of the diseases. Some of them had to be admitted to hospitals immediately. Others were able to stay at home while undergoing treatment. They had one feature in common: the ships' masters were unable to accept the responsibility for further treatment on board. It should be remembered that this occupational group consists of mainly young and healthy women who had passed a careful medical examination before they signed on.

The figures in Tables 3 indicate that the seven major categories – accounting for about 80% of the discharged – were diseases of the genito-urinary system, mental diseases, diseases of the musculoskeletal system, diseases of the respiratory system, diseases of the digestive system, complications of pregnancy and childbirth, and accidents, in that order. Hoiberg made a study of the health care needs of women in the (U.S.) navy, based on the hospitalization rates during the years 1966–1975 (Hoiberg [7]). They were young women selected for military service and under constant medical observation. Although these two groups are not quite comparable, it is interesting to note that there are many points of resemblance between them regarding the distribution of the main diagnostic categories.

It is no surprise that the Norwegian data showed that diseases of the genito-urinary system headed the list for the female seafarers, the rate of 15.2% being in accordance with the distribution in the general population (Fugelli [6]). Abortions and menstruation abnormalities were not recorded separately, but are, by experience, very common. In a study of 148 Wave (naval) recruits, Boehm and Salerno [3] report that 72 (48.6%) indicated that they had menstruation abnormalities: 60 amenorrhea 7 metrorrhagia and 5 metrorrhagia and amenorrhea. Normal menstruation resumed after 3–4 months on average. Michalk [12] reports that one-third of all female process workers in fishing vessels experienced similar irregularities on their first sea voyage. Irregularities of this kind occur rather frequently during stressful periods of adjustment.

Diseases of the genito-urinary system and complications of pregnancy and childbirth accounted for 25% of all women signed off sick.

The second largest category in the Norwegian study is mental diseases (diseases of the nervous system constitute a small fraction only of the total number). A division into four subgroups disclosed that neuroses and maladjustment were by far the largest and that diagnoses relating to personal disorders such as psychoses and alcoholism occurred less frequently. This was in sharp contrast to Norwegian male seafarers who presented a picture which was completely opposite. Schuckit and Gunderson [18] report in a study of psychiatric incidence rates for navy (US) women that the psychiatric hospitalization rate for enlisted women in the period 1966–1969 was four times higher than for enlisted men. The diagnostic distribution for both sexes corresponded to that of Norwegian seafarers referred to above. Discussing the disparity between the sexes, Schuckit and Gunderson [18] point to four possible explanations: selection of young single women who have a tendency to escape difficulties at home, the rigid life in the navy, certain inborn biological factors in women and a tendency to hospitalize even minor cases – and an interaction between the four. Obviously, there are some striking similarities between life and work in the navy and in the merchant marine.

Diseases of the respiratory, musculoskeletal and digestive systems are major categories, just as in the general population (Fugelli [6]). A substantial reduction of diseases of the digestive system has taken place during the period, while the other categories have remained fairly constant.

Accidents are less frequent among women because they work in more sheltered surroundings. Offer-Ohlsen [15] records that by far the greatest number of accidents occur on deck and in the engine room while only a small proportion happen in the catering department.

Skin diseases constitute a rather small but important group. Frequent contact with detergents may cause dermatitis and eczema which may finally result in unfitness for work at sea.

The remaining categories, including neoplasms and diseases of the circulatory system, are rare. This is not surprising. Women

Table 4. Data on the Norwegian females and males who signed off sick from ships in overseas service during the years 1964–1970

Year	Total males	Males signed off sick	Sick as % of total	Total females	Females signed off sick	Sick as % of total
1964	80211	9995	12.4	5581	1423	25.5
1965	78897	8851	11.4	6017	1299	21.6
1966	83349	9228	11.1	6755	1495	22.1
1967	78911	9114	11.6	6348	1456	22.8
1968	72135	9881	13.7	6198	1705	27.3
1969	62983	8227	13.1	5650	1421	25.1
1970	58882	7042	12.0	5432	1378	25.0

suffering from serious or chronic diseases should not be permitted to work at sea.

Any Differences Between the Sexes?

As indicated in Table 3, there are some striking differences between the sexes. Accidents and diseases of the digestive system account for more than 40% of the men who signed off sick, compared with less than 20% of women. Four times as many men were signed off sick from infectious diseases, including venereal diseases, and twice as many from diseases of the circulatory system. What happens to seafarers who fall sick on board? How many can be treated on board, and how many have to be signed off? Are there any differences between the sexes in this respect?

For the years 1964–1970, figures are available giving details of the total population on Norwegian ships in overseas service, as well as the number who signed off sick [1, 2]. The figures are recorded in Table 4.

As indicated in Table 4, women were signed off sick twice as often as men, 25% compared with 11%–13%. This is a striking difference. How can this disparity be explained? Certainly, there are at least two possible explanations. First of all: ships' masters are obviously less familiar with female than with male illness. Instruction and practice in gynaecology and obstetrics are typically inadequate and theoretical. The clinical examination of these patients is difficult and requires special equipment which is not available on board. One can understand the reluctance of masters facing the examination and treatment of these patients. Secondly, the women cannot easily be replaced in their capacities on board. This applies to radio officers as well as staff in the catering department. This observation seems to indicate that during this period women were signed off sick more frequently than men even if they suffered from minor disorders. Since the last decade, no statistical data have been available either from Norway or any other country. It is therefore not possible to draw any conclusions as to the general validity of this observation.

5.5.3.2 Fishing Vessels

Since 1960, the German Democratic Republic has employed women as process workers on fishing factory vessels owing to the shortage of male workers. In 1960, only seven were employed. The number reached a maximum of 120 in 1969 and then slowly decreased to 114 in 1970 and 107 in 1971 (Stiewe [19]). The work was hard: standing at process machines and conveyer belts, lifting, carrying and piling cases of about 15 kg at high speed. The working conditions were uncomfortable, the temperature low, the humidity high, the illumination below standard and the noise level very high. The movement of the ships, particularly in rough weather conditions, made work most stressful. The working days were 12 h in two shifts of 6 h each without pauses. The journeys lasted 2–3 months (Stiewe [19]; Michalk [12]; Marschall and Kersten [10]). The women employed belonged to the age group 18–35. Work physiology tests had indicated that women in this age group possessed the maximum work capacity (Stiewe [19]). Before they signed on they went through a careful medical (and gynaecological) examination.

The most frequent diseases among the female crew members were accidents and diseases of the musculoskeletal system, digestive system, skin and respiratory systems (Oschatz [16]; Müller [13]). They had a higher incidence of diseases than the men, and their average morbidity rate was 4.4 compared with 2.5 for the men (Kersten [9]). Their loss of working days was also higher (Stiewe [19]).

The men expressed dissatisfaction with the female workers. In case of sickness they had to be replaced by men who were able to do any type of work on board while the women could work only in the galley.

Some authors recommend, after 10 years' experience, that women should gradually be replaced by male workers. They consider the work to be too hard for them (Stiewe [19]; Marschall and Kersten [10]).

5.5.4 Medical Provisions

A ship must be self-supporting to a great extent and this includes the medical services. With a few exceptions, ships' masters are responsible for care and treatment of the sick and injured. They have at their disposal a medicine chest with a certain selection of medical equipment, bandages, drugs, etc. The contents of this chest are subject to regulations of the various national health authorities and vary a great deal.

Should the chest contain any equipment or drugs particularly for women? Typical female disorders are diseases of the genitourinary system and complications of pregnancy. The majority of these conditions are infections of different kinds. Medhus [11] examined the demand for health services on six ships with mixed crews. The majority of the cases were infections and, of 124 different drugs which were dispensed, 83, or 66.9%, were antibiotics. The medicine chest should therefore contain a suitable selection of these.

Of the special female disorders, vaginal bleeding is rather common either as a symptom of infection or organic disease of the internal genital organs or in connection with abortions. Stress situations may produce menstruation irregularities. Childbirth on board is rare. Ergometrine is the drug of choice to use in many of these cases and should be included in the medicine chest.

5.5.5 Standards of Fitness

Some maritime insurance companies had established their own standards of fitness (e.g. in Norway) before ILO passed Convention no. 73 dealing with the medical examination of seamen. At the end of 1981 28 countries had ratified this Convention. Among them are important maritime countries such as Argentine, Belgium, Canada, Denmark, Finland, France, West Germany, Italy, Japan, The Netherlands, Norway, Panama, Poland, Portugal, Spain, Sweden, the Soviet Union and Yugoslavia, but not Greece, Liberia, the United Kingdom or the U.S.A.

According to the rules of this Convention, every person who is going to sign on a ship must produce a medical certificate which states that he/she is fit for service at sea. He/she must not be suffering from a disease which can a) endanger the health of the other persons on board, b) be aggravated during the service or render him/her unfit for further work at sea.

A person serving on deck must have satisfactory colour vision, power of vision and hearing. A health certificate is valid for 2 years, a certificate for colour vision for 6 years.

The framework of the Convention is settled by ILO. It is left to the different countries to work out the details and their own standards of fitness. As a rule, women as well as men suffering from serious or chronic diseases should not be permitted to sign on. The following examples may serve as an illustration: personality disorders, psychoses (even after recovery), severe cases of neurosis, alcoholism and drug addictions, chronic polyarthritis, bronchial asthma and myocardial infarction. New applicants should be assessed strictly according to the rules while professional seafarers may be given an individual assessment.

It is particularly important that seafarers on modern ships have a satisfactory health standard. The crew is reduced to such a degree that there is no spare capacity and work is so specialized that a person can hardly be replaced. In the first ever published work-load study in seafaring personnel, Israeli et al. [8] found that the physical work-load in catering staff was unexpectedly high. Recently Rodahl [17] drew attention to the fact that women working in the catering department have a heavy work-load for extended periods, corresponding to 30%–50% of their maximum physical work capacity. A work-load test might have been desirable in these cases but was considered to be impossible to carry out. However, these women ought to be in good physical condition.

5.5.6 The Future

Greater changes in design and specialization have taken place during the last 2–3 decades than ever before. New technical equipment such as the computer have been introduced and have changed conditions on board fundamentally. Anti-collision systems and unmanned engine rooms have been in operation for some time.

During the last three decades, the size of the crew has been reduced from 50 to 20 and, in several countries, naval architects and engineers are busy planning the future ship with a crew of 10–12. Many companies have cut the sailing time to 2–4 months. In the near future, ships may be operated by two regular crews who relieve each other and have a sailing time of 1–2 months. In the offshore industry, the period of service is 2–6 weeks on and 2–6 weeks off according to the position of the vessel.

The seafarer will mainly be engaged in safety work and practically no maintenance work will be carried out. The days of hard physical work will nearly have come to an end, but on these ships there will be few opportunities for social activities – and the work at sea will be less attractive than it used to be.

What will the opportunities be for females on these future ships? They will certainly work in the catering department as they have done for decades, but we may expect to find them in greater numbers in other capacities as well, as navigators and as engineers. There is already a decline in the recruitment to the merchant marine in some countries and this fact may offer them an additional opportunity.

References

1. Aarsberetning for 1964–1980 for Direktoratet for sjömenn [Oslo]. Bergen: Reklametrykk 1965–1981.
2. Aarsmelding og regnskap 1964–1970. Trygdekassen for sjömenn i utenriks fart.
3. Boehm, F.H. and N.J. Salerno: Menstrual abnormalities in the Wave recruit population. Milit. Med. *138,* 30–31 (1973).
4. Female personnel aboard ship: Habitability design considerations (Report of FY 73 findings). Washington: Naval Ship Engineering Center. Department of the Navy 1974.
5. Fraser, S.: Nurse at sea. Can. Nurse *67,* 17–19 (1971).
6. Fugelli, P.: Helsetilstand og helsetjeneste paa Väröy og Röst. Oslo: Universitetsforlaget 1978.
7. Hoiberg, A.: Health care needs of women in the Navy. Milit. Med. *144,* 2, 103–109 (1979).
8. Israeli, R., M. Weinstein and D. Süssmann: Untersuchungen über die Arbeitsplatzanforderungen an Bord von Passagierschiffen. Neuzeit-

liche Gesichtspunkte bei Einstellungsuntersuchungen von Seeleuten. Arbeit und Leistung *21*, 8, 145–147 (1967).

9. Kersten, E.: Arbeitshygienische Beurteilung der Arbeitsanforderungen in der Schiffahrt unter besonderer Berücksichtigung der Beschäftigung von Frauen und Jugendlichen an Bord. Verk.-Med. *14*, 6, 203–219 (1967).
10. Marschall, B. and E. Kersten: Arbeitshygienische Betrachtungen zum Strukturwandel in der Hochseefischerei unter dem besonderen Aspekt der Frauenarbeit an Bord. Verk.-Med. *18*, 11, 481–491 (1971).
11. Medhus, M.: Kartleggning av helsearbeidet om bord paa skip. In: Sykdomsbildet hos sjöfolk – helsetjenesten til sjös. Ed.: Institutt for almenmedisin. Oslo: Norges Teknisk-naturvitenskapelige Forskningsraad 1980. pp. 68–99. (System for Sikkert Skip. Rapport 80/1)
12. Michalk, H.: Frauenarbeit auf See. In: Fragen der Schiffahrtsmedizin. Intern. Symp., Heiligendamm 28–31 March 1963. Medizinischer Dienst des Verkehrswesens II, pp. 42–51.
13. Müller, U.: Woman labor aboard ships. In: III International Symposiom on Marine Medicine, Leningrad 1968. Moscow 1969. pp. 69–70.
14. Münster, U.: Frauen an Bord. Was eine AG-Studentin dazu meint. Hansa *114*, 14, 1372–1375 (1977).
15. Offer-Ohlsen, D.: Skadebildet hos sjömenn i Wilh. Wilhelmsens Rederi 1976–1978. In: Sykdomsbildet hos sjöfolk – helsetjenesten til sjös. Ed.: Institutt for almenmedisin. Oslo: Norges Teknisk-naturvitenskapelige Forskningsraad 1980. pp. 15–54. (System for Sikkert Skip. Rapport 80/1)
16. Oschatz, R.: Die derzeitige Situation der Frauenarbeit an Bord der Fang- und Verarbeitungsschiffe. Dissertation, University of Rostock 1967.
17. Rodahl, K.: Arbeidsstress til sjös. Oslo: Arbeidsfysiologisk Institutt 1980. (System for Sikkert Skip. Rapport 80/2)
18. Schuckit, M. A. and E. K. E. Gunderson: Psychiatric incidence rates for navy women: implications for an all volunteer force. San Diego 1972.
19. Stiewe, M.: Eine kritische Einschätzung der Frauenarbeit in der Produktionsabteilung der Fang- und Verarbeitungsschiffe. Verk.-Med. *18*, 12, 521–528 (1971).
20. Vuksanović, P. and H. Goethe: Die Morbiditätsstruktur der Seeleute – ein internationaler Vergleich. In: Unfall- und Sicherheitsforschung Straßenverkehr. Kongreßbericht Jahrestagung 1981 der Dtsch. Ges. f. Verkehrsmed. gemeinsam m. d. Dtsch. Verkehrswacht. Hamburg, 7.–9.5. 1981. Ed.: Bundesanstalt für Straßenwesen im Auftrage des Bundesministers f. Verkehr. Braunschweig: Waisenhaus-Buchdruckerei 1981. pp. 57–66.

5.6 The Child at Sea

O. W. Tenfjord

5.6.1 Introduction

Throughout the ages children have been passengers on board ships and have usually been attended in sickness or in health by their mothers or members of their families. In former days the recreational and medical facilities for children were often sparse.

Modern passenger liners are equipped with kindergartens and have doctors and nurses on board together with the necessary facilities to deal with children of all ages in case of diseases or accidents.

Until quite recently members of the crew, with the exception of the master, have not, however, been permitted to bring their children with them. The position of the master on board is very special. Even in the era of sailing ships his living quarters were spacious with several rooms well suited to accomodate several persons. This gave him the opportunity of bringing his wife and children with him, even on deep sea voyages.

As long as the remaining crew members had to share cabins with each other, it was impossible for them to take any of their dependents with them on board. A satisfactory standard of living quarters was not attained by many maritime countries until after the Second World War. From the 1950s onwards, children tend to appear frequently on board with the permission and kindness of various shipping companies.

5.6.2 Children on Board: The Present Situation

As mentioned above, ships from many countries carry children on board today. To what extent does this occur and under what conditions? Is there any uniform practice? In order to obtain information about the different aspects of carrying children on board, colleagues from seven maritime countries and 13 Danish and six major Norwegian shipping companies were contacted and asked various pertinent questions. The answers received are set out below.

1. *Do seamen – officers as well as ratings – have permission to bring children with them on their sea voyages?*

In the USA, no company seems to allow children to accompany seafarers on a voyage. As passengers on freighters with accomodation for 12, children may travel and the minimum age is 1 year (Urner [8]).

In the UK, children are allowed on board ships belonging to large companies with mainly foreign-going vessels and to companies with mixed passenger and cargo vessels, but not on ships belonging to medium-sized companies and multinational oil companies. Children are never permitted on oil tankers. The permission to bring children on board extends to officers only, or officers and petty officers on company service contract (Watson [9]).

In Italy and the Netherlands, seafarers – officers as well as ratings – can bring children with them (Tortori-Donati [7]; Groeneweg [4]). The same practice applies to two of the large shipping companies in Sweden and a major navigation company in Israel (Lehmann [5]; Shani [6]).

In West Germany, the large oil companies do not permit children on board, but many other companies give such permission. One of the major companies extends this permission only to seafarers who have been on a contract for 6 months – officers as well as ratings. Excepted from this rule are cadets undergoing training and crew members of ships taking part in an 18-man crew project. The number of children on board must not exceed six (Backhaus [2]).

In Denmark, 12 of the companies, including all the major ones, permit children on board, the one exception being a salvage company. Seven of the companies grant this permission to officers and petty officers only, two to officers and ratings on company contract and three to all groups of seafarers.

The majority of Norwegian shipping companies gives permission to all seafarers, officers and well as ratings, but in some cases this is restricted to seafarers on company service contract only. Sometimes the final decision rests with the master.

It is generally understood that the children should be accompanied by their mothers. It is also requested that the wives of the seafarers make their beds, clean their cabins and give a helping hand when asked for. Additional people on board are an extra burden on the members of the catering department.

The children will usually have free board, but some companies charge a fee per day for food (Groeneweg [4]; Backhaus [2]).

2. *Are there any restrictions regarding the type of journey or time to be spent on board?*

In two of the countries referred to, there are no restrictions on the length of time children can stay on board. (Watson [9]; Shani [6]), but in all the other countries there is a time limit which extends from 2–3 months to 6 months. In a Dutch company the senior officers may keep their children on board for 26 weeks (Groeneweg [4]).

Seven of the Danish companies permit the children to stay on board 2–3 months; five have no restrictions at all.

A number of shipping companies do not permit children to take part in deep sea voyages, but on restricted ships only, e.g. coastal waters (Norwegian companies), North European waters (Norwegian companies) or the Mediterranean area (Tortori-Donati [7]).

3. *Is there any family accomodation on board?*

With one exception the answer was no. One of the major Norwegian tanker companies has two family apartments on each of their ships built later then 1975. As a rule, the wife and children will have to share the cabin of the seafarer.

4. *Is there a minimum age?*

There is a great deal of variation: 1 year (Shani [6], one Swedish company), 2 years (some Norwegian companies), 3 years (Tortori-Donati [7], Backhaus [2]), 4 years (Groeneweg [4], Lehmann [5], Backhaus [2]), 5 years (Watson [9]) and 6 years (Backhaus [2]). Five Danish companies stipulate no minimum age at all, the others 2–5 years. Some Norwegian companies stipulate no minimum age at all or no minimum age when the trip is restricted to coastal waters only. The final decision may rest with the master.

5. *Is a health certificate required?*

With a few exceptions the answer was no. The navigation company in Israel requires a health certificate and this must be issued by a paediatrician (Shani [6]), some British companies and the largest Danish company require a health certificate from the family doctor (Watson [9]) and a major West German company requires a health certificate issued by an approved seaman's doctor (Backhaus [2]).

As a rule the children must be properly vaccinated.

6. *Are there any stipulations on who should meet the cost of a) medical treatment and care in foreign ports, b) repatriation and c) deviation?*

Usually these costs will be covered by Marine insurance (Protection and Indemnity Club) and for some companies this is obligatory (Watson [9], Groeneweg [4], Shani [6] Backhaus [2]). If the national health insurance does not cover all the costs of medical treatment or repatriation, some Norwegian companies will debit the balance to the seaman involved; otherwise it is paid for by the companies themselves. The heavy costs of deviation will usually be paid for by the companies if they are not covered by the insurance. Two of the Danish companies require that all costs should be met by the seafarer himself.

5.6.3 Children on board: Health problems

The children are supposed to be healthy when they arrive on board and not suffering from any chronic disorders. Naturally, they may fall sick or be injured during a journey. What kind of medical problems may occur? It will mainly be a question of everyday medical disorders, but some special problems may arise, and these can appropriately be divided in the following five categories:

1. *Common children's diseases.* Many of these, such as diphtheria, polio and whooping cough, are rare today among children from the Western countries. Others, such as measles and chickenpox, run a mild course and should seldom give rise to any problems or complications of importance.
2. *Diseases of the respiratory system.* These occur rather frequently, particularly during winter; the common cold heads the list. Other important diseases or complications in this category are bronchitis, pneumonia, acute otitis media, laryngitis and, if the temperature runs high, fever cramps. Diagnosis and treatment may be difficult. These conditions are particularly dangerous for small children and infants.
3. *Diseases of the digestive system.* The disorder most feared is diarrhoea, which is particularly difficult to treat and serious for small children and infants.
4. *Accidents.* Children are liable to accidents on board as well as ashore. They may fall while on ladders and staircases and stumble and fall on loose objects on deck, particularly when the ship is rolling badly. Small children have a tendency to crawl all over the place, are quick and have a wide sphere of operation. At the age of 1–4 years they must be looked after properly, otherwise they may get on deck and run the risk of falling overboard.
5. *Tropical diseases.* The most widespread is malaria and this and a great number of other tropical diseases may present diarrhoea as the most important and dangerous symptom.

In addition to these five categories, emergencies of many types may arise.

5.6.4 The Future

A large number of companies in many maritime countries permit children to travel on their ships provided they are accompanied by their mothers. An increasing number of children may be expected on board in the years to come, from an increasing number of countries. There is a great difference between the companies concerning requirements as to minimum age, health certificates etc.

As discussed previously, many of the common diseases may be serious, above all for small children and infants. The masters are in charge of medical care and treatment. The responsibility for sick children is an extra burden on them and somewhat unfair because they have no instructions and no experience in dealing with this kind of patient. They may expect to be called upon by the mothers in everyday matters as well as in emergencies.

Certain steps should be taken to minimise the risks attendent upon having children on board. Some of these will be the responsibility of the companies themselves, because it is up to them to give the permission to join the ships, some will rest with the health authorities.

5.6.4.1 Minimum Age

Is it necessary to stipulate a minimum age and if so, what should the suitable age be? Five colleagues who are experienced company doctors were asked this question. One suggested that the minimum age should be 2 years compared with 1 year today in his company, the remaining four were in favour of 4, 5 or 6 years.

Twelve Danish companies were asked this question. One would not stipulate a minimum age at all, three were in favour of a minimum age of 2 years, one said 3 years and six said 4–5 years. One company did not answer this question.

A reasonable minimum age demanded by the companies should be at least 4 years for longer trips or deep sea voyages. At the age of 4 years, children are expected to be old enough to describe symptoms and to co-operate adequately in the treatment. In coastal waters with easy access to health services ashore, the minimum age may be reduced to 1–2 years.

If the seafarers are allowed to bring infants or small children with them, the mothers must be responsible for the supply of the necessary equipment for nursing them, such as suitable napkins, dusting powder, ointments and feeding bottles (Backhaus and Ziegenhagen [3]).

For the protection of small children, a playpen can be set up.

5.6.4.2 Health Certificate

A health certificate should be required for every child to ensure that the health condition is satisfactory upon arrival on board. Children on trips in coastal waters may be exempted from this requirement.

5.6.4.3 Family Apartments

This is a company concern and must be considered as part of its personnel policy.

Instruction to the Masters in Paediatrics

Masters should obviously receive instruction in paediatrics considering the increasing number of children who can be expected on board in the years to come; it should form part of the curriculum in medicine and first aid for the masters. Today, instruction in obstetrics is given although deliveries rarely or never take place on board cargo ships – just in case. It seems more reasonable to include paediatrics in the curriculum. The responsibility for the solution of this problem rests with the health authorities.

If it is accepted that masters should receive instruction in paediatrics, the Medical Guide should contain a chapter on this subject. Backhaus has written a useful guide to the officers of his own company with instruction about diagnosis and treatment of the most common children's diseases which may occur on board (Backhaus [1]).

5.6.4.4 Contents of the Medicine Chest

As inflammations and infectious diseases occur frequently among children the medicine chest should contain a suitable selection of antibiotics, and additional medical supply to meet disorders such as diarrhoea, poisoning etc. Doses of all medicines to be given to children vary according to age, and general instruction for the dispensing of these drugs should be available on board. The final pages of the new edition of the British Ship Captain's Medical Guide, published in 1982, are devoted to this subject.

5.6.4.5 Insurance

A comprehensive insurance policy should be provided for the children, covering medical care and treatment in foreign ports, repatriation and deviation. If the costs exceed the repayment of the insurance, the balance ought to be paid by the company as the children are on board by virtue of their permission.

Detailed rules for having children on board, such as a minimum age, a health certificate and vaccinations should be worked out by all shipping companies.

References

1. Backhaus, A.: Kinder an Bord von Seeschiffen. Hamburg 1971.
2. Backhaus, A. (Hafen- u. Flughafenärztl. Dienst, Hamburg): Personal information 1981.
3. Backhaus, A. and M.-L. Ziegenhagen: Raum für Mutter und Kind auf Passagier- und Fährschiffen. Hansa *109,* 21, 1966 (1972).
4. Groeneweg, J.J.P. (Regionale Bedrijfsgeneeskundige Dienst voor het Havengebied van Rotterdam en Omgeving, Rotterdam): Personal information 1981.
5. Lehmann, L. (Rederi AB. Transatlantic, Gothenburg): Personal information 1981.
6. Shani, E. (ZIM Israel Navigation Co., Haifa): Personal information 1981.
7. Tortori-Donati, B. (Finmare, Genoa): Personal information 1981.
8. Urner, Chr. (Lykes Bros., New Orleans): Personal information 1981.
9. Watson, E.N. (General Council of British Shipping): Personal information 1981.

5.7 Health Care of Passengers

P.O. Oliver

5.7.1 Introduction

Travel by sea has undergone considerable change over the past 20 years as a result of the ready availability of cheap, rapid air travel. With the decrease in the number of passengers using sea travel as a mode of transportation, the great passenger fleets of the past have disappeared to be replaced by purpose-built liners engaged in the holiday cruise business. Normally, the cruises are of 1–2 weeks' duration and are operated in areas where the climate is attractive and the seas calm. Nevertheless, a few passenger ships continue to operate popular world cruises of up to 3 months' duration. These can present their own particular problems as by their very nature they tend to attract an older clientele, often with pre-existing medical conditions.

With the increasing popularity of less expensive package tour cruising it is estimated that over 200000 passengers from the United Kingdom choose this type of holiday each year. Many of these cruises operate on a fly/cruise basis and it must, therefore, be remembered that fitness for sea travel must be considered in parallel with fitness for air travel. Those cruises which operate from and return to their own port of origin are obviously much less disruptive and are more suitable for those passengers with known disabilities. Long air-flights in order to join a ship overseas may involve significant disturbances of circadian rhythms, resulting in undue fatigue on arrival and aggravating pre-existing ill health. Sudden climatic changes from the winter cold of Western Europe to the hot humidity of the tropics can prove to be most demanding, especially for the elderly and infirm (Oliver [16, 17]).

Such people are often found on board cruise liners. Cameron [1] specifically dealt with the hazards of ocean cruises for elderly and infirm persons. It is the responsibility of both the family doctor and the hospital doctor to advise patients against sea voyages unless they are of reasonably robust health and adequate medical facilities are available on board.

Several authors have investigated the medical problems of cruises and the experiences of doctors aboard. Dahl [3] and Polonov [18] were of the opinion that diseases of the respiratory system were by far the most frequently diagnosed. It is evident from the figures given by Polonov that pharyngitis, motion sickness and gastro-intestinal diseases are the next most frequent illnesses.

In his survey of medical problems during package cruises, Carter [2] discussed emergencies requiring disembarkation. During 35 cruises, 12 patients had to be disembarked and admitted to hospital. The following diagnoses were listed:

4 myocardial infarctions
2 perforated peptic ulcers
1 melaena
1 haematemesis
1 pneumonia
1 hypercalcaemia
1 cerebrovascular accident
1 attempted suicide with aspiration of vomitus

Jones [12], Tortori-Donati [22], Tortori-Donati and Giannico [23] and Warncke [25] reported on experiences of doctors on board and the relevant preventive and therapeutic conclusions to be drawn. They all emphasized that, besides his occupational health knowledge, the doctor on board passenger vessels - particularly cruise ships - should be familiar with geriatric medical problems and the care of the disabled, which may present particular difficulties on board. Despite the awareness of special medical problems which may arise on board, there are always passengers who normally should have been advised against a sea voyage.

Jäger [8–11] dealt repeatedly with the problems of medical care on board passenger vessels at sea. He invented the term "cruise ship medicine". This author stressed the very high qualifications needed by a doctor on board a passenger vessel. He is usually on his own and has no specialist or emergency hospital facilities at hand.

Doctors recommending a holiday cruise for their patients should always ensure that they are provided with full medical documentation relating to their condition and details of any medication which they may be receiving. All too often patients in declining health are encountered, having mislaid their medication and without medical documentation. Such a situation can cause serious medical problems for the ship's doctor, whose diagnostic and therapeutic resources may be limited. Obviously, larger passenger vessels are more likely to provide more extensive medical facilities and this should be borne in mind by the family doctor when advising a patient to embark on a sea voyage.

5.7.2 Immunization

Despite the considerable progress that has been made by the World Health Organization in the eradication of contagious diseases world-wide, protective immunization against certain diseases is still strongly recommended for the majority of cruise passengers. Depending on the countries to be visited, typhoid, tetanus and cholera may all be indicated. Certain countries will require yellow fever inoculation, though fortunately smallpox vaccination is no longer necessary. Poliomyelitis should not be omitted and in special situations hepatitis inoculation may be advisable, especially in the Middle East and North Africa. Intending passengers should be advised to complete all inoculations well in advance of departure, preferably 2 weeks, so as to avoid the discomfort of any adverse reaction which may occur and which can all too easily spoil an otherwise pleasant vacation. Information regarding vaccination requirements can normally be obtained from the offices of the shipping company concerned. Correct documentation of vaccination certificates is essential if inconvenience by local health authorities overseas is to be avoided. Where it is known that there is a risk from malaria, appropriate prophylactic tablets should be recommended such as Paludrine (proguanil hydrochloride) 100 mg one tablet daily or Maloprim (pyrimethamine 12.5 mg, dapsone 100 mg) one tablet weekly. Dosage should be continued for at least 6 weeks after leaving a malarious area.

5.7.3 Passenger Facilities

A wide range of facilities are available to intending passengers, depending on the cost of the cruise, size of the vessel and nationality of the crew. At one end of the scale is the cheap package tour offering basic conditions with poor air conditioning, limited menus, absence of elevators and possibly low standards of food hygiene as well as minimal medical services. At the other end is the more expensive luxury cruise line providing high standards of catering and air conditioning as good as or better than any luxury hotel ashore, together with comprehensive medical facilities including electrocardiography and diagnostic radiography supported by experienced and well-trained medical staff. Passengers, especially if elderly or infirm, should give careful consideration to these factors before selecting an appropriate cruise or journey by sea. A modest additional expenditure may well ensure a more comfortable and safer vacation with the secure knowledge that good medical services are available should the need arise. Dental, physiotherapy and chiropody facilities can often prove of great value.

5.7.4 Gastro-intestinal Problems

Gastro-enteritis is a common complaint in passenger vessels. This is usually unrelated to poor food hygiene conditions but can be largely attributed to over-indulgence in food and alcohol and failure to observe safe eating habits ashore in foreign ports. Potable water, at one time a frequent source of gastro-intestinal infection, is now rarely the culprit as modern water supply systems are adequately chlorinated and subjected to frequent bacteriological examination to ensure potability.

In many publications the frequent occurrence of gastro-intestinal diseases on passenger vessels is related to the problems of sanitation and food hygiene aboard. It is not, however, always possible to isolate the pathogens.

Werner et al. [26] found that a gastro-enteritis outbreak on a cruise vessel was caused by *Salmonella infantis* and fortunately not by *Vibrio cholerae,* as originally suspected. Davies et al. [6] isolated *Salmonella typhi* during a typhoid epidemic on board. It was possible to stop the epidemic only by strict measures of sanitary hygiene. Merson et al. [15] traced *Shigella flexneri* as the cause of gastro-enteritis on board. During this epidemic, approximately 90% of the passengers and approximately 35% of the crew members fell ill.

In their survey report on 38 cruise vessels with 2445 passengers on board, Merson et al. [14] pointed out that gastro-intestinal diseases occurred in 92% of voyages, according to the medical logs. The actual incidence of gastro-intestinal illness determined by a questionnaire survey of passengers sailing on nine cruises was found to be at least four times as high as that recorded in the medical logs. A survey of the food-handling practices and water systems aboard selected ships demonstrated a significant potential for transmission of food-borne and water-borne disease. Also the Center for Disease Control, Atlanta, was concerned with the evaluation of the above-mentioned data. According to their findings the total rate of gastro-intestinal diseases was 50 per 1000 passengers (4%), and on approximately one-third of the 38 vessels these diseases occurred on board during the voyages.

Korcok [13] and also the Center of Disease Control in a "Survey of Environmental Sanitation on 12 Passenger Cruise Ships" [20] critically checked the sanitary and food hygiene facilities on board. They found that long years of education lead to partial improvement but that in some cases the situation leaves much to be desired as there is still a risk of outbreak of gastro-intestinal diseases.

In a survey of the incidence of gastro-intestinal illness on passenger cruise ships, the Center for Disease Control, Atlanta, stated that only 2 of 52 cruises on which at least 5% or more of the passengers became ill were reported to CDC Quarantine Stations. The incidence of gastro-intestinal illness overall was quite frequent [20].

Dannenberg et al. [4] reported on gastro-intestinal illness on passenger cruise ships between 1975 and 1978. A significantly high proportion of enteric disease outbreaks occurred on vessels that did not pass routine annual or semi-annual sanitation inspections. The cruise ship sanitation programme, developed with the cooperation of the cruise ship industry and the Centers for Disease Control, appears to have been successful in reducing the overall rate of outbreaks of enteric illness on cruise ships.

Travellers' diarrhoea, a well-recognized syndrome, is not uncommon and, although unresponsive to medication apart from symptomatic relief, usually resolves spontaneously after 48 h if dietary and alcohol abstinence is observed during this period. Diarrhoea, when persistent, responds satisfactorily to the administration by mouth of well-proven remedies such as kaolin and morphine mixture or Lomotil (diphenoxylate hydrochloride) or an electrolyte replacement preparation coupled with increased fluid intake to counteract the effects of dehydration. Antibiotics should be reserved for those cases where an infective element is apparent.

Diverticulitis and ulcerative colitis can produce unwelcome relapses at sea caused by changes in dietary habits and over-indulgence in alcohol. Changes in normal eating habits and the consumption of unfamiliar food and drink together with a change in social habits may aggravate a previously well-controlled colostomy. With shared cabin accommodation, obnoxious odours and toilet routine may cause considerable problems to such patients.

Peptic ulceration is an ever-present problem at sea with its danger of perforation or bleeding leading to haematemesis or melaena. Emergency surgery at sea, should conservative measure fail, can carry a high mortality. Blood transfusion on board can prove difficult and sometimes hazardous if cross matching and grouping procedures are not of the highest standard. The introduction of cimetidine has somewhat complicated the clinical picture. Many patients, especially those with duodenal ulcers, are now relieved of symptoms within a few weeks and embark on a cruise symptom-free and on a normal diet, with so-called healed ulcers.

Regrettably, cessation of treatment frequently results in relapse. It should be noted that cimetidine, apart from being very expensive, may not be obtainable on board or overseas. Normally patients should be advised not to undertake a long sea voyage until they have completed a full course of cimetidine treatment and have been free of symptoms for at least 3 months thereafter. Endoscopy to confirm satisfactory healing is a prudent procedure in such cases.

Appendicitis, once the scourge of seafarers, is now a less serious medical problem than in the past. The advent of conservative measures of treatment with antibiotics, intravenous fluid replacement and nasogastric suction has replaced the need for heroic surgery at sea with all its attendant dangers. It is of interest to note that the conservative management of patients presenting with acute abdominal pain is now standard practice in the U.S. and R.N. nuclear submarine patrols (Wilken [27]; Davies [5]). The ratio of non-specific abdominal pain (NSAP) to acute appendicitis rests largely with the skill of the examining ship's doctor, though the accurate diagnosis is unrelated to the outcome from conservative measures (De Dombal [7]).

5.7.5 Cardiovascular Disorders

With a disproportionate number of middle-aged and elderly persons travelling on holiday cruises, the incidence of cardiovascular accidents is high. A sudden acute cardiac ischaemic attack is the most common medical emergency encountered at sea. Fortunately in most modern passenger liners skilled medical assistance is readily available and transfer to the ship's hospital easily accomplished. Electrocardiographic and cardiac monitoring facilities, combined with defibrillation or anti-arrhythmic therapy, may prove life saving in this situation. It is essential that known cardiac cases carry with them full medical records of their condition and current medication so that the information is immediately available to the ship's doctor in an emergency.

Cerebral vascular accidents are relatively frequent in view of the high proportion of elderly passengers (many of whom are on hypertensive therapy) carried on board. Despite this fatalities are rare, a feature attributable to the high standard of medical and nursing care provided on many ships. Uncontrolled hypertension or a history of transient ischaemic attacks indicates a poor prognosis. The elderly or infirm should be advised to take care in choosing a cruise, especially of long duration, so as to ensure that high-quality medical services are available on board should the need arise.

Passengers with a residual hemiplegia should have no undue problems in coping with the shipboard environment provided they can attend to their own personal needs unaided and are not incontinent. Enquiries should be made to confirm that adequate elevators are available to all decks and that ship-to-shore gangways are conveniently available. Wheelchair assistance can be provided where necessary.

Subsequent repatriation or a return flight by air can cause serious problems following a cardiac or cerebral vascular accident, as airlines may impose their own criteria for fitness to travel.

5.7.6 Respiratory Disorders

In the confined shipboard environment, despite adequate air conditioning, upper respiratory infections are all too common and the opportunity for spread of infection is high. The majority of cases are viral in origin and response to antibiotics is poor. Ulewicz and Dolmierski [24] reported on an epidemic of pharyngitis on board a passenger ship. Such epidemics do not seem rare. From a total of 750 passengers and 300 crew members, 198 passengers and 84 crew members fell ill; they were treated with penicillin and tetracycline. After the voyage, serological examinations of some of the crew members showed high ASO and anti-M titres. Fortunately, no cases of legionnaires disease have been reported at sea. Effective antibiotic therapy of upper respiratory infection of bacterial origin has markedly reduced the incidence of complications such as bronchitis, pneumonia and pleural effusion. Radiographic facilities are normally available on most cruise liners so that early diagnosis can be established and complications recognized at an early stage. Asthma, particularly acute bronchospasm, is a dangerous condition at sea, especially where environmental conditions are poor, with small enclosed cabins and inadequate air conditioning. The wide range of medications on shore may not be available on board and oxygen therapy severely restricted. The situation can be further complicated by absence of elevators and lack of acclimatization to the heat and humidity of tropical climates. Patients should be advised to avoid such cruises unless their asthmatic condition is stable and well controlled with appropriate medication. Well-equipped ships's hospitals providing steroid therapy and supportive oxygen can deal adequately with asthmatic problems, although these facilities may not be available in smaller vessels.

Cases of pneumonia and acute bronchitis present no special problems at sea as recovery is normally complete following antibiotic treatment. Many passengers are on a fly/cruise programme and the prompt and effective treatment of pulmonary infection is essential if they are to be able to return home by air at the end of their vacation.

5.7.7 Mental Illness

Ships are poor places to suffer from a psychiatric illness. Contrary to popular belief, the depressive patient does very badly at sea and the expected improvement, resulting from a change in living conditions coupled with the relaxed and friendly atmosphere of shipboard life, does not occur. Inevitably the depression gets worse with further withdrawal from society and the ever-present risk of suicide by jumping overboard. The sea can hold a morbid attraction for such individuals. Patients with an endogenous depression or other psychotic illness should, therefore, not be allowed to embark on a prolonged sea voyage. Long days at sea, a warm sunny climate with consequent boredom often associated with increasing alcohol intake may all aggravate the condition. Unfortunately, individuals suffering from severe psychoneurotic illnesses are often encouraged to go on a holiday cruise under the mistaken impression that the change of environment will be of benefit. In practice nothing is further from the truth and subsequent deterioration is all too common. Patients with a psychotic illness such as schizophrenia present a serious problem at sea and should not be permitted to travel. Their behaviour is unpredictable and causes serious annoyance and alarm to other passengers, particularly if cabin accommodation is shared with strangers for weeks at a time. Serious immigration problems can arise if a passenger suffering from a mental illness is refused permission to disembark at his destination. In such circumstances the responsibility for repatriation rests with the shipping company concerned and may involve the provision of a medical escort with all its attendant problems. In contrast busy business executives suffering from mild anxiety and stress benefit greatly from a relaxing sea voyage, removed from their daily worries with the detached relaxation of the sea and the absence of telephones and sometimes world news – the cruise may produce a remarkable improvement in a short space of time.

Severe epilepsy at sea with frequent attacks is a serious hazard and however well controlled should always be viewed with caution. There are numerous dangers on board from falling overboard, collapsing on wet, slippery decks, or using stairs to open decks, sometimes in inclement and rough weather. Changes in social habits, overtiredness from late nights and excess alcohol may all precipitate a convulsion. Normally passengers with epilepsy, if adequately treated and with a history of infrequent convulsions, should present no problem. However, where there is any doubt it is prudent for such individuals not to travel alone.

5.7.8 Alcoholism

Alcohol dependence is an increasing problem in the Western World owing to rising standards of living and the ready availability of alcohol. It is estimated that there are currently 500000 alcohol-dependent persons in the United Kingdom and an equal number with alcohol problems.

Not surprisingly, this type of person is attracted to a holiday cruise with its convivial atmosphere, cheap alcohol and unrestricted bar hours. It is most unwise to advise an alcoholic patient to go on a holiday cruise with the high risk of deterioration, resulting in mental disorder or delirium tremens. Successful treatment with heavy sedation, vitamin B supplements and restriction of access to alcohol can sometimes be achieved although this places great responsibility on the shipboard medical staff. Many alcoholics suffer from severe anxiety problems in which the risk of suicide is high. Aggressive behaviour by male alcoholics, resulting from loss of libido, may precipitate physical assault on their consorts or other passengers. Restraint in such circumstances is usually violently opposed by the patient and can result in endless social and legal complications. Incarceration in a hospital ashore, where the language is not understood and social and religious cultures are very different, is to be avoided wherever possible.

5.7.9 Genito-urinary Problems

Acute urinary retention resulting from prostatic hypertrophy is a frequent medical emergency in passenger vessels. Catheterization under aseptic conditions usually relieves the condition, although where difficulty is encountered owing to spasm of the bladder sphincter supra-pubic puncture may be required. The retention of an indwelling catheter for the remainder of the voyage may be distressing and embarrassing to the patient. Patients with a pre-existing history of prostatic obstruction should be most carefully assessed before being permitted to undertake a long sea voyage. Recurrent urinary infection from partial urinary retention can prove troublesome as the range of urinary antibiotics may be limited and sensitivity tests unavailable.

Acute renal colic from the passage of renal calculi, frequently precipitated by a low fluid intake in tropical climates, may be a very painful and disabling condition requiring hospitalization on board and the administration of pain-relieving injections such as pethidine hydrochloride 100 mg combined with anti-spasmodics, like atropine sulphate 0.8–1.2 mg. Urinary obstruction from a calculus lodging in the urethra may precipitate an acute urinary retention.

Venereal disease is not uncommonly encountered in passenger vessels where the duration of the voyage is in excess of a week. The opportunity for sexual exposure from casual contacts, both on board and ashore, is high. Although syphilis is fortunately relatively rare, the reverse is true for gonorrhoea and non-specific urethritis. The need for correct diagnosis and complete treatment with appropriate antibiotics is essential, coupled with bacteriological examination of smears as appropriate. Blood examination to exclude syphilitic infection should be carried out before treatment is commenced, and the passenger advised of the result in due course. Regrettably, under seagoing circumstances diagnosis and treatment are all too often incomplete. Contacts on board should be identified as soon as possible so that spread of the disease can be prevented and treatment instituted wherever necessary. Much antibiotic drug resistance to gonorrhoea is encountered overseas, largely owing to incomplete treatment of the affected population. All penile sores and ulcers need the fullest investigation with appropriate dark ground illumination, and culture where indicated. Passengers contracting a sexually transmitted disease at sea should always be provided with a full medical report of the investigations and treatment so that this can be continued ashore until cure is complete.

5.7.10 Seasickness (Kinetosis)

The incidence of motion sickness has been dramatically reduced since the introduction of stabilizers in most modern passenger liners. However, in rough weather conditions, especially in the first few days, some cases usually occur. The most successful treatment is prevention, as once vomiting has commenced oral medication is of little value. A wide range of remedies are available, although the most effective and acceptable are promethazine compounds such as Phenergan or Avomine. Phenergan 25 mg orally taken at night and repeated two or three times the following day is beneficial and generally more effective than hyoscine hydrobromide, which causes considerable drowsiness. Phenergan 50 mg intramuscularly, repeated 6-hourly if necessary, the patient being instructed to lie down for 2–3 h following each injection, is usually successful. It is rare for a single 50-mg injection of Phenergan to fail. Alternative remedies such as hyoscine hydrobromide as Quick Kwells, cyclizine as Marzine and dimenhydrinate 50 mg as Dramamine are all of value. Recently Stugeron (cinnarizine 15 mg) has gained in popularity owing to its lack of sedative properties. Children respond well to Phenergan Elixir 5–10 ml according to age, with chlorpromazine (Largactil) in reserve. Suppositories of dimenhydrinate 50 mg (Dramamine) can be of value where oral medication is ineffective owing to vomiting and intramuscular injection is declined.

A new transdermal therapeutic system (TTS) was introduced some years ago in the treatment of motion sickness. It consists of a small gummed plate, 2.5 cm^2 in size, containing 1.5 mg scopolamine. This small plate is affixed to the skin in the retro-auricular area. According to the manufacturer it releases totally 0.5 mg scopolamine over a period of 3 days and this is absorbed transdermally. The achieved plasma level of the active substance is, presumably, in most cases sufficient to suppress kinetosis without showing the well-known side-effects of scopolamine (Price et al. [19]).

5.7.11 Sunburn

Most passengers on a holiday cruise in tropical climates suffer some degree of sunburn because of the overwhelming desire of most holidaymakers to acquire a glorious, romantic suntan and their neglect to adopt a programme of gradual acclimatization during the first few days of exposure. Many forget the serious dangers from reflected light which results from a clear sea and light sandy beaches. Failure to realize the dangers of exposure from an overcast sky with a warm dry wind may result in severe burns with constitutional signs of headache, general malaise, nausea and sometimes vomiting.

Sunburn can easily be prevented by adopting a programme of gradual exposure to the sun's rays from 30 min initially to 1 and then 2 h as the days progress. Avoidance of the mid-day sun, dark glasses and a sun hat, together with the judicious use of a good-quality sun screen or lotion can all help in avoiding sunburn of any severity. Some people may benefit from a course of Sylvasun taken orally twice daily for the first 2 weeks of their vacation. The action is based on the concept that vitamin A is an antagonist to vitamin D, which is concerned in the process of sunburning. Pre-exposure to UVA may be helpful to patients with sensitive skins.

Sunburn can be treated successfully with analgesics, bland lotions such as calamine together with added salt and fluid intake. Severe cases may require antihistamines by mouth, such as Fabahistin (mebhydrolin) 50 mg, or steroid preparations applied locally. Antihistamine creams are best avoided in view of the risk of skin sensitization. Many a holiday cruise can be spoilt, especially for fair-skinned people, by overexposure to sun in the early days and failure to adopt common-sense precautions.

5.7.12 Physical Handicap

Many vessels, particularly those in excess of 20000 gross tonnage, are unable to go alongside at some less well developed ports, especially in the West Indies, and this necessitates the movement of passengers ashore in launches or small boats, sometimes up to a distance of several miles. The physically handicapped may find this a serious problem, especially if disturbances of balance co-exist, unless they are accompanied by someone who can give them careful support. No passenger with a serious physical disability should embark on a cruise vacation or long sea voyage unless they are accompanied by a friend or relative or are physically independent and able to use the bathroom and toilet facilities without outside assistance. Wheelchair cases may be a difficulty as the standard size wheelchair will not pass through most cabin doorways and access to the bathroom may be restricted. Elevators, steps and stairs can be an obstacle to general mobility. A few passenger ships provide special facilities for the disabled but these are unusual. Blind persons or the partially sighted should not travel by sea unless accompanied, for reasons which are obvious. Those persons with serious errors of refraction requiring spectacles should always carry a spare pair with them and especially so if contact lenses are worn, as replacement overseas may prove difficult.

5.7.13 Miscellaneous

Passengers with well-controlled diabetes mellitus, whether on insulin or oral hypoglycaemic agents, present no particular problems at sea provided the ship's medical staff are aware of their condition. However, changes in diet and life-style together with climatic variations may upset the dietary balance or normal physiological rhythm. Prolonged sea sickness or gastro-intestinal upset with a disturbance in electrolyte balance and dehydration may lead to hypoglycaemic reactions or, alternatively hyperglycaemia may require an increase in insulin dosage. Diabetic coma can be a major hazard at sea where estimations of electrolytes are not available. The control of diabetes mellitus with insulin without the facility of accurate blood glucose estimations is a serious clinical situation. In many new world countries insulin may not be readily available and stocks on board limited, so diabetics should always carry with them sufficient supplies to deal with all emergencies.

Acute glaucoma, always a medical emergency, may present at any time amongst elderly passengers. Early diagnosis and prompt instillation of pilocarpine drops to reduce intra-ocular pressure are necessary to avert irreparable damage and loss of vision.

Women who are pregnant should plan to end their sea voyage by the 36th week if the complications of premature labour are to be avoided. Airlines do not normally accept passengers for travel after the 36th week, which presents an added complication to the journey home.

5.7.14 Medical Services

Surprisingly there is little legislation relating to the provision of medical services in passenger vessels. The United Kingdom Department of Trade regulations require a doctor to be provided on all vessels engaged in deep-sea trades in which there are more than 100 persons or 10 passengers. Hospital bed accomodation must be provided for the crew on the basis of one bed per 50 crew members, separate provision being made for the different sexes. There are no U.K. regulations regarding hospital facilities for passengers. A schedule of approved drugs is laid down for passenger vessels depending on the number of passengers and crew carried and this may be subjected to periodic inspection by shore officials. Other countries have special regulations regarding the medical equipment, the drugs to be carried and the medical accomodation for passenger ships, e.g. the Federal Republic of Germany. In general, most passenger vessels carry one doctor, a nurse and a dispenser/medical assistant where passenger numbers do not exceed 1000. In larger vessels an additional doctor is usually necessary together with supporting nursing staff. Shipboard medicine has changed significantly in the past decade as the demands of passengers for expert medical care have increased in parallel to that provided ashore. No cruise liner should be without full diagnostic, radiographic and electrocardiographic facilities. Cardiac resuscitation equipment in the form of a defibrillator and cardiac monitor is nowadays essential. Basic laboratory facilities should also be available. A fully stocked dispensary should be maintained not only to treat acute illness but to provide continuity of treatment for those passengers seeking advice for chronic illness whilst on board. It is suggested that a minimum of six beds be available in the ship's hospital in all passenger vessels irrespective of the numbers carried, separate facilities being provided for isolation of infectious diseases. With the mounting insurance claims by passengers for accidents and illnesses incurred on board, the need for defensive medicine is regrettably necessary as the threat of malpractice is ever-present. Shipping companies are well advised to provide well-equipped medical facilities on board together with permanent medical staff familiar with the problems of nautical medicine. The employment of a succession of relief doctors and nurses on a temporary basis, often ill paid and without senior officer status, is to be deprecated. Medical staff should possess a sound knowledge of emergency, accident and resuscitative procedures and have some expertise in carrying out basic laboratory procedures.

Passenger vessels engaged on short sea voyages such as ferries do not normally carry medically qualified personnel on board, despite the fact that passenger numbers may exceed several hundred. In these circumstances a sufficiently well-stocked medicine chest together with resuscitation equipment should be available for use by a doctor passenger should he be called upon to deal with a sudden emergency. This should be in addition to the normal first aid medical supplies and dressings available for use by the crew.

References

1. Cameron, D.C.: The hazards of ocean cruises for the elderly and infirm. Scot. med. J. *17*, 168–171 (1972).
2. Carter, J.W.: Shipboard medicine on package cruises. Brit. med. J. 1, 553–556 (1972).
3. Dahl, E.: Almenpraksis til sjos. Medisinske erfaringer fra en jordomseiling. T. norske Laegeforen. *99*, 6, 327–330 (1979).
4. Dannenberg, A.L., J.C. Yashuk and R.A. Feldman: Gastrointestinal illness on passenger cruise ships, 1975–1978. Amer. J. publ. Hlth *72*, 5, 484–488 (1982).
5. Davies, D.M.: Medical experience in nuclear submarines. J. roy. nav. med. Serv. *57*, 3, 136–141 (1971).
6. Davies, J.W., K.G. Cox, W.R. Simon et al.: Typhoid at sea: epidemic aboard an ocean liner. Can. med. Ass. J. *106*, 877–883 (1972).
7. De Dombal, F.T.: Acute abdominal pain – An OMGE survey. Scand. J. Gastroent. *56*, 14, 29–43 (1979).
8. Jäger, H.: Ärztliche Versorgung auf See. Kreuzfahrt – medizinische Erfahrungen. Fortschr. Med. *97*, 27, 1191–1194 (1979).
9. Jäger, H.: Kreuzfahrtmedizin. Ärztliche Betreuung von Besatzung und Passagieren auf See. Z. Allg. Med. 56, 942–948 (1980).
10. Jäger, H.: Kreuzfahrtmedizin. Bordärztliche Erfahrungen auf modernen Passagierschiffen. Ther. d. Gegenw. *118*, 4, 616–631 (1979).
11. Jäger, H.: Schiffsarzt – immer noch ein Abenteuer. Praktische Erfahrungen bei Kreuzfahrten. Ärztl. Prax. *30*, 95, 3248–3250 (1978).
12. Jones, H.A.: Health problems in cruise ships. Canad. Pac. Steamship Ltd., 10 pp.
13. Korcok, M.: Follow-up report on cruiseships: have sanitation standards improved? Canad. med. Ass. J. *121*, 7, 998–1012 (1979).
14. Merson, M.H., J.M. Hughes, B.R. Wood et al.: Gastrointestinal illness on passenger cruise ships. J. Amer. med. Ass. *231*, 7, 723–727 (1975).
15. Merson, M.H., J.H. Tenney, J.D. Meyers et al.: Shigellosis at sea: an outbreak aboard a passenger cruise ship. Amer. J. Epidem. *101*, 2, 165–175 (1975).
16. Oliver, P.O.: Health problems of passengers at sea. Practitioner *219*, 1310, 204–210 (1977).
17. Oliver, P.O.: Medical hazards at sea. Brit. J. Hosp. Med. *22*, 6, 615–618 (1979).
18. Polonov, K.: Characteristics of morbidity among passengers during voyages with hotel-class ships. In: Fourth International Symposium on Marine Medicine. Oct. 15–17, 1970, Varna. Varna 1972. pp. 298–303.
19. Price, N., L.G. Schmitt and J.E. Shaw: Transdermal delivery of scopolamine for prevention of motion-induced nausea in rough seas. Clin. Therapeutics *2*, 4, 258–262 (1979).
20. Survey of environmental sanitation on 12 passenger cruise ships operating in the Caribbean. Ed.: U.S. Department of Health, Education, and Welfare. Public Health Service, Center for Disease Control. Atlanta, Georgia 1974.
21. Survey of incidence of gastrointestinal illness on passenger cruise ships. Ed.: U.S. Department of Health, Education, and Welfare. Public Health Service, Center for Disease Control. Atlanta, Georgia 1974.
22. Tortori-Donati, B.: La attrezzatura ed il funzionamento del reparto sanitario di grandi transatlantici stranieri. Lav. e. Med. *20*, 3, 105–118 (1977).
23. Tortori-Donati, B. and L. Giannico: Practice of medical profession on board passenger ships, remarks on equipment and activity of the medical department of the liners and on morbidity on board. In: III. International Symposium on Marine Medicine, Leningrad 1968. Moscow-Leningrad 1969. pp. 189–196.
24. Ulewicz, K. and R. Dolmierski: Pharyngitis epidemic on a passenger ship. Bull. Inst. mar. trop. Med. Gdynia *27*, 1, 105–108 (1976).
25. Warncke, J.: Gesundheit, Sicherheit und Bequemlichkeit des Reisenden aus der Sicht der Schiffahrtsmedizin. Verk.-Med. *15*, 4, 133–146 (1968).
26. Werner, S.B., M.P. Hudgins, F.R. Morrison et al.: Gastroenteritis on a cruise ship – a recur-

ring problem –. Publ. Hlth Rep. *91,* 5, 433–436 (1976).

27. Wilken, D. D.: Significant medical experiences aboard polaris submarines. A Review of 360 patrols during the period 1963–1967. [Connecticut:] Submarine Medical Res. Laboratory. 1969.

Additional References

Levy, S. and A. G. Stoner: An offshore medical service at the Cape of Good Hope. S. Afr. med. J. *51,* 14, 476–480 (1977).

Turner, A. C.: Travel medicine. Edinburgh, London, New York: Churchill Livingstone 1975.

5.8 The Sea Pilot

J. M. Harrington

5.8.1 Introduction

Seafaring is a noble, ancient and potentially dangerous occupation. The hazards of going to sea have always been great though the true toll in mortality and morbidity has frequently been underestimated (Schilling [11]). Whereas the dangers faced by ocean-going seamen are obvious, the intricacies and perils of coastal water sailing have frequently been overlooked by investigators. The problems inherent in guiding ships safely in and out of port are often related to the peculiarities of the inshore sea bed as much as to the navigability of the vessel. Thus there has been a long-standing need for mariners familiar with the locality to be on hand to assist ships' captains in the berthing of their vessels.

The British pilotage service received a Royal Charter from Henry VIII for the establishment and operation of Trinity House (London) in the sixteenth century, whilst in the Federal Republic of Germany the Hamburg pilotage authority was established in 1656. As an aside, it is interesting to note that these two pilotage routes are perhaps the most tortuous and complex in Western Europe and thus it is not surprising that they should have been recognised early as important routes for official control.

Commercial developments in maritime trade have been enormous, particularly since the Second World War, with not only an increase in vessels piloted but also in gross tonnage moved. Furthermore, data from the United Kingdom have shown a steady increase in the proportion of foreign ships handled in pilotage acts [4] as well as a separate but even more significant rise in the size of single vessels handled. These very large vessels in excess of 200000 tonnes dead weight are equipped with highly sophisticated navigational aids but present special pilotage problems in view of their long delays in ship response to pilotage input. The cargoes are frequently highly flammable and can present catastrophic dangers in the event of a collision with either another vessel or the berthing facilities.

The progressive growth in size and complexity of pilotage operations is mirrored in the size of the pilot population. In the United Kingdom, for example, Trinity House (London) more than doubled its pilot population between 1946 and 1970. The 522 pilots employed in 1970 (one-third of the United Kingdom total) piloted an average of 117 ships per year with an average tonnage per ship of 2648 (Harrington [6]).

The percentage of foreign ships doubled in the same post-war period. By contrast the port of Milford Haven has experienced a 50-fold increase in tonnage handled since the port became an oil terminal in 1960 (Cook [2]).

In the Federal Republic of Germany, approximately a third of the 1000 pilots work in the Hamburg region, piloting ships through the difficult 110 km down the Elbe from Hamburg to the Kiel Canal and beyond to the North Sea. Although pilots operate in and out of major ports throughout the world, few such operations are as long or difficult as the Thames or Elbe. In West

Africa, for example, the process of pilotage is often a relatively simple task of escorting a vessel directly from the open sea to the harbour berthing.

5.8.2 The Pilotage Operation

The wide diversity in skill required for various pilotage procedures is reflected in the training and experience necessary to be a pilot in various ports. For example, apprentices are trained to guide vessels in the Liverpool/Manchester port complex whereas on the Elbe and the Thames, a pilot must be at least 30 years old and hold a valid master mariner's ticket. The induction period is then, long intensive and often poorly paid. The German pilots on the Elbe operate to and from the Kiel Canal either seawards or towards port, but in the Thames estuary, a pilot operating from Gravesend, for example, is either licensed to pilot a vessel in or out but rarely both.

The time involved in piloting may be an hour or so for a straightforward job into an open sea harbour, up to 6 h from Gravesend to the North Sea in good weather. Thus the length of time away from the pilot station may be as long as 36 h on the Elbe or the Thames. Bad weather can considerably extend the length of the tour and may even prevent the sea-going pilot from disembarking. Indeed, the vagaries of time, tide and vessel movement can involve the pilot in considerable periods of waiting for a ship. The prolonged period of inactivity may be rapidly followed by a vertical climb of perhaps 20 m to reach the bridge. There the pilot may be confronted with a bewildering array of modern navigational equipment aboard a foreign vessel. Given such working conditions it would not be surprising to discover some occupational health sequelae.

5.8.3 The Health of Sea Pilots

It is not uncommon for occupational health problems to be brought to light by the work-force itself. Such was the case regarding British sea pilots. In 1970, at the time of the mortality study of English Channel Pilots (Harrington [5]), no other published investigation of sea pilot mortality was extant. Indeed, only two studies of sea pilot morbidity were available, both from Sweden (Dahlmann [3], Kilbom [8]). Both studies noted an excess incidence of peptic ulcer morbidity which was considered by the authors to be related to the work-load. Dahlmann considered that the gastric disorders were due to the "exacting duties of the pilot service with irregular working hours and meals and increased duties during and after World War Two". In this respect, the effects, if real, are organisational rather than truly occupational. Shift working, though much maligned, has been shown to cause few incontrovertible health effects other than gastric disorders (Harrington [7]), and the irregular hours of work with scant regard for time of day could similarly be responsible for the pilots' digestive disorders.

Mortality studies have implied other hazardous effects. A study of 393 English Channel pilots for the period 1956–1968 showed a statistically significant excess of coronary artery deaths, particularly in the younger pilots aged 35–49 years (Harrington [5]). Extensions of this study to Manchester and Liverpool showed similar though statistically insignificant results and the same picture emerged from an investigation of Humber pilots (Kywe [9]). A study of 525 deaths in pilots who worked on the Elbe, Weser and Kiel Canal noted a 5.5-fold excess of coronary artery deaths compared with urban male populations and, once again, this excess occurred in the younger pilots (31–50 years old) and in the pre-1960 period (Zorn et al. [13]). Erikssen et al. [4a] found a significant difference between Norwegian pilots and the male Oslo population regarding ECG and exercise performance and other indicators of coronary heart disease: the pilots seemed to be more prone to coronary artery disease.

Each of these studies suggests that the stress of the job and the work-load involved could be at least partially responsible for the excess mortality from coronary artery disease. However, there is anecdotal evidence of heavy cigarette smoking and high alcohol consumption amongst pilots, the former habit when on duty, the latter almost exclusively off duty.

However, the latent period for atherosclerotic change is likely to exceed the length of pilotage experience for this young population, and their Merchant Navy experience could well be involved as an additional, if ill-defined, risk factor.

Attempts to test these hypotheses have met with some methodological difficulties. A study of catecholamine excretion as a measure of so-called stress was undertaken on five volunteer pilots over three separate pilotage operations (Zorn and Seifert [14]). The results showed a statistically significant rise in urinary catecholamines during all pilotage operations.

As a direct consequence of these studies, a full-scale work-load investigation was undertaken (Shipley [12]). In a random sample of 55 London based pilots, 36% were noted to have a health impairment on routine examination. When more stringent health criteria were adopted, the percentage of "failed" pilots rose to 55%. A comparison with business executives suggested that significant health impairment was twice as common in the pilots. Moreover, the pilots showed higher prevalences of abnormal liver function, excess tobacco consumption and hypercholesterolaemia.

Questionnaire surveillance of 800 pilots (55% of the total United Kingdom population) suggested that they reported half as much sickness absence as the general male population, with approximately 6% reporting work-related injuries. These were mainly falls during embarking or disembarking. The commonest reported diseases were musculoskeletal disorders (39%), haemorrhoids (27%) and varicose veins (14%). No comparisons were made with referent land-based populations.

Direct work-load studies were undertaken using portable instruments for measuring heart rate. Higher pulse rates were noted in pilots handling very large crude carriers (VLCC) (104.5 per minute versus 77.8) and this was particularly in evidence during the procedure of "swinging" these vessels as compared with forward movement. Heart rates in excess of 150 beats/minute were recorded during manoeuvring vessels in restricted waters though there was little difference between day and night time operations. Nor, surprisingly, did the size of the vessel seem to correlate well. It appears that the act of manipulating any vessel in a restricted place is a stressful situation. Boarding a vessel could also produce heart rates twice the resting level. In this respect, such episodes of tachycardia compare with those noted in racing car drivers but were far in excess of rates observed in business executives and air traffic controllers "under stress".

Nevertheless, at times of peak activity, heart rates in excess of 120 beats/minute are not necessarily hazardous and thus although a pilot's work-load may be high, such a conclusion does not necessarily imply a dangerous situation. To that extent, pre-existent heart disease may create a potentially dangerous state but the work related "stress" then becomes a contributory rather than an underlying risk factor for myocardial damage.

In a later human factor study the fatigue of pilots was especially investigated (Cook and Shipley [16]) by means of ambulatory-monitored electrocardiograms and intermittent measurements of oral temperature, skin conduction, reaction time, and self-ratings of subjective feelings. The main conclusions were that the sea pilots experience considerable challenge to their alertness, and are extremely tired after "long haul" pilotage, particularly at night. Their body rhythms are those of normal day workers, and they must frequently need to rely on an effort of will to maintain adequate vigilance when on watch during uneventful passages.

There is clearly room for more extensive studies of pilotage activity, preferably with data collected from other countries and a variety of working conditions. The cause(s) for the pilots' seeming predilection for coronary artery disease has not been satisfactorily elucidated though that should not prevent measures being taken to diminish the risk factors discovered thus far.

5.8.4 Prevention and Control of Occupational Ill Health

Measures to protect the health of pilots fall into two broad groups: procedures to ameliorate the work-load factors, and measures to monitor the health of pilots both before and during employment.

5.8.4.1 Work Practices

The current, relatively haphazard, monitoring of pilot duties could be considerably improved. The aim should be to make more efficient use of on-duty hours by diminishing the time spent on standby and by ensuring that, once the pilotage is over, the pilot is either transported rapidly back to base or provided with clean, quiet and comfortable rest facilities at the place of disembarkation. Although the arrival of vessels in the pilotage area is subject to considerable variability due to weather, sailing times and tides, the present short notice given to pilots is unacceptable and unnecessary. A longer notice of the need for a vessel to require a pilot is feasible and this would lead to more predictable duty periods.

Although accident and illness rates as a whole appear to be comparatively low, the current working arrangements of many pilots would militate against their taking time off for any but the most serious illnesses or injuries. Improved design of pilot cutters and the methods of ascent and descent from the vessel piloted would reduce the injuries caused by slipping on wet or dangerous surfaces. Such accidents are occasionally fatal. There is also a need, on behalf of mariners as well as pilots, for improvements in the ergonomic design of bridge controls (Brigham [1]). For example, a VLCC must be brought into contact with a jetty at a speed frequently less than 0.12 m/s. Direct perceptions required by the pilot or master to achieve such a manoeuvre are frequently below psychophysical thresholds. The strategic positioning of buoys would greatly aid such delicate manipulations of a vessel. Such external devices would need to be supplemented by improved on-vessel electronic equipment, such as computer-assisted simulations of planned manoeuvres, and international agreement should be sought concerning the minimum navigational requirements for a given vessel berthing at a given port. In addition, greater uniformity of equipment design is needed to ensure that a pilot boarding a foreign vessel is at least not faced with unfamiliar navigational equipment.

5.8.4.2 Pilot Health Monitoring

In the early 1970s it was clear that no major European pilotage authority was operating any efficient monitoring of pilot health. The confirmation of excess coronary artery disease mortality and morbidity has encouraged considerable changes in the occupational health surveillance of British pilots.

In 1975, a new set of health standards was proposed to Trinity House for pre-employment health screening and this has been applied since 1976 (McLean [10]). All new entrants are required to complete a detailed medical history questionnaire and all are subsequently required to pass a full clinical examination. Electrocardiography and serum biochemistry are also performed. In order to pass, a pilot must be demonstrably fully fit in terms of life assurance and permanent health assurance standards. The information collected is confidential to the examining doctor, though Trinity House are provided with a statement of "up to required standard" or "not up to required standard". Visual acuity standards are those laid down for Merchant Navy navigating officers. It appears that such entrance requirements are now more stringent and more effectively imposed than for other European pilotage authorities.

Subsequent periodic medical reviews are less well established and the problems concerning pilots who become temporarily or permanently disabled have yet to be sorted out. There are good reasons for this delay. Firstly, the pilotage authorities are in a state of flux both organisationally and financially. Secondly, a decision was made recently to introduce a new set of medical standards for maritime shipping which is likely to be promulgated as Government regulations in July 1983. When these regulations have come into force, the pilotage authorities are likely to follow suit.

Therefore, in the near future, the health monitoring of Trinity House pilots is expected to approach the desiderata of a well-organised factory-based occupational health service with appropriate pre- and post-employment health screening combined with contingency planning for temporary and permanent disablement from the job. There remains, however, a need for some Europe-wide standards which could be profitably extended to other pilotage authorities world-wide.

5.8.5 Conclusions

The occupation of sea pilot is an ancient and skilled one which in recent years has been the subject of some medical scrutiny. It appears that although the work-load is, at times, heavy, the majority of pilots are capable of coping with the rigours of the job. Nevertheless, research in several European countries has demonstrated an excess mortality and morbidity from coronary heart disease and possibly gastro-intestinal disorders which, at least in part, may be due to the job or the previous Merchant Navy life-style. Little attention had been paid to the provision of an occupational health surveillance programme for pilots until the mid 1970s, but in the United Kingdom, at least, some progress has now been made in the recognition of their specific needs and the development of a formal programme of health monitoring is underway. Less satisfactorily, much work remains to be done to improve the rostering of pilot duties and the establishment of efficient and uniform procedures for the work these men do whilst on the bridge.

References

1. Brigham, F.R.: Ergonomic problems in ship control. Appl. Ergonomics *31*, 14–19 (1972).
2. Cook, T.C.C.: A study of pilotage in a U.K. oil port including workload monitoring. Dissertation, University of London 1977.
2a Cook, T.C. and P. Shipley: Human factors studies of the working hours of UK ship's pilots. Appl. Ergonom. *11*, 2, 85–92 (1980) and *11*, 3, 151–159 (1980).
3. Dahlmann, T.: Incidence of peptic ulcer and gastritis amongst Swedish sea pilots. Brit. J. industr. Med. *10*, 157–162 (1953).
4. Economics and marine pilotage. London: Her Majesty's Stationery Office 1973. (Department of Trade Report)
4a Erikssen, J.A., Höiem Johansen and K. Rodahl: Coronary heart disease in Norwegian sea-pilots; part of the occupational hazard? Acta med. Scand. (Suppl. 0) *645*, 79–84 (1981).
5. Harrington, J.M.: A mortality study of English Channel pilots (1956–1968). Dissertation, University of London 1972.
6. Harrington, J.M.: Mortality from coronary artery disease of English Channel and Hamburg pilots. Trans. Soc. occup. Med. *22*, 19–23 (1972).
7. Harrington, J.M.: Shift work and health – A critical review of the literature. London: Her Majesty's Stationery Office 1978. (Health and Safety Executive [Employment Medical Advisory Service] Monograph)
8. Kilbom, A.: Pilots and piloting. Stockholm: Arbetsmedicinska Institutet 1969.
9. Kywe, K.M.: A mortality and morbidity study of Humber maritime pilots (1956–1972). Dissertation, University of London 1973.

10. McLean, A.: Personal information 1981.
11. Schilling, R. S. F.: Hazards of deep-sea-fishing. Brit. J. industr. Med. *28,* 27–35 (1971).
12. Shipley, P.: A human factors study of marine pilotage. London: Dept. of Industry. Ship and Marine Technology Requirements Board 1978.
13. Zorn, E. W., J. M. Harrington and H. Goethe: Ischemic heart disease and work stress in West German sea pilots. J. occup. Med. *19,* 11, 762–765 (1977).
14. Zorn, E. and R. Seifert: Catecholamine excretion by marine pilots in action. Agressologie *18,* 5, 269–272 (1977).

5.9 Extreme Conditions Aboard Ship

B. Tortori-Donati

This chapter deals with situations which are uncommon during a voyage. They assume the feature of an emergency, which means an unlikely event. An emergency does not follow any foreseeable rule; therefore it is impossible to give general instructions which may be considered valid for every case. Shipwreck, extremely long working hours without rest, extreme stress for long periods or at frequent intervals and extremes of temperature are discussed in this chapter.

5.9.1 Shipwreck

Shipwreck with the loss of the ship is a rare event. The International Maritime Conventions bring up to date safety measures designed to improve the safety of ships and of human beings on board.

It is difficult to outline precisely how one should behave in a shipwreck because this can happen for different reasons and behaviour has to change according to the pattern of events.

On board a ship which is about to be abandoned, the medical personnel usually have to cope with the traumas due to the dramatic event which almost always exacerbate any previous chronic ill-health. In addition, very frequently first aid medical activity is hampered by the listing of the ship and the inaccessibility of medical equipment. Moreover, the passengers and crew are frightened and anxious to an extent which impedes satisfactory treatment.

There is no doubt that psychological training of seafarers is one of the most important factors in ensuring that the rescue operations are successful. The ship's personnel must be aware that, during any voyage, a shipwreck can happen, even if this is a very rare occurrence. The crew members must receive careful instructions on what to do in the case of an emergency, with the aim of improving the chances of survival (Tortori-Donati [15]).

Life boats, rafts and all other life-saving equipment must be checked periodically. Giving instructions only once on a lengthy voyage is useless; regular, repeated instructions including practical training in the handling of all of the equipment is necessary. There must be fixed rules and exercises for all emergency procedures including fire fighting drills, manning of boats in the proper dress and rescue operations. There must be well-known and practised rules regarding the additional supply of boats and rafts with clothing, blankets, water, food, first aid and medical supplies etc. In emergency situations under adverse conditions only procedures which have been well practised will prove successfull and life-saving. Otherwise panic reactions will worsen the shipwreck disaster, adding to the danger to the lives of passengers and crew.

5.9.2 Extreme Length of Working Hours Without Rest

The working activity aboard ships is organized in watches; therefore, normally, the work/rest cycle allows the seaman to recuperate physically and mentally. However, it can happen that during a voyage the aforesaid organization of work must be cancelled and the seaman continues to work without being relieved for several hours. In these cases, fatigue ensues because of the intensity and the length of the work and influences the psychological and physical balance (Granati and Melino [11]).

Fatigue is not easy to define or measure. It is the sensation of being tired during prolonged efforts. It cannot be measured specifically and it is subjectively expressed as an impairment of the working capacity. Whether acute or chronic, general or localized, it produces a diminution of the functional efficiency of the body and, consequently, of work performance and concentration. Fatigue develops when the working activity is immoderate, either in rhythm, length or intensity. These factors have no absolute value, but they are related to individual sensitivity and to environmental conditions (Brown [3]).

Obviously, the more the working environmental conditions are influenced by adverse climatic factors or by pollution, or the more the quality of the work is psychologically stress producing, the more rapid is the onset of fatigue with subsequent malaise for the worker. As to the influence of climatic factors in the onset of the fatigue, it is easy to understand the importance of this link in the activity of seafarers, who, during the voyage, have to work under climatic conditions quite different from those to which they are accustomed. In addition, psychological stress is a constant component of the working activity aboard ships and seafarers therefore frequently undergo this upsetting experience (Moreigne [13]).

The situation is worse on newly built ships, which have a high degree of automation; this calls for greater concentration and results in more fatigue and monotony (Drummer [8]). Furthermore, modern research on the sociological organization of the work has emphasized the harmful consequences of the working shifts: frequent alteration of the biological rhythms, of the relationship between sleep and being awake and of living habits. These changes adversely influence the physical and psychological integrity of the shift worker, producing dissatisfaction and anxiety. Physical reaction to that anxiety may include the onset of dyspepsia, bowel malfunction and even peptic ulcer [1]. Moreover, when physical or psychological overloading results from both the quantity and the quality of work (excessive working hours, unsatisfactory type of work, extreme responsibility, frequent arguments while working etc.) there is a particularly adverse influence on the cardio-circulatory system which can predispose to the onset of hypertension, ischaemic heart disease or coronary heart disease.

5.9.3 Extreme Stress or Responsibility

Aboard ship, every seaman carries a certain degree of responsibility. This is especially true on the newly built ships with refined technologies, which result in a progressive reduction of manual work and, as already stated, an increase of activities which requirs a high degree of professional training and concentration. The degree of professional training varies according to the rank of the seafarer, being directly proportional to the importance of the type of work carried out on board. It can happen that, because of some very particular climatic conditions encountered during a voyage or, for example, because the ship has to pass through very dangerous waters, the load of responsibility becomes extreme and prolonged without allowing adequate periods of mental relaxation and physical rest. As a consequence of this stressful rhythm of activity, some seamen, particularly those who feel deeply a sense of responsibility in their work, undergo mental strain which can be followed by anxiety or even, later on, by anguish, these being the three degrees of severity of a particular emotional condition of an unpleasant nature (Dolmierski [7]). This progression of unpleasant feelings, which can have a damaging influence on the physical health of those who are subjected to it, happens inside the unconscious mind. The anxiety state especially when prolonged, induces a group of somatic troubles, among which the most frequent are tachycardia, polyuria, profuse sweating, vasomotor troubles, changes in the blood pressure and angina-like syndrome (Cesena et al. [4]).

Usually the conscious mind is in order and lucid but, without doubt, in the most serious cases it can be impaired, with a decline of critical powers and the presence of an abnormal psychological reaction amounting to panic. This is more apparent when affecting a senior officer who is forced to take an important decision too quickly when the ability to analyse the dangerous situation and choose the right solution may be impaired. (Matsevich and Poroshenko [12]). It is evident that in emergencies there is a physical and mental overload which reduces the effectiveness of the sufferer (Paslaru [14]). Man, when facing a critical situation, behaves in an unpredictable manner, which is frequently independent of his background of physical and mental resistance.

5.9.4 Extremes of Temperature Aboard Ship

A ship, during a voyage, passes from one climate to another in a relatively short time. However, in newly built ships the air conditioning system greatly reduces the possibility of the extremes of temperature encountered during a voyage becoming harmful to the seamen.

Human beings possess a remarkable thermoregulatory capacity, which allows the body to maintain, within certain limits, a constant core temperature, even when great external thermal ranges are present. Only when the outside temperature reaches a particularly high or low degree and this is accompanied by other climatic components with potentially harmful effects, such as humidity and movement of the air, without there having been a sufficient period of acclimatization, is it possible that the physiological mechanism of thermoregulation will become inadequate, with consequent damage to the human body.

5.9.4.1 Extremes of Cold (see also Chap. 5.10)

Exposure of a person to cold weather for prolonged periods produces two harmful effects: a) damage to the part of the body directly exposed (cold injury) and b) a negative influence on the core temperature (hypothermia).

Cold injury is due mainly to vascular damage in the exposed tissues, with decrease of the blood circulation and resulting hypoxia.

The damage is directly proportional to the degree of cold, to the length of exposure, to the presence of some aggravating factor such as humidity or wind, and to the extent to which the body is protected by suitable clothing. Cold injury is divided into four degrees according to the seriousness of the symptoms and the importance of the sequelae.

1st degree: hyperaemia and oedema
2nd degree: hyperaemia and blister formation
3rd degree: necrosis of the skin and of the subcutaneous tissues, with ulcer formation
4th degree: deep necrosis with loss of tissue

The degree of a cold injury cannot be ascertained immediately after the accident, but only in retrospect, when the evolution of the lesion is complete [5].

For the onset of hypothermia it is necessary to take into account several factors, which may be a) general, such as the degree of cold and the length of exposure, together with the presence or absence of other environmental factors such as humidity and wind, or b) individual, such as age, sex, race, physical constitution, previous health conditions, presence of fatigue and incidence of trauma (Glaser and McCance [10]). When the physical and chemical thermoregulation is inadequate to counteract the influence of the cold weather, the core temperature falls. When the core temperature reaches 34 °C, general hypothermia, which can be fatal, sets in. Four degrees of this very serious syndrome have been described corresponding to the extent to which the internal temperature is lowered. General hypothermia can thus be mild (core temperature between 35 °C and 32 °C), moderate (between 31 °C and 28 °C), deep (between 27 °C and 25 °C) or profound (below 25 °C). When the core temperature falls to around 24 °C the patient dies from unsatisfactory oxygenation of the tissues, lack of glycogen and consequent accumulation in the tissues of lactic and carbonic acid, so inducing terminal acidosis.

The symptoms of general hypothermia are, in the beginning, sudden blanching of the skin, fatigue, indifference, sleepiness, reduction of eyesight and of hearing, pronounced hypotension and bradycardia followed by cardiac arrhythmia. If the patient is not immediately and adequately treated, with the aim of raising the core temperature to normal levels, he will die, because, after the cortical centres, the bulbar centres are involved. Generally, death is due to a cessation of function of the respiratory centre.

5.9.4.2 Extremes of Heat (see also Chap. 2.4)

Frequently, ships are employed in geographical areas characterized by high temperature and a high degree of humidity. Usually, the ships, particularly the newly built ones, have a system of air conditioning which allows the crew to enjoy good conditions of life and of work on board. Therefore, it is unlikely that heat exhaustion and, especially, heat stroke due to the influence of the high temperature on the human body, will take place. The most exposed among the seamen are those who work in the engine room and in the galley, because, in addition to the outside heat, they have to work in premises with several sources of radiant heat.

Particularly important for the understanding of the effects on the human body of exposure to extremely hot environments are the experiments performed to discover the objective criteria by which it is possible to foresee an imminent heat collapse.

As has been underlined when discussing extremes of cold, there exists an individual level of tolerance of heat, which is separate from the other general criteria of evaluation such as age, sex, race, previous health condition, fatigue and intoxication, with particular emphasis on alcohol. Moreover, it must be remembered that of importance in addition to the air temperature are the degree of humidity, the movement of the air, the quality of the work, the clothing and, most importantly, the degree of acclimatization of those exposed. Therefore, seamen who are "first trippers" are particularly liable to thermal stress.

The human body, in an attempt to keep the internal temperature constant in the face of high thermal radiation, increases the loss of heat through sweating, cutaneous vasodilatation and pulmonary hyperventilation. When these mechanisms become inadequate, a multiform symptomatology develops, characterized by general malaise, asthenia, headache, vertigo, nausea and vomiting, pseudo-angina syndrome, hallucination, incoherence, mental confusion, reduced concentration, memory defects and irritability or depression. It is easy to understand that this mental impairment can be very dangerous on board a ship, because it can provoke in those seamen who have responsibility for navigation, a psychological inability to cope with their task (Collins [6]; Walters and Bell [16]).

Heat collapse can be foreseen in the presence of the following objective data: a) raising of the internal temperature above 39 °C; b) remarkable increase of the pulse rate (more than 150 beats per minute), which becomes arrhythmic; c) onset of general tiredness, nausea, vomiting, sleeplessness and psychological troubles; and d) dehydration caused by an excess of sweating with muscular cramps and a tendency to heart failure. The increase of sweating produces, besides the loss of water, a loss of the Cl^-, Na^+ and K^+ ions, which are very important for the maintenance of the chemical and physical condition of the protoplasma colloids, to which the tendency to heart failure and the onset of cramp are closely related (Bell et al. [2], Eismont [9]). The increased thermodispersion through which the human body tries to mitigate the consequences of thermal stress requires a wastage of energies, which only the organism in good general condition can tolerate.

Beside the previously described heat exhaustion, under particular circumstances during a trip in tropical zones a crew member may undergo an acute episode of heat stroke, which has dramatically serious symptoms and requires urgent therapeutic measures to prevent the death of the patient.

Heat stroke is an acute rise in the body temperature owing to inadequate thermodispersion when the environmental temperature and humidity are very high. Individual sensitivity and predisposing factors, such as impairment of the cardio-circulatory system or of the kidney or liver function, together with the presence of harmful climatic condition, are of the greatest importance in precipitating the onset of heat stroke. The mechanism of thermodispersion, through which the human body defends itself against thermal stress, passes from a condition of excitement (hyperhydrosis) to a condition of depression or paralysis (anhydrosis). Consequently, the body temperature quickly rises above 41 °C with loss of consciousness, hallucinations and the possibility of convulsions. The nervous system is so compromised that coma can occur. The face of the patient is red, the skin is dry because sweating has stopped, the breathing is rattling, the pulse rate is very high, the blood pressure is low and the urinary output is much reduced or even stopped. Death can be a question of a few hours or even less (fulminating heat stroke). Probably the pathogenesis of death from heat stroke can be seen as a cessation of function of the cerebral thermoregulator centres owing to the environmental high temperature and humidity in a person who is particularly predisposed by general and/or particular sensitivity. When a case of heat stroke occurs, it is necessary to start correct therapy immediately, with the aims of: a) reducing hyperthermia by cooling down the body until sweating starts again; b) improving the dehydration by intravenous infusions of salt solution; c) supporting the circulation in order to prevent cardio-circulatory collapse, which is frequent and extremely serious; and d) calming down the nervous system.

References

1. Lavoro e turni, cronobiologia e protezione della salute. Atti simposio nazionale, Verona 15 marzo 1980. Verona: Zendrini 1980.
2. Bell, C. R., M. J. Crowder and J. D. Walters: The prediction of safe exposure times for men working in thermally severe environments. Ed.: Medical Research Council. Royal Naval Personnel Research Committee. ES 5. London 1970.
3. Brown, I. D.: Measurement of fatigue in abnormal physical environments. In: The effects of abnormal physical conditions at work. Ed.: C. N. Davies, P. R. Davis and F. H. Tyrer. Edinburgh: Livingstone 1967. pp. 168–178.
4. Cesena, G. C., R. Zanettini, R. Curti et al.: Stress e patologia cardio vascolare. Med. d. Lavoro *1*, 3–12 (1981).
5. Cold injury. TB MED 81, NAVMED P-5052-29, AFP 161-11. Ed.: Departments of the Army, the Navy, and the Airforce, Washington, D.C. Washington U.S. Government Printing Office: 1976.
6. Collins, C. P.: Health and efficiency in men of the Royal Navy under thermal stress. J. roy. nav. med. Serv. *41*, 199–217 (1955).
7. Dolmierski, R.: Neurosen und Verhaltensstörungen bei Seeleuten. In: V. Internationales

Symposium über Schiffahrtsmedizin, Rostock, 19–21 Oct. 1972. Rostock 1973. pp. 25–30.
8. Drummer, H.: Physical, psychic and sociological effect and problems affecting the crew as a result of automation. Bull. Inst. mar. Med. Gdańsk *25*, 2-3-4, 378–381 (1974).
9. Eismont, V.: The problem of acclimatization in the torrid zone on the basis of the research conducted at the marine medicine institute. In: International symposium on marine medicine, Leningrad, 1968, Vol. 3. Moscow 1969. pp. 78–83.
10. Glaser, E. M. and R. A. McCance: First report on arctic survival trials. Ed.: Medical Research Council. Royal Naval Personnel Research Committee. London 1950.
11. Granati, A. and C. Melino: Aspetti medico-sociali del lavoro marittimo. Rome: Istituto Italiano di Medicina Sociale 1976.
12. Matsevitch, L. M. and A. S. Poroshenko: The influence of the duration of a voyage on the functional state of a seaman's body. Bull. Inst. mar. Med. Gdańsk *25*, 2-3-4, 443–446 (1974).
13. Moreigne, E.: Fatigue opérationelle dans la marine. Rev. Path. gén. 415–422 (1960).
14. Paslaru, V.: Study of stress in seamen during prolonged voyages for labour evaluation and on improvement of socio-hygienic conditions on board of vessels. In: VII International symposium on marine medicine, Odessa 23–30 September 1976. Moscow 1976. p. 294.
15. Tortori-Donati, B.: Activity of the medical profession on the occasion of a disaster at sea. The tragedy of the Andrea Doria witnessed by the ship's doctor. J. roy. nav. med. Serv. *66*, 1, 63–70 (1980).
16. Walters, J. D. and C. R. Bell: The prediction of imminent heat collapse in extremely hot environments. J. roy. nav. med. Serv. *60*, 22–27 (1974).

Additional References

Goethe, H., E. Zorn, R. Herrmann et al.: Die psycho-physische Belastung des Personals moderner Seeschiffe als aktuelles Problem der Schiffahrtsmedizin. Zbl. Bakt. Hyg., I. Abt. Orig. B *166*, 1, 1–36 (1978).

Gorbulevitch, J.: Growth of neurosis among fishermen during deep sea fishing. In: Abstracts of the Int. Symp. Mar. Med. Varna, 1970. p. 79.

Low, A. and H. Goethe: Hypothermiebehandlung eines Besatzungsmitglieds nach Untergang eines Küstenmotorschiffes. Med. Welt *32*, 803–838 (1981).

Polonov, P.: Neurological and vegetative changes during long voyages in tropical conditions. In: Abstracts of the Int. Symp. Mar. Med., Varna, 1970. p. 96.

Prosetzky, P. A., J. M. Stenko, E. S. Simhovitch et al.: Some aspects on crew social psychology. In: Abstracts of the Int. Symp. Mar. Med., Varna, 1970. p. 97.

Schadewaldt, H.: The pathophysiological and pathopsychological observations of the surgeon Jean-Baptiste-Henri Savigny during the shipwreck of the "Méduse" in 1816. Bull. Inst. mar. Med. Gdańsk *17*, 3, 443–456 (1966).

Shafran, L. M. and N. V. Pavlov: Certain biochemical mechanisms of adaptation of the organisms of seamen in the tropics. In: Int. Symp. on Mar. Med., Vol. 3, Leningrad, 1968. Moscow 1969. pp. 83–86.

Simhovich, Z. M. and J. M. Stenko: Time perception and work capacity stimulation of fishermen during long voyages. In: Abstracts of the Int. Symp. Mar. Med., Varna, 1970. p. 103.

Steimatsky, A. R.: The influence of monotonia on the working capacity in skippers. In: VII Int. Symp. on Mar. Med., Odessa, 23–30 Sept. 1976. Moscow 1976. p. 296.

5.10 Search and Rescue Medicine – Survival at Sea

J. C. Duffy

In all the annals of man's adventure on the world's seas, no more chilling a subject can be found than "shipwreck". Popular literature has recounted tales of survival after shipwreck involving weeks and months. Tragically, all too often these stories were the exception and not the rule. The vast majority of seamen died, many owing to a phenomenon only recently understood – hypothermia.

Perhaps no other working environment can present the extremes that may confront the seafarer and challenge his ability to survive. The research on the physiology of survival systems of "search and rescue" from a medical point of view, and practical approaches to survival techniques for seamen will be reviewed in this chapter.

The British Royal Navy and its Survival-at-sea Subcommittee reviewed the variety of physiological parameters in survival at sea.

Although isolated individuals from the time of Herodotus onwards had recognized the importance of cold as the primary threat to life of men immersed in water, only in the 1940s did this come to be generally recognized (Critchley [4]; McCane, et al. [16]; Molnar [17]). Mention must be made also of the experiments carried out by the Nazis on prisoners at Dachau, which, although totally repugnant morally, established a number of facts about immersion hypothermia that subsequent work has confirmed (Alexander [2]; Hervey [9]). Molnar [17] showed particularly clearly that progressive fall in body temperature occurs in nearly all people immersed in water at any temperature below about 20 °C, i.e. in seas anywhere outside the tropics. The temperature of the sea along the Atlantic routes and around the coasts of Great Britain, Northern Europe and North America is never much higher than 15 °C (Hutchins and Schaarf [13]); thus most people immersed in the sea outside the tropics and not rescued will die within 1–6 h, depending on the latitude and time of year. Even after a survivor has boarded a conventional ship's boat or life-craft, McCance et al. [16] showed that the cold hazard remains. During short voyages in such a craft at sea temperatures below 5 °C, the death rate was between 20%–30%, whereas it was less than 1% on voyages of similar length when the sea temperature was over 20 °C. "Immersion foot", moreover, was always a serious risk even in a conventional life-craft because occupants often had to sit for long periods with their feet in the water (Ungley et al. [22]). These problems were largely solved as a result of the research into equipment referred to above and it was found that in the newly designed inflatable covered life-craft, clothed men lying in close proximity tended to generate enough heat to keep themselves and the air inside the raft sufficiently warm for survival even when the external air temperature was at freezing point (Glaser and McCance [8]).

Survivors are still at risk when they are picked up, particularly if they have low body temperatures. During the Battle of the Falkland Islands in the First World War, most of the 200 survivors from the *Gneisenau* died on board the rescue ships (Scott-Daniel [19]). After the sinking of the

Lusitania in 1915, some of the survivors died on board the fishing vessels which picked them up (Hoehling and Hoehling [10]). During the Second World War, both the Allies and the Germans became aware that some survivors who were alive when they were rescued from cold water died shortly afterwards. The Nazi's SS (Schutz-Staffel) was responsible for the notorious Dachau experiments, reported by Alexander [2], in which some subjects removed from cold water while still alive died shortly afterwards and usually within 30 min. McCance et al. [16] found that 17% of survivors rescued from water at 10 °C or less died within 24 h, whereas none of the 210 survivors rescued from water above 20 °C died. Critchley [4] reports that of ten men who spent 30 min. in water at −1 °C, nine died immediately after rescue.

The best research available for treatment of hypothermia may be summarized as follows:

A. The evaluation and treatment of hypothermia, whether wet or dry, on land or water, is essentially the same. Therefore, the following discussion does not specifically distinguish between chronic and acute, or wet and dry hypothermia.

B. In the cold patient, a rectal temperature is one of the vital signs. In terms of the ABCs, think:
   A – Airway
   B – Breathing
   C – Circulation
   D – Degrees

C. "Low reading" thermometers are important in the care of the hypothermia patient. Regular thermometers are useless and probably dangerous in this setting.

D. Obtaining a temperature reading is important and useful when treating hypothermia. However, there is considerable variability in individual physiological responses at specific temperatures. In addition, there will be times when a low reading thermometer is not available. Therefore, these guidelines are not based on the patient's measured temperature.

E. Axiom: With the hypothermia patient, *think heat*.
   1. No cold intravenous (iv) fluids.
   2. No cold ventilation therapy.
   3. No cold treatments of any kind.

F. Unheated oxygen should not be used for the hypothermia victim because it will add cold to the victim. Attempt to administer warm, moist oxygen if possible.

G. We must, at least, *prevent further heat loss at the core*. This can be done only by insulating the entire patient, plus adding heat to the "core areas" (head, neck, chest and groin).

H. *Add heat* gradually and gently:
   (The term "add heat" is used rather than "rewarm" because often the patient is not actually any warmer with the addition of heat, but rather only a further decrease in core temperature is minimized).
   1. Apply external warm objects to the head, neck, chest and groin. Use:
      a) Hot water bottles
      b) "Warm packs" (chemical heat packs must be used with great care so as not to burn the patient's skin, e.g. wrap in a towel and watch carefully)
      c) Warm rocks wrapped in towels
      d) Warm bodies
   2. Administer warm, moist air or oxygen.

I. Never try to cool the extremities or use tourniquets, or other occlusive dressings.

J. Be wary of statements or actions while working on patients who are "unconscious" or require cardiopulmonary resuscitation (CPR). These patients frequently remember what is done and said and severe psychological problems may result. This applies equally to warm and cold patients.

If hospital facilities are available, the staff should understand the special requirements of these patients. A total approach is required by the hospital staff.

A. *Some General Points*
  1. Treat to the level of your ability as your hospital equipment, staff and skills dictate.
  2. All patients should be stabilized before any transport to another facility. The patient should be kept in the sending hospital until the condition is stable.

B. *Evaluation*
  1. Initial attention to the airways, breathing and circulation (ABC) and to CPR.
  2. Vital signs, including rectal temperature.
  3. Brief history.
  4. Brief physical examination:
     a) Feel for skin coldness or warmth
     b) Level of consciousness
     c) Cardiopulmonary examination
     d) Associated trauma
  5. Suggested laboratory and X-ray evaluation, depending on available staffing and equipment:
     a) Chest X-ray
     b) 12-lead electrocardiogram
     c) Urine: sediment, pH, glucose, protein, ketone, sodium and osmotic concentration (osmolarity)
     d) Blood: complete blood count including platelets, blood-urea nitrogen, creatinine, electrolytes, sugar, prothrombin time, liver function tests, amylase
     e) Arterial blood gases
     f) Weight

C. *Monitoring and Treatment*
  1. Basic treatment is the same as that indicated for pre-hospital personnel in these guidelines.
  2. Cardiopulmonary monitoring.
  3. An iv and/or central venous pressure line (in the superior vena cava, not the right heart), with D_5W at 75 cc per hour. The iv fluid and rate of infusion will vary depending on the patient's level of hydration and laboratory data.
  4. Urinary bladder catheter.
  5. Nasogastric tube, if the patient is unconscious and the airway is protected.
  6. Endotracheal/nasotracheal tube is indicated in the deeply unconscious patient with lack of spontaneous reflexes after carefully checking the cervical vertebrae for possible damage.
  7. Daily weights: intake and output.
  8. Always ventilate with warm, moist air or oxygen. [Typical unwarmed ventilation is approximately 72 °F (22 °C).]
  9. Sodium bicarbonate administration is based on arterial blood gases.
  10. Continue monitoring until stable and warm.

D. *Adding Heat*
  1. The recommended possibilities include:

External methods	*Internal methods*
a) Gradual spontaneous rewarming	a) Warm steam inhalation/ventilation
b) Warming blankets, warming mattresses etc.	b) Peritoneal lavage
c) Tub bath	c) Warm iv fluids
	d) Extracorporeal circulation (Atrioventricular shunt)

  2. Regardless of the method chosen for adding heat, the patient must be under total physiological control, to allow you to deal with his metabolic needs.
  3. Tub bath is one of the most rapid methods and requires *immediate* lab-

oratory results and extremely close physiological monitoring to maintain control of the situation.

4. Do not compromise extremity circulation by using tourniquets, pneumatic antishock garments or ice packs.
5. The recommended temperature is about 105°–110 °F (40°–43 °C) for all methods.
6. *For severe hypothermia without signs of life (requiring CPR)*
   Warm the core as rapidly as you can, using one or more of the methods (e.g. warming mattress, warm steam inhalation *and* peritoneal lavage), trying to get the patient warmer than approximately 85 °F (30 °C).
7. *For severe hypothermia with signs of life*
   Use your judgment, using one or more of the methods.

E. *Most Common Problems*
   Note: Drug therapy should be moderated because in cold patients medications are both inefficient and poorly metabolized.
   1. *Arrhythmias* – these are usually atrial arrhythmias:
      a) If patient is very cold, these atrial arrhythmias will usually convert spontaneously with rewarming.
      b) If the temperature is rising and the arrhythmia does not convert, you may want to use the usual antiarrhythmic medication.
      c) If the treatment is not working, add more heat.
      d) Ventricular fibrillation in the very cold patient is treated with CPR, adding heat, and cardioversion after the temperature reaches approximately 85 °F (30 °C).
      e) In the patient whose temperature is rising, the standard treatment for ventricular fibrillation should be utilized (American Heart Association, others).
   2. *Dehydration:* Monitor and treat accordingly.
   3. *Hyperkalaemia:* Monitor and treat accordingly.
      (Do not infuse potassium in iv fluids).
   4. *Hyperglycaemia:* Monitor and treat accordingly.

Much can be done to reduce the consequences of hypothermia by educating the seafarer on what he can do in a practical way to improve his survivability. Such education should include the following information directed at his level of understanding.

5.10.1 The Human Body

An understanding of how the body reacts to cold air or water exposure and knowing the steps that can be taken to help the body delay the damaging effects of cold stress, will help in the struggle to stay alive in the event of cold water exposure.

Nature requires that the body core be kept at an ideal temperature of 98.6 °F (37 °C). A network of blood vessels running through the core and the outer layer of the body picks up the heat produced by the "furnace" within the core, and distributes that heat throughout the body. Nature also gives the body a very accurate system to regulate automatically the core temperature at 98.6 °F (37 °C). For example, if the surrounding temperature conditions are high, as on a warm day or in a hot boiler room, the blood vessels near the skin of the body enlarge, allowing more blood to flow to the skin area and give off greater amounts of body heat. This is to keep one comfortable and to keep the core temperature 98.6 °F (37 °C) from rising. However, if the surroundings are cool, the body will constrict the blood vessels at the skin surface and keep that valuable body heat from being lost too rapidly.

5.10.2 Hypothermia

The loss of body heat is one of the greatest hazards to the survival of a person in the sea. The rate of body heat loss depends on water temperature, the protective clothing worn and the manner in which the survivor conducts himself. An abnormally low body core temperature can be recognized by a variety of symptoms. Very early during exposure, the body tries to combat the excessive heat loss both by constricting its surface blood vessels (to reduce heat transfer by blood to surface) and by shivering (to produce more body heat). However, if the exposure is severe, the body is unable to conserve or produce enough heat. Its core temperature begins to fall, creating a condition known as "hypothermia". As the body core temperature approaches 95 °F (35 °C), it starts to fall more rapidly. By then discomfort, tiredness, poor coordination, numbness, impaired speech, disorientation and mental confusion appear. As the internal temperature decreases into the 80s (below 32.2 °C), unconsciousness may result, as well as a blue tinge of the skin, collapse of the veins in the skin, enlargement of the pupils, and muscle stiffness.

The heart becomes irregular and the pulse barely detectable. Although death may occur whenever the core temperature is below 90 °F (32.2 °C), it is very difficult to be sure whether the patient is alive or dead when the body core temperature is below 85 °F (29.4 °C). Death is then defined as failure to revive on rewarming.

Survival procedure in the event of a ship sinking should be preplanned to increase the chance of a successful rescue. Records show that ship sinkings, even in the worst cases, usually require at least 15–30 min for the vessel to fully submerge. This affords valuable time for preparation. Here is some sound advice that should be remembered in a situation of this type:

1. Put on as much warm clothing as possible, making sure to cover head, neck, hands and feet.
2. If an immersion (exposure) suit is available, put it on over the warm clothing.
3. If the immersion (exposure) suit does not have inherent flotation, put on a lifejacket and be sure to secure it correctly.
4. All persons who know that they are likely to be affected by seasickness should, before or immediately after boarding the survival craft, take some recommended preventive tablets or medicine in a dose recommended by the manufacturer. The incapacity caused by seasickness reduces the chance of survival; vomiting removes precious body fluid while seasickness in general makes one more prone to hypothermia.
5. Avoid entering the water if possible. Board davit-launched survival craft on the embarkation deck. If davit-launched survival craft are not available, use overside ladders, or if necessary lower yourself by means of a rope or fire hose.
6. Unless it is unavoidable, do not jump from higher than 5 m (16.4 ft) into the water. Try to minimize the shock of sudden cold immersion. Rather than jumping into the cold water, try to lower yourself gradually. A sudden plunge into the cold water can cause rapid death or an uncontrollable rise in breathing rate may result in an intake of water into the lungs. On occasions it may be necessary to jump into the water; if so, you should keep your elbow at your sides, cover your nose and mouth with one hand while holding the wrist or elbow firmly with the other hand. One should not jump into the water astern of the life-raft lest there is any remaining headway on the ship.
7. Once in the water, whether accidently or by ship abandonment, orientate yourself and try to locate the ship, lifeboats, life-rafts, other survivors or other floating objects. If you were unable to prepare yourself before entering the water, button up clothing now. In cold water you may experience violent shivering and great pain. These are natural body reflexes that are not dangerous.

You do, however, need to take action as quickly as possible before you lose full use of your hands; button up clothing, turn on signal lights, locate whistle, etc.

8. While afloat in the water, do not attempt to swim unless it is to reach a nearby craft, a fellow survivor or a floating object on which you can lean or climb. Unnecessary swimming will "pump" out any warm water between your body and the layers of clothing, thereby increasing the rate of body-heat loss. In addition, unnecessary movements of arms and legs send warm blood from the inner core to the outer layer of the body. This results in very rapid heat loss. Hence, it is most important to remain as still as possible in the water, however, painful it may be. Remember, pain will not kill you, but heat loss will!
9. The body position you assume in the water is also very important in conserving heat. Float as still as possible, with your legs together, elbows close to your side and arms folded across the front of your life-jacket. This position minimizes the exposure of the body surface to the cold water. Try to keep your head and neck out of the water. Another heat-conserving position is to huddle closely to one or more persons afloat, making as much body contact as possible. You must be wearing a life-jacket to be able to hold these positions in the water.
10. Try to board a lifeboat, life-raft or other floating platform or object as soon as possible in order to shorten your immersion time.

    Remember, you lose body heat many times faster in water than in air. Since the effectiveness of your insulation is seriously reduced by water soaking, you must now try to shield yourself from wind to avoid a wind-chill effect (convective cooling). If you manage to climb aboard a life-boat, shielding can be accomplished with the aid of a canvas cover or tarpaulin, or an unused garment. Huddling close to the other occupants of the lifeboat or raft will also conserve body heat.
11. Do not use "drown-proofing" in cold water. "Drown-proofing" is a technique whereby you relax in the water and allow your head to submerge between breaths. It is an energy-saving procedure to use in warm water when you are not wearing a life-jacket. However, the head and neck are high heat loss areas and must be kept above the water. That is why it is even more important to wear a life-jacket in cold water. If you are not wearing a life-jacket, tread the water only as much as necessary to keep your head out of the water.
12. Keep a positive attitude about your survival and rescue. This will improve your chance of extending your survival time until rescue comes. Your will to live does make a difference!

5.10.3 Man Overboard

Any man overboard is probably not prepared and off his guard. Some useful advice to follow for preventing this situation and being better prepared is:

1. Always wear a life-jacket when safety regulations require it or when you have to go on deck for any reason in poor weather.
2. Use extreme care when walking along decks, up and down ladders, and across gangways.
3. Grip firmly any rails and other support devices. Do not lean on rails or lifelines.
4. Be alert when moving around the main deck of the ship and especially around cable and rope. Keep hands out of pockets, free to grab for support if you fall.
5. Be particularly careful at night or in fog. Poor visibility increases both the chances of accident and the difficulties in locating you in the water.

6. If possible, avoid walking on an open deck in poor weather or rough conditions.
7. Inform someone of your plan to go on deck, especially if the weather conditions are poor.
8. Walk or work in pairs, if possible. Try not to be alone.
9. Common sense says dress appropriate to the weather, but some care in selection of clothes can make a difference in survival. If possible, wear many layers of clothing, including a waterproof outer layer. Make certain that the neck, wrist and ankle portions of the clothing are snug-fitting. This will reduce the exchange of water within your clothing should you go into or under water. Also, woollen clothes are better insulators than cotton, especially when wet.
10. Carry at least one reliable distress signal with you at all times. Preferably, this should be in the form of a good quality battery-powered light or chemical light stick and a whistle.
11. Wear an outer garment that is bright in colour. As an alternative, sew strips of reflective tape on upper portions of your outer garment. Reflective tape is available at drug, sporting goods or auto-supply stores.

5.10.4 Distress Signals

The immediate need of both men-overboard and ship casualty victims, once in the water, is to be rapidly located and rescued. Since water entry may occur at any time of day or night and in various degrees of fog and visibility, it is important that some distress signal should be carried at all times. Types of signals that can be easily carried include whistles, chemical lights, battery lights, mirrors and even a white handkerchief. It should be remembered that batteries have a limited service life and require regular replacement; consequently a high-quality battery should be used. Another point to remember is that cold temperature reduces the effectiveness of even a fresh battery. Therefore, the light and battery should be given a little body warmth to improve the battery performance.

High-visibility outer clothing (luminescent) or reflective tape sewn to the outer garment will reflect the beam of a rescue searchlight and prove to be a valuable detection aid on a dark night. And, of course, the waving of outstretched arms or splashing of the water is an effective and simple signalling technique, but one which should be used only when rescue is nearby. If one has a light source, moving it will enhance detection.

5.10.5 Rescue

Rescue of survival victims in the water or afloat in a lifeboat or life-raft may come about in several ways. A surface vessel may sight the victims and help them aboard. Rescue may also come in the form of a helicopter. The most popular retrieval device in use for hoisting a water survivor is a mesh-screened rescue basket. The use of the basket is rather obvious; it has an open top and all that is required of the survivor is to climb in and stay put as he is raised to safety. Although some services have a variety of "pick-up" devices, ones commonly used for non-military situations are the rescue sling (horse collar) and the rescue net. The rescue sling is a padded belt that is wrapped around the back and under the arms of the survivor. The two ends of the sling are attached by their looped rings to a hook at the end of the helicopter cable. The Navy rescue net is a rope-like cage with an open side for the survivor to enter and be seated while being raised to safety. No matter which approach is used, rescuers will enter the water and offer assistance in getting into the retrieval device if a victim is not able to help himself.

5.10.6 Treatment of Hypothermia

The treatment of hypothermia will, of course, depend on both the condition of the survivor and the facilities available. Generally speaking, survivors who are rational and capable of recounting their experiences, although shivering dramatically, merely require removal of all wet clothes, replacement with dry clothes or blankets and rest in a warm environment.

In more serious cases, where the victim is semiconscious, unconscious or apparently dead, contact should be made immediately with a ship or shore medical facility for detailed information on the care and handling of the victim. While awaiting medical instructions, the following first-aid care should be administered immediately:

1. Remove the victim from the cold; rescue and carry him if possible only in a horizontal position; do not move him unnecessarily and be sure to avoid rough handling; check for the presence of breathing and heartbeat.
2. Take the victim to a sheltered place; remove his clothes with a minimum of movement of the victim's body; cut the clothes away with scissors or knife, if necessary. Do not massage.
3. Lay the unconscious or semiconscious victim in the recovery position. Be sure to check the victim's breathing and heartbeat frequently. One must be prepared to give cardio-pulmonary resuscitation if breathing and heartbeat stop.[1]
4. If available, administer warm, humidified oxygen by face mask. The oxygen will not only benefit victims if they are having difficulty breathing or have a low respiratory rate, it will also provide some core rewarming.
5. Insulate the victim from further heat loss by warming him in a blanket. Do not attempt to aggressively rewarm the unconscious victim. Severe hypothermia is a true medical emergency, but rewarming the victim can be associated with many complications. Definitive rewarming should be attempted in a hospital. The main goal in providing first-aid is to prevent the victim from getting colder.
6. If there will be a long delay in getting the victim to a hospital, gentle rewarming techniques may be used:
   a) Apply heating pads or hot-water bottles under the blanket, to the victim's head, neck, chest and groin. Keep the victim wrapped in the blanket.
   b) Apply body warmth by direct body-to-body contact with the victim. A blanket should be wrapped around both people to conserve the heat being supplied.
7. In no case should the victim be given alcohol. Unconscious victims should be given nothing to eat or drink.

It should be kept in mind that the techniques of rescue procedures including the treatment of hypothermia differ very widely from country to country. Especially the appropriate treatment of hypothermia is still under discussion, and even specialists have different opinions in rewarming techniques.

5.10.7 Motion Sickness

Motion sickness is an age-old problem for seafarers. In the development of the tented inflatable life-craft it became evident early on that this is a particularly seasickness-inducing craft. The crew are enclosed without any horizon and the raft is flexible and adheres to the surface, so that its floor follows the contour of even the smallest wave.

It is most important that motion sickness should be prevented in raft occupants. Seasick men lying immobile in the bottom of a craft are much more likely to become casu-

---

1 It should be accepted that even a doctor might have difficulty in detecting a pulse or breathing movements in a severely hypothermic patient. The patient is particularly prone to the onset of serious cardiac irregularity. In consequence there are considerable differences of opinion on the administration of CPR.

alties from hypothermia. Sickness can lead to loss of morale and so to failure to perform essential actions such as closing down and bailing, searching for further survivors, tying rafts together, and so forth. Vomiting causes loss of body fluids and so accelerates death from dehydration.

Holling et al. [11] tackled the problem on behalf of the Armed Forces and carried out some of the first systematic and realistic experiments on prevention of motion sickness. They began by investigating the proprietary "seasick medicines" of the day, and found "Mother Siegal's Soothing Syrup" the most effective. This contained hyoscine, which they then studied systematically. They found that doses of 0.6 or 1.2 mg were highly effective, provided the drug was given well before the onset of motion. Some of the test subjects complained of dryness of the mouth, but the authors did not regard this as a serious disadvantage. They stressed the difficulty of performing satisfactory trials at sea, where the motion was never the same from day to day, and suggested that some form of machine might be built to simulate wave motion. They obtained some results with a swing, but did not consider this adequately simulated a ship.

In the United States, Tyler and Bard [20] wrote an important review of motion sickness. The discovery by Gay and Carliner [6] that Dramamine was an effective treatment received publicity, but their work was not well controlled and this drug has since become less popular. Chinn et al. [3] investigated a large number of remedies. Glaser [7] studied the side-effects of hyoscine, promethazine hydrochloride and diphenhydramine hydrochloride in subjects on land. He concluded that the side-effects were proportional to the drugs' ability to prevent motion sickness, and might reflect a common hyoscine-like action. Tolerance was acquired after administration for 4 days. He also noted that the experimental procedure without drugs sometimes provoked the "side-effects".

Considerable further work has been done on motion sickness, with some advance in fundamental understanding. A particularly important contribution was by Johnson et al. [15] and Johnson and Mayne [14], who demonstrated convincingly the importance of Coriolis Force as a factor in the causation of motion sickness. Although it is difficult to relate it to the survival-at-sea situation, the development of de-conditioning treatment in the RAF by Dobie [5] was an important therapeutic advance. The study of brain-stem neurotransmitters opens up the possibilities of a better understanding of the physiological processes which produce motion sickness, and may eventually lead to a new rationale for seeking preventive drugs. Money [18] has published an excellent review of the natural history and pathogenesis of motion sickness.

5.10.8 Water

A survivor who has reached a life-craft has also to face the hazards of dehydration. A man's water requirements vary considerably with a) the environmental temperature, wind and sun, b) his clothing and micro-environment, c) his physique and physical activity, d) the past and present nature of his food and e) his renal efficiency (Adolph, et al. [1]). The physiology of the urge to drink and the problem of water lack have been collated by Wolf [23].

Although water carried in containers is relatively heavy, it is a sure source of supply and makes the minimum demands on effort by an exhausted man (Holt [12]). Chemical desalting kits are not favoured as they are expensive and troublesome to operate. These kits give about a five-fold gain in terms of space or weight and have application where these are not the all-important factors as, for example, in one-man dinghies. A solid-fuel still which was tested during the Singapore trials produced lethal concentrations of carbon monoxide (0.2%)

inside the raft in 5 min, before any water had been distilled, and the value of this type of still in inflatable life-rafts seems a very remote possibility. Solar stills, on the other hand, have shown much promise. The advantages of being able to collect rainwater have led to catchment arrangements being used in the design of the modern covered life-raft.

On no account should survivors drink seawater or mix it with fresh water when rations are short. Seafarers with plenty of fresh water and good prospects of replenishing their supplies may use a little seawater in their cooking, but the amount of salt consumed in this way should not exceed that taken in normal life ashore.

All rain catchment areas and collecting utensils must be maintained in a good state of cleanliness and free from salt. A solar still and desalting apparatus should be used if provided, and a distilling plant should be improvised if facilities are available. Dew should be collected at night: if clothes are hung in the rigging, they can then be placed over the face and the drops sucked in. Dew may also be collected on cold surfaces in the boat.

In ice regions, it must be remembered that icebergs, glaciers and old sea-ice consist of fresh water. Old sea-ice is distinguished from young sea-ice by its smooth corners, bluish colour, glossy surface and ease of splintering when struck. Young sea-ice has angular corners, a milky colour, a tough texture and is difficult to splinter. Pieces of sea-ice piled up for 2 or 3 days lose their salt. The pools which form on ice in summer are fresh: those should be selected which are remote from possible contamination by salt sea spray. Where heating apparatus is available, ice should be used rather than snow – it is more economical on heat.

References

1. Adolph, E. F. et al.: Physiology of man in the desert. New York: Interscience 1947. Chaps. 14, 17.
2. Alexander, L.: The treatment of shock from prolonged exposure to cold especially in water. Combined Intelligence Objectives Sub-committee, Item No. 24, File No. 26–37.
3. Chinn, H. I., W. K. Noel and P. K. Smith: The prophylaxis of motion sickness. Arch. intern. Med. *86,* 810–822 (1950).
4. Critchley, M.: Shipwreck survivors. A medical study. London: Churchill 1943.
5. Dobie, T. G.: The treatment of airsickness in aircrew by means of a spin-table. 41st Annual Scientific Meeting. Aerospace Med. Ass., St. Louis, 1970.
6. Gay, L. N. and P. E. Carliner: The prevention and treatment of motion sickness. Bull. Johns Hopkins Hospital *84,* 470–487 (1949).
7. Glaser, E. M.: Experiments on the side-effects of drugs. Brit. J. Pharmacol. *8,* 2, 187–192 (1953).
8. Glaser, E. M. and R. A. McCance: First report on Arctic survival trials. (Tromso Febr.–March 1950). Ed.: Medical Research Council, Royal Naval Personnel Committee 1950. (Report No. RNP 50/591).
9. Hervey, G. R.: Physiological changes encountered in hypothermia. Proc. roy. Soc. Med. *66,* 10, 1053–1058 (1973).
10. Hoehling, A. A. and M. Hoehling: The last voyage of the Lusitania. London: Longmans, Green 1957.
11. Holling, H. E., B. McArdle and W. R. Trotter: The prevention of sea sickness by drugs. Lancet *1,* 127–129 (1944).
12. Holt, W. J.: Recent developments in naval life-saving equipment. Transact. Inst. nav. Architects *97,* 331–352 (1955).
13. Hutchins, L. W. and M. Schaarf: Maximum and minimum monthly sea surface temperatures charted from the world atlas of sea surface temperatures. Sears Foundation J. Mar. Res. *6,* 3 (1947).
14. Johnson, W. H. and J. W. Mayne: Stimulus required to produce motion sickness. J. Aviat. Med. *24,* 400–411 (1955).
15. Johnson, W. H., R. A. Stubbs, G. F. Kelk et al.: Stimulus required to produce motion sickness. J. Aviat. Med. *22,* 365–374 (1951).
16. McCance, R. A., C. C. Ungley, J. W. L. Crosfill et al.: The hazards to men in ships lost at sea. 1940–1944. London: Her Majesty's Stationery Office 1956. (Medical Research Council Special Report Series No. 291).
17. Molnar, G. W.: Survival of hypothermia by men

immersed in the ocean. J. Amer. med. Ass. *131*, 1046–1050 (1946).
18. Money, K.E.: Motion sickness. Physiol. Rev. *50*, 1, 1–39 (1970).
19. Scott-Daniel, D.: World War I: an illustrated history. London: Benn 1965.
20. Tyler, D.B. and Ph. Bard: Motion sickness. Physiol. Rev. *29*, 4, 311–369 (1949).
21. Ungley, C.C.: The immersion foot syndrome. Advanc. Surg. *1*, 269–336 (1949).
22. Ungley, C.C., G.D. Channell and R.L. Richards: The immersion foot syndrome. Brit. J. Surg. *33*, 17–31 (1945).
23. Wolf, A.V.: Thirst – physiology of the urge to drink and the problems of water lack. Springfield: Thomas 1958.

5.11 Life-Saving Appliances

R. Herrmann

In spite of rapid progress in the technology of ship construction and navigation, the problem of developing the best possible life-saving appliances to ensure certain survival for seamen in all weather conditions and in every distress situation still has not been solved.

Technical publications deal exhaustively with this problem. As early as 1947 Sweger [28] examined the question, "What have you done for the fleet sailor's life?" in a report entitled *Advances in Shipboard Life-saving Equipment.* He outlines the history of life-saving appliances, reports on the currently available life-saving appliances and speculates on future developments in the expectation of nearing an optimum. He presents a few answers to his question; however he adds, "But to carry on even more effectively it is time for the U.S. Navy to recognize the need and dedicate men, money and resources to the successful implementation of a complete and co-ordinated programme designed to protect and save the lives of our men." From this sentence we may infer that the author thought at the time that more must be done in that direction.

Holt [10] described the development of life-saving appliances, giving special attention to life-jackets and different sorts of inflatable life-rafts, immersion suits and distillation apparatus.

Nicholl [19] detailed, in 1960, in his work *Survival at Sea,* under the headings "History", "Application" and "Technology", the problems posed by different life-saving appliances ranging from life-jackets and life-rafts through to water distillation systems. The contents of the book record the construction and practical application in addition to dealing with future construction forms. In conclusion the author indicated the full extent of the difficulties. In December 1972 in *The Standard Specifications for Merchant Ship Construction* of the Maritime Administration [27], the standards of individual and collective life-saving appliances are described.

Haag and Jacobi [4, 5, 6, 7] described the extent and use of different types of life-saving appliances. The details of their use in certain emergencies are given, together with defects which have been found in practice. Comment was made on the guidelines which are to be found in the recommendations and instructions issued by the See-Berufsgenossenschaft and other marine authorities. The authors emphasize that the suggested improvements are technically possible and could be achieved if properly funded.

The different life-saving appliances may be categorized as follows:

1. Individual life-saving appliances
2. Collective life-saving appliances
3. Life-saving appliances designed to rescue the shipwrecked of other ships.

This chapter deals with the first two types, as well as discussing cold protection suits.

5.11.1 Individual Life-Saving Appliances (Life-jackets)

When ships are abandoned and also in other shipping emergencies, it may be necessary to spend relatively long periods immersed in water. It is important to explain a few physical principles which throw light on the question of which protective measures are suitable to enable man to survive in the medium of water.

The weight reduction of bodies immersed in water is equal to the amount of displaced water. This phenomenon is called buoyancy. Bodies with a specific gravity *higher* than water displace a smaller volume of water than their own weight and therefore sink. Bodies with a specific gravity *equal to* water displace an amount of water corresponding to their weight and therefore remain, in the absence of other factors, afloat but not necessarily on the surface. All parts are immersed in water. Bodies with a specific gravity *lower* than water displace a greater amount of water than their corresponding weight. The ensuing buoyancy is greater than the displacement volume. In the absence of other factors these bodies stay afloat on the surface, whereby a part of the mass is not immersed in water.

The human body must also be considered in separate parts if the steps in the process are to be understood.

In experiment, if the head, the trunk (torso) and the extremities are immersed in water separately, the head and the extremities slowly sink to the bottom on account of their higher specific gravity. The trunk remains afloat and even protrudes above the surface, i. e. its specific gravity is lower than that of the water. When the parts are rejoined the specific gravity of an average person with partially deflated lungs corresponds to that of the water; the body will therefore remain afloat. With fully deflated lungs the body will slowly sink to the bottom because its specific gravity will then be slightly higher than that of the water. Buoyancy can be affected by variations of weight and build, i.e. specifically in the case of extremely light people who do not sink in spite of deflated lungs, the opposite being true of especially heavy people.

With partially deflated lungs, therefore, man is able to keep his nose and mouth just above water-level without swimming or additional buoyancy aids. It is necessary only to make movements to adjust his balance and in this way survival is possible (Fig. 1). Unfortunately any small disturbance of the water (waves, current etc.) may upset this equilibrium so that the face is submerged. Swimming action, if executed with enough strength, leads to an increased dynamic buoyancy and in most cases enables a person to survive longer. But this cannot be guaranteed in distress and rescue situations. It is quite possible that a man who has fallen into the sea after an accident will not have enough energy to make the necessary movements (owing to fear, panic, hypothermia, injuries, exhaustion and fatigue).

Figure 2 shows a person in a vertical floating position with his face under water. In the case of weakened or unconscious persons the head will automatically fall forwards. The very high specific gravity of the head will cause the body to shift forwards and over. The relatively high specific gravtiy of the arms will cause a similar effect in the same direction. The trunk causes a reverse effect but this is counteracted by the particularly high specific gravity of the legs. The body will then, irrespective of the degree of inflation in the lungs, automatically come to rest in the well-known position "face below water" whilst floating on the surface or slowly sinking in this position (Fig. 3). There is no hope of survival.

The paramount aim of the life-jacket must be to support the head of a person safely above water without any exertions on his part.

Generally speaking the total body minus head has a positive buoyancy quotient of 1.5 kp (15 N). The head has an average quotient of 6 kp (60 N), which demonstrates that the difference between these two forces is approximately 4.5 kp (45 N). With an additional lift of 4.5 kp (45 N) a safe level of buoyancy is reached (Fig. 4). A buoyant appliance attached in a favourable position would let the body re-emerge

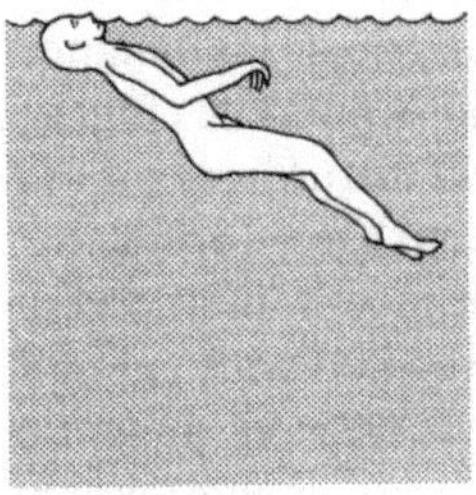

Fig. 1.

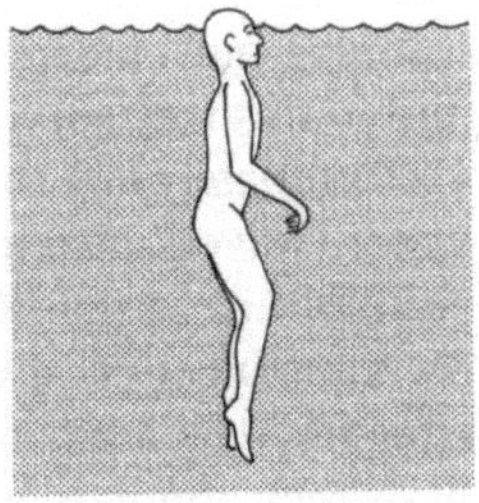

Fig. 2.

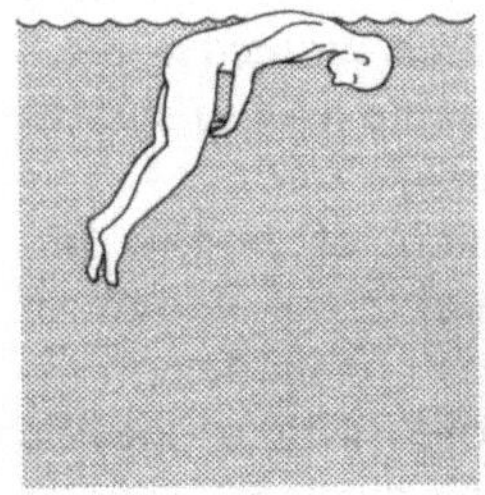

Fig. 3.

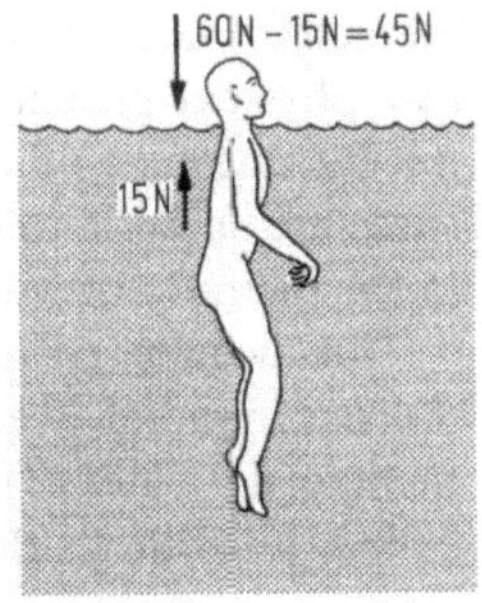

Fig. 4.

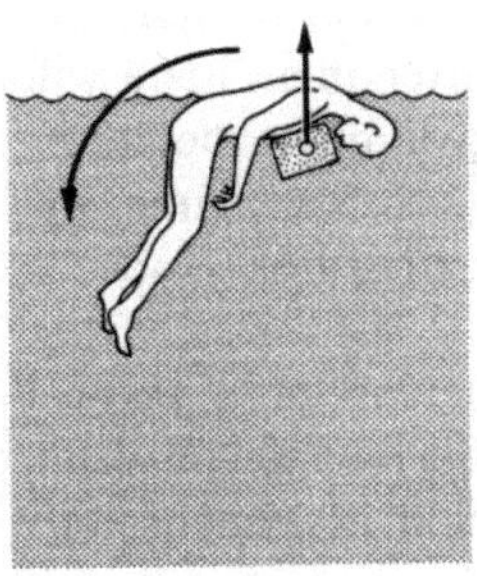

Fig. 5.

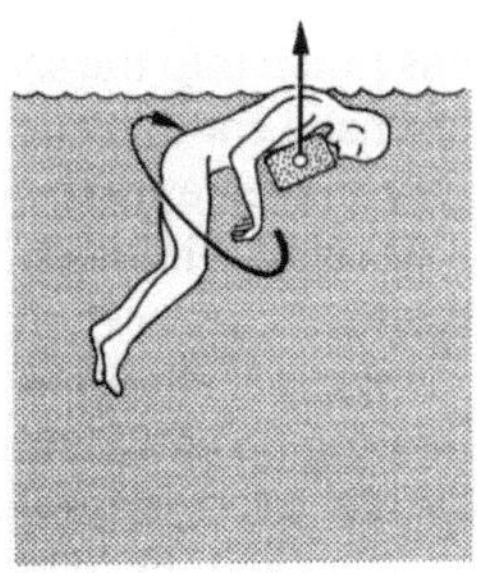

Fig. 6.

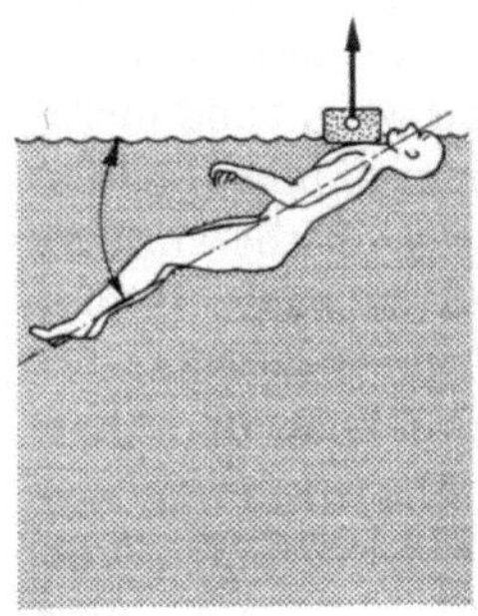

Fig. 7.

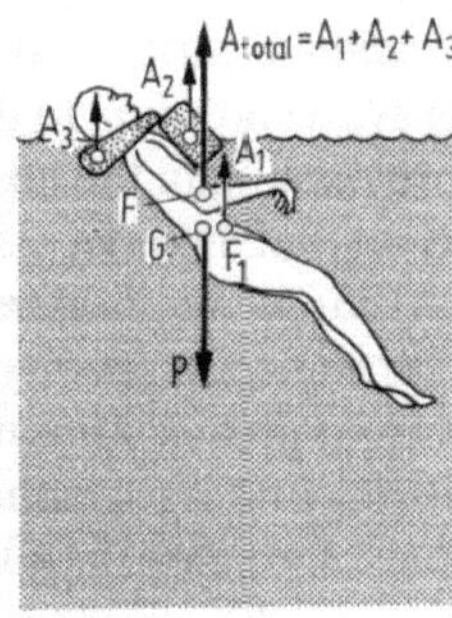

Fig. 8.

(Fig. 5), turn it on its back (Figs. 6, 7) and maintain it in this position. However, the head would automatically sink backwards; in order to counteract this effect an additional buoyant appliance should support the head from behind. Measures should also be taken to prevent sideways tilting.

These measures will require a higher buoyancy than the above-mentioned 4.5 kp (45 N) in order to bring about the best positioning in the water.

In accordance with the different possible uses, the volume of a life-jacket varies from 10 to 16 dm^3 (sports sailing) up to 16 dm^3 (professional shipping). The life-jacket's surplus buoyancy volume protruding above the surface stabilizes the whole system and counteracts submersion of the face when the sea becomes rough. Thus the person is enabled to make the necessary movements to stay afloat. The now completely serviceable life-jacket is shown in Fig. 8, whereby the buoyancy of the human body (A1) acts at its centre of gravity (F1), and the buoyancy of the life-jacket (A2 and A3) acts at its flotation points (F2 and F3). The stability of the whole system depends on the distance between the point (F) – the centre of gravity – and the point (G) – the buoyancy capacity of the whole system. The greater the distance between (F) and (G), the more stable is the whole system. It is important that (F) lies above (G). The system shown in the last diagram is the one most commonly used in shipping today. However, the author's investigations have shown that considerable problems arise in rough seas. The inertia of the human body in water delays its movement in the waves even when a life-jacket with a greater volume is worn. This results in the face of a person floating in the sea being periodically and unavoidably under water at a wave-height of 60–80 cm. The life-jackets approved of by merchant shipping do not prevent this happening at a frequency of 15–20 per minute, the duration lying between 20% and 30% of the total immersion

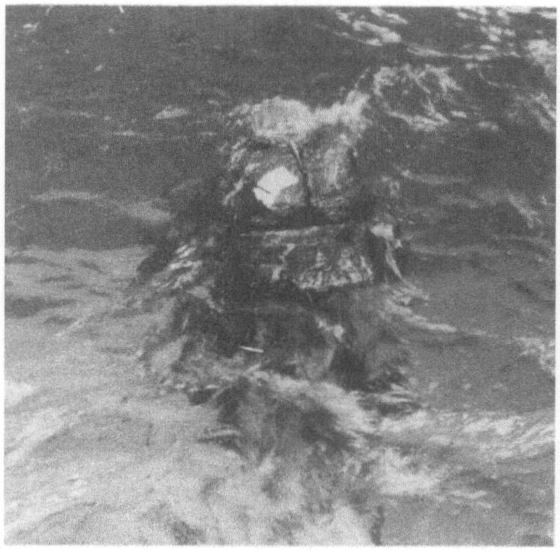

Fig. 9.

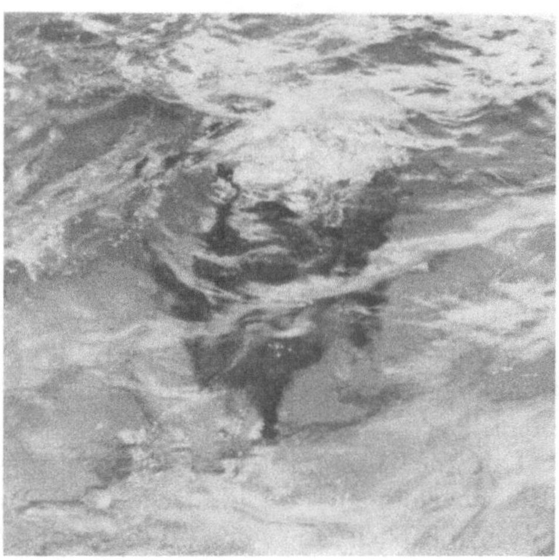

Fig. 10.

time. This constitutes a considerable danger to the chances of survival (Figs. 9, 10).

Wind and sea factors cause a person wearing a life-jacket to float with his face against the wind, looking towards the oncoming waves. Water channels form on the life-jacket which prove especially dangerous because of the splashing effect (Figs. 11, 12). These channels are illustrated in the photographs lettered "A". Such water channels are always found when recovering floating bodies. Just as dangerous are

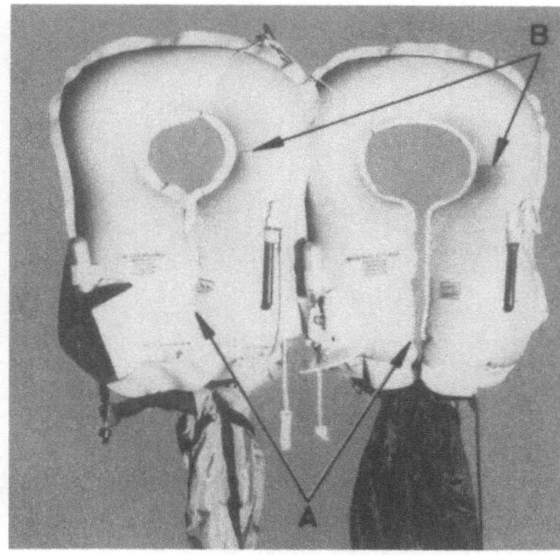

Fig. 11.

the flat buoyant components of the life-jacket which lie sideways against the face (Figs. 11 and 12, lettered B). Water can splash into the nose and mouth when the body is lying sideways. The best jackets are those without water channels in the chest area and with little lacing at the sides of the head. The ideal would be a life-jacket with an additional facial guard of transparent film (Fig. 13). This guard must contain ventilation holes to ensure an adequate air intake while keeping water out. A slight increase of CO_2 in the inspired air does not represent a danger.

The temperature of the air under the facial guard rises to 1°–2 °C above the exterior air temperature; therefore the survival chances are marginally increased by the retained heat. Life-jackets with facial guards are not generally in use; they have been used in only some navies and on pleasure craft. They should without doubt be carried for use in merchant ships.

Many authors have dealt with the problem posed by individual life-saving appliances, but these works have rarely been based on actual comprehensive experimental studies. The following publications present a wide-ranging insight into developments made in this area.

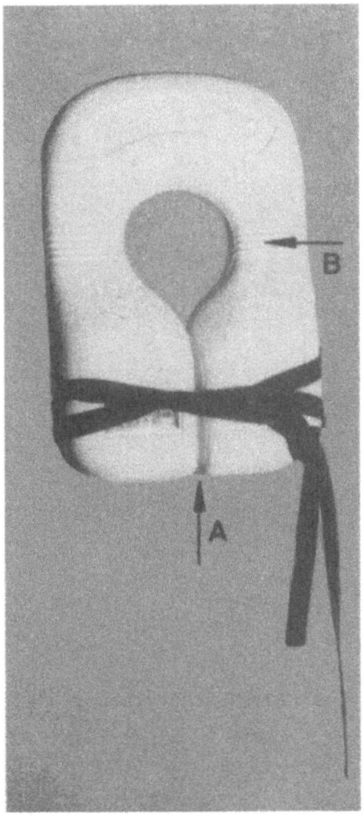

Fig. 12.

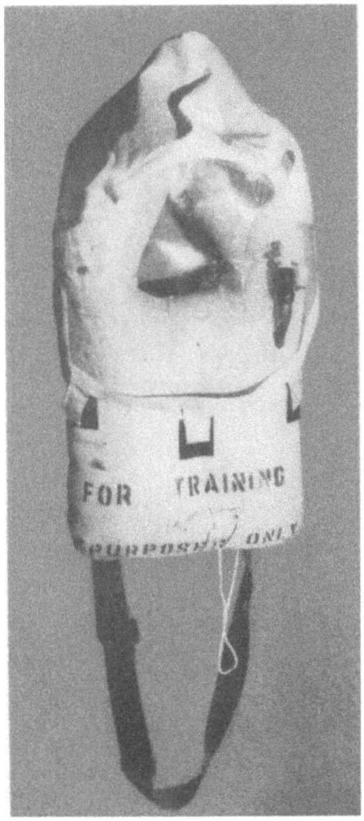

Fig. 13.

Macintosh and Pask [16] were the first to report on methods of testing life-jackets. The authors describe the technique of intubation anaesthesia which enables the experiments to be done on unconscious subjects – in this case, anaesthetized persons. The most important result of this rather heroic test was the discovery that the best floating position of the human body could be reached at an angle of 45° to the surface.

Bernhardt [1] describes the physical aspects of the human body in relation to swimming. Based on the physical properties of the body, he offers some constructional suggestions on how to design the best life-jackets. These propositions are presented in diagram form, backed up by physical and mechanical laws and formulae.

A detailed standardization of regulations for life-jackets on merchant ships was published in 1974 in the international agreement for safety on ships [11]. Nearly all national regulations conform to this agreement.

Lauckner [13, 14, 15] describes the historical development of life-jackets, man's physical capacity to swim and the stability of the body in relation to the life-jacket. The physical principles of appliances for individual life saving are clearly defined by means of sketches and formulae.

Pask [22] gives an insight into the problems of life-jackets in practice. He also reports on experiments with anaesthetized persons. In his opinion such experiments are impracticable for the future. He recommends conducting such experiments with immersible dummies which should function in a way as near as possible to persons swimming. In conclusion he gives the criteria which lead to the development of such dummies and describes first experiments with the appliance. The results were judged to be valid; however, Pask thought that the dummy was unnecessarily complicated in design. He suggested that much simpler dummies should be tested to compare the results with those produced by the more sophisticated prototype.

The same author described the construction of a medium-sized dummy in another publication [21]. The design is shown by means of tables and pictures. He believes the device will be of use in the design and testing of individual life-saving appliances.

The technical requirements for currently approved life-saving appliances for merchant vessels are detailed in the testing and approval conditions for life-jackets of 25 October 1977 of the See-Berufsgenossenschaft in Hamburg [24].

The Minister for Transport in the Federal Republic of Germany published guidelines for the manufacture and testing of life-jackets for pleasure craft [26], including constructional and functional requirements for life-jackets. At the moment a DIN-standard is in development, but has yet to be published.

5.11.2 Cold Protection

One of the greatest hazards of immersion in cool seas is hypothermia. Hypothermia claims a large proportion of the victims of disasters at sea. In temperate latitudes or in areas with an extremely cold climate the chances of a person surviving in the sea are slim and range from a few minutes to a few hours depending on the degree of cold (Fig. 14). An efficient life saving appliance can prevent death by drowning but will do nothing to hinder death by hypothermia.

The obvious solution would be to provide a garment which will keep heat in and water out. Insulation suits to protect against hypothermia have been developed but they are not in general use. Differing designs of suits are available but all possess considerable disadvantages which counteract their advantages.

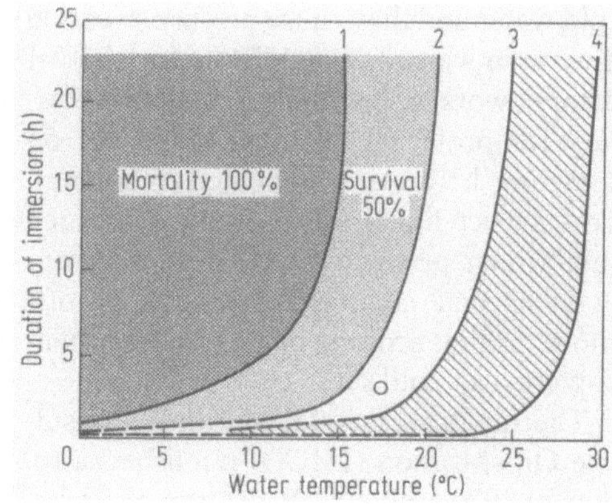

Fig. 14. Contrast between the tolerance times of fat (curve 3) and thin (curve 4) nude men immersed in water at various temperatures and the survival rates for well-clothed men according to Molnar (1946) (curves 1 and 2). The survival time of victims of the Lakonia disaster is indicated by the o.

Curve 1: fat persons } well clothed
2: thin persons
3: fat persons } nude
4: thin persons

o: survival time of victims of the Lakonia disaster (Maclean and Emslie-Smith [17])

The most usual design is a suit made from thin waterproof plastic material or coated fabric which is worn over either normal clothing or added thick warm clothes. The purpose of the suit is to provide temporary protection against hypothermia in the period between leaving the ship and reaching the life-craft. The protection given is for short-term only and it is not suitable for longer periods in the sea. All insulation suits are supposed to prevent water penetrating to the clothing underneath but this is not always possible. However, water that has leaked into the suit is warmed by the body and provided that it does not leak out, heat exchange between the body and the sea will be reduced. These non-insulated suits have been used by a few merchant fleets.

The need to increase the survival period has resulted in the production of more sophisticated suits which incorporate a heat insulating system. These suits have been designed for periods spent in extremely cold water and they cause profuse sweating if worn in warm surroundings, especially if there is work to be done. It is often necessary for protective clothing to be put on sometime before an anticipated emergency. This aspect limits the usefulness of such suits which, up to now, have been worn only in special circumstances such as offshore drilling projects or on transport helicopters over cold seas.

The Intergovermental Maritime Consultive Organization (IMCO) published a report in 1970 entitled "Prevention of Hypothermia" [23] in which the various aspects are examined in detail. This report deals with the physiological processes of the body under the influence of such factors as age, drugs, alcohol and clothing and their relation to consequent symptoms and indications of hypothermia. The treatment of persons suffering from hypothermia and the changes in their condition are described. The subcommittee thinks that still more should be done to prevent hypothermia and recommends that the following points be taken into consideration in future studies:

1. To investigate the criteria of selection, training and acclimatisation;
2. To improve the specific treatment of complications of hypothermia;
3. To define the nature of the best cold protection (sort of clothing, use of oil or other material).

Golden [3] gives a detailed report on the problems of immersion and comes to the following conclusions:

1. All immersion casualties should be admitted to hospital for observation. If water has been inhaled and there are clinical signs in the chest they should be admitted to an intensive treatment unit.
2. Attempts at resuscitation should always be made in apparently dead hypothermic immersion victims and only abandoned if unsuccessful after rewarming has occurred.
3. Always consider the possibility that an underlying pathological disturbance caused the incapacitation that led to the immersion incident.
4. If ventilatory support is required, PEEP should be instituted as soon as possible.

Keatinge [12] writes in his book *Survival in Cold Water* about the physiology and treatment of immersion hypothermia and of drowning. The mechanism of body temperature control and the effect of the clothing and fitness on body temperature are considered. The author suggests points in the treatment of hypothermia immersion victims when the factors of age, drugs, alcohol and acclimatization have influenced the core-temperature regulation of the body.

Maclean and Emslie-Smith [17] published their book *Accidental Hypothermia* in 1977. This can be considered as the most comprehensive work on hypothermia and its treatment.

Hayward et al. [8] describe the effectiveness of 23 different cold protection suits, including a few diving-suits. Experiments with and without cold protection suits are compared.

The Finnish Board of Navigation published in 1981 *Testing of Immersion Suits* [29], in which nine cold protection suits from Finland, Norway, the U.S.A. and Canada are examined in extensive testing reports in relation to their cold protection effectiveness.

5.11.3 Collective Life-Saving Appliances

The function of collective life-saving appliances is to offer protection to fairly large numbers of people after the ship has been abandoned. There are different systems, but each system has its own drawbacks and advantages. Life-boats have the advantage of easy manoeuvrability, which means, firstly, that survivors floating about in the sea can be systematically rescued, and secondly, that the boat can be steered. The disadvantage is their vulnerability in rough seas. Unfortunately it often happens that the boat is so badly damaged by the rough weather before the disaster that it is no longer seaworthy when required. It is also not always possible to lower the boat when the ship is listing. The danger of hypothermia is also present in the case of open boats sailing in bad weather as the clothing of the people on board is constantly soaked, resulting in a considerable evaporative cooling due to high winds.

Rigid life-rafts are less easily damaged but it is just as difficult to get them into the water. Covered rafts help prevent hypothermia. All life-rafts are difficult to manoeuvre or steer in comparison with a lifeboat. The currently used system allows inflatable life-rafts to be floated without any damage ensuing. But the danger remains that they will drift in high winds. These rafts are therefore attached to the ship by a cord which must have a specific breaking point so that the sinking ship does not pull the life-raft down with it. But as high winds may cause similar tension there is a danger that the cord will snap at the specific breaking point and the raft would then drift away before the crew can climb in. Unfortunately, inflatable life-rafts capsize fairly often when set into water or inflated and they may be difficult to right in bad weather. Inflatable life-rafts offer good protection against the weather, and hypothermia is not to be feared if an adequate number of people are on board.

Currently, some countries are investigating methods whereby life-saving appliances can be launched when the ship is floating in an abnormal position, e.g. listing. Ideally, any new system should be installed in the superstructure of the ship and be approachable from the emergency assembly point without it being necessary to cross the dangerous open decks. The crew should be able to launch the capsule from shipboard sitting inside the capsule. Once these survival capsules are in water, they should give the crew the best possible protection.

Survival chances are greatly endangered if the supply of water on a lifeboat is not sufficient. Most lifeboats contain only enough water to provide half a litre a day per person for a period of 1 week.

One danger exists in every collective life-saving appliance, especially the covered inflatable life-rafts, namely a higher risk of motion sickness. Apart from the general physical and mental weakening of the affected person, the loss of fluid which accompanies motion sickness is extremely dangerous when coupled with the limited water supply on board. It is therefore extremely important to provide the crew with medication against sea sickness at least 1 hour before the expected abandonment of the ship. Simultaneously the crew members should put on cold protection suits if such suits are available. Failing this warm, insulating clothing should be worn.

It is clear that at present conventional lifeboats and inflatable life-rafts do not offer the best solution. For this reason controversial views are common in many technical publications.

Müller et al. [18] treat the problem of drinking water conservation in lifeboats. Among other things they describe conservation experiments. Drinking water from a public water supply was used to fill polyethylene cans with a volume of 30 litres each. After being treated with 0.1 mg per litre Ag (silver colloids), the cans were stored for 3 years and were frequently examined for bacteriological and chemical state. The results showed the water had no objectionable properties even when some cans had been kept under tropical conditions. The possibility of contaminating water reservoirs in lifeboats has always been very high and means of preventing this should be introduced.

Herrmann and Stöver [9] describe bacteriological examinations of drinking water from lifeboats on ships under German and other flags. There were no serious hygienic differences between water from home and foreign ships.

Drinking water that had been frequently changed was prone to bacteriological contamination. It is clear that this contamination of the water had been brought about in most cases during the exchange of the new water for the old. In order to avoid diarrhoea among the crew members during long periods in life-boats the authors recommend that pure drinking water be stored for at least a year and an approved water disinfectant be added. Because of the favourable long-term effect the authors recommend colloidal silver treatment in preference to other disinfecting processes.

In Hansa [2] a report appeared in 1977 on the first self-stabilizing, self-bailing lifeboats for effective use. These boats are not completely covered, which makes the self-bailing design necessary. The boats were tested by the See-Berufsgenossenschaft on their self-bailing and -righting capacity. When fully flooded the boat bails itself out completely in approximately 20 s. When the boat was forced to keel over it righted itself in about 6 s. The water which poured into it as the boat was stabilizing itself (about 20% of the inner volume of the boat) had run out after 7 s. The engine, which automatically shuts down if the boat capsizes, could be started immediately after the boat was upright.

In another publication [30] other types of boats are reported on. These were introduced by Watercraft Ltd., Boat Building Company. Of glass-fibre manufacture, these boats are completely covered and are for use on tankers, including gas-tankers, and also in a modified version on offshore oil-rigs, production platforms and drilling ships. These boats should enable the crew to leave a danger area consequent upon any and every imaginable hazard. This boat's crew is completely independent of the exterior atmosphere. Fire safeguards fixed to the outer boat, i.e. spraysystems, protect the whole surface for up to 10 min in case of fire. This means a distance of 1 mile at a speed of 6 knots. Compressed air is available in the boat to maintain the interior atmosphere. A positive pressure builds up within the boat, preventing the penetration of vapours and gases.

Hansa [25] reports on a Swedish study made on life-saving appliances carried out by the Kockums Shipyard. They developed a type of survival capsule that acts as a shelter and control room from which measures to save the ship can be taken. The capsule should be placed as near to the accomodation quarters as possible and, being accessible from the free deck and stairway, serves as the main assembly point in an emergency. Other features were a gimballed structure to retain its usefulness even if the ship listed, fire proofing, adequate ventilation and the ability to remain afloat even if the ship should sink. When floating, the deck of the capsule was supposed to act as a helicopter touch-down pad.

Zander [31] makes recommendations for self-rescue measures for the crews of merchant ships. A newly developed life-saving appliance should be constructed to be easy and safe when put into action, to have sheltered access and to have prolonged attachment to the ship until its sinking becomes inevitable. The appliance should be optimally designed so as to allow for self-rescue in all circumstances, e.g. fire and sinking. Developmental considerations are described in as much detail as the early planning stage allows.

The appliance is a so-called survival capsule, which can be entered by the crew directly from the assembly point in emergencies. The appliance must be able to withstand fire on board for a period before it is launched. The crew should be able to launch it at any time without additional help.

Överaas [20] describes the results of a Scandinavian research project which also deals with a survival capsule. In contrast to the ones in the aforementioned excerpts from the literature, this capsule is not attached to the superstructure of the ship. However, it can be launched in any position the ship might take. Freefall from heights of 20 m, pitching angle of up to 15° and a listing position of up to 30° should be possible. If the ship sinks, automatic release is planned. This life-saving appliance has already been tested in practice.

References

1. Bernhardt, J.: Der Mensch im Medium Wasser. Ein Beitrag zur Problematik der Schwimmweste. Schiff und Hafen *11*, 3, 244–247 (1959).
2. Die ersten selbstaufrichtenden selbstlenzenden Rettungsboote für den praktischen Einsatz. Hansa *114*, 19, 1715–1716 (1977).
3. Golden, F. St. C.: Problems of immersion. Brit. J. Hosp. Med. *23*, 4, 371–383 (1980).
4. Haag, R. and H. Jacobi: Art, Umfang und Einsatz von Rettungsmitteln. Einzelrettungsmittel. Part 1. Hansa *116*, 17, 1311–1314 (1979).
5. Haag, R. and H. Jacobi: Gruppenrettungsmittel. Part 2. Rettungsboote. Hansa *116*, 19, 1473–1476 (1979).
6. Haag, R. and H. Jacobi: Gruppenrettungsmittel. 2. Teil: Rettungsflöße. Hansa *116*, 20, 1569–1571 (1979).
7. Haag, R. and H. Jacobi: Gruppenrettungsmittel. Schluß: Fremdrettung. Hansa *116*, 21, 1657–1658 (1979).
8. Hayward, J. S., P. A. Lisson and M. L. Collins: Survival suits for accidental immersion in cold water: Design concepts and their thermal protection performance. Ed.: University of Victoria. Victoria 1978.
9. Herrmann, R. and A. Stöver: Seenot-Trinkwasser. Hansa *115*, 15/16, 1311–1314 (1978).
10. Holt, W. J.: Recent developments in naval lifesaving equipment. Transact. Institut. nav. Architects *97*, 331–352 (1955).
11. Internationales Übereinkommen von 1974 zum Schutz des menschlichen Lebens auf See (SOLAS 74). BGBl. Teil II, 8 (1979).
12. Keatinge, W. R.: Survival in cold water. The physiology and treatment of immersion hypothermia and of drowning. Oxford: Blackwell 1969.
13. Lauckner, G.: Überleben in Seenot. I. Die Schwimmweste – "Eyn gar nuetzlich Geraet" – Kleiner Streifzug durch die Geschichte. Kommodore *3*, 198–204 (1963).
14. Lauckner, G.: Überleben in Seenot. II. Ein Kapitel über "Schwimmphysik". Kommodore *4*, 262–265 (1963).
15. Lauckner, G.: Überleben in Seenot. III. Stabilität des Körpers und der Einheit Körper-Schwimmweste. Kommodore *5*, 323–326 (1963).
16. Macintosh, R. R. and E. A. Pask: The testing of life-jackets. Brit. J. industr. Med. *14*, 168–176 (1957).
17. Maclean, D. and D. Emslie-Smith: Accidental hypothermia. Oxford: Blackwell 1977.
18. Müller, G., Th. Kempf, H. Goethe et al.: Trinkwasserkonserven für Rettungsboote. Forum Städte-Hygiene *28*, 2, 33–34 (1977).
19. Nicholl, G. W. R.: Survival at sea. The development, operation and design of inflatable marine lifesaving equipment. London: Coles, Harrap; New York: de Graff 1960.
20. Överaas, S.: Die Entwicklung neuer Rettungsmittel. Schiff und Hafen *29*, 9, 838–841 (1977).
21. Pask, E. A.: The design of life-jackets. Brit. med. J. *11*, 1140–1142 (1961).
22. Pask, E. A.: Prüfung des Individuellen Rettungsmittels in physiologischer Hinsicht. Mitt. Dtsch. Ges. Verkehrsmed. *15*, 21–31 (1964).
23. Prevention of hypothermia. Note by the Secretariat. IMCO. Sub-Committee on Life-Saving Appliances. 11th Session. Agenda item 5. Geneva, 22 April 1977.
24. Prüfungs- und Zulassungsbedingungen für Rettungswesten. 25 October 1977. Hamburg: SBG Hamburg 1978.
25. Rettungsmittelstudie aus Schweden. Hansa *115*, 5, 417 (1978).
26. Richtlinien für die Herstellung und Prüfung von Rettungswesten für die Sportschiffahrt. Bundesanzeiger No. 140, 30 July 1977.
27. Standard specifications for merchant ship construction. Springfield: U.S. Dept. of Commerce, Maritime Administration 1972.
28. Sweger, G. A.: What have you done for the fleet sailor's life today? Advances in shipboard lifesaving equipment. Washington: Association of Senior Engineers of the Naval Ship Systems Command. Department of the Navy. 1974.
29. Testing of immersion suits. Finnish Board of Navigation 1981.
30. Watercraft enclosed lifeboats. Schiff und Hafen *28*, 10, 991 (1976).
31. Zander, A.: Überlegungen zur Eigenrettung von Handelsschiffsbesatzungen. Schiff und Hafen *33*, 12, 74–76 (1981). Dtsch. Küstenschiffahrt *11*, 322–324 (1981).

5.12 Offshore Medicine

R. A. F. Cox

The term "offshore medicine" covers all health matters which arise in connection with the exploration for and production of hydrocarbons from beneath the sea. Such activities now take place on most of the world's continental shelves in water depths to 1 000 m, often in extremely hostile conditions and sometimes in areas remote from medical services of any sort. Offshore work falls into one of three phases – exploration, development and construction, and production. During the first phase, drilling is conducted from isolated mobile structures which usually have 75–100 men on board. In the second phase there is pipelaying and heavy engineering and construction taking place from various specialised vessels which may have crews of up to 350 or 400 men. Diving is a prominent activity during this period. In the third phase the oil and gas is in continuous production and the main activities are those of control, monitoring and maintenance. Throughout the life of a field, which averages 12–20 years, medical support must be provided at the site and on shore to cover environmental hygiene, day-to-day health care of the workers, major disasters and occupational health.

The various functions are discharged by appropriately trained nurses or sick berth attendants (known as medics) on the installations themselves and by properly organised supporting services from doctors and hospitals on shore. The offshore medics need suitably designed and equipped hospitals or sick bays from which to work. By ensuring that all offshore employees meet certain basic medical standards before they are allowed offshore, the incidence of major medical problems is minimised.

The medical examination for offshore work is designed to detect conditions which would be a danger to the employee or to others in the remote, offshore environment where the only source of immediate medical assistance is the medic. From time to time offshore installations may be completely isolated by bad weather, perhaps for several days. Fog, for example, may prevent any movement of helicopters while evacuation by sea may take 48 h or more.

Drillings rigs and barges do not have spare quarters or reserve crew and, therefore, anyone sick or injured and unable to work for more than about 24 h must be sent ashore. Not only are such evacuations expensive, they may also be dangerous. When a sick man needs to be evacuated in bad weather conditions, the helicopter crew may well be endangering their own lives. At least one helicopter with all its crew, including a medical team, has been lost during a medical evacuation in the North Sea.

The medical policy concerning standards of fitness must, therefore, take account of these factors and no person should be allowed offshore with any detectable medical condition which could deteriorate or become complicated and require urgent medical intervention within 48 h. The policy must also take account of infectious or contagious diseases which could be a danger to others and of disabilities which may be a liability to the person affected or to others should an emergency arise which may be serious enough to require evacuation of the rig.

The examining doctor should be aware of the fact that the financial rewards of the offshore industry are so attractive that some potential employees will go to great lengths to conceal their disabilities. The examiner should take a very detailed medical, personal and occupational history and the examination itself should be no less thorough. Routine ancillary investigations are not necessary, though a chest X-ray is usually advisable and an audiometry will provide a permanent record of the employee's hearing, which is important as offshore structures may be noisy. Most companies will supply detailed forms for recording the results of the examination.

In some countries, Norway for example, the examinations are legally required and official forms must be completed by the examining doctor, who must also be approved by the Norwegian Health Directorate. In other countries, such as the U.K., there is, at present, no statutory requirement although it is accepted by the responsible Government agencies that such examinations are necessary and they have approved the medical standards of fitness which have been compiled by the industry. These standards are contained in the book *Recommended General Medical Standards of Fitness for Designated Offshore Employees* [6] published by the United Kingdom Offshore Operators Association (UKOOA) and obtainable from that organisation at 192 Sloane Street, London SW1X 9QX. It is suggested that any doctor called upon to examine an offshore employee should first consult this document. The standards have been compiled primarily to cover persons working in the North Sea but the principles embodied apply to offshore locations anywhere in the world. A more detailed discussion of offshore medical fitness can be found in *Offshore Medicine* [5].

Apart from their pre-placement examinations, offshore employees should be re-examined every 2 or 3 years to determine their continued fitness for offshore employment. In all cases where fitness for offshore work is confirmed, the employee should be furnished with a written statement to that effect. Many companies and some Government agencies will require this to be entered on an official document.

5.12.1 The Medics

The term "medic" deserves a little explanation. It is in common use throughout the offshore industry to describe the appointed person, irrespective of his qualifications, who is responsible for all medical and health matters. The term "nurse" does not adequately describe this more highly qualified status, while "paramedic" is usually applied to an American type of medical auxiliary whose functions are rather different. "Emergency medical technician" is too cumbersome and pretentious while the term "medic" has a friendly connotation about it and its exact meaning is clearly understood by all who work offshore.

The medic is the key to the provision of good offshore medical care. He will cope with the day-to-day minor complaints of the crew as well as being the source of skilled first aid and immediate primary care in the event of single or multiple major accidents. He must be able to examine a patient, accurately assess his clinical condition and convey his findings precisely and objectively to the supporting doctor on shore, under whose direction he will be working. He is, in short, the eyes and ears of the shore-based doctor, who depends entirely upon the medic for reaching his clinical decisions until he arrives on site himself.

Apart from their purely medical functions, the medics also have other duties, including maintaining all medical and first aid equipment on board, making regular hygiene inspections and writing reports, first aid training, participation in safety meetings and counselling, as well as various non-medical clerical duties.

Most offshore medics are registered nurses or equivalent or military sick berth attendants with additional training and experience. There is now an increasing tendency to employ only registered nurses (SRN in the U.K.), partly to ensure that they have the essential basic training and partly because the professional status conferred by such an official qualification confers medicolegal protection both on the medic and on the doctor from whom he is taking instructions. The responsibilities of a medic, and the difficulties of training and up-grading persons with lesser qualifications, are such that anyone lacking a full nursing qualification should be considered for employment only in the most exceptional circumstances.

Having acquired his or her basic nursing qualification, the potential medic will need several years post-qualification experience, especially in departments such as accident and emergency, ophthalmology, otolaryngology, dermatology and venereal diseases.

The technical skills he must acquire are the setting up of intravenous infusions, simple suturing, cardio-pulmonary resuscitation and endotracheal or oesophageal obturator intubation, gastric lavage and bladder catheterisation. He must also develop his diagnostic skills and have a good knowledge of therapeutics. Above all, he must have the necessary knowledge, skills and confidence to act independently and without direct supervision. At the same time he must be aware of his professional limitations.

In order that he can maintain all these attributes and skills he must regularly attend practical refresher courses at appropriate hospitals. Such courses last for about 4 weeks and should be repeated every 2 or 3 years. Only in this way will the medic be adequately prepared to cope with any medical emergency which may occur.

In order that the closest possible rapport can be established between the medics and the supporting doctors ashore, it is a great advantage if the latter can participate in the medics' training and refresher courses.

Though most offshore medics are male, there are now an increasing number of female nurses being employed and this is likely to rise in the future as more women in other jobs are employed offshore.

The medic can expect to perform about 6 new consultations per day for every 100 men on board, and, on average, about 3 people per 2000 are sent ashore daily for medical reasons.

Doctors are permanently stationed offshore in some operations where there may be more than 1500 people living. In these circumstances some operators claim that the additional cost of a doctor is balanced by the saving in the reduction of medical evacuations and lost working time. However, at the present time, doctors offshore are the exception rather than the rule.

5.12.2 Back-Up Services

All offshore operations are dependent upon shore-based medical services for support. This may be in the form of advice furnished to the medic by radio, the reception on shore of patients evacuated for medical reasons or the despatch of a doctor or specialised medical team to the offshore location in the event of a major incident.

In most areas ashore medical support is organised in two tiers; a primary care team usually consisting of local general practitioners, and a specialist team for major disasters.

It is necessary to have a doctor permanently on call so that he can give radio advice to the medics or can fly offshore immediately in an emergency. It is usually most convenient to equip the "on call" doctors with pocket radios, to keep them on call and avoid restricting their mobility. The members of the specialist team usually work full time in the local hospitals and so are readily obtainable by telephone. There is also less urgency in mobilising a specialist team.

Both the primary doctors and the specialist team must be properly equipped with all necessary drugs, dressings and equipment, as well as personal protective and survival clothing (dry immersion suits will be needed in all but tropical climates).

All members of the medical teams must be familiar with the offshore environment and each member must visit the offshore installations and understand the activities which go on there. They must appreciate the logistics of helicopter and supply ship operations and be fully familiar with all the channels of communication which they may need to use. They must also be fully trained and experienced in the technique of being winched from a helicopter as they will, not infrequently, find themselves called to casualties on vessels which have no helicopter landing facilities.

The frequency of calls to the doctors ashore is variable. It is highest during the exploratory phase of the operation and especially from rigs with new or inexperienced crews. It should be emphasised that any advice tendered to a medic, even by radio, may have serious medicolegal consequences, and careful notes of all such conversations should always be kept. Where possible all instructions should be confirmed by telex.

Specialist assistance from the shore will be essential when major disasters occur. The most likely causes of major disasters are blowout (the uncontrolled emission of gas or oil), fire, collisions or the foundering of a rig in a storm. In any of these events, total evacuation of the installation will be necessary and the number of people involved may vary from 20 to 300 or more with an equally variable number of casualties.

Plans for such a disaster must be carefully formulated in advance. The important features of such plans, which should be written into a manual, are as follows:

1. The provision of at least three primary care doctors who can be immediately mobilised to proceed to the site of the incident.
2. An adequate stock of drugs, dressings and equipment to be held on every offshore installation.
3. The designation of the nearest unaffected installation for the reception of casualties for triage.
4. The provision of adequate space on every installation for the performance of triage.
5. The organisation of a properly trained and equipped team of specialist doctors from shore hospitals who can be rapidly mobilised to fly to the rig.
6. The integration of the offshore disaster plan with other plans which may, or should, have been made for handling local disasters.
7. The local police, hospital and other emergency services must be fully incorporated into the offshore disaster plan.
8. Adequate and additional communication channels must be provided.
9. Administrative procedures for the proper documentation and accounting of casualties and survivors must be established.
10. A senior, knowledgeable and experienced industry doctor must be located in the disaster control room where he can advise the controllers on all medical matters and especially on priorities.
11. All major disaster procedures must be rehearsed from time to time.

A detailed description of the organisation required for the planning of major disasters appears in *Offshore Medicine* [5] and in the *Practitioner 1970* (Cox [1]).

5.12.3 Medical Facilities

Some sort of first aid room or hospital is necessary on all manned offshore structures irrespective of their location or distance from the shore. Any facility must be designed and equipped to accommodate patients for 48 h. It must also be sufficiently equipped not only for the normal complement of workers on the installation but also for the additional maintenance contractors and other workers who are frequently on board. It must be capable of acting as a designated reception place for survivors from any adjacent rig.

The size of the room will vary according to the size of the vessel or installation but, on most rigs, a room of about 18 m^2 is adequate. To comply with Norwegian regulations, the hospital, if a single room, must be 20 m^2. The hospital should be located with easy access to elevators and the helideck and close to a large room which, in a major emergency, can be quickly cleared of all furniture, to receive a large number of casualties for triage. A messroom, lounge or recreation room is often convenient. The hospital must have a sink with elbow-operated taps and an adjacent waterproof work surface of adequate size. It will also need a separate toilet, washbasin and shower and the bathroom should contain a standard bath for the immersion treatment of cases of hypothermia.

There should be at least two free-standing beds allowing access from all sides. Only on the very largest installations are more beds necessary. Bunks are not suitable. An examination couch and, preferably, a minor operating table will also be required. Good lighting with a shadowless light over the table is essential.

Plenty of storage space for stretchers, intravenous fluids, blankets, resuscitators, drugs, dressings and general equipment is required, along with lockable storage cabinets for medical records. A small refrigerator and a steriliser or autoclave should also be provided, and some form of incinerator for the disposal of dirty dressings is valuable.

It is essential that there should be a radio link extension in the hospital so that the medic can speak directly to the doctor on shore without leaving the patient. There must also be a call system between the hospital and the medic's cabin. It is not permissible for the medic to live and sleep in the hospital, in spite of current practices on some rigs.

A more detailed description of offshore medical facilities can be found in *Offshore Medicine* [5] and *Offshore Services and Technology* (Cox [2]).

Lists of suitable medical stores for offshore hospitals may be found in *Offshore Medicine* [5], *U.K. Statutory Instrument Number 1019* [4] and the Norwegian regulations regarding medical facilities on offshore installations [3].

5.12.4 Special Problems

Most of the medical problems associated with offshore drilling and production arise from the geographical isolation and the hostile environment in which the activities are conducted and trauma is the commonest reason for medical intervention. However, there are a few specific problems which should be mentioned:

5.12.4.1 Hydrogen Sulphide

This so-called sour gas may occur in varying concentrations but in some parts of the North Sea it may be as high as 500 parts per million (ppm). It may be encountered unexpectedly during drilling, when uncontrolled release of gas may occur. It may also occur in the stagnant water which accumulates in oil storage reservoirs, oil water separators and the legs of offshore platforms and semi-submersibles. Respirators must be worn whenever the concentration rises above 8 ppm.

5.12.4.2 Methane

Methane is the principal constituent of natural gas, of which it constitutes about 85% by volume. It is non-toxic but will cause asphyxia in high concentrations.

5.12.4.3 Methanol

Methyl alcohol is used in gas production to prevent the formation of hydrates which may freeze and obstruct the pipelines. For practical purposes it is only toxic if ingested and offshore workers can therefore be reassured that they will not be exposed to any risk during their normal handling of the material.

5.12.4.4 Ethylene Glycol

This is used to absorb water during gas production and, like methanol, is only toxic when ingested.

5.12.4.5 Drilling Mud

The chemically variable and complex material used to lubricate the drilling bit, remove rock fragments from the well and counteract the pressure of hydrocarbons by a hydrostatic counterpressure is known as mud. The dry constituents are compounded in the mud room and then mixed with water or oil before injection into the well. Common constituents of mud are bentonite (a clay from volcanic ash), barytes (barium sulphate), asbestos fibre, cellulose polymers, carboxymethyl cellulose, ligno-sulphonates, diatomaceous earth and various caustic materials.

If the operators do not handle drilling mud with care, wearing protective clothing all the time and respirators when appropriate, they may suffer serious effects on the skin, eyes and respiratory tract according to the particular constituents. Many dermatological and other problems occurring in offshore workers can be traced to contact with drilling mud.

5.12.4.6 Noise

Noise can be a serious problem, particularly on the older structures, causing insomnia, stress and, in some cases, hearing loss. The highest noise levels occur in compressor houses and pump rooms, where ear defenders must be worn, but there may be a high background noise level in the accommodation areas of some installations. In these circumstances, where it may cause stress and interfere with normal conversation, it may create a safety hazard by interfering with communication. With the greater realisation of the potential dangers of noise, steps have been taken to reduce it on modern installations and it is less of a problem than it used to be. Nevertheless, offshore structures will never be as quiet as most work-places on shore and there should be a hearing conservation programme in operation for all offshore workers.

5.12.4.7 Psychological Disturbances

When offshore exploration and production first began in the North Sea in the mid-1960s, psychological disturbances were common. Those most likely to suffer from this problem have now "selected themselves out" of the general pool of offshore workers. Nevertheless, it is a problem in new areas or when new, inexperienced crews are recruited. The offshore environment is an isolated, rough, tough world where the mental balance of any person who is not completely stable may well be disturbed. Conditions on many drilling rigs are far from comfortable, there is a lack of privacy and a mixed community of people very different socially and intellectually. There is constant noise and intense, arduous work interspersed with periods of great boredom. The people most likely to develop psychological symptoms, usually of anxiety or depression, are the more intelligent, professional types, such as engineers and geologists. Some may have a real fear of flying and the weekly helicopter ride may be a cause of severe stress. This has been particularly noticeable after helicopter crashes.

Occasionally a patient may develop an overt psychosis which can pose a difficult management problem. He must be sedated and confined until the arrival of a doctor who will then need to sedate him very heavily for the helicopter journey ashore.

5.12.4.8 Diving

The medical problems associated with diving also figure prominently in the practice of any doctor associated with the offshore industry but they are dealt with in another chapter of this book.

5.12.4.9 Summary

Offshore drilling for oil and gas is a heavy arduous job, usually conducted in a harsh and hostile environment. Proper medical support is an essential part of the operation but it imposes upon those who provide that support physical and professional challenges which they will not find in many other aspects of medical practice.

References

1. Cox, R. A. F.: An emergency plan for an offshore disaster. Practitioner *205*, 663–670 (1970).
2. Cox, R. A. F.: Offshore hospitals need better design and expert advice. Offshore Services and Technology, July 1982.
3. Norwegian Royal Decree of 25th November 1977, relating to hygiene, medical equipment and medicines, etc., on installations for production of submarine petroleum resources, etc. Oslo: Sosialdepartmentet 1977.
4. Offshore installations (Operational Safety, Health and Welfare) regulations 1976. London: H. M. S. O. 1976.
5. Offshore medicine. Ed.: R. A. F. Cox. Berlin, Heidelberg, New York: Springer 1982.
6. Recommended general medical standards of fitness for designated offshore employees. Ed.: UKOOA. London 1983.

Additional References

Medical aspects of North Sea oil (editorial). Brit. med. J. *3*, 576–580 (1975).

Offshore Medicine (editorial). Lancet *2:* 751 (1977).

Proctor, D. M.: Medicine and the North Sea – hospital support in offshore emergencies. J. Soc. occup. Med. *26*, 50–52 (1976).

Rawlins, J. S.: Medical problems in support of the offshore oil industry. Trans. med. Soc., London *94*, 25–32 (1977–1978).

Medical problems of oil development in Shetland (editorial). Scott. med. J. *20*, 146–147 (1975).

Shepherd, F. G. G.: Medicine and the North Sea – emergencies for the general practitioner. J. Soc. occup. Med. *26*, 50–52 (1976).

Training of offshore sick bay attendants (rig medics). Ed.: Health and Safety Executive. London: H. M. S. O. 1978. (H and S Exec. Guidance Note MS16).

Offshore construction health, safety and welfare guidelines. Ed.: Health and Safety Executive. London: H. M. S. O. 1980. (HS (G) 12).

Offshore installations' emergency procedures regulations. London: H. M. S. O. 1976. (S1 no. 1542).

Bustin, H. E.: Environmental health guidelines for offshore installations. Ed.: UKOOA. London 1980.

5.13 Underwater Medicine and Diving

A. Low

5.13.1 Introduction

Water covers approximately 70% of our planet's surface, and the oceans reach a maximal depth of 11.2 km. Water has always attracted man, be it through sailing, swimming or diving. With time, we have determined the physical properties of this liquid medium: the specific gravity is 1.0–1.03, the density is 1, the speed of sound in water is 1320 m/s, there is a vertical linear pressure increment of 1 atm/10 m, the thermal conductivity is approximately 24 times greater than that in dry still air of the same temperature, there is usually a non-linear vertical temperature decrease (distinct temperature strata occur), and there is optical disortion because the refraction index is different from that in air, i.e. objects appear nearer and larger than they really are. The absorption of light energy in water is 1000 times greater than in air so that only one quarter of our daylight reaches a depth of 5 m and one eighth a depth of 15 m. Colour is absorbed in a certain order – red first and blue last (see Table 1).

Table 1. Properties of water of interest for divers

Property	
Density	1 g/cm^3
Specific gravity	1.0–1.03
Refraction, air vs water	1:1.333
Compressibility	Non-compressible
Thermal conductivity	24 times that of air
Sound velocity	Approx. 1320 m/s
Pressure increase	Linear, 1 atm/10 m
Temperature range	– 1.9 °C to approx. + 30 °C
Vertical temperature drop	Non-linear
Light energy absorption	1000 times of that of air
Colour absorption	First red, then orange, yellow, green and blue
Transparency	Max. 60 m horizontally and 450 m vertically
Viscosity	1.8 cP (0 °C) to approx. 0.8 cP (30 °C)

The history of man's attempts to dive and to live underwater goes back countless centuries. Probably the first skin diving was undertaken in order to retrieve something of value that had fallen overboard and sunk. Certain drawings, paintings and friezes from ancient Greece, the Roman Empire and even Assyria show people preparing to dive and in the process of diving using primitive means. Table 2 gives a brief chronological review of the development of the art of diving from ancient to present times.

It is understandable that when the depths reached and the times spent underwater increased through the use of more sophisticated technology, new problems and ailments of the human body began to occur. Divers and caisson workers complained, for instance, of ear pains, headaches and pains in their joints. Gradually, physicians became more involved in these problems, investigating not only their causes but also suitable therapies and prophylaxes. Symptoms of decompression sickness (DCS) were first mentioned in 1841 [6] and two physicians started investigating them in 1854. Green, in 1861, mentioned nitrogen narcosis occurring at a depth of 50 m (Bennett and Elliott [2]). In

Table 2. Brief history of development of diving (Adapted from Bennett and Elliott [2]; [6])

Approx. date	Milestones, achievements or inventions
330 B.C.	Alexander goes underwater in a "diving bell"
1535	de Lorena develops first true "diving bell"
1620	von Driebel makes first submarine
1640s	von Treileben's primitive bell descends to 132 ft (40 m)
1690–91	Halley builds first modern diving bell, descends to 60 ft (18 m)
1715	1-atm diving suit made by Letheridge
1774	Freminet develops a helmet-hose-pump system and stays at 50 ft (15 m) depth for 1 h
1790	Smeaton's diving bell with air pump
1819	Siebe (London) rivets a copper helmet to a leather jacket and air hose
1837	Siebe makes a waterproof suit bolted to a breast-plate and helmet with valves and air-exhaust valves
1879	Fluess develops first scuba with oxygen
1913, 1920	1-atm diving suits
1926	Le Prieur patents a scuba
1930	First use of swim fins
1933	1-atm diving suit
1943	Cousteau/Gagnan introduce their aqualung (demand regulator)
1945	Browne makes a lightweight triangular diving mask for descents of up to 90–100 ft (27–30 m)
1962	First underwater saturation diving habitats
1972	Development of a 1-atm armoured suit "Jim" usable to a max. depth of 1 000 ft (300 m) (31 atm)

1878 Bert, a pioneer high-pressure researcher, proved that gas bubbles appeared during quick decompressions and found oxygen to be toxic at elevated pressures ($pO_2 > 2$ atm). Haldane developed his now famous decompression tables for compressed air work in about 1908 and End dived to a depth of 420 ft (127 m) breathing a helium/oxygen mixture in 1937. 1945 saw the release of new US Navy decompression tables that were soon to be used worldwide [20]. And finally, the medical principles of saturation diving were investigated between the mid-1950s and 1962, opening new horizons for long sojourns, i.e. days or weeks, under pressure on the seabed ([20]; Ruff et al. [24]).

Historic milestones in the conquest of the deep are thus of a medical as well as of a technical nature, the foremost of these being in the author's opinion Haldane's decompression tables (1908) and Cousteau/Gagnan's aqualung (1943). They have made diving on a worldwide scale possible.

5.13.2 Diving

5.13.2.1 Means and Methods of Diving

In principle, there are four means of diving from which all others have evolved: skin diving with no aids; diving with a mask, snorkel and fins; scuba (= *s*elf-*c*ontained *u*nderwater *b*reathing *a*pparatus) diving; and finally, caisson/bell diving. Several methods of diving exist and are used/applied according to the work, task, estimated duration etc. underwater. The most frequent method is diving from the surface with and without scuba gear. The next most frequent methods are partial saturation diving from the surface in a bell and saturation diving, e.g. from underwater habitats, with or without excursion dives to greater depths. Finally, in recent years, mini-submarines with 1-atm internal pressure or pressurisable to the ambient pressure and 1-atm armoured diving suits have been used increasingly.

Diving is performed by many hundreds of thousands of people, by many governmental agencies and also by the military for a great variety of reasons, but basically diving can be subdivided into sports-recreational-leisure diving, professional diving and scientific/research diving, in that order of frequency (Table 3). Sports diving can take place in inland waterways, i.e. rivers and lakes, and also along the coastlines of seas and oceans. Professional divers in

Table 3. Classification of diving and maximal depths

Personnel	Type of diving	Max. depths
Civilian	Sports/recreational	< 60 m
	Commercial/professional	< 450 m+
	Scientific/research	≦1600 m+
Government	Fire brigade, police, life-saving/rescue groups etc.	< 60 m
Military	Navy, army, air force and military research (research and development = R & D)	≦2000 m+

small and large diving companies (national and international) perform a multitude of sophisticated jobs in predominantly dangerous environments in rivers, harbours, lakes and in ever increasing numbers in our seas and oceans, especially in the offshore oil and gas industries with their drilling rigs, submarine pipelines and seabed installations (Low [18]).

5.13.2.2 Types of Underwater Work

At least 25 different skills are demanded of the professional diver, for example, salvaging, demolition, inspection and repair, underwater construction, welding, cutting and rivetting, maintenance, search and rescue, underwater surveying and mapping, photography, plumbing, archeology, derusting and preserving of ship hulls and underwater structures, and bomb and mine raising and/or deactivating. This list is by no means complete.

5.13.2.3 Diving Equipment

Within the last 3 decades, a great variety of makes, types and models of diving equipment have appeared on the market. The minimal gear necessary for skin diving is a mask, snorkel and fins. Masks can be bought integrated with one or two snorkels (dangerous!) and covering eyes, nose and mouth; so-called full-face masks or, more commonly, mask and snorkel are acquired as separate items. In this case, the mask only covers the eyes and nose. In scuba diving, further equipment is required: one or two compressed air cylinders (often called "tanks"), each of 7–12 litres and pressurisable to 200–300 atm (2940–4410 psi). The cylinders are attached to a back-harness and a lung-demand regulator (aqualung) with one or two hoses leading to a mouthpiece through which air is breathed automatically adjusted to the same pressure as the surrounding depth of water. A belt with lead weights and a quick-release buckle is needed to compensate for the lift of the cylinders and thus reduce the muscular energy otherwise necessary to counteract the undesired lift. A diver's knife is a vital requirement in case of entanglement; also important are a water- and pressureproof watch and a depth meter (see 5.13.5: Decompression).

Normally, scuba gear works as an open-circuit system, in which exhaled air is not reprocessed but passes on into the water as large bubbles. The equipment can, however, be designed as semiclosed and as closed-circuit systems. Semiclosed means that exhaled air passes through a CO_2 scrubber (baralime), which eliminates metabolic CO_2. Oxygen either alone or with N_2 is automatically or manually added as required to make up for the loss, and any excessive pressure build-up in the breathing bag is vented into the water. In a closed-circuit system, no gas is vented at all (Haux [13]). Instead of carrying all their compressed air equipment on their backs, many professional divers are linked by air-supply hoses to the surface in predominantly open systems having only a small emergency compressed air cylinder with them, should surface airflow suddenly stop.

To enable safe deep diving beyond a depth of 50 m, i.e. without N_2 narcosis, mixed-gas diving systems have been developed. In these, the diver breathes He/O_2 or $He/N_2/O_2$ in predetermined mixture ratios depending on his working depth. In principle, these systems are basically the same as the above-mentioned compressed air gear – open, semiclosed or closed circuit. Owing to the increasing price of helium, great efforts are at present being made to re-use the exhaled He. Thus, most interest is in closed-circuit systems. Due to the great depths (50–500 m) involved in offshore diving, the majority of mixed-gas diving is done via a hose connection between the surface gas supply/reprocessing unit and the diver far below, either directly or using the diving bell as an intermediate (Haux [13]).

Oxygen diving equipment consists of a closed-circuit breathing system and it has been in use for many years by the military. Because of the danger of O_2 poisoning (100% O_2), it is only permitted for depths no greater than 8–10 m and its use requires extensive special training. Oxygen diving gear is not obtainable on the commercial market.

5.13.2.4 Diving Suits

With depth, water temperatures become progressively colder. It is obvious that man has to be protected against cold and general hypothermia. During the last 2 centuries, five types of diving suits (Table 2) have been designed and further developed to high standards – wet (neoprene) suits, dry vulcanised rubber constant volume suits, dry foam suits, helmet diving suit combinations (copper or plastic) and 1-atm armoured suits. Depending on the design, they protect against cold, marine plants/animals, injuries, environmental poisons and contamination (e.g. radio-active or toxic/allergic substances), and against the surrounding hydrostatic pressure (e.g. 1-atm armoured suits).

5.13.2.5 Logistics/Surface Support

In commercial diving, especially when conducted in the open seas at depths beyond 50 m, complex surface support facilities on the shore, on oil rigs and on special diving mother ships or tenders are mandatory. Depending on the working depth, planned overall working time, gas mixtures and whether partial saturation or saturation techniques (see 5.13.5) are used, the composition of the logistic system can vary. Basically, it consists of: cranes for raising and lowering the diving bells, personnel transfer chambers (PTCs), deck transfer chambers (DTCs), deck decompression chambers (DDCs), portable DDC, mixed-gas supply, monitors for the divers' breathing gas and for the DDC, He-recycling equipment, a diving supervisor, reserve divers and a paramedic qualified in diving medicine. All chambers and PTCs should be able to interlock hermetically with each other to ensure no pressure drop when divers are transferred, for instance, from the PTC into the DTC at say 16 atm (Bennett and Elliott [2]).

5.13.2.6 Pathways to the Deep

As mentioned earlier, several methods are at hand to enable divers to reach the depths necessary for their underwater work. The choice depends on various factors, e.g. water temperature, currents, visibility, pressure/depths and estimated duration of the job. These methods are: free descent with scuba, hose or mixed gas; descent in a 1-atm bell (PTC) with external manipulators; descent in a pressurised bell (PTC) with opening of hatch at depth and exit of hose-connected diver; and descent in work/mini-submarines without or with lock-out capabilities, the latter enabling divers to leave the submarine via a built-in pressure chamber with an airlock.

In theory, access to stationary habitats on the seabed is possible with all four methods. Regulations, however, only permit compressed air diving to a maximum depth of 50–60 m. Therefore all offshore diving, down to the greatest current operational depth of 450 m or 46 atm (by the Comex Company in 1977), is done with He/O_2 or $He/N_2/O_2$.

5.13.2.7 Working in the Deep

Once at his place of work, either at some predetermined level, e.g. for inspection of a ship's hull, or on the seabed, the compressed-air diver works for up to several hours, in part depending on his depth and the decompression table (see 5.13.5.2) he plans using; he is then hoisted to the surface or ascends himself after giving a prearranged signal on his safety line or by phone to the surface. The mixed-gas diver, being far deeper, works up to approximately 100 m from the diving bell, either at the same depth, slightly above or at a maximum of 50 m below it, and is connected to it by a gas supply and heating hose, a phone cable and a safety line, i.e. the "umbilical". For reasons given below (see 5.13.5.2), upon completion of his task the bell diver returns to the bell, closes the hatch and is hoisted to the surface while the same pressure is maintained within the bell as at the site of work. It is then connected to a DDC and decompression begins (Haux [13]). Divers or aquanauts working from underwater habitats adhere, in principle, to the same rules as bell divers except that they live at the bottom of the sea for days or weeks [20].

Caisson workers differ from divers insofar as they work in a dry and not in a wet hyperbaric environment at a maximum depth of 30 m (4 atm), have a 6-h working day under pressure and return to the surface dry, usually decompressing in a chamber at the top. A caisson is used for underwater bridge support construction, for the building of underwater tunnels and even for the archeological retrieval of sunken ships (Wünsche and Scheele [27]).

5.13.3 The Diver

5.13.3.1 Skin and Sports Diver

Skin and sports divers come from every age group from children to the elderly. As there are no compulsory laws for pre-dive medical check-ups in most countries, these people can be found in all states of health, even with such ailments that would automatically ban them from diving from a doctor's point of view. They also range from extremely lean to grossly obese individuals.

5.13.3.2 Professional Divers

Within the category of professional divers, the picture is a different and more favourable one. Their ages lie between 20 and 45 years in general and retirement from active diving is usually around 55 years at the latest. Their personality structure is such that many tend to be loners and experts responsible to and trusting primarily only themselves. Their motivation to work in harsh environments can be regarded as high, knowing that work at depth can be both mentally and physically extremely demanding (Low [18]).

The health status of these several thousand professional divers is on average good to very good, especially in those performing mixed-gas and saturation diving. This is because the offshore industry, for example, employing 2000–2500 divers worldwide, performs a thorough medical check of these men as disablement during an underwater deep sea mission would be very expensive for the oil company. Professional divers often have an athletic build and are not too tall. Their jobs are mainly manual and it is usually essential that they have learned a craft before commencing diving training.

Most of the highly developed countries have special training schools for civilian professional divers encompassing 1- to 6-month courses in normal and even advanced diving techniques, e.g. in Aberdeen. Germany, unfortunately, has no facilities of this type. Professional divers are usually very well paid. Their salaries vary according to the depth, duration of dive and inherent dangers at particular locations. An example of the dangerous tasks that are performed is diving in the cooling system of an atomic reactor to repair a defective valve.

5.13.3.3 Diver Health Certificate

It is obvious from the above that prerequisites for safe diving are or should be good health, average weight, stable personality, physical strength, good work-load tolerance and the ability to work independently and calmly in extreme situations. Since different types of diving (skin diving, scuba, diving bell, caisson etc.) involve different particular stresses, several types of diving health certificates (DHCs) are used by doctors. A sports diver, for instance, does not encounter the same dangerous deep-sea environments that bell divers do, and caisson workers stay in dry hyperbaric surroundings. Thus, DHCs have been modified (with time). Bell divers going to extreme depths as well as saturation divers must, understandably, comply with the most stringent medical health standards (Ehm and Seemann [7]; [20]).

Definition

A DHC is a document from a qualified doctor, preferably with a knowledge of diving medicine, stating that a certain person is medically fit or healthy enough to pursue a particular type of diving. It is also an important document in the event of a diving accident to prove that a diver had no ailment that could have led to the accident or injury and thus will entitle him to health/accident insurance benefits. Diver health certificates are issued with a 1-, 2-, or 3-year validity period. In sports diving, DHCs are often valid for 3 years up to the age of 40 years and must then be renewed annually. In offshore, bell, saturation and scientific diving, it is becoming more usual for annual diving medical check-ups to be demanded, independent of the diver's age. For these extreme forms of diving, X-ray pictures of the large joints taken at regular intervals are compulsory so that any aseptic bone necrosis may be detected early (Harvey [12]; McCallum et al. [19]). Should a diver become ill or have an operation or accident within the period of the DHC validity, he is required to see his doctor and if need be go through a new medical check-up prior to commencing diving again.

Table 4. Some current diving health certificates and standards

Name	Required for
Physical Standards for Scuba Divers (USA)	Sport scuba divers (approved by Undersea Medical Society)
CMAS[1] (Europe)	Sport scuba divers
NOAA[2] (USA)	Research divers, aquanauts
Taucherarbeiten VBG 39 (Federal Republic of Germany)	Commercial divers, research divers, aquanauts

[1] Commission Mondiale des Activités Sous-marines
[2] National Oceanic and Atmospheric Administration

Unfortunately, DHCs are not yet standardised internationally, although efforts are being made in this direction. Therefore, many countries have their own DHCs. Military divers, of course, adhere to specific health regulations. Table 4 lists a few current DHCs and standards.

When Is a Diver Unfit for Diving?

A doctor examining divers should be well-acquainted with underwater conditions to understand why a number of ailments, diseases and physical abnormalities, either inherited or acquired, bar a person permanently or temporarily from diving. The most important of these are: obesity and underweight; intestinal hernias (due to the possible danger of incarceration); diabetes; hyper- and hypotension; coronary and lung diseases; tendency to spontaneous pneumothorax; epilepsy; disturbances of equilibrium; nervous and vegetative disorders; stomach, liver and spleen disorders; history of kidney colic; and eye and ear, nose, and throat (ENT) diseases, especially perforated eardrums and otitis media and externa (Ehm and Seemann [7]; Linaweaver [17]; [20]). A physician must realise that he takes on a great responsibility when asked to issue a DHC and should weigh the pros and cons objectively.

5.13.4 Diving Medicine

5.13.4.1 Definition

Diving medicine, also known as underwater and/or hyperbaric medicine, investigates, researches and treats medical problems associated with man diving below the surface of the water. It differs from traditional medicine in several fundamental aspects since a number of physiological parameters taken for granted at sea level, i.e. at a pressure of 1 atm, change to other values according to depth and the time spent at depth. Courses on diving medicine for doctors are given at certain universities and by the navies of various countries.

5.13.4.2 Scope of Diving Medicine

The theoretical and practical curriculum of diving medicine encompasses many medical, chemical and physical fields, such as: inert gas physiology – N_2, He, Ar, Ne, Xe, N_2 narcosis; gas toxicity – CO, CO_2, O_2, N_2; hyperbaric physiology and its effects on the body, e.g. positive- and negative-pressure barotraumas of the sinuses and lungs, the high-pressure nervous syndrome (HPNS); hyperbaric biochemistry; ENT problems, surgery and internal medicine; effects on and efficiency of drugs administered at high pressures; neurological alterations of the CNS associated with depth (EEG), psychomotor changes; and decompression and therapeutic recompression techniques.

Occupational medicine, an accepted special discipline on land, is also a necessity underwater with factors and complications like work-load, hypothermia, currents, hyperventilation, panic, equipment failure, entanglement and injuries affecting divers to be taken into account and dealt with. A knowledge of orthopaedics is desired as decompression sickness (DCS) can lead to aseptic bone necrosis with damage to the large joints, for instance, hip, shoulder or knee joints. Finally, diving medicine deals with chronic ailments of disabled or prematurely pensioned former divers, such as deformed major joints, arthrosis, accelerated decline in hearing (often caused by incorrect pressure equalisation in the middle ear over a period of many years), mental decay and sequelae of thorax squeeze (Bennett and Elliott [2]; [6]).

5.13.4.3 Necessity of Diving Medicine

Now the reader will begin to understand why more and more emphasis is being put on diving medicine worldwide. Diving medicine is becoming an integrated part of diving in sport. In non-professional diving, underwater-medical doctors have worked with scientific and research projects for many years, whereas in commercial diving this has become so primarily since the advent of offshore diving. Divers employed by government agencies – in fire brigades, police departments, life-saving and rescue groups etc. – usually contact specialists in hyperbaric medicine only for DHC renewals. In the military services, doctors specialised in diving medicine are assigned to navy, army and air force units, though primarily to the navy, and are also employed in research and development institutes.

5.13.4.4 General Tasks of Physicians in Diving Medicine

These tasks may be summarised as follows: DHC examinations and renewals; supervision of diving excursions; experiments on land (in high-pressure chambers) and at sea; acting as consultant to divers and diving companies; development of prophylactic measures and of alarm and rescue plans for diving missions; providing hyperbaric first-aid training; treatment of diving casualties on the surface and underwater; and theoretical and practical diving medical research.

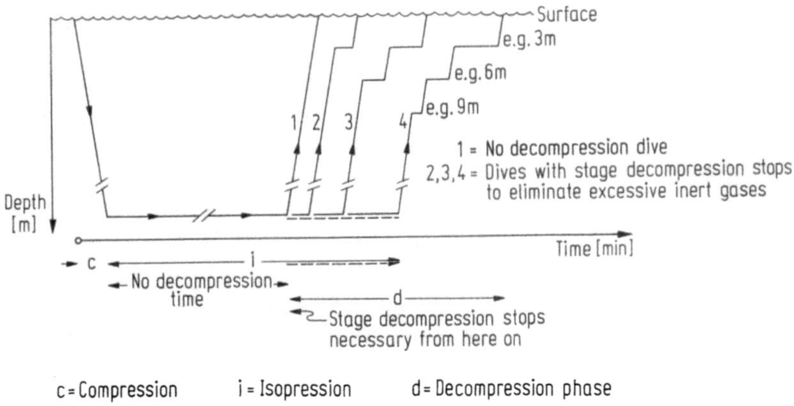

Fig. 1. Basic diving and decompression profiles (depth and time dependent).

5.13.5 Living and Working Underwater

From a medical point of view, every dive consists of three phases: compression, isopression and decompression. Each phase affects the body physiologically in different ways. These must be understood to avoid dangers and injuries (Fig. 1).

Compression. Increase in external pressure leads to barotraumas of the rigid air-filled sinuses, the middle ear, teeth with incorrect fillings and the thorax if pressures are not or cannot be equalised. This causes increasing pain, blood pooling, haemorrhages and burst blood vessels and, in the chest, can lead to lung oedema, heart dilatation and death (negative barotrauma or "squeeze"). Compression can cause N_2 narcosis (>40 m), He tremor, HPNS (> 200 m) and O_2 toxicity (>2–3 atm O_2) (Bennett and Elliott [2]).

Isopression. This term means that the external or ambient pressure stays constant, i.e. the working depth has been reached. Immediate factors confronting the diver are high pressure, darkness, cold water and currents. As time goes on, hypothermia can gradually commence, lowering the core temperature. More and more compressed gas (air or He/O_2) goes into solution in all the various body tissues, which become saturated either rapidly (pressure equilibrium) or more slowly, depending on their perfusion and diffusion rates and their gas-storage capacities (so-called short or long half-time values), hence the expressions partial saturation and saturation. For example, the saturation time for nitrogen in human tissues is approximately 100 h. If pO_2 is higher than 0.5 atm for several days, O_2 intoxication of the lungs along with a drop in vital capacity and possibly pneumonia will occur. If the pO_2 rises above 2 atm, twitching, neurological symptoms, cerebral seizures and eventually death will take place (Rister and Baehner [22]).

Decompression. This refers to external pressure reduction or ascent. If the air-filled sinus passages become blocked, e.g. by mucus or because of a sore throat, excessive pressures cannot escape and will cause a positive barotrauma with increasing pain the higher a person ascends. Should a laryngospasm inhibit the exhaling of air, the lungs will overinflate and finally tear, causing gas embolism and/or pneumothorax with gas bubbles reaching the heart, viscera and cerebrum. Death can occur quickly if gas emboli reach the vital cerebral centres. Unequal pressure decrement in the middle ear causes alternobaric vertigo, and a sudden loss of hearing has been noted in divers coming up from great depths (Roydhouse [23]). Depending on the depth and time spent underwater, a diver must give his body ample time to eliminate the hyperbarically dissolved N_2 or He in his tissues by making several exactly predetermined stops on the way up (decompression tables). If he fails to do so and ascends too fast, he will suffer from decompression sickness (DCS), either mildly or severely, and can even die. Decompression sickness can occur as tingling, joint and extremity pains, chokes and CNS symptoms. It is important that an incorrect or missed decompression be immediately treated by recompression in a DDC at the surface with ensuing decompression to avoid possible DCS. Hypothermia can affect gas elimination speed and necessitate longer decompression schedules (Fig. 1).

Underwater, a diver perceives a reduction in weight or even weightlessness; there is an increase in the speed of sound but a person is incapable of pinpointing its source. Falling objects have a decreased velocity, the diver's breathing gas mixture has an increased density and the boiling point of water is higher.

5.13.5.1 The Effects on Humans

Greater gas densities and viscosities lead to a change in the pitch of the human voice and in the intelligibility of the spoken word, to alterations in the senses of taste and smell, to different grades of subtle euphoria and to a slower pace of work than expected. This has especially been noted in underwater habitats (Goeters [10]; Ruff et al. [24]).

The adaptation time for the body to adjust to hyperbaric conditions, e. g. for aquanauts in underwater habitats, is dependent on the depth and gas mixture and can take 1–3 days. The mental drive is slower under hyperbaric conditions and a shift in the ambient comfort temperature zone towards higher temperatures, $\lesssim 35\,°C$, occurs as a result of the greater thermal conductivity of helium (Low [18]). The increased relative humidity (60%–95%) leads to a softening of the skin, making it more susceptible to mycosis and injuries, and accelerates a shift from Gram-positive to Gram-negative bacteria in the external auditory canal and on the body's surface (Alcock [1]).

Hypothermia can make a diver more prone to colds and infections, decrease his manual dexterity and reduce his mental capabilities. High pressure seems to reduce or augment the effects of medicines depending on which drug is given. However, as yet, little is known about the latter. The raising of the boiling point of water from 100 °C to 120 °C and even higher, under hyperbaric conditions has, for instance, accidentally led to internal and external scalds and burns.

5.13.5.2 Working from Diving Bells, from Underwater Habitats and in Caissons

Divers working underwater have to cope with some or all of the seven major problems common to such conditions – depth (i. e. hydrostatic pressure), strong currents, semi or total darkness, time, hypothermia, dangerous and painful external ear infections, and accidents. Most of these can, if protective measures are not taken, easily reduce the efficiency and performance of divers in the aqueous environment and rapidly endanger their lives. These problems, together with the difficulties they may bring about, are listed in Table 5. As can be seen, most of these difficulties are of a medical nature.

In addition to leading to *hypothermia*, diving at depth can cause several disorders, such as HPNS, N_2 narcosis, toxic oxygen effects on the lungs and CNS, and DCS.

It is erroneous to assume that in most places in which professional divers work the water is clear. On the contrary, in almost all rivers and estuaries the *visibility* is zero on or not far below the water surface. In the North Sea, usually hardly anything is discernible below 30 m. Visibility can be greatly impaired by plankton and sus-

Table 5. Major problems for divers and possible difficulties and dangers

Major problems	Possible difficulties
Depth/pressure	Positive and negative barotraumas, N_2 narcosis, impaired pulmonary function, HPNS, increased diuresis, DCS
Darkness	Disorientation, entanglement, panic, death
Currents	Increased work-load, decline in performance, faster fatigue, entanglement, disorientation
Time	Hypothermia, decline in performance, more gas goes into solution→partial or full saturation, DCS
Hypothermia/ cold	Increased metabolism, increased diuresis, decrease in dexterity, performance and efficiency, rapid cooling through helium breathing, DCS, euphoria, drowning, death
Otitis externa	Contagious, rapidly worsening ear pain, reduced ability or inability to dive, early termination of underwater missions (high expenses)
Underwater accidents	Injuries, unconsciousness, drowning, death

pended microdebris. Divers must, therefore, depend to a great extent on their sense of touch. Deep-sea divers are connected to the bell or habitat by air-hose and telephone cable, which are a means of finding the way back should danger arise. Owing to the possibly fatal risk of DCS, the endangered diver must first of all always try to reach the bell/habitat and not ascend to the surface.

At rest, O_2 uptake is approximately 0.5 litres/min. It rises to 1.2–3.5 litres/min. for divers wearing heavy lead boots. When swimming against strong *underwater currents* with fins, O_2 uptake increases to between 2.5 and 4 litres/min. Metabolism is accelerated greatly and glycogen stores are depleted faster, in addition to an earlier onset of hypothermia. Work-loads increase several fold, fatigue sets in and performance declines. Current velocities of up to 2 m/s and more are commonplace underwater in rivers and in the sea (Ruff et al. [24]).

The total *time* spent underwater is an important medical factor in diving. The longer the time underwater, the greater the amount of inert gas, N_2 or He, that is absorbed by the aqueous and fatty tissues of the body. N_2 is absorbed by fat and water in a 5:1 ratio, whereas the ratio for He is 1.2:1. Therefore, the longer a diver remains at depth, the more inert gas is dissolved in his body (partial saturation, then saturation) and so decompression becomes lengthier, hours or days, in order that these excessive quantities of gas can be slowly exhaled via the lungs without harming the diver. Failure to adhere to the decompression rules can or will lead to severe DCS with multiple micro and macro gas emboli, often combined with hemi-, para- or tetraplegia and perhaps immediate death. Time is also a factor contributing to hypothermia and decreased performance [6].

Cold, or *hypothermia,* is one of the most detrimental factors influencing human efficiency underwater. Hypothermia depends on the depth, length of dive, water temperature, thickness and material of suit, and the breathing gas mixture, i.e. its helium content. The pressure increase with depth compresses the diver's suit, reducing its thickness and thus its insulating properties. Water has approximately 25 times the thermal conductivity of dry still air of the same temperature and 1000 times its specific heat. These factors together with the observation that hypothermia is accelerated in correlation with the volume percentage of He in the breathing mixture (through its having five to six times the thermal conductivity of air) make a cooling of the diver via the skin surface and the respiratory tract likely if no protective measures are taken. Below a certain depth, heat loss through the airways becomes greater than increased metabolism is able to cope with. Thus, the diver's core temperature will inevitably begin to drop. As it does so, O_2 uptake and metabolic rate increase, while manual dexterity deteriorates and with it job efficiency and performance. Cold-induced diuresis leads to a voiding of latent heat stores; mental sluggishness and euphoria can finally occur and drowning becomes very probable (Hanson [11]). Two methods of avoiding or at least minimising hypothermia in deep diving conditions have been utilised with good results: (a) heating the wet (Neoprene) or dry diving suit, either electrically or by conducting hot water (40 °C) from the surface to the diver via a hose and thence through underwear of an interwoven plastic tube design; (b) preheating the breathing gas mixture in accordance with the underwater work-load and depth, and carefully monitoring it from the surface (< 45 °C gas temperature).

Otitis externa in divers is usually caused by *Proteus vulgaris, Pseudomonas aeruginosa* and *Staphylococcus aureus* either singly or in combination. The ear becomes very tender and painful, and a watery to thick greenish-yellow pus is found in the auditory canal. Outer ear infections are encountered much more frequently in deep-sea saturation diving, in which the divers remain under pressure for days or weeks, than in short duration shallow-water diving or sports diving. In diving teams living and working together in hyperbaric environments (increased pO_2, relative humidity and temperature), otitis externa can be very contagious and if prophylactic measures (see 5.13.7) are not strictly adhered to, most of the divers will be incapacitated and unable to dive for a few days. Doctors in diving medicine and hygienists have been working on this problem for many years (Alcock [1]; Jones and Davis [14]).

With regard to underwater accidents, the reader is referred to the section 5.13.6.

5.13.5.3 Supervision of Divers Underwater

Sports and commercial divers are taught the importance of diving supervision and of keeping a watch on their diving companion(s) as the underwater world is a hostile environment for the human being and a dangerous situation can develop very quickly. For this reason, sports divers should never dive alone. Before commencing a dive, the proposed duration, depth and location should be told to the surface personnel and recorded. Monitoring of the divers can take place either from the surface or underwater or both:

1. From the surface, by diving supervisor, reserve diver, signalman, diving paramedic or diving doctor.
2. Underwater, by a diving companion visually and/or connected by "buddy-line" (wrist to wrist) or by a second diver in a bell, habitat or minisubmarine.
3. Combined, by a diver in a bell, habitat or minisubmarine, who can also be and usually is in contact with surface control.

Several technical means are at our disposal to improve communication with the diver. The oldest and most frequently used method is a signal line attached to the diver's waist along which messages can be passed. Underwater telephones built into the diver's helmet and running to the surface in waterproof cables have been in use for decades. This telephone link can also be between diver and bell, bell and surface etc. Underwater ultrasonic communication is a relatively new development, liberating divers from cables which can hamper their movements. Underwater television cameras can also be mounted in bells and habitats and even be carried by divers, the corresponding monitor screens being installed where appropriate.

The problem of monitoring physiological parameters under high pressure has led to the development of new systems and sensors (Oser and Wegmann [21]). Heart frequency, breathing, EEG, ECG, core temperature etc. can be monitored and registered in open-sea dives and in simulated hyperbaric chamber dives to depths of approximately 2000 m (201 atm) (Bennett and Elliott [2]; Walsh [26]). Breathing and breathing frequency are indirectly monitored via the telephone affixed to the diver's helmet, which is constantly kept switched on in the one-way direction from diver to surface or to bell. Thus, it is possible to discern whether the diver is breathing regularly, hyperventilating (e.g. due to excessive work-load, rise in CO_2 or panic) or not breathing at all. It is impractical to monitor physiological parameters in commercial deep diving, however, as the support team on the surface usually does not have the medical experience to be able to analyse immediately abnormal ECG or EEG curves and to take the appropriate first-aid or rescue measures.

Voice distortion through He in deep diving has often led to support teams not being able to understand what the diver below is saying. This can be tragic if the diver is in great danger, ill or injured and urgently needs help. A variety of He unscramblers have been developed in several countries, e.g. USA, France and Germany, in an effort to solve this problem. Current models now provide an intelligibility level of 80%–90%, thus giving deep divers greater psychological assurance while on the seabed.

5.13.6 Accidents, Sickness Underwater and Rescue

5.13.6.1 Accidents

Accidents are caused by a number of factors, each in itself usually not dangerous, interacting with one another and sometimes leading to disastrous or fatal results, especially when occurring underwater. Prime factors influencing accidents are sea and weather conditions, individual skills, training standards, health status and technical and equipment malfunctions.

Sports Diving

Accidents and injuries can happen on the water surface owing to strong currents, bad weather or rough surf regions, underestimation of one's strength and overexertion. Incorrect swimming and diving techniques in the surf zone may lead to difficulties and give rise to panic. Nausea with vomiting caused by waves can incapacitate a swimmer or diver down to about a depth of 5 m. Hyperventilation, a technique often used by snorkel divers to remain longer underwater or to dive a greater horizontal distance, has caused numerous cases of unconsciousness (drop in arterial pO_2) and death upon ascending, usually just below the surface. The majority of sports diving accidents occur at weekends and frequently in areas where immediate first aid and a recompression chamber are not available. Swimming and diving after meals and consumption of alcohol have caused death in healthy individuals, alcohol raising the N_2 narcosis level to a depth of approximately 10 m in extreme cases (Bennett [3]).

Medicines taken for various reasons by divers, e.g. tranquillisers, analgesics and anti-emetics, may have side-effects such as drowsiness or decrease in concentration and perceptive faculties, which, acting together with increased pressure, can greatly endanger divers. Ear barotraumas can occur during descent through incorrect pressure equalising in the middle ear (Valsalva manoeuvre) and on ascending; the latter causes alternobaric vertigo with nausea. In sports diving, the increasing number of cases of DCS – comprising "niggles", bends, chokes, spinal cord lesions or CNS symptoms – as well as cases of gas embolism through overextended or burst lungs are causing concern (see 5.13.5: Decompression). An important rule in diving is "never dive alone", i.e. the "buddy" system. This functions well if both parties trust each other and have had the same training. If not, mistakes with grave consequences can occur.

Professional Diving

Here, the scope of underwater activities is different and thus the spectrum of possible accidents and injuries changes. Injuries, for example, through blasts, welding accidents, suction devices, explosions and entanglement, occur in addition to those through equipment malfunction at depth or in surface support facilities. An example may illustrate the dangers involved: In January 1976, two divers had been working for 1 h at the bottom of the North Sea at a depth of 78 m, one inside and one outside a diving bell. The latter returned to the bell but before he could close the hatch, the ground-weight of the bell detached itself. The bell shot to the surface in 42 s, rapidly losing interior pressure. One of the divers died immediately through a massive lung overpressure trauma, whereas the other, deeply unconscious, was recompressed to a pressure level of 81 m in a very short time and survived (Frankel [9]). The training standards of professional divers also affect accident probability, bearing in mind the extremely hostile surroundings they often have to work in (Biersner et al. [4]).

5.13.6.2 Rescue

When a diver is injured or otherwise incapacitated underwater, the obvious reaction is to bring him out of the hostile environment and to the surface as fast as possible. Yet what seems simple on land may often be difficult in diving. For example, it is usually easier to bring a disabled diver up from shallow depths – unless he is trapped – than from greater ones without additionally endangering him.

In shallow waters, rescue should, in principle, be: Dive to the casualty, free the airways, administer compressed air (if necessary), release the weight belt, inflate the buoyancy collar (or personal flotation device) and ascend to the surface with the casualty, checking that he exhales on the way up to avoid a possible and often lethal lung overextension. Continue cardiopulmonary resuscitation on the surface if necessary and treat any wounds. Determine whether DCS symptoms are present, transfer to the next decompression chamber, preferably in a recumbent position, either by road or in a very low-flying airplane (< 300 m) and recompress the patient in accordance with the therapeutic tables [20].

Deep-water rescue raises more problems due to the increased pressure and the greater amount of dissolved inert gas in the diver's body tissues. If an accident occurs at a depth of say 200 m, the diver in the bell must notify surface control at once and then go out and try to retrieve the injured diver, bring him through the 60- to 80-cm circular entrance hatch into the bell, close the hatch and, while remaining at working depth pressure, be hoisted to the surface, giving cardiopulmonary resuscitation if necessary (Fisher [8]). Topside, the bell is connected to a large DDC in which first aid can be given by diver paramedics as the DDC is slowly (hours or days) decompressed to 1 atm. If a rapid ascent without slow decompression were to be made, e.g. in panic, death would follow within minutes. Sending a paramedic down to a disabled deep-sea diver (depth > 150 m) is theoretically possible but impractible because he would have to be compressed slowly in order to maintain his mental capabilities and avoid the HPNS (Fisher [8]).

5.13.6.3 Decompression Sickness and Its Symptoms

If a sports or professional diver, irrespective of the reason, ascends too fast for the time spent at a certain depth or decompresses incorrectly, i.e. incorrect duration of predetermined stops on the way up, he can easily suffer from DCS. It usually commences minutes to hours after surfacing or even while the diver is still underwater, depending on the amount of N_2 rapidly changing from the dissolved state to the gas-bubble state and the location of such bubbles in the body. Table 6 summarises possible DCS symptoms that could confront a doctor or layman.

Table 6 progresses from mild to very severe DCS or even death, i.e. from dermal to cerebral symptoms. In the current medical literature on diving, DCS with skin sen-

Table 6. Types of decompression sickness and the symptoms

Name	Symptoms
Skin symptoms	Transient rashes and itches, tingling, burning feeling
"Niggles"	Slight pains in limbs
Bends	Severe pain in muscles and joints
Bends in the vertebral column	Seldom, involves CNS and leads to paralysis of limbs
Chokes	Chest pain, stemming from lungs and increasing with inspiration. If severe, can cause shock and collapse
Cerebral effects	Examples: visual disturbances, vertigo, deafness (death)
Staggers	Type of vertigo

sations and muscle or joint pains only is called type I DCS and the severe forms with neurological effects and traumas, type II DCS.

5.13.6.4 Therapeutic Recompression

This term refers to returning someone with suspected or manifest symptoms of mild or severe DCS to high pressure. It is the only method known for treating DCS and air embolism with 100% success if applied correctly and at the right time. Any inert gas bubbles in the body tissues can only be reduced in size and go back into solution, i.e. the DCS symptoms disappear, by increasing the external pressure. In therapeutic recompression, this is done by putting the patient into a one- or multiseated hyperbaric chamber, raising the pressure to the level ($\leqq 6$ atm) prescribed for treating his specific symptoms, keeping him there until these symptoms vanish and then carefully decompressing the patient in stages while observing his condition. About six different tables for hyperbaric treatment with compressed air exist *(US Navy Diving Manual)*. Over the past 15 years, these have gradually been combined with and finally superseded by four short-durational and very efficient recompression tables (known as Tables 5, 5A, 6 and 6A) using 100% O_2 breathing ($\leqq 2.8$ atm) alternating in part with short intervals of compressed-air breathing [6]. The 100% O_2 breathing eliminates the dissolved N_2 and N_2 in the bubble state much faster than compressed-air breathing, owing to the greater N_2 gradient.

Recompression is necessary for tissue and bone or joint inert gas bubble (emboli) symptoms originating from:

- Too rapid ascent in sports, professional and saturation diving
- Correct decompression in very cold water or in cases of obesity
- Incorrect stage decompression
- Overextension or rupture of lungs with gas emboli
- Cerebral gas emboli
- Flying shortly after scuba diving (omitting the advised 24-h interlude)
- DCS of caisson or tunnel workers
- Air in veins with subsequent coronary or cerebral emboli due to incorrect infusions or artificial kidney malfunctions in hospitals
- Anaerobic gas gangrene

As described elsewhere untreated inert gas emboli can lead to permanent tissue or joint damage and even to death (Wünsche and Scheele [27]).

5.13.6.5 Internal Medical and Surgical Treatment Under High Pressure

During therapeutic recompression, situations can occur that necessitate surgical or internal medical treatment by a doctor or a diving paramedic inside the hyperbaric chamber. For this purpose, they would enter the chamber via an airlock. Such cases may, for example, be gastric pains or ulcers, kidney pains or colic, heart and chest ailments. Any of these, commencing suddenly underwater, might have been the prime reason for a too rapid ascent or missed decompression in the first place, thus causing DCS and requiring recompression. When serious, injuries, wounds and fractures sustained while diving may have to be treated by a surgeon in the DDC, i.e. before the chamber has again reached sea-level pressure.

In hospitals, there is an increasing tendency to establish hyperbaric units or departments for coronary surgery (e.g. of "blue babies"), gas gangrene casualties, cases of carbon monoxide poisoning, and other emergencies, usually with remarkable and rapid success previously impossible.

5.13.6.6 Possible Problems in Medical Treatment in Diving

When a disabled diver is recompressed for treatment he may be conscious or unconscious. In the latter case, he would not be able to equalise the pressure in his middle ear in accordance with the rising chamber pressure and thus his eardrums could easily rupture (at an increase in pressure $\geq$ 0.5 atm). To avoid this, doctors sometimes carefully puncture each eardrum (paracentesis). If a diver with a burst lung (gas emboli) together with pneumothorax is recompressed, a dangerous tension pneumothorax may develop, requiring immediate medical action. Using infusions in rigid glass bottles is potentially dangerous during compression and decompression phases with their pressure gradients. Blood can be sucked up into the drip bottle or excessive air in the bottle can be forced into the venous blood stream, leading to multiple gas emboli. Implosions of bottles have also occurred in DDCs. These dangers are non-existent when infusions in soft sterile plastic bags are used.

The behaviour of drugs and medicines administered under pressures >1 atm is very complex and depends on many factors. According to Walsh [26], there appears to be a complete void in the literature as to the toxicity and interaction of medicines with compressed air between 2 and 7 atm, which also spans the range of current recompression pressures. A doctor should bear in mind that the sea-level properties of a medicine need not be valid at higher pressures; it may be necessary to increase or decrease the dose. Anaesthetic drugs often alter in hyperbaric environments, leading to the question of which of them is best suited for operations in high-pressure chambers. Cox and Robinson [5] found that ketamine is least altered in its effects in comparison with propanidid and thiopentone, of which the doses have to be increased with increased pressure. Owing to the danger of contamination of the chamber atmosphere, lumbar or intravenous anaesthesia should be given preference over inhalation anaesthesia.

5.13.7 Frequent Diseases in Diving

Sports as well as professional divers, predominantly engaged in activities in a wet and cold environment, are prone to various diseases beside those caused by barotrauma and DCS, which have been dealt with elsewhere. These are mostly nose and throat ailments and colds. The usual remedies and nasal decongestants bring relief. The use of nose drops, however, should not become a habit for the diver. Various skin diseases of an allergic origin (jellyfish), fungal (pH shift and softening of the skin), traumatic (underwater rocks and corals), animal (eel, shark bites) or toxic (stonefish, catfish) origin can and do occur and must be treated appropriately ([6]; Ehm and Seemann [7]).

Skin wounds tend to heal slower in divers owing to the salt water contact. Contact of the external auditory canal with a high relative humidity or with water for a period of days often causes excessive cerumen production. This, together with noise from air compressors and incorrect Valsalva manoeuvres, can lead to transient or even long-lasting hearing decrements or losses. Otitis externa is a frequent and painful bacterial infection known to divers worldwide. Caused, among other reasons, by high relative humidities or water entering the ear, it is best healed by abstaining from diving and using antibiotic eardrops, if possible in conjunction with an antibiogramme (Alcock [1]).

Infections of the urogenital system can be seen in the northern latitudes owing to the colder waters giving rise to hypothermia. Kidney and bladder pains should be a warning sign for divers to see their doctor. Diving puts a certain strain on the kidneys owing to immersion-induced as well as cold-induced diuresis, as has been found in recent research.

Myalgia and rheumatic pains through overexertion and cold are also quite often encountered among divers.

5.13.8 Prevention of Diving Accidents

Diving medicine incorporates diving accident prophylaxis, although this is also a part of diving technology and support. Accident prevention underwater, though not completely possible, can be achieved to a high degree by adhering to the following precautionary measures:

1. A thorough medical check-up (once a year)
2. A very good training in sports or professional diving, i.e. in courses or diving schools
3. Education in underwater and DCS first aid
4. Sufficient protection against hypothermia
5. Medical prophylaxis against colds and otitis externa
6. Exact adherence to appropriate decompression tables
7. Knowledge of recompression tables
8. Never diving alone, after meals, with residual alcohol in body or when not feeling well
9. Terminating dive before exhaustion
10. Wearing manually activated buoyancy vests to assist in emergency ascents
11. Having an adequate life-support system:
    a) *Sports divers,* large enough gas cylinders with reserve compressed-air supply
    b) *Professional divers,* emergency compressed-air cylinder and perhaps a second regulator
12. Making medical emergency and transportation plans to next DDC before commencing a dive.

5.13.9 Future Trends in Modern Diving and Diving Medicine

Progress in diving has been enormous over the last 100 years (Table 2). The next decade will bring advanced ideas, new knowledge and new equipment to the diver and to diving in general. Spectacular breakthroughs, however, are not to be expected. Theoretical and practical diving medical research will continue in an attempt to make shallow and, in particular, complex deep diving safer and will increase, step by step, the operational working depth. For instance, six men recently spent 35 days at a simulated depth of 500 m (51 atm) in Norway [25].

5.13.9.1 Diving Medicine

Research into the causes of pulmonary and cerebral oxygen toxicity at high pressures and its avoidance will continue (Rister and Baehner [22]). High-pressure inert-gas physiology, especially of the CNS, will remain important, as will the interactions and effects of drugs on the CNS and their changes in efficiency under high pressure (Walsh [26]). New gas mixtures (bimix, trimix – mixture of three gases) resulting from such research will be of benefit to the diver. Current decompression tables for sports divers will be subtly improved where they are still not ideal, and efforts to standardise them internationally will be pursued. The tables used in commercial offshore deep diving – and often regarded as confidential by the companies (time is money) – will be streamlined. The protection of commercial deep divers from hypothermia as well as the treatment thereof is still a subject of great importance, considering that the comfort temperature zone rises and becomes progressively smaller with increasing depth (Hanson [11]). Investigation into the possibilities and potentials of liquid breathing originally begun by Kylstra et al. [15] many years ago may be resumed.

5.13.9.2 Diving Technology

In diving technology, an emphasis on reducing the breathing resistance in scuba gear and the development of electronic decompressiometers can be expected. Research into electronic gas-sensor-controlled semiclosed- and closed-circuit gas-mixture breathing equipment will be pursued. Inert gas recovery systems, especially for helium, will be used more and more in order to decrease the enormous costs of deep, and offshore diving (Low [18]).

References

1. Alcock, S.R.: Acute otitis externa in divers working in the North Sea: a microbiological survey of 7 saturation dives. J. Hyg. (Lond.) *78,* 395–409 (1977).
2. Bennett, P.B. and D.H. Elliott: The physiology and medicine of diving. London: Ballière Tindall 1975.
3. Bennett, P.B.: Nitrogen narcosis. In: Diving medicine. Ed.: R.H. Strauss. New York: Grune & Stratton 1976.
4. Biersner, R.J., M.L. Dembert and M.D. Browning: Comparisons of performance effectiveness among divers. Aviat. Space environ. Med. *51,* 11, 1193–1196 (1980).
5. Cox, J. and D.J. Robinson: Anaesthesia at depth. Brit. J. Hosp. Med. *23,* 2, 144, 147, 150–151 (1980).
6. Diving medicine. Ed.: Richard H. Strauss. New York: Grune & Stratton 1976.
7. Ehm, O.F. and K. Seemann: Sicher Tauchen. Stuttgart: Müller 1965.
8. Fisher, J.M.: Immediate care pack for the diver. In: Proceedings of the 3rd International Conference on Disaster Medicine, Monaco, 6–10 April 1979. Geneva: International Society on Disaster Medicine 1980.
9. Frankel, H.L.: Paraplegia due to decompression sickness. Paraplegia *14,* 306–311 (1977).
10. Goeters, K.M.: Die Beeinflussung der geistigen Konzentrationsfähigkeit durch Überdruck unter Berücksichtigung der zusätzlichen Belastungsfaktoren Arbeitsbeanspruchung und Isolation. Ed.: Deutsche Forschungs- und Versuchsanstalt für Luft- und Raumfahrt. Köln/Porz 1978. (Deutsche Luft- und Raumfahrt. Forschungsbericht 78-12)
11. Hanson, R.deG.: Working in cold environments – lessons to be learned from diving. Ann. occup. Hyg. *21,* 193–198 (1978).
12. Harvey, C.A.: Dysbaric osteonecrosis in divers: a survey of 611 selected US Navy divers. Undersea biomed. Res. *3,* 1, A 41 (1976).
13. Haux, G.: Tauchtechnik. Ed.: Drägerwerk. Lübeck 1968.
14. Jones, D.M. and P. Davis: Upper respiratory tract and aural flora of saturation divers. J. clin. Path. *31,* 721–723 (1978).
15. Kylstra, J.A., C.V. Paganelli and E.H. Lanphier: Pulmonary gas exchange in dogs ventilated with hyperbarically oxygenated liquid. J. appl. Physiol. *21,* 177–184 (1966).
16. Lemaire, C. and E.L. Murphy: Monitoring the heart rate and core temperature of divers to signal dangerous levels of cooling or overheating. Undersea biomed. Res. *3,* 1, A 45 (1976).
17. Linaweaver, P.G. jr.: Physical examination requirements for commercial divers. J. occup. Med. *19,* 12, 817–818 (1977).
18. Low, A.: Medizinische Probleme des modernen Taucherwesens, besonders im Offshore-Bereich. In: Unfall- und Sicherheitsforschung Straßenverkehr. Kongreßbericht Jahrestagung 1981 der Dtsch. Ges. f. Verkehrsmed. gemeinsam m. d. Dtsch. Verkehrswacht, Hamburg, 7–9 May 1981. Ed.: Bundesanstalt f. Straßenwesen, Bereich Unfallforschung, Köln, i. Auftrage d. Bundesministers f. Verkehr. Braunschweig: Waisenhaus-Buchdruckerei 1981. pp. 52–56.
19. McCallum, R.I., D.N. Walder and V.B. Thickett: Bone necrosis in commercial divers. Undersea biomed. Res. *3,* 1, A 41 (1976).
20. NOAA Diving Manual. Washington: U.S. Government Printing Office 1975.
21. Oser, H. and H.M. Wegmann: Die Ausscheidung von Katecholaminen und 17-Hydroxycorticosteroiden bei 5 Aquanauten während des Aufenthaltes im Unterwasserlabor "Tektite II". Ed.: Deutsche Forschungs- und Versuchsanstalt für Luft- und Raumfahrt. Köln/Porz 1978. (Deutsche Luft- und Raumfahrt. Forschungsbericht 74-02).
22. Rister, M. and R.L. Baehner: Neue Aspekte zur Toxizität des Sauerstoffs. Dtsch. med. Wschr. *103,* 23, 977–981 (1978).
23. Roydhouse, N.: Sudden deafness and scuba divers. N. Z. med. J. *93,* 678, 131 (1981).
24. Ruff, S., H.D. Fust, H. Oser and A. Low: Unter-

wasserlaboratorium Helgoland. Ed.: Deutsche Forschungs- und Versuchsanstalt für Luft- und Raumfahrt. Inst. f. Flugmedizin. Bonn-Bad Godesberg 1971. (Deutsche Luft- und Raumfahrt. Forschungsbericht 71-63).

25. Taucher in 500 m Wassertiefe. Hansa *119,* 1/2, 106 (1982).

26. Walsh, J. M.: Drugs in diving. In: Diving medicine. Ed.: R. H. Strauss. New York: Grune & Stratton 1976.

27. Wünsche, O. and G. Scheele: Röntgenologische Untersuchungen bei Druckluftarbeitern. Köln, Opladen: Westdeutscher Verlag 1973. (Forschungsbericht d. Landes NRW. No. 2351).

5.14 Forensic Nautical Medicine

W. Naeve

5.14.1 Forensic Medicine

Forensic medicine is a special branch of medicine because of its peculiar problems and their interpretation by means of specific methods. It concerns itself with research into and clarification of such questions as arise in practical legal administration which can be answered only with the help of medical and scientific knowledge. The medical questions resulting from a legal case have to be debated according to viewpoints foreign to general as well as nautical medicine.

In the majority of countries the working methods of forensic medical specialists are essentially similar. The limits of their fields of work, however, vary considerably. In some countries their activity is restricted to the field of forensic pathology as being the basis of forensic medicine. In other countries close connections exist between forensic medicine and occupational medicine, social medicine, insurance medicine, criminology and forensic psychiatry and they often overlap. A generally valid definition of the branch "forensic medicine" is therefore not possible. In addition, the regulations, the legal definition of facts and the requirements for objective proof vary from state to state.

In general, the forensic medical specialist submits his authoritative judgement according to his own views and findings, which are in accordance with the legal requirements of the country in which the examination is carried out and the judgement made. An exception to this procedure which arises from time to time is when findings were made in other places in accordance with different legal requirements or when forensic or medical findings are not available at all because of prevailing circumstances. Should, however, the forensic questions have to be authoritatively answered after incidents on ships which were either at sea or in foreign ports at the time of occurrence, then this exception becomes the rule.

5.14.2 Forensic Nautical Medicine

The specific points of forensic nautical medicine are based on the following:

1. In most of the expert opinions submitted by forensic medical specialists of the native country the important pathological findings which are necessary for establishing the cause of death will have been made abroad and are therefore not always compiled in compliance with the laws valid in the native country,

   or

   a partial autopsy, or none at all, has been carried out abroad and the corpse brought to the home country more or less appropriately preserved (embalmed),

   or

   medical findings were not made at all (sea committal),

   or

   the deceased has been transferred to the home country under unfavourable storage conditions: this makes the pathological and toxicological findings more difficult due to more or less serious changes caused by putrefaction.

2. To clarify a case of accident, or for the penal judgement of bodily injury or homicide, it is often important to know whether the injured person or the victim of a crime or the perpetrator was under the influence of alcohol. A test to determine the alcohol level in the body may not be made in certain circumstances:
   a) The body has been buried at sea
   b) The incident took place at sea where facilities for the examination were not available
   c) Testing was not the custom or it was thought to be unnecessary

   It must also be accepted that the methods of testing for alcohol and the specific requirements vary between countries. Unsatisfactory preservation of the corpse may make testing for alcohol in the blood or tissues at a later date almost impossible.

3. In the case of persons having suffered bodily injury by accident, injury by others or self-mutilation abroad or at sea, as a rule only a few indications are available to the forensic medical specialist for making a judgement (i.e. whether a wound is open or closed; depth of injury; alcohol intoxication of the person injured accidentally, the victim of a crime or the perpetrator).

4. The living and working conditions on board ships and in foreign ports differ in many ways from those of the evaluator's home country. A basic knowledge of nautical medicine is required for forensic medical evaluation.

5. Also to be judged are cases of death and incidents on board ships which at the time of occurrence were in other climatic zones than that of the native country. In this connection, the tropics and the subtropics are significant. A basic knowledge of tropical medicine and tropical pathology is then required for an evaluation. When necessary, an expert in tropical medicine or a pathologist with a knowledge of tropical pathology must be consulted.

6. In cases of death at sea or in foreign ports, the order for autopsy is often issued by the shipping agent when the authorities do not demand it. The doctor's attention is at times not called to the specific points in question, including the legal requirements of insurance companies. Quite often the examination has to be delegated to doctors who have no, or very little, pathological-anatomical and forensic medical knowledge and experience.

7. Sometimes the crew cannot be questioned for facts by the doctor until months after the incident at sea. Then it is often found that the incident is made light of or details are concealed because of camaraderie. Also it is often the case that crew members who could contribute to the forensic medical clarification of the case by their statements have already left the ship and cannot be found.

These observations on the difficulties with which the forensic medical specialist can be confronted when professionally evaluating incidents on board ships were compiled on the basis of more than 30 years' activity and experience as a forensic medical specialist in a seaport (Naeve [14], Naeve [16]). The resulting conclusions about the problems, the kind of evaluation data and the sources of error in forensic nautical medicine form the basis of this chapter.

In reviewing the literature some collated information can be found on the field of forensic nautical medicine (forensic pathology and toxicology) as well as statistical data about the influence of alcohol on seamen having had an accident at sea or while working in ports. There is, however, no comprehensive study presenting the specific problems of forensic nautical medicine.

5.14.3 Forensic Medical Examination and Evaluation of Fatalities in Seafaring

In practice the need for clarification of unexplained fatalities in seafaring depends very much on the country in which the examination is carried out and whether the ship on which the case occurred is registered at home or abroad. If it is not obvious homicide, then sometimes nothing further is determined and a post-mortem examination to establish the cause of death does not take place. Should the examination, however, be carried out in a country, or for authorities of a country, where the penal and social laws and regulations are very sophisticated, then pathological-anatomical examinations, including histological and toxicological findings, are inevitable. In some countries, therefore, there are practically no problems in forensic nautical medicine whereas in others such evaluations are made more difficult or even impossible because of findings which are either lacking or have been made abroad.

An unexplained death at sea or abroad which requires forensic medical inquiry should be examined in the native country, if at all possible. Only there can it be guaranteed that the special requirements which differ so greatly in the various countries will be observed from the beginning. Autopsy can take place after transferral of the deceased by ship or air. Any alterations due to putrefaction will influence the expert evaluation less than inadequate descriptions of findings of an autopsy made somewhere else and sometimes incompetently.

The legal stipulations regarding transfer of corpses into foreign countries also vary considerably. Embalming is often required but instructions concerning the method of embalming exist in only a few countries.

Embalming, which derives its name from scented resinoids formerly applied to preserve a corpse, is carried out today – if done at all competently – mainly by injecting antiputrefactive liquids into the blood vessels of the corpse. Embalming can be done with or without opening the body cavities. Numerous techniques have been developed. The composition of the preserving liquid differs. A formalin solution of about 5% is best suited for preservation under seafaring conditions. Water or alcohol (approx. 70%) is used as a solvent. As additives, small amounts of glycerin (0.5%), sodium chloride (10%) and carbolic acid (5%) are recommended but not necessary. In cases where the body cavities have not been opened, the full amount of preserving liquid (approx. 5 litres) can be injected into a single blood vessel (arteria femoralis).

Incomplete or incompetent embalming will in general not essentially affect a subsequent autopsy. It is, however, vital that, when embalming, no organs be removed from the corpse without anatomical findings having been compiled. When investigating and evaluating an unexplained death it is, as a rule, important to establish whether alcohol had been taken and, if so, the amount. Therefore a blood sample for determination of alcohol content should be taken before embalming the corpse and also when opening it. The blood sample should be taken if possible from an upper thigh vein using a sterile needle or, if this is unavailable, a skin cut. About 8–10 ml blood should be withdrawn into a sterile test tube or suitable glass vial. The container should be sealed securely, then labelled with the full name of the deceased and the time and place of withdrawal. Never use needles or glass containers which have been sterilised in either alcohol or fluids containing alcohol. Ensure refrigeration of the blood samples until the examination can be made. It is appropriate to examine the blood according to the usual methods of the country in which the cause of death is to be evaluated. If possible send the blood sample by airmail. Even after refrigeration of the blood sample for days or weeks in a securely sealed test tube, results suitable for evaluation can be obtained. Even if a corpse is already in a state of putrefaction when being embalmed or preserved (death at sea, death by drowning in port), results suitable for evaluation can still be expected by applying special methods of examination. When decay has set in, one blood sample should be taken from each of two or three blood vessels separately (i.e. right and left upper thigh vein, upper arm vein).

The examination of blood changed by decay and the critical assessment of results of analyses should always be delegated to a forensic medical specialist experienced in this special field. When available, in addition to blood samples from decayed corpses, a urine sample (8–10 ml or less) should be kept for an alcohol test. Sometimes it is not possible to withdraw a blood sample from decayed corpses, not even from the heart (blood from the heart is less suitable for alcohol determination). In any particular case alcohol may diffuse from the stomach after death, thus raising the amount which would be found there at post-mortem examination. If no blood can be withdrawn, the alcohol concentration of the urine alone can indicate the presence of alcohol influence. If neither blood nor urine are available for samples, an attempt should be made to withdraw fluid from either the eye chambers or the knee joints. If that fails, a rough estimate of the influence of alcohol may be obtained from examination of tissues such as brain or skeletal muscle. Preservation and storage of these should be as described for "blood samples". In some countries death from natural causes can under certain circumstances be recognised in law as qualifying for compensation. The histological findings in such a case are indispensable. Unfortunately, an autopsy carried out in a different country may be restricted to deciding only on death from natural or violent cause and histological findings may not have been either made or recorded. The general post-mortem findings made by a doctor called upon only occasionally to perform an autopsy must also be evaluated critically and with reservation. If the corpse is sent to the home country, a second autopsy is often necessary to obtain specimens for histological examination. The organs removed at the first autopsy are rarely retained or forwarded to the home country.

Personal observations: a) Death at sea. Coronary thrombosis and infarction given as cause of death by examiner. Further examination: no coronary thrombosis, coronary arteries not incised. Cause of death histologically proved: chronic myocarditis. b) Partial autopsy abroad. Cause of death: angina tonsillaris – sepsis. Further autopsy including histological examinations: cerebral form of an acute malaria tropica. c) Death at sea, autopsy abroad. Cause of death: lung oedema after previous protozoal infection. Further autopsy including histological examination. Cause of death: recurrence of malaria tropica, acute cerebral form.

Serious occupational poisoning resulting almost exclusively from inhalation of poisonous gases or vapours is not rare in seafaring. The same holds true for death by suffocation while in parts of the ship in which there were actually no toxic substances but where the oxygen content of the air was substantially reduced (storage rooms). Some of these cases of death are, according to the facts, indisputable as far as the cause is concerned – poisoning or suffocation – and do not necessarily require a medical examination. In some cases, however, doubt may exist as to the cause of sudden death. Natural death, poisoning or suffocation may be the cause. Sometimes there has been an attempt by others to conceal some deficiency, such as a defective respirator, which is an offence against existing safety regulations. In the same way others may have deliberately or subconsciously attributed a natural death to an accidental cause. A good example of this is death resulting from acute poisoning while working (pension claim).

The clarification of questionable causes of death by poisoning in seafaring can be associated with the greatest of difficulties because findings in suffocation are uncharacteristic. They also occur in connection with cardiac death. Without question a macroscopic and microscopic anatomical examination should be sougtht. As far as existing circumstances permit, an attempt to obtain chemical-toxicological proof should be made in cases of questionable poisoning by inhalation. From practical experience, such examinations prove successful only if the organs and body fluids to be examined are obtained properly and soon after death and when the analysis is made at an institute where suitable facilities for examination are at hand.

Organs and body fluids (lung, brain, blood, urine) which are designated for toxicological examination must be placed in a securely closed container immediately after withdrawal, kept cool and examined soon thereafter. In the practice of forensic nautical medicine, however, such chemical-toxicological examinations can hardly ever be carried out under the necessary conditions because of the circumstances peculiar to seafaring.

In connection with questionable poisoning by inhalation at sea, an attempt is generally made to either prove or exclude a natural death by means of an autopsy including histological findings. Anatomical alterations of the respiratory tract and the lungs are not frequent in cases of intoxication by inhalation. If they occur these alterations are more or less characteristic, even though not specific, and may indicate poisoning by inhalation. When medical judgement is made according to the legal penal point of view, such cases of death often remain "doubtful", because intoxication cannot be proved from the anatomical findings alone with the assurance required by criminal law. From this it can be seen that medical findings alone are not sufficient to clarify such deaths if this is required. It is indispensable that, outside the field of medicine, a technician or a chemist should make an objective examination and judgement of the scene of the accident in question and of the equipment possibly used. Carbon monoxide intoxication must always be considered in cases of unexplained death (blood withdrawal, quantitative examination of blood for carbon monoxide content).

Sudden and unexpected death from natural causes may give reason to suspect accidental death from exterior violence or intoxication. In general, the forensic significance of these deaths is based on the fact that, as a rule, their cause is unknown and cannot be clarified without further examination. It has proved convenient for the interpretation of findings made during the autopsy in such cases to classify them in three degrees of severity. The first group includes findings which in themselves, on the basis of their degree of severity and their localisation, make death self-explanatory (i.e. infarction, apoplexia cerebri, pericardial tamponade after cardiac rupture by infarction, bleeding to death from peptic ulceration, internal bleeding after rupture of an aortic aneurysm, massive pulmonary embolism). In the second group of cases of sudden death, changes in organs are found which may explain death but from which, however, a cause for a sudden and unexpected death cannot be recognised. In most cases it is a matter of chronic diseases (general arteriosclerosis, coronary sclerosis, hypertension, valvular heart disease). Death occurs mostly from an induced cause or from special predisposing factors. The third group includes cases of death where no positive cause of death can be proved in spite of comprehensive and careful examination. Undoubtedly the number of such medically unsolved cases depends on the quality and exactness of the examinations (Janssen and Naeve [8]).

The deaths in the second and third groups often cause one to connect fatalities with working conditions in seafaring. Anatomical findings alone are not sufficient to decide whether external effects were the essential reason for death. The evaluation of such cases is made especially difficult by anatomical findings made in a foreign country without the possibility of a second autopsy or preservation of organs used for histological examination during the first autopsy. Among the external conditions which may be a cause of death or may be the precipitating factor in death from an existing illness, minor accidents, abnormal bodily stress, extreme climatic conditions (Kutz [10], Tromp [19]) and extremely acute mental strain are especially important. At times the question arises whether death or inducement of natural death was brought about by animals via allergic reactions or toxic effects (Banner [1]; Russel [18]), by consumption of incompatible or poisonous plants or parts of plants with the food (Morton [12]) or by consumption of contaminated food.

An occupational illness of seamen, malaria, is often overlooked (Haas et al. [5]). Malaria must always be considered when establishing the cause of death of seamen. Death from malaria can be pathologically-anatomically proved even if the organs to be examined are in a state of advanced putrefaction (Naeve [13]).

Among the natural causes of sudden death at sea, the relevant statistics show that coronary diseases outnumber all others (coronary sclerosis with or without coronary thrombosis and with or without morphologically proved infarction).

Formerly the assistance of a doctor was seldom considered necessary when judging a homicide. "The methods of killing were rough and could easily be ascertained from external findings. It was not uncommon for a captain to be murdered in the times of sailing ships. In the times of the big passenger liners the following three groups gained prominence: killing in fighting and in sexual excitement among the crew, murder in connection with insurance deception and the murdering of passengers not by members of the deck crew but by other members of the crew" (v. Hentig [6]). Nowadays it is exclusively homicide which occurs in the course of an act of violence among members of the crew, at least as far as the cases are known at all. As a rule the perpetrator and the victim are under the influence of alcohol. For the most part death is caused by knife stabbing or by punching and kicking. Of 29 cases of homicide among crew members on ships examined in recent years in Hamburg, 13 involved stab wounds, 7 severe blows (fist or blunt instrument), 4 shooting, 3 being thrown into the water, and 2 being pushed down stairs or thrown into a cargo hold. Notably, there were no deaths by strangulation (choking, strangling). About half of these homicides occurred at sea, the others on board ships lying in port.

Where there is evidence of external force, autopsies on persons having died at sea are carried out whether it is a matter of homicide or the result of an accident. These examinations refer especially to skull-brain injuries. Personal experience has shown that, especially in deep sea fishing, accidental skull injuries may occur which, at first, cannot be distinguished from the effects of a blow made by an attack with a blunt instrument. Together with a careful autopsy, knowledge and consideration of the existing working conditions are required for clarification of this kind of case (Knight [9]). Forensic medical evaluations are especially a problem in cases where it is a question of unproved guilt and the deceased was buried without autopsy at sea or abroad.

If it is a matter of legal consequence, suicides on board ship are seldom a forensic medical problem. This is not the case when judging such fatalities for social accident insurance or private insurance. It is of importance for this kind of evaluation, depending on the type of insurance, whether the effects of working conditions (accident, extreme climatic conditions, extreme physical or mental stress), organic diseases (fever), endogenous mental illnesses, chronic alcoholism (also alcoholic delirium), acute alcoholic intoxication or medicine/drugs were present. It is also of importance in cases of suicide where the balance of the mind is disturbed. Without exact case histories and anatomical as well as chemical-toxicological examinations, some of these cases of suicide at sea remain unclarified with regard to aspects of insurance. In most cases only possibilities, at most probabilities, can be presented for purposes of evaluation.

It is common experience that not a few fatalities on board ships, viewed critically from a forensic medical standpoint as to their cause, remain unsolved in the end. The explanation for this lies in the peculiarities of seafaring. It is better for the medical administration of justice to accept this fact rather than to construct a hypothetical cause of death.

When evaluating death at sea for purposes of forensic medicine, the question must at times be answered whether death of the injured or sick seaman would have, in all probability, occurred under conditions ashore, i.e. with regular medical care. Such questions, of course, can be answered only after a pathological-anatomical examination. Similar problems occur in evaluating the question of a lack of effort to help when, because of the ship's schedule or other reasons, a sick or injured seaman was not attended by a doctor although that would have been a possibility. The following questions would then have to be taken into account: Could a complication of an illness, or the fatal development of such, have been prevented by medical help, obtained by calling at a port? Which diagnostic and therapeutic possibilities would have existed in the ports which could have been reached within reasonable time? How much time would have elapsed between the decision to call at a port and the arrival of the ship in the harbour? Would there have been a possibility for the officer in charge to obtain radiomedical advice? What signs and symptoms were evident on examination of the injured or sick person? Should a layman have recognised the severity of the existing illness or injury with his basic medical knowledge gained in connection with his professional training?

Each of these questions present added difficulties. No generally valid guidelines can be laid down. Pure theoretical-medical evaluations of such cases do not do justice to all circumstances. The manifold peculiarities of seafaring must be taken into account, and a theoretical and practical basic knowledge of nautical medicine is a prerequisite.

5.14.4 Identification in the Realm of Forensic Nautical Medicine

A forensic medical specialist may be asked to identify a dead person when the methods used by the police and criminologists fail or can no longer be applied. This task is usually made very difficult by bodily changes caused by fire, explosion or prolonged immersion in the sea. The loss of limbs and facial deformities can add to the difficulties. It may be necessary to consult other specialists such as radiologists, dental surgeons and anthropologists (Hunger and Leopold [7]).

Should several corpses be found floating on the water after a mishap on board ship then it is not only a matter of identifying missing crew members but also a question of whether persons not belonging to the crew were on board and lost their lives at the time of the incident. Such investigations of identity regarding the positions where the individual corpses were found on board ship may sometimes make it essential to establish the cause of a mishap. In addition to identification, the cause of death as well as other findings are of significance: determination of carbon monoxide in the blood of burned corpses to clarify the question of whether the effects of the burns occurred during life or after death; confirmation or exclusion of death by drowning in reference to corpses recovered from the water; the influence of alcohol etc. Unless it has been reported previously that a seafarer is missing, a corpse recovered from the water may be difficult to identify, especially if there have been decomposition changes. When searching, one must consider that, under special current or weather conditions, corpses are carried far out to sea within a few days or can be carried far upstream from the sea when in tidal waters.

It is not possible here to go into details and discuss techniques which could be used in connection with forensic medical examinations for the purpose of identification. However, three categories of identifying features were distinguished by Grüner and Helmer [4]:

1. Classification as to sex, body size, age and race. These findings alone do not guarantee a certain identification.
2. Features or peculiarities of the body present from birth or acquired: illnesses, results of illness, scars, amputations, tattoos. These identifying marks do not in every case lead to positive decisions.
3. Dactyloscopy, X-ray identification (Graham [3]; Evans et al. [2]) and identification by the specific features of the dentures (Luntz and Luntz [11]).

Dactyloscopy and X-ray identification (X-rays of the skeleton or parts of such and comparing them with X-rays of the missing person) lead to exclusion or proof of identity provided that comparable X-rays are at hand.

Special techniques make it possible to obtain useful fingerprints for purposes of comparison even after extreme distension of the calloused skin of the fingers and the palm or removal of this layer of skin. Tattoos on corpses found in the water can be made visible again and photographically recorded by special techniques, even if they are only faintly recognisable as a result of putrefaction changes.

5.14.5 Evaluation of Crimes in Connection with Alcoholic Influence

In several chapters in this handbook, attention has been called to the dangers of bodily or psychological harm to seamen who occasionally or by habit drink alcohol to excess. The forensic medical expert, when dealing with living persons, is concerned primarily with persons who, because of alcohol abuse, have not so much exposed themselves but rather others to considerable danger or have done bodily injury or have damaged or endangered objects (i.e. a ship or port facilities).

From forensic medical experience, seafarers and especially the younger ones who go ashore under the influence of alcohol are often liable to harm themselves or others. One of the most frequent causes of fatal accidents among crew members is falling into water when returning to the ship from ashore. Even more frequent is the incidence of prosecution by police after drunken seamen have been involved in violence (Naeve [17]).

For the most part it is a matter of minor offences. The forensic medical specialist ordered by the court to make an evaluation should not base his judgement on a "degree of drunkenness" ascertained by breath or blood analysis alone, but should take into account the conditions of the individual case peculiar to seafaring: this involves race, unaccustomed climatic conditions, the type of alcohol consumed, alcohol prohibition on the ship of the involved person and drinking habits and alcohol availability in the native country. Practice does show that (a) seamen from countries in which obtaining alcohol is difficult because of high taxes or in which the consumption of high percentage alcohol is not common and (b) seamen on ships prohibiting alcohol, often drink alcohol in intolerable amounts when going ashore in foreign ports. Abnormal reaction to alcohol and abnormal degrees of drunkenness, sometimes with low concentrations of alcohol in the breath or in the blood, can be the result. Cases of drunkenness while the ship is underway are judged and prosecuted quite differently in individual countries. The exact assessment of the degree of drunkenness during navigation is an additional difficulty. Such cases of drunkenness come to light in practice only when navigating in coastal waters and rivers and during manoeuvres in port.

Forensic medical observations about the effect of drunkenness while navigating on the high sea are not known. The demands on the psychological and sensor efficiency while navigating a ship on the high seas are essentially less than, for instance, in coastal waters. However, emergencies such as failure of important instruments of navigation, damage to engine, sudden climatic changes, breaking out of fire or expelling of toxic gases on board ship may arise at anytime and anywhere. In considering all the possible eventualities it is clear that for the deck crew a high blood alcohol level is inconsistent with safe and competent navigation. From personal observations, 64 cases of drunkenness while navigating in coastal waters and ports were evaluated (Naeve and Klages [15]). The largest group consisted of persons who navigated a ship or played an essential part in the navigating. Forty-five incidents involved 51 persons: 42 cases involved the ship's senior officer or the captain, while 8 cases involved other navigational personnel. In one case an engineer made a mistake in the engine operation, resulting in a collision. It was necessary to take a sample of blood for alcohol estimation in 22 incidents which had resulted in collision. In the remaining incidents a blood sample was taken after abnormal steering of the ship, or sudden collapse of a crew member who was drunk. At the time of withdrawal the blood alcohol concentration was between 1.1‰ (110 mg per 100 ml) and 4.04‰ (404 mg per 100 ml); the average value of all individual examinations was approximately 2.3–2.4‰ (230 mg–240 mg per 100 ml).

A peculiarity in shipping is that drinking while navigating is possible, and when making a legal judgement, uncertainties often arise as to which crew member was in command of the ship at the critical moment. The demands on a ship's navigator in present-day traffic in harbours, on rivers or in coastal waters are very high. In the described cases of evaluation a change of personality resulting from alcohol was often considered responsible for the incompetent navigation of a ship, given the prevailing circumstances.

References

1. Banner, A. H.: Hazardous marine animals. In: Forensic Medicine, Vol. 3. Philadelphia, London, Toronto: W. B. Saunders 1977. pp. 1378–1436.
2. Evans, K. T., Knight, B. and D. K. Whittaker: Forensic Radiology. Oxford, London, Edinburgh, Boston, Melbourne: Blackwell Scientific Publications 1981.
3. Graham, D.: The use of X-ray techniques in forensic investigations. Edinburgh, London: Churchill Livingstone 1973.
4. Grüner, O. and R. Helmer: Identifizierung. In: Gerichtliche Medizin, 2. ed., Vol. 1, Berlin, Heidelberg, New York: Springer 1975. pp. 156–206.
5. Haas, I., Mohr, W. and W. Dennig: Malaria bei Seeleuten. Zbl. Verkehrs-Med. *14,* 234–240 (1968).
6. Hentig, H. von: Der Schiffsmord. Hamburg: Kriminalistik-Verlag 1967. (Kriminologische Schriftenreihe aus der deutschen Kriminologischen Gesellschaft, Vol. 25.)
7. Hunger, H. and D. Leopold: Identifikation. Berlin, Heidelberg, New York: Springer 1978.
8. Janssen, W. and W. Naeve: Der plötzliche Tod aus natürlicher Ursache. In: Gerichtliche Medizin, 2nd ed., Vol. 1. Berlin, Heidelberg, New York: Springer 1975. pp. 248–304.
9. Knight, B.: Hazards of the fishing industry. In: Forensic Medicine, Vol. 3. Philadelphia, London, Toronto: W. B. Saunders 1977. pp. 1167–1171.
10. Kutz, H.-E.: Hitzeschäden. Ein Überblick über Pathogenese, Klinik und Therapie. Z. Tropenmed. Parasit. *10,* 178–231 (1959).
11. Luntz, L. L. and P. Luntz: Handbook for Dental Identification. Philadelphia, Toronto: J. B. Lippincott 1973.
12. Morton, I. F.: Poisonous and injurious higher plants and fungi. In: Forensic Medicine, Vol. 3.

Philadelphia, London, Toronto: W. B. Saunders 1977. pp. 1456–1567.
13. Naeve, W.: Zum histologischen Nachweis einer akuten Malaria tropica an fäulnisveränderten Organen. Z. Rechtsmedizin *69*, 210–216 (1971).
14. Naeve, W.: Forensische Schiffahrtsmedizin. Z. Rechtsmedizin *73*, 321–324 (1973).
15. Naeve, W. and U. Klages: Trunkenheit bei der Führung eines Schiffes. Blutalkohol *11*, 357–385 (1974).
16. Naeve, W.: Gerichtsmedizinische Obduktionen und Begutachtungen von Todesfällen auf See. Acta medicinae legalis et socialis *24*, 961–964 (1975).
17. Naeve, W.: Bedeutung des Alkohols bei tödlichen Unfällen an Bord und im Hafen. Blutalkohol *13*, 27–38 (1976).
18. Russel, F.: Terrestrial and marine venomous snakes. In: Forensic Medicine, Vol. 3. Philadelphia, London, Toronto: W. B. Saunders 1977. pp. 1437–1444.
19. Tromp, S. W.: Influence of the physical environment on accidents, crime, suicide and disease of man. In: Forensic Medicine, Vol. 3. Philadelphia, London, Toronto: W. B. Saunders 1977. pp. 1627–1642.

Sources of Information

A variety of cross-references to various sources of literature appear in the contributions to this Handbook. In this way it is hoped that the user may more readily gain access to further material. However, it must be added that in practice the acquisition of such material presents a great deal of difficulty. To aid the reader in his quest for information we would like to point out that the following institutes active in the field of nautical medicine have libraries at their disposal:

- Instytut medycyny morskiej i tropikalnej w Gdyni
  (Institute for Maritime and Tropical Medicine in Gdynia),
  Ul. Starowiejska 50,
  81-356 Gdynia, Poland

- Maritime Labour Research Institute,
  4-5-1 Kojimachi, Chiyoudaku,
  Tokyo 102, Japan

- Medizinischer Dienst des Verkehrswesens der DDR
  (Medical Service for Traffic of the GDR),
  Dehmelstr. 23,
  2500 Rostock, German Democratic Republic
  Main library in:
  Medizinischer Dienst des Verkehrswesens der DDR,
  Zentrale Leitung, Abt. Information/Dokumentation,
  1080 Berlin, P.O.B. 1280, German Democratic Republic

- Nauchno-issledovatelskiy institut gigieny vodnogo transporta (NIIGVT)
  (Research Institute for Water Transport Hygiene),
  Leningradskoe Chaussee 95 a,
  Moscow 125195, USSR

- Transporten meditsinski institut
  (Transport Medical Institute),
  G. Dimitrov 110,
  Sofia 1233, Bulgaria

In addition to these civilian institutions, some naval medical institutions administer similarly orientated libraries:

- Centre d'Etudes et de Recherches biophysiologiques appliquées á la Marine,
  H. I. A. Sainte Anne, B. P. 610,
  83800 Toulon Naval, France

- Department of the Navy/National Medical Center,
  Bethesda, Md 20014, USA

- Institute of Naval Medicine,
  Alverstoke, Hampshire PO122DL,
  United Kingdom

- Institut za pomorsku medicinu
  (Maritime Medicine Institute),
  Krizine 66,
  58002 Split, Yugoslavia

- Schiffahrtmedizinisches Institut der Marine
  (Medical Institute of the Navy),
  Kopperpahler Allee 120,
  2300 Kiel-Kronshagen, Federal Republic of Germany

A specialised collection of literature on nautical medicine and related fields (nautical medical literature documentation) is to be found at the following institute:

- Bernhard-Nocht-Institut für Schiffs- und Tropenkrankheiten,
  Abteilung für Schiffahrtsmedizin,
  (Bernhard-Nocht-Institute for Nautical and Tropical Diseases,
  Department of Nautical Medicine),
  Bernhard-Nocht-Straße 74,
  2000 Hamburg 4, Federal Republic of Germany

Nearly all excerpts and quotations which appear in the different chapters of this Handbook as well as further reading material mentioned in the references can be found in this collection. A "Bibliography Nautical Medicine", vol. I published in 1977, presents a complete survey of the documentation undertaken in the field of nautical medicine. The second volume, published in December 1982, contains a guide to all publications registered in the catalogue since 1977. The bibliographies, as well as the whole documentation catalogue, are subdivided by key words specially chosen for the field of nautical medicine. This simplifies the task for those seeking access to such publications. An index of the authors of all publications is also provided.

The collection of material on nautical medicine is open to all interested parties; they may study the material at their leisure in the reading room at the Bernhard-Nocht-Institute. A limited number of photocopies may be made at the individuals' own cost.

Subject Index

A

B

F

G

H

I

J

* In 1981/82 this organization was renamed from "Intergovernmental Maritime Consultative Organization" (IMCO) to "International Maritime Organization" (IMO).

K

L

M

Q

R

S

T

W

X

Y

Z

MIX
Papier aus verantwortungsvollen Quellen
Paper from responsible sources
FSC® C105338

If you have any concerns about our products,
you can contact us on
ProductSafety@springernature.com

In case Publisher is established outside the EU,
the EU authorized representative is:
Springer Nature Customer Service Center GmbH
Europaplatz 3, 69115 Heidelberg, Germany

Printed by Libri Plureos GmbH
in Hamburg, Germany